ADVANCES IN BIOMIMETICS

Edited by **Anne George**

INTECHOPEN.COM

Advances in Biomimetics
Edited by Anne George

CBS, Edition **2016**

Published by InTech

Janeza Trdine 9, 51000 Rijeka, Croatia

Publishing Process Manager Ivana Lorkovic

Technical Editor Teodora Smiljanic

Cover Designer InTech Design Team

Additional hard copies can be obtained from orders@intechopen.com

Advances in Biomimetics, Edited by Anne George
p. cm.
ISBN 978-953-307-191-6

INTECH

open science | open minds

Contents

Preface

Biomimetics is the science of emulating nature's design. In nature, living organisms synthesize mineralized tissues and this process of biomineralization is under strict biological control. It involves the interactions of several biological macromolecules among themselves and with the mineral components. Generally, natures design principles are based on a "Bottom-Up" strategy. Such processes lead to the formation of hierarchically structured organic-inorganic composites with mechanical properties optimized for a given function. A common theme in mineralized tissues is the intimate interaction between the organic and inorganic phases and this leads to the unique properties seen in biological materials. Therefore, understanding natures design principles and ultimately mimicking the process may provide new approaches to synthesize biomaterials with unique properties for various applications. Biomimetics as a scientific discipline has experienced an exceptional development. Its potential in several applications such as medical, veterinary, dental science, material science and nanotechnology bears witness to the importance of understanding the processes by which living organisms exert an exquisite control on the fabrication of various materials. Despite several breakthroughs, there exist only a limited number of methods for the preparation of advanced materials. Consequently, precisely controlling the architecture and composition of inorganic materials still remain enigmatic. Biological organisms have the extraordinary ability to fabricate a wide variety of inorganic materials into complex morphologies that are hierarchically structured on the nano, micro and macroscales with high fidelity. The next generation of biologically inspired materials fabrication methods must draw inspiration from complex biological systems.

The interaction between cells, tissues and biomaterial surfaces are the highlights of the book "Advances in Biomimetics". In this regard the effect of nanostructures and nanotopographies and their effect on the development of a new generation of biomaterials including advanced multifunctional scaffolds for tissue engineering are discussed. The 2 volumes contain articles that cover a wide spectrum of subject matter such as different aspects of the development of scaffolds and coatings with enhanced performance and bioactivity, including investigations of material surface-cell interactions.

Anne George
University of Illinois at Chicago,
Department of Oral Biology,
Chicago,
USA

1

A Cultural Perspective on Biomimetics

Bernadette Bensaude-Vincent
Université Paris 1Panthéon-Sorbonne/IUF
France

1. Introduction

Gecko's feet, lotus leaves, blue butterfly wings, spider's silk, fireflies, mother-of-pearl.... All these wonders of nature, which traditionally filled the pages of natural history magazines have attracted the attention of materials scientists over the past decades. They have often been presented as models to design and engineer optimal structures. And this renewed interest in natural systems has undoubtedly brought about innovating strategies in chemistry, materials science and nanotechnology.

But what exactly does mimicking nature mean? Can we really transfer nature's "technology" to human projects? Does talking about "nature's technology" even make sense?

The view of technology copying nature is as fascinating as it is deceiving. We all know that in aeronautics, repeated attempts to mimic birds' flight have led to spectacular failures. Hence the basic principles of modern technology are anything but inspired by nature: The mechanical machines, metallic alloys, combustion engines, jet engines, direct synthesis of ammonia, etc… have no equivalent in nature. They proceed from the fundamental laws of physics, thermodynamics, and aerodynamics rather than from imitating nature. At the other end of the spectrum, we all know a few examples of successful inventions, such as the Velcro, which was inspired from cocklebursclinging to socks or dog's fur after a hike in the hills. Yet failures to imitate nature by far outnumber the rare successful biomimetic inventions. (Vogel, 1998) Does this mean that biomimicry strategies are generally doomed to fail?

This chapter will consider the current biomimetic trends from a broad historical perspective. Its aims are to pin-point what prompted the renewed interest in biological structures and processes in the field of high-tech materials, and to clarify what kind of relations exist between nature and artefacts in emerging technologies. Finally, it will make the case for a paradoxical use of mimicry strategies.

2. Challenging nature

First of all, it is important to keep in mind that chemistry is the subject of a number of strong and deeply rooted stereotypes in our culture. The image spread by Goethe's Faust and Shelley's Frankenstein of the alchemist mixing mysterious liquors in a dark laboratory, trying to rival Nature , has prompted the association of chemistry with the mythical figure Hubris, or even Man's original sin of pride. Chemistry thus ends up irresistibly connoting the idea of boundary transgression.

This stereotype is reminiscent of the philosophical disputes raised by medieval alchemists' attempts to make gold. They were blamed for counterfeit, because according to the prevailing scholastic culture, there was literally an essential difference between natural gold and alchemist's gold. The latter could only be an imitation of the real thing. Artificial gold may have looked like its natural counterpart, but it had to be deprived of the 'substantial form' inherent to natural gold. (Emerton,1994) This argument was based on Aristotle's view of technology (*technê*) as imitation of nature (*physis*). The view that artefacts were necessarily deprived of inner movement or 'substantial form' was propagated in medieval times by the scholastic tradition, and constituted an obstacle to technological advances . Alchemical and mechanical arts were blamed for being 'against nature'. (Newmann, 1989)

The resilience of the cultural stereotype seeing chemistry as being against nature, is the symptom of the values attached to the cultural boundary between nature and artefact, as well as between inanimate and animate matter. Throughout history, the culture of chemistry has been associated with the promotion of artificial over natural. Significantly, early attempts to produce in the laboratory natural products normally made inside living organisms - such as urea -, were used for metaphysical purposes to fight against vitalism rather than for technological purposes. The claim that Wölher's synthesis of urea in 1828 destroyed the metaphysical belief in the vital force is a legend forged by nineteenth-century chemists wanting to demonstrate that life was merely a set of physico-chemical phenomena. (Brooke, 1968, Ramberg, 2000) The urea mythology is still alive today in chemists' communities.

Indeed, such metaphysical challenge was an integral part of Marcellin Berthelot's defence of chemical synthesis. He planned to synthesize all the compounds made by living organisms, using only elements and the range of molecular forces. (Berthelot, 1860) Starting with the four basic elements—carbon, hydrogen, oxygen, and nitrogen—and proceeding systematically from the most simple to the most complex compounds, he boasted that chemists would synthesize the most complex compounds and dissipate the mystery of life.

Such attitude made it easy for physiologists such as Claude Bernard, to retort to arrogant chemists that synthesizing a product from its elementary principles did not mean getting the properties of living beings. (Bernard, 1865) Bernard also emphasized that the synthetic agents used by chemists in their laboratories were very different from those created by organisms. (Bernard 1866) In brief, chemists could imitate nature's structures but they could not emulate its processes and properties.

Should we consider the revival of biomimetism at the turn of the twenty-first century a new challenge to Bernard's defence against ambitious chemists? Are we now in a position to emulate natural processes and properties, and consequently to blur the boundaries between natural and artificial?

3. Looking for technological solutions in nature

The recent biomimetic trend in materials design seems to proceed from quite different and more pragmatic motivations. In the context of the fierce competition in space and military technologies that marked the Cold War period, conventional materials such as wood, metal, paper, ceramic, and polymers were deemed no longer relevant to making missiles and rockets. Hence chemists and materials scientists were encouraged to design high-performance materials with unprecedented combinations of properties for example materials as light as plastic, with the toughness of steel and the stiffness or heat-resistance of ceramics. This goal was achieved through the development of a new approach, known as "materials by design". (Bensaude-Vincent, 1997) For instance, starting from the functions of a particular airplane's wing, the best structure combining the set of properties required to perform those functions could be designed. The corresponding list of requirements thus translated into a list of performances, then a list of properties and finally into a structure. Thus function became the priority in the design process, while material became the outcome.

The design of materials-by-design relies heavily on the technology of composites. In contrast to conventional materials with standard specifications and universal applications, composites created for aerospace and military applications were developed with the functional demands, and the services expected from the manufactured products in mind. Such high-tech composite materials, designed for a specific task, in a specific environment, are so unique that their status becomes more like that of biological structures than standard commodities.

Therefore modest creatures such as insects, molluscs, butterflies, spiders or even protists became the subject of intense interest for materials chemists who had to design high-performance composite structures for space or military programs. Paradoxically, such materials-by-design came to replace materials extracted from the natural world, even as chemists and materials scientists came to realize that high-performance, multi-functional materials already existed in nature. As Stephen Mann -a natural scientist who entered the field of materials science- wrote: "We can be encouraged by the knowledge that a set of solutions have been worked out in the biological domain". (Mann et al., 1989, p. 35)

Amazing combinations of properties and adaptive structures can be found in the merest of creatures. Sea-urchin or abalone shells, for example, are wonderful bio-mineral structures made out of a common raw material, calcium carbonate: They present complex morphologies and assume a variety of functions. Spider webs are made of a an extremely thin and robust fiber, which offers unrivaled strength-to-weight ratio. Marine biologists were invited to apply the structure and performance concepts and methods of materials science to studying mollusc shells. Biomineralization thus emerged as a new research field which could "teach many lessons" to materials scientists. (Lowenstam H.A. and Weiner S., 1989; Mann, Werbb,Williams, 1989).

Plant biologists also started applying a materials perspective to their traditional objects of investigation. Not only are any plants currently being re-evaluated as potential sources of environmentally safe raw materials (biodegradable polymers or biofuels), but wood, the oldest and most common construction material, is now being described as 'a composite material with long, orientated fibers immersed in a light ligneous matrix, presenting a complex structure with different levels of organization at different scales'.

The complex hierarchy of structures in biomaterials is what biomimetic chemists most envy nature. Each different size scale, from the angström to the nanometer and micron, presents with different structural features. The remarkable properties of bio-materials, such as bone or tendon are the result of such complex arrangement at different levels, where each level controls the next one. (National Advisory Board, 1994) In other words, here is a level of complexity far beyond any of the complex composite structures that materials scientists have been able to design.

Another feature of biomaterials that scientists try to achieve in their own man-made materials is their adaptability to the environment. Designing responsive, self-healing structures was one the major objectives of materials research in the 1990s. To this end, programs on smart or intelligent materials were launched. On a basic level, intelligent materials are structures whose properties can vary according to changes in their environment or in the operating conditions. For example, materials whose chemical composition varies according to their surroundings are used in medicine to make prostheses. Some materials, whose structure varies according to the degree of damage caused by corrosion or radiations, are able to repair themselves. At the heart of the problem is the creation of in-built intelligence. It requires to have at least some embedded sensors (for strain, temperature, or light) and actuators, so that the structure becomes responsive to external stimuli.

Yet, materials chemists have been impressed by more than the elegance and the performances of biomaterials. Over the past decades, their attention has turned not only to composite and multifunctional structures but to nature's building processes themselves. Self-assembly, (i.e. the spontaneous arrangement of small building blocks in ordered patterns) is ubiquitous in living systems. In nature, the mortar and the bricks of biominerals are made simultaneously and self-assemble through the use of templates while the process is tightly controlled at each level. Self-assembly is the ultimate dream for materials designers. Such processes are crucial for designing at the nanoscale, where human hands and conventional tools are helpless. In addition self-assembly is extremely advantageous from a technological point of view, because it is a spontaneous and reversible process with little or no waste and a wide domain of applications. (Whitesides & Boncheva, 2002, Zhang 2003 , *MRS Bulletin*, 31 January 2006) Thus self-assembly appears as the holy grail of twenty-first century materials science:

> "Our world is populated with machines, non living entities assembled by human beings from components that humankind has made.... In the 21st century, scientists will introduce a manufacturing strategy based on machines and materials that virtually make themselves; what is called self-assembly is easiest to define by what it is not."(Whitesides, 1995)

How can we make machines and materials build themselves without active human intervention? To reach this fascinating goal, two contrasting strategies are being developed: The former which can be labelled 'soft chemistry' brings about deep changes in chemical culture; the latter which can be labelled 'hybrid technology' tends towards the substitution of biotechnology for chemical technology.

4. Two alternative strategies

On the chemical side, many processes are being explored with the aim to make variants of nature's highly directional self-assembly. The challenge for chemists is to achieve the self-assembly of their components and control the resulting morphogenesis, without relying on instructions from the genetic code. To meet this challenge, chemists have mobilized all the resources available from physics and chemistry: Chemical transformations in spatially restricted reaction fields, external solicitations such as gravitational, electric or magnetic fields, mechanical stress, gradients and flux of reagents during synthesis. They take advantage of all sorts of interactions between atoms and molecules. Instead of using covalent bonds traditionally used in organic chemistry, they rely on weak interactions such as hydrogen bonds, Van der Waals and electrostatic interactions. Chemists also use templates surfactants mesophases to build such as mesoporous silica, or conduct synthesis in compartments. They make self-assembled monolayers using microfluidics and surfactants, which in turn enables the move from atomic and molecular level structures to macroscopic properties.

To imitate nature's processes of self-assembly, chemists have developed a new "chemical culture" for which Jacques Livage coined the phrase "chimie douce" (soft chemistry) in 1977. Whereas conventional synthetic chemistry usually takes place in extreme conditions which are costly in terms of energy, uses large quantities of organic solvents and produces undesirable waste products, biomimetic chemistry relies on chemical reactions taking place at room temperature in rather 'messy', aqueous environments. Such approach using quasi-physiological conditions, generating only the renewable, and biodegradable by-products associated with nature's synthetic processes, is used to make new materials at the low cost. The development of soft chemistry has led to the use of increasingly complex raw reagents, including macromolecules, aggregates and colloids. The 'Supramolecular chemistry', promoted by Jean-Marie Lehn in 1978, makes extensive use of hydrogen bonds in an attempt to reproduce the receptor-substrate interaction specificity, itself a hallmark of biology. Thanks to these forms of molecular recognition and assembly mechanisms, building blocks can self-assemble to form supra-molecular structures, and even generate macroscopic materials.

As self-assembly relies on spontaneous reactions between building blocks, it presupposes that the instructions for assembly are either an integral part of the material components themselves, or that they are the product of their interactions. Although inanimate matter is deprived of a genetic program, it is not viewed as a passive receptacle upon which information is imprinted from the outside. Molecules have an inherent activity, an intrinsic *dunamis* allowing the construction of a variety of geometrical shapes (helix, spiral, etc). This dynamic is not an obscure and mysterious vital force; nor is it an algorithm or a set of instructions embedded in a machine. It is instead a blind process of creation using combinations and selection without an external designer. Although chemists often use the paradoxical phrase 'we self-assemble molecules', the process takes place without human involvement. The subject "we" just initiates the process of self-assembly by securing the necessary agencies and appropriate conditions.

By contrast, in hybrid biotechnology strategies, natural structures and processes are truly 'engineered', or at least 're-engineered'. Such strategies are often seen to be more promising than biomimetic attempts. It can seem more reasonable to make use of the exquisite structures and devices selected by biological evolutionary processes in order to achieve our own goals, rather than to try and imitate them. In particular, it is rather tempting to use biological devices of molecular recognition to move along the path prescribed by the so-called Moore's law, to build smaller and smaller electronic circuits that assemble without human manipulation. In 2003 Erez Braun, a biophysicist from Technion at Haïfa announced that he used the complementarity of DNA strands to make nanotransistors. Now the use of DNA strands is routine practice in the laboratory, and is awaiting applications on an industrial scale.

5. Technomimetism

Synthetic biology develops a radical program to rewrite the genetic code formerly deciphered by molecular biology and genomics over the past decades. It aims to synthesise artificial organisms beyond what nature has created. In addition to the synthesis of new functional sequences, synthetic biology includes the design of gene circuits analogous to electrical components and circuits, with oscillators, switches, etc.... Another goal is to make up a minimal genome - deprived of all superfluous functions but able to support a self-replicating organism. Such minimal genomes could be used as 'chassis' on which desired functions could be grafted in the same way synthetic chemists used to graft functions on a benzene ring.

Hybridizing and synthetic biology strategies rest on the view that living systems are collections of devices that can be abstracted from their environment decoupled from other functions and put at work in artificial machines. They are treated like parts in a clock. The designer of artificial machines borrows the specific material or devices "invented" by biological evolution regardless of their specific environment. The fact is that traditional technologies have been doing just that for centuries. They extracted resources such as wood, bone, or skin and processed them to make a variety of artefacts. Similarly, nanotechnology and synthetic biology extract a number of small units, which are as close as possible to the building blocks of living systems (DNA, bacteria,..), in order to build artefacts from the bottom-up. Bio-molecular systems are broken down into elementary units, redefined as functionalities, and abstracted from their own environment. Furthermore, these elementary units can be processed and modified through genetic engineering to perform specific tasks in an artificial environment.

Synthetic biology is explicitly aimed at creating bio-systems operating along the principles of engineering. Instead of making artefacts mimicking nature, synthetic biologists synthesize living organisms modelled after machines. Synthetic biology can therefore be seen as a technomimetism, an alternative strategy to biomimetism, which is consequently dismissed as a poor amateurish strategy:

> "If biological engineering were aviation, it would be at the birdman stage: some observation and some understanding, but largely naive mimicry. For the field to really take flight, it needs the machinery of synthetic biology. [...] At the turn of the last century, the Wright brothers achieved manned flight not by mimicking natural systems, but by applying the principles of engineering and aerodynamics. Similarly, synthetic biology allows us to dispense with biological mimicry and design life forms uniquely tailored to our needs. In doing so, it will offer not only fundamental insights into questions of life and vitality but also the type of exquisite precision and efficiency in creating complex traits that genetic engineers could previously only dream of. » (anonymous editorial, 2009)

Unlike biomimetism, technomimetism is a kind of engineering which consists in implementing the rationality of machines in natural systems. Biosystems have to be redesigned along the principles of engineering because they are too complex or have not been optimized by evolution for human purposes. Synthetic biologists like Drew Endy are proud to apply the engineering approach to biosystems. His main purpose is to "make routine the engineering of synthetic biological systems that behave as expected". (Endy, 2005) The emphasis is on constructing reliable artefacts that get rid of all the messiness and unpredictability of natural systems. Standardization of the bioparts is the first requirement for the design of technomimetic biosystems. The Registry of Standard Bioparts created in Berkeley is meant as a catalogue of the standard parts bioengineers can compile into a physical structure once they have targeted their system's specifications.

A number of synthetic biologists go beyond the ambition of redesigning life according to the basic principles of engineering. Their purpose is to make life as it could be, rather than as it is. In order to create living organisms as different as possible from all existing life forms, they aim to synthesize unnatural DNA. Steven Benner for instance insists that the four-base DNA code might not be the only way to reproduce and pass on genetic information. Consequently he has made up an alien DNA, which contains two artificial nucleotides in addition to A-G-C-T, and which is already licensed and marketed by a company called EraGen-Bioscience. Benner's ambition is to expand the genetic information system to twelve bases. Owing to the difficulty of confining genetically modified organisms to laboratories, his "alien genetics" is promoted as a way to circumvent the risks of contaminating the environment, and possibly as a way to support life on other planets, to create new parallel forms of life.

6. A reciprocal mimesis

Is it a mere coincidence that a strong movement of technomimetism runs parallel to an equally strong movement of biomimetism? In a famous study of machines and organisms, French philosopher Georges Canguilhem noticed that organisms have often been described in technological terms, even though there is no reason why *a priori,* this analogy between organisms and machines should not work the other way round. (Canguilhem, 1947) In fact a quick glimpse at history suggests that the analogy works both ways.

While Aristotle, in his *Physics,* claimed that technology imitates nature in his biological works, he described nature according to the model of technology. Human arts provided a lot of images that helped clarify how nature worked in living beings. They served as models to understand that all natural beings were end-directed. "As *technê,* so *phusis*" was a conviction that informed Greek medicine. (Von Staden, 2007).

By contrast, when modern science emerged in the seventeenth century, nature was conceived according to the model of machines, and described as a passive, rigid, precise clock mechanism. Descartes' theory of animal machines spread a mechanical understanding of life, with the mind being the exception. Later, eighteenth-century materialist philosophers repudiated Descartes' separation between mind and body, and claimed that all human functions were mechanical processes. It is against this philosophical background that Jacques de Vaucanson or Pierre Jaquet-Droz created their famous automata. (Riskin, 2007) These ancestors of modern robots were used to test the mechanical views of mind and body as much as for entertainment.

In the course of the twentieth-century, our representation of nature and life has been reconfigured again and again. First the mass production of polymers by synthetic chemists brought about what is called the "plastic age". It encouraged the view that nature was rigid and limited, in contrast to the plasticity and indefinite potentials of artefacts. (Bensaude-Vincent, 2007). Since the mid-twentieth century, our understanding of the brain and of living cells have been deeply transformed by cybernetics and information technology. Significantly, it was in the 1960s, when cybernetics raised great enthusiasm, that biomimetism became its own field of research. It was then named "bionics", a term coined in 1958, and defined by Jack Steele of the US Air Force as "the science of systems whose function is based on living systems, or which have the characteristics of living systems, or which resemble these". (quoted in Vogel, 1998, p. 250) Bionics was thus centred on systems, while biomimetics was more concerned with mechanics. According to Waren Mc Culloch in 1962, biomimetics encompassed all areas in which organisms may copy each other. It included technological inventions as much as, for example, the mimetic behaviours displayed by some insects.

In the 1960s, computer technology provided the conceptual framework for molecular biology. From the metaphor of the program, which prevailed through "the century of the gene" to the more recent metaphor of "genetic circuitry" used in synthetic biology, information technology has continuously inspired our understanding of life at the molecular level. (Fox Keller, 1995, 2002) And molecular biology, in turn, inspired nanotechnology, at least if we assume that Richard Feynman's famous 1959 lecture at the meeting of the American Institute of Physics actually foretold the future. His celebrated vision that "there is plenty of room at the bottom" was explicitly inspired by the then recent discovery of DNA's structure and function by Francis Crick and James Watson. The storage of huge amounts of information in DNA macromolecules persuaded him that it may be possible to store the entire Library of Congress on the pin of a needle.

Nanotechnology illustrates well the self-reinforcing interaction between technological paradigms and views of nature. According to the definition given in the US National NanoInitiative, nanotechnology is: "Working at the atomic, molecular and supra-molecular levels, in the length scale of approximately 1 - 100 nm range, in order to understand, create and use materials, devices and systems with fundamentally new properties and functions because of their small structure." (Roco, Bainbridge, Alivastos, 2000, p.3)

Having access to the nanoscale blurs a number of boundaries, which had been already challenged by chemistry and materials science. On the one hand, nanoscientists argue that at the nanoscale, the boundary between inanimate and living matter no longer makes sense. DNA for example, is seen as a chemical macromolecule made up of four pairs of bases which does not enjoy any privileged status such as witholding "the secret of life". On the other hand, the boundary between science and technology is also blurred, the ultimate constituents of inorganic and organic systems are viewed through engineering lenses. The building blocks of matter and life are considered as devices or machines. Atoms, molecules, micelles, DNA, proteins and neurons, all natural entities are viewed as functional units capable of performing interesting tasks. They are characterized by what they perform rather than by what they are made of. Living systems are viewed as molecular manufactures and the analogy is often used as proof that a particular project can be achieved - in other words, if nature can do it, so can we.

Simultaneously, biologists describe the molecular components of cells as tools or machines operating at the macromolecular level: Ribosomes are assembly lines for proteins, myosin fibers are motors, polymerases are copy machines, membrane proteases are electric fences, and so on. Even though biologists generally agree with the idea that living systems are the results of blind and random evolution rather than of design, they still describe them as devices designed for specific tasks. In the past, descriptions of organisms and cells as little factories were occasionally used for teaching or popularizing purposes. But following the introduction of the genetic code in the early times of molecular biology, these metaphors became more than expository tools. They started providing heuristic models, and guidelines for research and design.

Eric Drexler, one of the champions of nanotechnology, took the metaphor of the cell machinery for granted and promoted his "molecular manufacture" as a biomimetic manufacture. The main feature he retained from biology was that bio structures are built from bottom-up, molecule-by-molecule rather than carved from bulk material. He could then contrast two styles of technology: the conventional style, which prevailed from prehistoric flint-choppers to micro-electronic chips works from the top down, and generates waste, pollution and many nuisances. Molecular manufacturing, which shapes artefacts atom-by-atom, would open a new era of clean, efficient, energy saving manufacturing. Thanks to universal assemblers modelled after ribosomes, we should be able, in his view, to pick and place atoms and dispense with dirty and messy chemical manufactures.

Thus, between nature and technology exists a two-way traffic of concepts, images and models. As French philosopher Maurice Merleau Ponty pointed out in 1956: "We cannot think about nature, without realizing that our idea of nature is permeated by artefacts". (Merleau Ponty, 1956, p. 120). Nature and artefacts are mutually defined by an ambivalent relationship of connivance and rivalry.

7. How to deal with mimicry?

If nature and technology are continuously reconfigured in a process of mutual mimesis, we may feel like we are trapped in a circle. All circles however are not necessarily "vicious". Indeed, analogies and attempts to mimic can prove extremely fruitful. Ironically though, their heuristic power does not so much rest on analogies as it does on differences. I will argue that mimicry is more interesting as a differentiation strategy than as attempts to copy or emulate a model.

In particular, Drexler's assumption that 'bio is nano' prompted many criticisms, and emphasised the differences between our vision of machines and the "biological machinery". In an essay entitled *Soft Machines,* Richard Jones's argued that the 'machines' found inside living cells work on principles which are quite different from those of conventional machines. (Jones, 2004) Firstly, living systems unlike organic chemistry do not use rigid molecules: Proteins, for example, can readily change their shape and conformation. Secondly, instead of channelling the traffic of materials by means of tubes and pipes, living systems take advantage of Brownian motion, which moves molecules and continuously bombards them with nano-objects. In addition, at the molecular level where bio-machinery operates, inertia is no longer a crucial parameter, while surface forces, particularly viscosity, determine whether or not nano-objects will stick together.

From a chemical perspective, the differences between the strategies used in the evolution of life and laboratory procedures are also striking. Funnily enough, nature was never taught laboratory procedures and laboratory procedures require conditions that are far from common in nature such as high temperature, pressure, or vacuum. Chemists have been taught how to work with pure and homogenous substances, which have stable compositions. They can control reactions carried out at the bench, by limiting the number of parameters involved. In contrast, natural substances are chemically impure and riddled with faults; most of them are mixtures or composites. In addition, nature never uses metals as structural material. Nature operates along lines, which look unorthodox to the eye of ordinary chemists, at ambient temperature, and in the presence of a whole range of perturbations.

The constraints in nature differ from the constraints met by chemists and materials engineers in the laboratory. Through trial and error, nature spent billions of years designing and perfecting high-performance structures capable of sustaining life. Life itself, according to the Darwinian evolution, generated a great variety of species and selected the beneficial variants. Engineers work in quite different conditions to evolution, which require projects, planning, anticipation and selective pressures coming from time, money, safety, and security. Despite its strong power of attraction, the view that nature is the perfect standard for design is misleading. In fact, so great is the gap between human design and nature's processes of fabrication, that any project of 'technology transfer' from nature to factory would be totally inadequate.

Nature cannot provide a model for human technologies, because the same performance criteria cannot be applied. Let us for a moment try to evaluate nature's performances along our criterion of optimization: What does optimization even mean for biosystems? Is it more efficient devices? Our notion of efficiency rests on the principle of *maximum de minimo*: For instance getting the highest resistance from the lowest quantity of matter, or getting a maximum amount of benefits at minimum costs. (Quintinilla & Lawler, 2000) Obviously, this kind of economical rationality does not even register in natural systems. Should we therefore adopt a more qualitative definition of efficiency, such as being a match between means and end? No sooner would we do this than we would stumble upon a new obstacle to determine what the ends of nature may be. As long as we assume that biological evolution is not a teleological process, it would be arbitrary to decide whether its ends are reproduction, or survival, or adaptation for example; or whether these ends should concern individuals or populations etc..

8. Conclusion

Simply copying nature is out of the question. Strictly speaking, nature does not teach anything. It does not deliver either lessons or recipes, which could be applied to technological projects. Nature is basically inexorable, indifferent to our projects and concerns. Living organisms may be seen as holding the answers to questions arising from biological evolution, but they cannot meet our needs resulting from military and economic competition, or societal concerns (for instance health, energy saving or pollution…).

Taking inspiration from nature is a more relevant attitude, and often results in a better understanding of the differences between nature and technology. Bio-inspired designers having to elucidate the principles at work in biomaterials, have to sort out the main variables and constraints operating in the natural world and are gradually able to confront them with the variables and constraints of technological design. In reality, we take inspiration from our understanding of nature, which in itself is inspired from the dominant technological paradigms of our time. The main merit of bio-inspiration is to emphasize the differences between nature and technology and to restore the polarity, which technomimetic strategies have tended to blur.

9. References

[anonymous] editorial (2009) Unbottling the genes, *Nature Biotechnology*, 27, 12, Dec 2009, 1059.

Bensaude-Vincent B. (2007) Reconfiguring nature through syntheses: From plastics to biomimetics, In: *The Artificial and the Natural. An Evolving Polarity*, B. Bensaude-Vincent , W.R. Newmann eds, p. 293-312, MIT Press, Cambridge Mass.

Bensaude-Vincent, B.; Arribart, H.; Bouligand, Y. & Sanchez, C. (2002), Chemists at the School of Nature, *Journal of European Chemistry*, 26, January 2002, 1-5.

Benyus, J.M. (1998), *Biomimicry, Innovation inspired by Nature*, Quill edition, New York.

Bernard, C. [1865] *Introduction à l'étude de la méthode expérimentale en médecine*, Flammarion, Paris, 1984.

Bernard, C. [1878] *Leçons sur les phénomènes de la vie communs aux animaux et aux végétaux*, Vrin, Paris, 1966, p. 202-229.

Berthelot, M. (1860), La *chimie organique fondée sur la synthèse*, Alcan, Paris.

Brooke, J. H. (1968) Wöhler's Urea and its Vital Force - A Verdict from the Chemists, *Ambix*, 15, 84–114.

Canguilhem, G. [1947] Machine et organisme, In: *La connaissance de la vie*, Vrin, Paris, 1971, p. 101-127.

Emerton, N. (1994)*The Scientific Reinterpretation of Form*, Ithaca, Cornell University Press.

Endy D (2005) Foundations for engineering biology. *Nature*, 438, 25 November, 449-453.

Fox Keller, E. (1995) *Refiguring Life. Metaphors of Twentieth century Biology*, Columbia University Press, New York.

Fox Keller, E. (2002) *The Century of the Gene*, Harvard University Press, Cambridge Mass.

Merleau-Ponty, M. [1956-57] *La Nature. Notes. Cours du Collège de France*, Editions du Seuil, Paris, 1995.

Jones, R (2004) *Soft Machines*, Oxford University Press, Oxford, New-York.

Lowenstam H.A.; Weiner S. (1989) *On Biomineralization*, Oxford University Press, Oxford, New York.

Mann, Stephen, Werbb John and Williams, Robert J.P. eds (1989) *Biomineralization , Chemical and Biological Perspectives*, VCH, Weinheim:.

National Advisory Board (1994), *Hierarchical Structures in Biology as a Guide for New Materials Technology*, National Academy Press, Washington DC.

Newman, W. (1989) Technology and alchemical debate in the late middle ages, *Isis*, 80, 423-445

Quintanilla M.; Lawler D. (2000) El concepto de eficiencia técnica, In: Denegri, G.M. & Martinez, G.E. eds, *Topicos actuales en filosofia da ciencia. Homenagem a Mario Bunge en su 80° aniversario*, p. 203-24, Universidad nacional de Mar del Plata, Mar del Plata.

Ramberg, P. (2000) The Death of Vitalism and the Birth of Organic Chemistry: Wölher's Urea Synthesis and the Disciplinary Identity of Chemistry, *Ambix*, 47, 170–195.

Riskin, J. (2007) Eighteenth-century wetware, In: B. Bensaude-Vincent , W.R. Newmann eds, *The Artificial and the Natural. An Evolving Polarity*, pp. 239-274, MIT Press, Cambridge Mass.

Roco, M.C.; Bainbridge W. & Alivastos, P. (2000), *Nanotechnology Research Directions*. IWGN *Interagency Working Group on Nanoscience Workshop Report*, Kluwer, Dordrecht, Boston.

Vogel, S. (1998) *Cats' Paws and Catapults. Mechanical Worlds of Nature and People*, Norton & Company, New York, London.

Von Staden, H. (2007), Physis and technê in Greek Medicine, In: B. Bensaude-Vincent , W.R. Newmann eds, *The Artificial and the Natural. An Evolving Polarity*, p. 21-49, MIT Press, Cambridge Mass.

Whitesides, G. M.; Boncheva, M.(2002) Beyond molecules: Self-assembly of mesoscopic and macroscopic components, *Proceedings of the National Academy of Science*, 99, April 16, 2002, 4769–4774.

Whitesides G.M.; Grzybowski B. (2002) Self-assembly at all scales, *Science*, 295, March 19, 2002, 2418-21.

Zhang, S. (2003) Fabrication of novel biomaterials through molecular self-assembly, *Nature Biotechnology*, 21, 10, Oct 2003, 1171-78.

2

Biomineralization and Biomimetic Synthesis of Biomineral and Nanomaterials

Ming-Guo Ma and Run-Cang Sun
Institute of Biomass Chemistry and Technology,
College of Materials Science and Technology,
Beijing Forestry University
P. R. China

1. Introduction

Biominerals and biomaterials with unique microstructure are mainly consisted of organic and inorganic materials, and exhibit excellent biological and mechanical properties. The formation mechanism of biomineral indicated that the organic matrixes have an important influence on the morphology and structure of the inorganic matrix material in the process of biomineralization. However, the biomineralization mechanism research of biomineral is still in the initial stage, many phenomena need to be further explored, such as the effect of organisms on the different morphologies and polymorphs of biominerals, the biomineralization mechanism of the formation process of the biomineral in the existence of organic matter. Biomineralization and biomimetic synthesis of biomineral and nanomaterials have been receiving considerable attention. Biomineralization is the formation process of mineral by organisms. Biomimetic synthesis is simulation of biomineralization, using the mechanism of biomineralization, to achieve biomineral and materials with special structure and function. In a word, biomimetic synthesis is learning from the mineralization of organisms and learning from nature. Therefore, we should understand the concepts, process, and mechanism of biomineralization, which was briefly reviewed in section one.

Biomineral including calcium phosphate, hydroxyapatite (HA), calcium silicate, calcium carbonate, and calcium sulfate, are important calcium-based inorganic biodegradable materials and have been widely used in biomedical field. Biomineralization is the mineralization of biomineral. Biomimetic synthesis was first used in the fabrication of biomineral. So it is necessary to provide an overview of the biomimetic synthesis of biomineral. This chapter summarizes our recent endeavors on the biomimetic synthesis of biomineral including HA, calcium silicate, $CaCO_3$, $BaCO_3$, and $SrCO_3$, etc.

Biomineral synthesis includes morphology, structure, and function biomineral synthesis. It is well known that the structure determines property and the morphology is the external display of structure. Here, we intend to review recent progress in biomineral synthesis of other nanomaterials.

2. Biomimetic synthesis of calcium-based inorganic biodegradable nanomaterials

2.1 Background

The biomineral in nature with different composition and specific biological functions formed from the body of bacteria, microbes, plants, and animals has more than sixty kinds of species. Among the half of the biomineral, calcium-based inorganic biodegradable nanomaterials (CIBNs) including calcium phosphate, hydroxyapatite (HA), calcium silicate, calcium carbonate, and calcium sulfate, etc, are important materials and have been widely used in biomedical fields such as bone cements (Islas-Blancas et al., 2001), drug delivery (Kim et al., 2004), tooth paste additives (Oktar et al., 1999), dental implants (Gross et al., 1998), gas sensors, ion exchange (Yasukawa et al., 2004), catalysts or catalysts supports (Venugopal & Scurrell, 2003), and host materials for lasers (Garcia-Sanz et al., 1997). Compared to biomedical polymer materials, CIBNs have received considerable attention due to their excellent osteoconductivity, biocompatibility, bioactivity, biodegradablity, chemical stability, and mechanical strength (Hing, 2004; Boskey et al., 2005; Wahl & Czernuszka, 2006; Dorozhkin, 2007). CIBNs have some solubility, bonding ability between biological tissues, releasing innoxious ions on the body and can promote repairment in tissue. However, the traditional biodegradable materials mainly refer to polymers with biodegradable ability such as poly(lactic acid) and poly(amino acid). So strengthen the research of CIBNs as the expansion of biodegradable materials will do a favor to exploiting the applications of biomedical materials.

For a long time, CIBNs have been considered as a kind of bioactivity materials. CIBNs, for example bioactive glass, bioactive cement, HA, etc, have been found to have some solution and absorption in the organism, and they had calcium and phosphorus element in their composition, which can be replaced in the body's normal metabolism pathway through the hydroxyl groups bonding to human tissue. The defect sites could be completely replaced by new bone tissue after the implantation of CIBNs, while the CIBNs were only used as temporary scaffolds. Some of CIBNs even took part in the formation of new bone. β-tricalcium phosphate (β-TCP) porous materials were fabricated by Getter et al. in 1972, and they also made use of β-TCP as bone graft in 1977 (Cameron et al., 1977), and made clinical bone fill experiment in 1978. Using β-TCP in bone regeneration experiment was first reported in 1981 (Groot & Mitchell, 1981). In recent years, it was found that β-TCP is a good tissue engineering scaffold material in biomedical field. This type of material has some advantages including the gradual degradation in the organisms' metabolic process, the process of replacement and growth of new bone, without prejudice to newly grown bone in material substitution process.

It is well known that the naturally tooth and bone are organic/inorganic composites with the ingredients including calcium phosphate, HA, calcium silicate, and calcium carbonate. Especially, HA is similar in composition to bone mineral, has been found to promote new bone formation when being implanted in a skeletal defect, and has been used in clinical bone graft procedures for about 30 years. However, its poor tensile strength and fracture toughness make it unsuitable for practical applications. It was discovered that naturally derived tooth HA did not differ from synthetic ones (Oktar et al., 1999). A nanostructured HA was thermally sprayed on Ti-6Al-4V substrates via high velocity oxy-fuel, and a uniform layer of apatite was formed via immersing the coating in a simulated body fluid (SBF) for 7 days (Lima et al., 2005). Thian *et al* (2006). fabricated nanocrystalline silicon-substituted HA thin coatings with enhanced bioactivity and biofunctionality applied to a titanium substrate via a magnetron co-sputtering process. An increase in the attachment and growth of human osteoblast-like (HOB) cells on these coatings was observed throughout the culture period, with the formation of extracellular matrix. Biomedical nanocomposite fibers of HA/poly(lactic acid) with homogeneous structure were synthesized by electrospinning (Kim et al., 2006). Initial cellular assays indicated excellent cell attachment and proliferation. In this section, we briefly review the interrelated papers concerning the biomimetic fabrication, mechanism, and future development of CIBNs. The chapter also provides an overview about the potential application of nanotechnology in biomedical field (Ma & Zhu, 2010).

2.2 Fabrication of calcium-based inorganic biodegradable nanomaterials

Some successful methods including precipitation, hydrothermal, microemulsion, sol-gel, biomimetic synthesis have been employed for the synthesis of CIBNs. The liquid phase precipitation method is one of the earliest methods for the synthesis of CIBNs. In recent years, the system such as $Ca(OH)_2$-H_3PO_4-H_2O, $Ca(NO_3)_2$-NH_4NO_3-$NH_3 \cdot H_2O$, $CaCl_2$-K_2HPO_4-KOH, and $CaHPO_4$-$Ca_4(PO_4)_2O$-H_2O has been adopted in the preparation of HA (Tarasevich et al., 2003; Lu & Leng, 2005; Kanakis et al., 2006). However, impurities were also observed as the byproducts. Some successful strategies including chemical mechanical vapor deposition (Chi, 2010), mechano-chemical process (Tofighi & Rey, 2010), dual nozzle spray drying techniques (Chow & Sun, 2010), high alumina fly ash (Zhang et al., 2009), have been also employed for the synthesis of CIBNs.

HA and calcium silicate are the typical examples among the CIBNs. HA has a composition and structure analogous to the bone apatite and shows high bioactivity (Suchanek et al., 2002; Landi et al., 2004 ; Sun et al., 2009). Calcium silicate is used in drug delivery and bone tissue regeneration due to its good biocompatibility, bioactivity, and degradability (Matsuoka et al., 1999; Oyane et al., 2003; Cortes et al., 2004; Li & Chang, 2005; Jain et al., 2005; Kokubo et al., 2005). Recently, the key point of the present research aims to the synthesis of HA (Rudin et al., 2009) and calcium silicate nanostructures by novel methods. Liu *et al* (2005). fabricated HA nanoribbon spheres by a one-step reaction using the bioactive eggshell membrane as a directing template in the presence of ethylenediamine. The authors indicated that spheres can be modified with fluorescein to obtain a fluorescent probe material with strong luminescence. HA nanorods were formed by the liquid-solid solution method reported by Wang *et al.*(2006). The bubble-template route is also employed to synthesize flower-like porous B-type carbonated HA microspheres (Cheng et al., 2009). Using double emulsion droplets as microreactors, mesoporous HA could be fabricated (Shum et al., 2009). The size and the geometry of the droplet microreactors can be tuned by using capillary microfluidic techniques. We reported the synthesis of hierarchically nanostructured HA hollow spheres using $CaCl_2$, NaH_2PO_4, and potassium sodium tartrate via a solvothermal method at 200 °C for 24 h in water/*N,N*-dimethylformamide (DMF) mixed solvents, HA microtubes using $CaCl_2$ and NaH_2PO_4 in mixed solvents of water/DMF by a solvothermal method at 160 °C for 24 h (Fig. **1**) (Ma et al., 2008; Ma & Zhu, 2009).

Currently, the research of CIBNs has been focus on β-tricalcium phosphate (β-TCP), $CaSO_4$, calcium silicate, and some natural materials such as natural coral (primarily composed of $CaCO_3$) and its composite materials. These materials are mainly used in bone substitute materials, or scaffolds for tissue engineering. The drug loading and releasing materials are mostly made of the biodegradable polymers. With the development of CIBNs, their application can also be extended to controlled drug delivery system.

Using HA and calcium silicate in drug delivery and other biomedical applications has become a key topic regarding CIBNs' application. A novel magnetic HA nanoparticles can be used as non-viral vectors for the glial cell line-derived neurotrophic factor gene by the treatment with iron ions using a wet-chemical process (Wu et al., 2010). Yuan *et al* (2010). investigated the effect of the particle size of the HA nanoparticles on the anti-tumor activity, apoptosis-induction and the levels of the apoptotic signaling proteins in human hepatoma HepG2 model cells. The experiments indicated that the size of HA and thereby the cellular localization had predominant effect on the HA-induced cytotoxicity, apoptotis, and the levels of the apoptotic proteins in HepG2 cells. HA nanoparticle-coated micrometer-sized poly(L-lactic acid) microspheres were fabricated via a "Pickering-type" emulsion route in the absence of any molecular surfactants, which can promote the cell adhesion and spreading (Fujii et al., 2009).

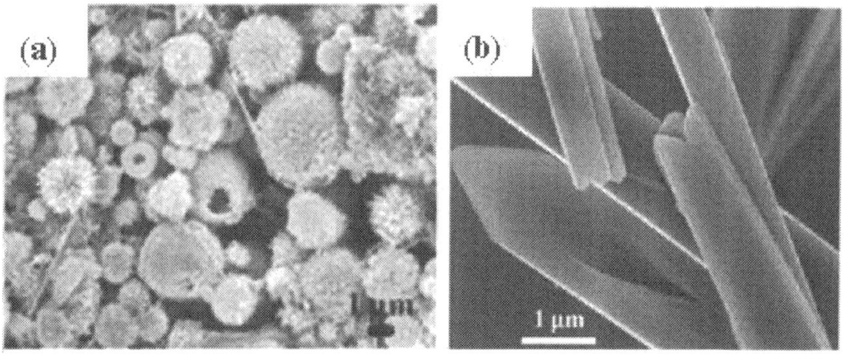

Fig. 1. (a) SEM micrograph of the hierarchically nanostructured HA hollow spheres, (Reproduced with permission from Eur. J. Inorg. Chem. **2009**, 5522. Copyright **2009** *VCH.*) and (b) TEM micrograph of the HA microtubes. (Reproduced with permission from Mater. Lett. **2008**, *62*, 1642. Copyright **2008** *Elsevier*)

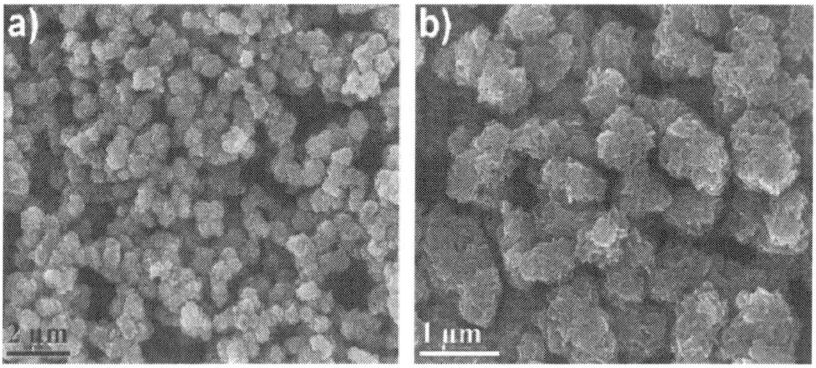

Fig. 2. SEM images of hierachically nanostructured mesoporous spheres of calcium silicate hydrate, prepared by the surfactant-free sonochemical synthesis. Reproduced with permission from Adv. Mater. **2009**, *22*, 749. Copyright **2009** *VCH.*

In the past decades, calcium silicate materials have drawn growing attention on their potential applications in the bone tissue engineering field (Rodríguez-Lorenzo et al., 2009; Wei et al., 2009). Nanosized calcium silicate and poly(epsilon-caprolactone) nanocomposite for bone tissue regeneration using calcium silicate slurry, other than dried calcium silicate powder, was fabricated by Wei *et al* (2009). in a solvent-casting method. The results suggested that the incorporation of calcium silicate could significantly improve the hydrophilicity, compressive strength, and elastic modulus of calcium silicate/poly(epsilon-caprolactone) composites.

Some studies have been carried out on calcium silicate transformation to bonelike apatite/HA, but few have extended their applications in drug delivery systems (Jain et al., 2005; Li & Chang, 2005). Recently, Wu *et al.* (2009) reported the low-cost and surfactant-free sonochemical synthesis of hierachically nanostructured mesoporous spheres of calcium silicate hydrate with well-defined 3D network structures constructed by nanosheets as building blocks (Fig. **2**). The calcium silicate hydrate has the advantages of large specific surface area, large pore volume, extremely high drug-loading capacity (2.29 g IBU is loaded in per gram carrier), adjustable drug-release rate, good bioactivity, and fine biodegradability. Moreover, calcium silicate hydrate can entirely transform to HA after the drug release in simulated body fluid, implying the good bioactivity and biodegradability. Besides the hierachically nanostructured mesoporous spheres of calcium silicate hydrate, they also prepared HA and calcium silicate nanostructured porous hollow ellipsoidal capsules, which were constructed by nanoplate networks using the inorganic $CaCO_3$ template (Fig. **3**) (Ma et al., 2008). $CaCO_3$ ellipsoids were synthesized via the reaction between $Ca(CH_3COO)_2$ and $NaHCO_3$ in water and ethylene glycol mixed solvent at room temperature. The drug loading and release behavior of HA hollow capsules indicated that HA hollow capsules had a high specific surface area and high storage capacity. Calcium phosphate (CaP)/PLGA-mPEG hybrid porous nanospheres were synthesized by a facile room-temperature method, which can be applied as DNA vectors for DNA loading and in vitro transfection (Wang et al., 2010).

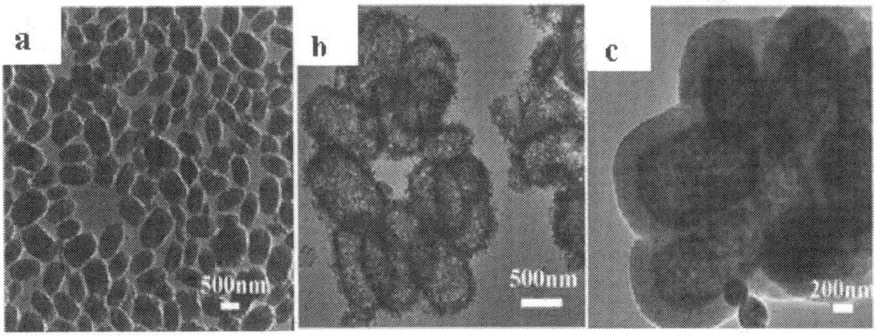

Fig. 3. TEM micrographs of (a) $CaCO_3$ cores, (b) HA nanostructured hollow ellipsoidal capsules, (c) calcium silicate nanostructured hollow ellipsoidal capsules. Reproduced with permission from J. Mater. Chem., **2008**, *18*, 2722. Copyright **2008** *RSC.*

In addition, the synthesis of calcium phosphate (Lee et al.,2009; Matsumoto & Nakasu,2010)., dipterinyl calcium pentahydrate (Moheno & Pfleiderer, 2010), calcium phosphate pasty material (Lacout et al., 2009), and HA calcium phosphates (Godber & Leite, 2009) has been also reported. Calcium sulfate was aseptic, biocompatible and biodegradable, which was an ideal substitute of bone transplantation material (Mirtchi et al., 1990; Sato et al., 1998; Nilsson et al., 2002; Bohner, 2004), and antibiotic-carrier material (McKee et al., 2002; Rauschmann et al., 2005).

A single component of CIBNs has some limitations such as too fast or too slow degradation time, low mechanical properties. However, compared to the individual components, nanocomposites provided the possibility for the enhancement of multifunctional properties due to interaction between the counterparts. Therefore, to develop new CIBNs-based nanocomposites with the control over the crystal phase and morphology is of great importance for broadening applications of CIBNs.

There are a few reports about CIBNs-based nanocomposites (Sotome et al., 2009; Furuzono et al., 2009; Yaszemski et al., 2010). Chitosan-HA nanostructured biocomposite films with high volume fraction were prepared by solvent casting their hybrid suspensions using biomimetic synthesis method (Kithva et al., 2010). HA-coated zirconia-magnesia composite for protein separation was also be prepared by biomimetic technique (Li & Feng, 2009). An invention patented by Ding *et al.* (2009) has provided a sol-gel method for synthesizing calcium silicate-based composite cement, which provided a novel mixture for bone tissue repairment. Bioactive bone-repairing materials with mechanical properties analogous to those of natural bone can also be fabricated through the combination of calcium silicate with polyetheretherketone (Kim et al., 2009).

As the most abundant renewable material and natural polysaccharide found on earth, cellulose becomes one of important biodegradable materials owing to its unique properties such as chemical stability, mechanical strength, biocompatibility, biodegradation (Iguchi et al., 2000; Gindl & Keckes, 2004; Shoda & Sugano,2005). The cellulose-calcium silicate nanocomposites are considered to have potential applications in biomedical field with such striking features as high mechanical properties and excellent biocompatibility. We fabricated the cellulose-calcium silicate nanocomposites with calcium silicate nanoparticles homogeneously dispersed in the cellulose matrix using cellulose solution, $Ca(NO_3)_2{\cdot}4H_2O$ and $Na_2SiO_3{\cdot}9H_2O$ in ethanol/water mixed solvents at room temperature for 24 h (Fig. **4a**) (Li et al., 2010). Cellulose-HA nanocomposites were also obtained using microcrystalline cellulose, $CaCl_2$, and NaH_2PO_4 in *N,N*-dimethylacetamide solvent by microwave-assisted method at 150 °C (Fig. **4b**) (Ma et al., 2010).

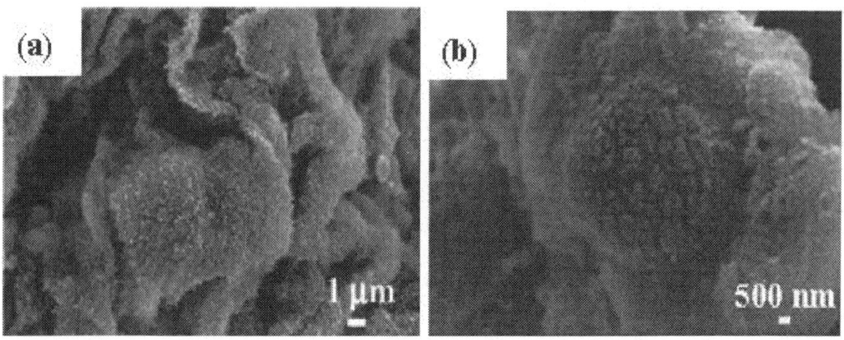

Fig. 4. SEM micrographs of (a) the cellulose-calcium silicate nanocomposites and (b) the cellulose-HA nanocomposites. Reproduced with permission from Carbohydr. Polym. **2010**, *80*, 270 and Carbohydr. Res., **2010**, *345*, 1046. Copyright **2010** *Elsevier*.

In view of the recently research of the fabrication of CIBNs and CIBNs-based nanocomposites, development of simple, low-cost, and high yield methods for the synthesis of CIBNs with complex microstructure and complex components is of great importance for broadening and improving their industrial applications. For example, one can combine the advantages of two or more kind's methods such as sol-gel-hydrothermal, microwave-hydrothermal, electrospinning-hydrothermal methods to fabricate CIBNs. The CIBNs with hierarchically nanostructure and/or pore microstructure have high surface area and can be promisingly used in biomedical fields. It is worth pointing out that the main challenge associated with making effective and functional nanocomponents of CIBNs is related to their homogeneous dispersion within a polymer matrix. Although rapid progress has been made in the past years, the strategies for the fabrication of CIBNs-based nanocomposites need to be further explored.

2.3 Degradation mechanism of calcium-based inorganic biodegradable nanomaterials

The degradation of CIBNs had two routes: the dissolution by body fluids, and phagocytosis and absorption by cells (mainly macrophage), except that calcium sulfate was relatively easy to dissolve in the body. As fluid contained a number of acidic metabolites such as citrate, lactate and acid hydrolysis enzyme in the implants, which provided acidic environment for dissolution of the material, CIBNs were split into particles, molecular or ion. The degradation process of macrophages on CIBNs can be divided into intracellular and extracellular degradation.

Particles were split into ions after phagocytosis by macrophages under the effect of cytoplasmic and lysosomal enzymes, and then the degradation products such as Ca^{2+}, PO_4^{3-}, CO_3^{2-}, SO_4^{2-}, etc, can be transferred to extracell. In addition, macrophages contained rich acid hydrolase including lysosomal enzyme and acid phosphatase enzymes, which can secrete H^+ to the area of extracell and induce the formation of acidic environment. If the diameter of β-TCP particles was bigger than the size of macrophages (14~20 μm), macrophages may extend small protuberances, covering and closely attaching to their surface, and forming a closed cell-material area. At the same time, the dissolved enzyme of cytoplasm of macrophages can release in this areas. The CO_2 and H_2O in macrophages form carbonate under the action of carbonic anhydrase, and then decomposed into HCO_3^- and H^+. H^+ induced the high-acid environment at cell-material area, which cause the degradation of β-TCP particles. For example, the extracellular degradation process of calcium phosphate can be expressed by the following formula:

$$CO_2 + H_2O \xrightarrow{CA} H_2CO_3 \xrightarrow{CA} H^+ + HCO_3^-$$

$$Ca_3(PO_4)_2 \xrightarrow{H^+} Ca^{2+} + 2CaHPO_4 \xrightarrow{H^+} 3Ca^{2+} + 2PO_4^{3-}$$

The degradation product, Ca^{2+}, can enter the blood through the blood circulation to the organs and tissues, to participate in metabolism, and be excreted through feces and urine from liver and kidneys. The other part is stored and used when needed, without causing organic damage and pathological tissue calcification. The CIBNs can be degraded and absorbed. Its metabolites can participate in the formation of new bone, thus completing the transform from inorganic materials to organism.

The considerable changes of the HA implants displayed in surface morphology caused by leaching, corrosion, and active resorption by osteoclasts cells was reported in 1990 by Muller-Mai *et al.* (1990) using scanning electron microscopy (SEM) and transmission electron microscopy (TEM) tracking transverse fractures in the interface. The effect of osteoclasts cells on the degradation mechanism of CIBNs was further research by Wenisch *et al*, (2003) who reported that osteoclasts were localized immediately beneath the ceramic surface after 6 weeks of implantation by simultaneous resorption and phagocytosis, and were capable of phagocytosing the resorbed CaP crystals. Recently, the effect of osteoclastic sodium-bicarbonate co-transporter (NBCn1) on the degradation of HA was investigated in vivo and in vitro (Riihonen et al., 2010). They discovered that down regulation of NBCn1 both on mRNA and protein level inhibited bone resorption and increased intracellular acidification in osteoclasts.

The bone formation around HA blocks was observed by using HA as a space filler in surgically created bone defects of seven cases due to curettage of bone tumours or removal for bone grafts (Yamaguchi et al., 1995). After that, the differences of bone bonding ability and degradation behaviour in vivo were observed between amorphous calcium phosphate (ACP) and highly crystalline HA coating by implantation in the tibiae of rabbits and rats (Nagano et al., 1996). The HA coating benefits to coating longevity, while the ACP coating may be in favor of the osteoconducive property of calcium phosphate coating for initial fixation of porous materials. The ratio of crystalline and amorphous contents also has an effect on the degradation (Gross et al., 2002). A high amorphous content provides fast resorption, while the amount of crystalline particles increased at the distal location of the stem and the threads of the acetabular shell. The Ca/P ratio is another important key factor (Wang et al., 2003). It was indicated that the relatively small amount of CaO was more susceptible to degradation and the TCP-containing ceramic exhibited slightly higher resistance to degradation than HA. The HA-coated AZ31 alloy with good bioactivity, which was prepared by a cathodic electrodeposition method and post-treated with hot alkali solution (Wen et al., 2009), slowed down the degradation rate and effectively induced the deposition of Ca-P-Mg apatite in simulated body fluid (SBF).

The intrinsic mechanism of CIBNs needs to be further explored due to the complexity of biochemistry process. Deep understanding of the degradation mechanism can instruct the synthesis of CIBNs and improve the applications of CIBNs. The intrinsic degradation mechanism will be gradually discovered with increased level of awareness and testing technology.

2.4 Current & future developments

In recent years, rapid progress has been made in the preparation of CIBNs nanostructures, the understanding of mechanism of CIBNs, and exploration of their extensive biomedical applications. So far, inorganic biodegradable materials have been widely used for bone or bone substitute materials, dental filling materials, scaffold materials for temporarily replacing injured skeleton and promoting new tissue formation. However, the practical application research of CIBNs has just started; therefore there are many unknown things that need to be explored, such as the interaction mechanism of inorganic nanoparticles and cancer cells, the biological effects from nanoparticles, and so on. Using nanoparticles in cell separation, cell staining, special drugs and new antibodies for the locally oriented therapy is currently in the initial stage.

Using biodegradable nanomaterials as carrier material in drug delivery system is still limited to organic biomaterial. There have been only a few reports using CIBNs as drug delivery carrier materials. These new fields need to be explored. For example, radiation therapy is a useful method for the cancer surgery, but at the same time a large area of radiation will harm normal cells, especially the bone marrow stem cells with the hematopoietic and immune function. The research discovered that apatite nanoparticles can inhibit a variety of cancer cells and has promising potential applications in various fields. HA nanoparticles had no effect on normal cell activity in cell culture experiments in 1992 (Li et al., 1992). HA crystallite can inhibit the growth of cancer cells in 1994 (Kano et al., 1994). It was found that the cytosolic Ca^{2+} concentration of W-256 carcinosarcoma cells increased under HA microcrystals. Sakai *et al.* (1994) also reported the Ca^{2+} concentration of tumor cells increased in the experiments of photo-excitation TiO_2 nanoparticles. It indicated the death of tumor cell because of important physiological functions of Ca^{2+} on the cells. Of course, the intrinsic and detailed restraining mechanism of Ca^{2+} to cancer cell growth needs to be further explored.

In addition, the fast development of tissue engineering brings forward high requirements on biomedical materials. CIBNs adapt to the standard of biomedical applications. CIBNs can be gradually degraded or dissolved under physiological condition, and was absorbed by the body metabolism. Moreover, the units or their degradation products of the majority composition of CIBNs are small molecules or ions in vivo and have good biocompatibility and safety, compared to non-degradable material.

3. Biomimetic synthesis of $CaCO_3$, $BaCO_3$, $SrCO_3$ and $BaCrO_4$

$CaCO_3$ is a typical biomineral that is abundant in both organisms and nature and has important industrial applications. $CaCO_3$ has six polymorphs: vaterite, aragonite, calcite, amorphous, crystalline monohydrate, and hexahydrate $CaCO_3$ (McGrath, 2001). Therefore, to develop new synthesis methods for the control over the crystal phase and morphology are of great importance for broadening applications of $CaCO_3$. Moreover, $CaCO_3$ is sensitive to the synthesic condition. The biomimetic synthesis of $CaCO_3$ with various unusual biomimetic morphologies, such as pumpkin-like, olive-like, sphere-like, willow-leaf-like, flower-like, cauliflower-like, polyhedron-like, etc, was reported by one-step base- and microwave-assisted method using $CaCl_2$, $(NH_4)_2CO_3$ or Na_2CO_3, basic additives (urea, hexamethylenetetramine ($(CH_2)_6N_4$, HMT), ethylenediamine ($C_2H_8N_2$, EDA) and NaOH), poly(vinylpyrrolidone) (PVP)) in a polyol solvent (Fig. 5) (Ma et al., 2010). The experimental results indicated that the heating temperature, heating time and the type of the basic additive has significant effects on the morphology and the polymorph of $CaCO_3$ crystals. This microwave-assisted heating method is simple, fast, low-cost and may be scaled up for large-scale production of $CaCO_3$ with various unique morphologies.

Using $(NH_4)_2CO_3$ without any basic additive at 130 °C, the pumpkin-like morphology of aragonite with sizes of about 1 μm (Fig. 5a). The low magnification view of SEM in Fig. 5a shows relatively uniform sizes of pumpkin-like aragonite. The insets of Fig. 5a show typical aragonite pumpkins at high magnification. Each pumpkin-like microstructure consisted usually of four parts (the right-upper inset of Fig. 5a), and was open at both ends (the left-bottom inset of Fig. 5a).When Na_2CO_3 was used instead of $(NH_4)_2CO_3$ as the CO_3^{2-} source and without any basic additive at 130 °C, the shape of $CaCO_3$ was irregular instead of the pumpkin-like morphology in the case of $(NH_4)_2CO_3$. Even when the temperature was increased to 180 °C, the shape of $CaCO_3$ was still irregular (Fig. 5b). In this case, the main phase of $CaCO_3$ prepared was calcite, other than aragonite in the case of $(NH_4)_2CO_3$. From Fig. 5b, some irregular cube-like morphologies, which are typical morphologies for the calcite phase. The different results obtained by using Na_2CO_3 and $(NH_4)_2CO_3$ may be due to the different pH of the solution. Na_2CO_3 is more basic than $(NH_4)_2CO_3$.

The $CaCO_3$ prepared using $(NH_4)_2CO_3$ and urea at 150 °C consisted mainly of crystalline aragonite phase with an olive-like morphology (Fig. 5c). The inset of Fig. 5c shows a typical olive-like morphology at a high magnification. We also carried out the preparation at 180 °C, however, no product was obtained. This was due to the decomposition of $(NH_4)_2CO_3$ at 180 °C. The olive-like morphology was formed by the assembly of $CaCO_3$ nanoparticles. If Na_2CO_3 and urea were used at 180 °C, the sample prepared consisted mainly of aragonite with the porous willow-leaf-like morphology (Fig. 5d). Cross-willow-leaf-like morphology was also observed. This porous willow-leaf-like morphology of aragonite prepared by the present method is quite different from the spherulite morphology of vaterite prepared using $CaCl_2 \cdot 2H_2O$ and urea in a polyol solvent under solvothermal condition (Li et al., 2002) and also different from the needle-like aragonite prepared by aging the solution of $CaCl_2$ in the presence of urea in ultrasonic bath at 90°C (Wang et al., 1999).

When using $(NH_4)_2CO_3$ and hexamethylenetetramine as a basic additive, $CaCO_3$ spheres assembled from nanoparticles of the vaterite phase were formed (Fig. 5e). The inset of Fig. 5e shows a typical sphere with the diameter of about 600 nm. If Na_2CO_3 instead of $(NH_4)_2CO_3$ was used, the cuboid-like morphology of calcite was obtained (Fig. 5f). When ethylenediamine was used as an additive, spherical nanoparticles of amorphous $CaCO_3$ were obtained using $(NH_4)_2CO_3$ as the CO_3^{2-} source (Fig. 5g). Using Na_2CO_3 instead of $(NH_4)_2CO_3$ as the CO_3^{2-} source and ethylenediamine, one can see the flower-like morphology of aragonite (Fig. 5h). It is well known that the ethylenediamine is a bidentate ligand and the strong coordination ability. NH_4^+ ions may have an influence on the coordination between ethylenediamine and Ca^{2+}. When a strong alkali NaOH was used instead of a weak base such as urea, hexamethylenetetramine and ethylenediamine, different morphologies were obtained. The flake congeries of vaterite were obtained using $(NH_4)_2CO_3$ as the CO_3^{2-} source (Fig. 5i). Kojima et al. (1993) reported the formation of spherical vaterite by dipping spherical particles of amorphous $CaCO_3$ in NH_4Cl aqueous solution, the spherical amorphous $CaCO_3$ was synthesized in the reaction system of $CaCl_2$-Na_2CO_3-NaOH. This indicates that NH_4^+ ions favor the formation of the vaterite phase. Using Na_2CO_3 as the CO_3^{2-} source and NaOH, the cauliflower-like morphology of calcite was obtained (Fig.5j). The morphology and polymorph of $CaCO_3$ obtained by the present method is completely different from the previous reports by Kojima et al. (1993) and by Koga et al. (1998), who prepared amorphous $CaCO_3$ through reacting a mixed solution of Na_2CO_3-NaOH with a $CaCl_2$ solution at room temperature, respectively. From the above discussions, one can see that there is a tendency to form spherical or near-spherical morphology when using $(NH_4)_2CO_3$ as the CO_3^{2-} source. When the basicity of the basic additive increases, the sizes of $CaCO_3$ structures decrease. However, there seems a tendency to form assembled complex morphology when using Na_2CO_3 as the CO_3^{2-} source. There results shows that the source of carbonates has a significant influence on the morphology of $CaCO_3$.

When using Na_2CO_3 as the CO_3^{2-} source and NaOH as an alkali additive by microwave heating at 180 °C for 20 min in 1,4-butanediol instead of EG, a completely different shape (polyhedral) of $CaCO_3$ was observed. In comparison, as discussed above, cauliflower-like shape was formed when using ethylene glycol as a solvent. These results indicate that the polyol solvent played an important role in the control of the morphology of $CaCO_3$.

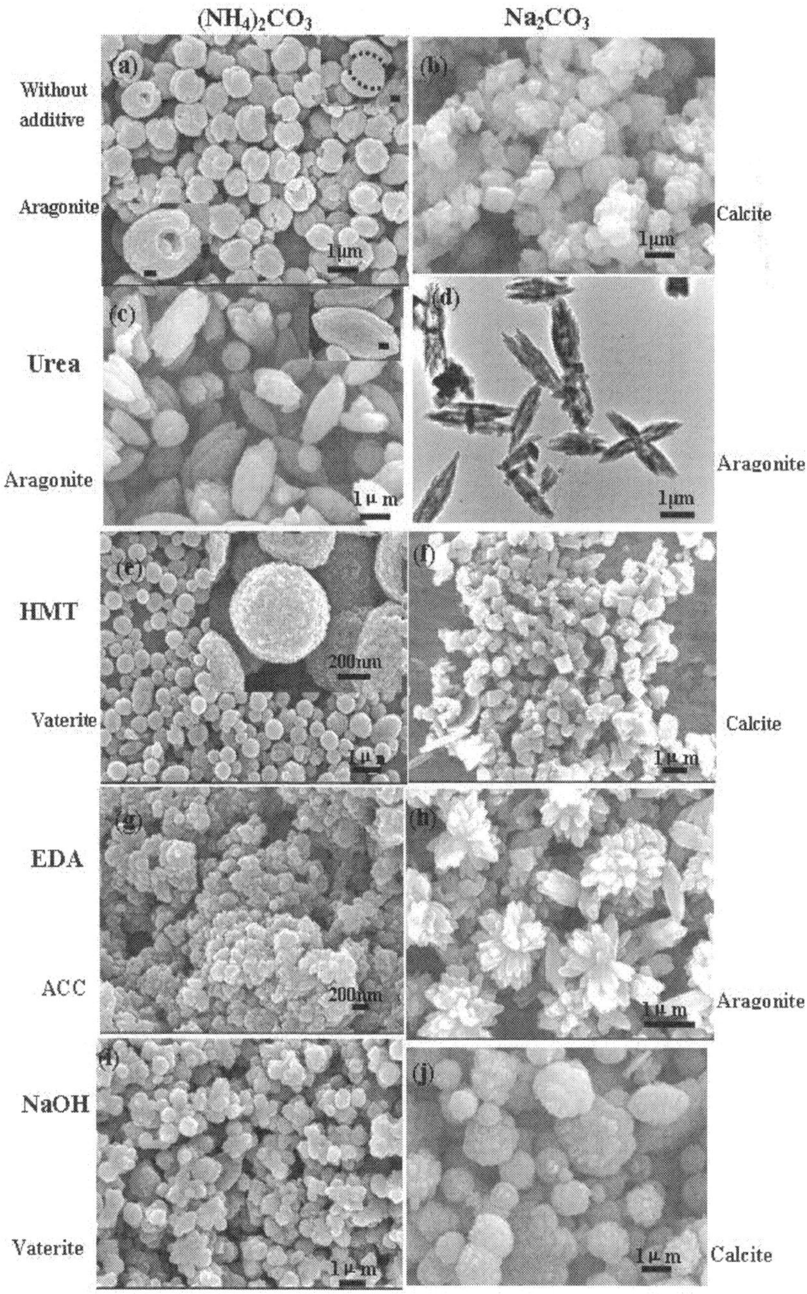

$(NH_4)_2CO_3$
Na_2CO_3
(a)
(b)
Without additive
Aragonite
Calcite
1μm
1μm
(c)
(d)
Urea
Aragonite
Aragonite
1 μ m
1μm
(e)
(f)
HMT
Vaterite
Calcite
200nm
1 μ m
(g)
(h)
EDA
ACC
Aragonite
200nm
1 μ m
(i)
(j)
NaOH
Vaterite
Calcite
1 μ m
1 μ m

Fig. 5. SEM micrographs of samples prepared using different CO_3^{2-} source and basic additive in EG by microwave heating for 20 min (except (j) for 1 h). (a,c,e,g,i) using $(NH_4)_2CO_3$ as the CO_3^{2-} source at 130 ºC (except (c) at 150 ºC); (b,d,f,h,j) using Na_2CO_3 as the CO_3^{2-} source at 180 ºC. (a,b) without an basic additive, (a) shows pumpkin-like morphology of aragonite phase of $CaCO_3$, the insets of (a) show typical pumpkin-like morphology, scale bar = 200 nm, (b) shows cuboid-like morphology of calcite phase; (c,d) using urea, (c) shows a typical olive-like morphology of the aragonite phase, the inset of (c) shows a typical olive-like morphology, scale bar = 200 nm, (d) TEM micrograph showing the porous willow-leaf-like morphology of the aragonite phase; (e,f) using hexamethylenetetramine (HMT), (e) shows a sphere-like morphology assembled from nanoparticles of the vaterite phase, the inset of (e) shows a typical assembled sphere, (f) shows cuboid-like morphology of calcite; (g,h) using ethylenediamine (EDA), (g) shows spherical nanoparticles of amorphous phase of $CaCO_3$, (h) shows flower-like morphology of aragonite; (i,j) using NaOH, (i) shows the flake congeries of the vaterite phase, (j) shows cauliflower-like morphology of the calcite phase. Reproduced with permission from Adv. Mater. Res. **2010**, *92*, 139. Copyright **2010** *TTP*.

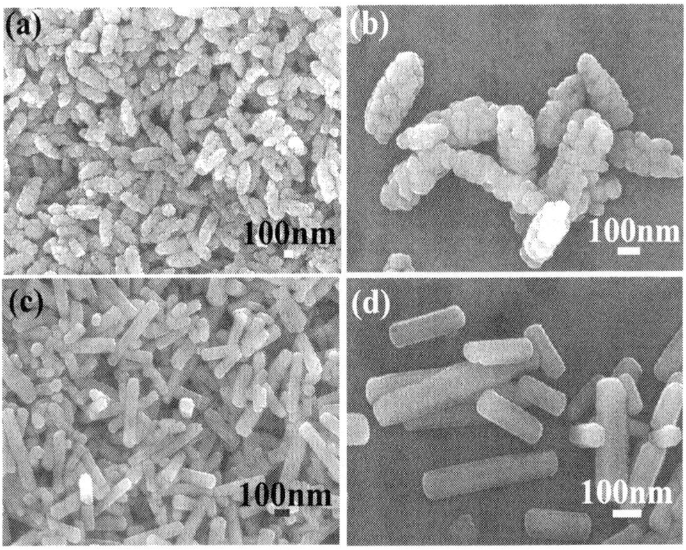

Fig. 6. SEM micrographs of $BaCO_3$ prepared by microwave heating at 90 ºC for 40 min in ethylene glycol. (a,b) using NaOH, (c,d) using hexamethylenetetramine. Reproduced with permission from Chem. Lett. **2006**, *35*, 1138. Copyright **2006** *CSJ*.

The above experimeatl results implied that the various basic additives and the temperature provide more possibilities for the control over the morphology and the polymorph of $CaCO_3$. However, the intrinsic and detailed biomimetic formation mechanism of $CaCO_3$ with various unusual biomimetic morphologies needs to be further explored.

Barium carbonate ($BaCO_3$) is an important material used in the production of glasses and ceramics industry (Gutmann & Chalup, 2000). $BaCO_3$ nanorods (Ma et al., 2006) can be synthesized by the microwave-assisted method using $Ba(NO_3)_2$ and $(NH_4)_2CO_3$ in the presence of NaOH or hexamethylenetetramine ($(CH_2)_6N_4$) in ethylene glycol (Fig. 6). Fig. 6a,b shows SEM micrograph of the sample synthesized by microwave heating in the presence of a strong alkali NaOH at 90 °C for 40 min in ethylene glycol, from which one can see $BaCO_3$ nanorods assembled from nanoparticles. $BaCO_3$ nanorods had relatively uniform sizes with the diameters of about 200 nm and the lengths of about 450 nm. The influence of the weak alkalescent additive (hexamethylenetetramine) on the morphology of $BaCO_3$ was also investigated (Fig. 6c,d), from which one can see nanorods with a hexagonal cross section. This indicates that the base has a significant influence on the morphology of $BaCO_3$. $BaCO_3$ nanoparticles formed and selfassembled into nanorods in the presence of a strong basic NaOH. However, nanorods with a hexagonal cross section were obtained when using a weak basic hexamethylenetetramine.

The heating method also had an influence on the morphology of $BaCO_3$. The aggregates of irregular nanoparticles were formed in the presence of NaOH by heating in an oil bath, in contrast to the nanorods assembled from $BaCO_3$ nanoparticles prepared by the microwave heating. However, the needles with two sharp ends were produced in the presence of hexamethylenetetramine by heating in the oil bath.

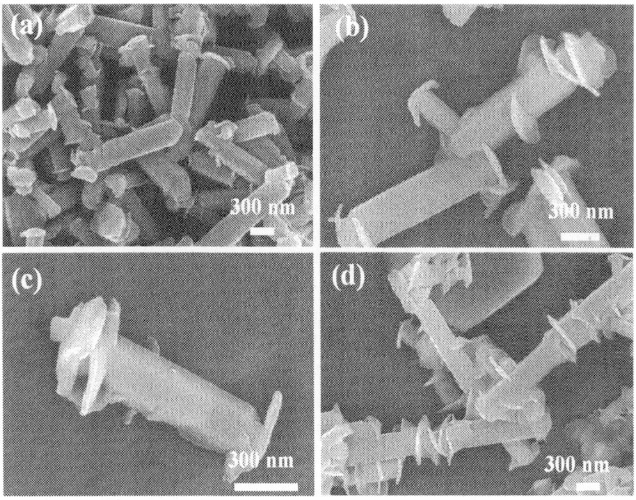

Fig. 7. SEM micrographs of $BaCO_3$. Reproduced with permission from Mater. Lett. **2007**, *61*, 5133. Copyright **2007** *Elsevier.*

However, Barium carbonate ($BaCO_3$) nanorods (Ma et al., 2007) with the nanosheets grew perpendicularly on the nanorods were synthesized using $Ba(NO_3)_2$ and $(NH_4)_2CO_3$ in the water/ethylene glycol (EG) mixed solvents by oil bath heating at 80 °C for 30 min (Fig. 7). The molar ratio of water to EG had an effect on the morphology of $BaCO_3$. $BaCO_3$ nanorods with diameters of about 250 nm and lengths of about 1μm. It is interesting that the nanosheets grew perpendicularly on the nanorods, as shown in Fig. 7b-d. The sizes of $BaCO_3$ nanorods were relatively uniform. In contrast, the aggregates of irregular nanoparticles were formed using a basic additive sodium hydroxide in a single solvent of ethylene glycol.

The liquid phase precipitation method is one of the earliest methods for the synthesis of inorganic particles. Lamer et al. (1950) reported the synthesis of monodisperse colloidal sulfur in ethanol/water mixed solvents in 1950. The precipitation reactions involve the nucleation, growth, ripening, or agglomeration processes. The separation of nucleation and growth is the key step for the preparation of high quality crystals. The growth mechanism, such as Ostwald ripening (Dadyburjor & Ruckenstein, 1977; Sugimoto, 1978; Marqusee & Ross, 1983) and aggregation especially oriented attachment (Penn & Banfield, 1999; Banfield, 2000), will dramatically affect the size, morphology, and properties of the products. In Ostwald ripening process, the larger particles will grow at the expense of the smaller ones. The "oriented attachment" mechanism was reported by Penn and Banfield (Penn & Banfield, 1999; Banfield, 2000). Although some theories have been established, it is necessary to provide more experimental examples for better understanding of these mechanisms. $BaCO_3$ rods with diameters of about 250 nm and lengths of about several micrometers (Ma et al., 2008) were obtained using $Ba(NO_3)_2$ and $NaHCO_3$ as the $CO_3{}^{2-}$ source at room temperature in water (20 mL) for 30 min (Fig.8). Fig. 8a-c shows TEM micrographs of the sample using $NaHCO_3$ as the $CO_3{}^{2-}$ source, from which one can see $BaCO_3$ rods with diameters of about 250 nm and lengths of about several micrometers. Fig. 8b shows a typical individual nanorod. The corresponding SAED pattern of an individual rod (the up inset of Fig. 8b) indicates the single-crystalline structure of the rod, which shows that the preferential growth direction of the nanorod was along the [100] zone axis of $BaCO_3$. We also found that $BaCO_3$ rods were not stable under electron beam irradiation and changed from single crystalline to polycrystalline structure after exposure to the electron beam (the down inset of Fig. 8b). A similar phenomenon that one-dimensional structures changed under electron beam irradiation was reported for $PbCrO_4$ rods (Wang & Zhu, 2005), $Ag_6Mo_{10}O_{33}$ rods (Cui et al., 2004), and Bi nanotubes (Li et al., 2001). They all could transform into polycrystalline structure under electron beam irradiation.

It is interesting that the rod assembled from nanoparticles was observed in a few cases, as shown in Fig. 8c. One can clearly observe the nanoparticles and the boundary between the particles. The corresponding SAED pattern of the rod indicates the oriented aggregation of nanoparticles (the inset of Fig.8c), implying that the growth of $BaCO_3$ rods followed the oriented attachment mechanism. It is possible that this polycrystalline rod was an intermediate product. The oriented attachment-based self-assembly and crystallization were also reported for ZnO (Pacholski et al. 2002) and $CaCO_3$ (Zhan et al., 2003). The understanding of the formation mechanism is the key point for the realization of controlled synthesis of one-dimensional nanomaterials.

In order to understand the formation mechanism of $BaCO_3$ rods, the sample was synthesized at room temperature for 30 s, while the other reaction conditions were the same (Fig. 8d-h). All the rods were assembled from nanoparticles. A typical single rod assembled from nanoparticles was shown in Fig.8h. This result conformed that the growth of $BaCO_3$ rods followed the oriented attachment mechanism.

When using $(NH_4)_2CO_3$ as the $CO_3{}^{2-}$ source, a completely different shape (bundle and flower) of $BaCO_3$ was observed (Fig. 9a-b). These $BaCO_3$ bundles and flowers were assembled from nanosheets. We also investigated the effect of the surfactant on the morphology of $BaCO_3$. When P123 was used, more dense flowers were observed (Fig.9c) compared with those shown in Fig. 9a-b. When SDBS was used (Fig.9d-e), the major morphology was bundle-like, and some fragments were also observed as a minor morphology. When CTAB was used, the loosely assembled flowers were obtained (Fig. 9f). Therefore, the type of the surfactant has an effect on the morphology of $BaCO_3$.

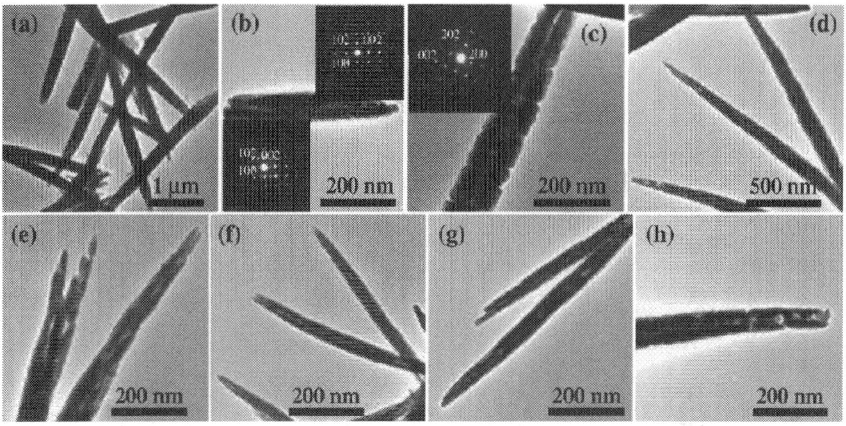

Fig. 8. TEM micrographs of the sample prepared using $NaHCO_3$ as the CO_3^{2-} source for different time: (a-c) 30 min; (a) A typical TEM micrograph; (b) an individual nanorod and the corresponding SAED pattern of the individual nanorod before and after exposure to electron beam irradiation, respectively; (c) the rod assembled from nanoparticles and the corresponding SAED pattern. (d-h) 30 s. Reproduced with permission from Mater. Lett. 2008, *62*, 3110. Copyright 2008 *Elsevier.*

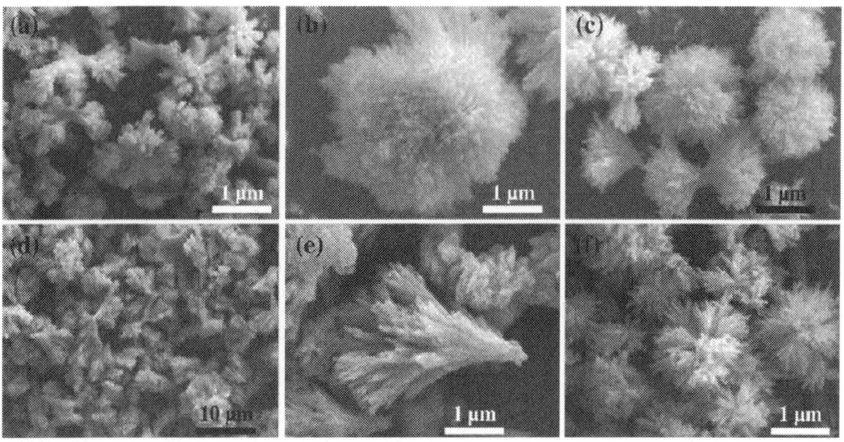

Fig. 9. SEM micrographs of the sample prepared using $(NH_4)_2CO_3$ as the CO_3^{2-} source. (a) A typical SEM micrograph; (b) an individual flower-like structure. (c) using 20 mL 2.9 g/L P123; (d, e) using 20 mL SDBS (25.090 g/L); (f) using 20 mL CTAB (9.100 g/L). Reproduced with permission from Mater. Lett. **2008**, *62*, 3110. Copyright **2008** *Elsevier.*

$SrCO_3$ is a simple mineral that has only one polymorph, the study of crystallization process of $SrCO_3$ may be useful to help understand the formation of the isostructural $CaCO_3$ phase (aragonite) and the mineralization process of other biominerals. $SrCO_3$ is an important reactant in the production of glass for color television tubes and ferrite magnets for small

DC motors (Bastow, 2002), and also used in the production of iridescent and special glasses, pigments, driers, paints, pyrotechnics, catalysts and chemical sensors (Zeller, 1981; Griffiths, 1985; Erdemoğlu & Canbazoğlu, 1998; Owusu & Litz, 2000; Shi et al., 2002).

The microwave-assisted method was also used for the synthesis of $SrCO_3$ with an olive-like or flower-like morphology (Ma & Zhu, 2007) using $Sr(NO_3)_2$ and $(NH_4)_2CO_3$ in ethylene glycol or water. The olive-like morphology was obtained in ethylene glycol (Fig.10). From Fig. 10c one can see that the olive-like $SrCO_3$ structures were formed by the assembly of $SrCO_3$ nanoparticles. The sizes of olive-like $SrCO_3$ were relatively uniform. The width of the olive-like structures was about 160 nm and the length was about 500 nm. However, the flower-like (majority) and bundle-like (minority) morphology was prepared using water as the solvent instead of ethylene glycol (Fig. 11). Each flower-like or bundle-like microstructure was formed by the assembly of nanosheets. Interestingly, a hollow was observed in the central bottom of the flower-like morphology (Fig. 11c). Figs. 11b and 11c show the typical flower-like morphology of $SrCO_3$. Fig. 11e shows a typical bundle-like $SrCO_3$ assembled from nanosheets.

The heating time has an effect on the morphology of $SrCO_3$. When the heating time was 30 s (Fig. 12a), low-symmetry bundle-like $SrCO_3$ structures were observed as a major morphology and the degree of assembly was low. Flower-like morphology was formed as a minor product. When the heating time was increased to 1 min, the flower-like morphology consisted of nanosheets dominated although some bundles still existed (Fig. 12b).

It is well known that ethylenediamine is widely used as a chelating ligand in inorganic chemistry and coordination chemistry (Cotton et al., 1999). The syntheses of II-VI semiconductor 1-D nanostructures by a solvothermal process using ethylenediamine as a coordination molecular template have been reported (Gao et al., 2002). The influence of EDA on the formation of $CaCO_3$ in various reaction systems were reported (Sugihara et al., 1997). One-dimensional $SrCO_3$ nanostructures assembled from nanocrystals (Ma & Zhu, 2008) can be successfully synthesized by a microwave-assisted aqueous solution method at 90 °C using $Sr(NO_3)_2$, $(NH_4)_2CO_3$ and ethylenediamine ($C_2H_8N_2$) for 20 min (Fig. 13). When the microwave heating time was 5 min, the hexagonal cone-like structures of $SrCO_3$ were observed as majority morphology and some nanoparticles as a minor morphology were also observed (Fig. 14). Fig. 14b shows some nanoparticles surrounding the hexagonal cones. Fig. 14c shows the top view of the hexagonal cone, from which one can clearly see the six crystal planes. A typical hexagonal cone is shown in Fig. 14d, from which one can see hexagonal cylinder with cones at two ends.

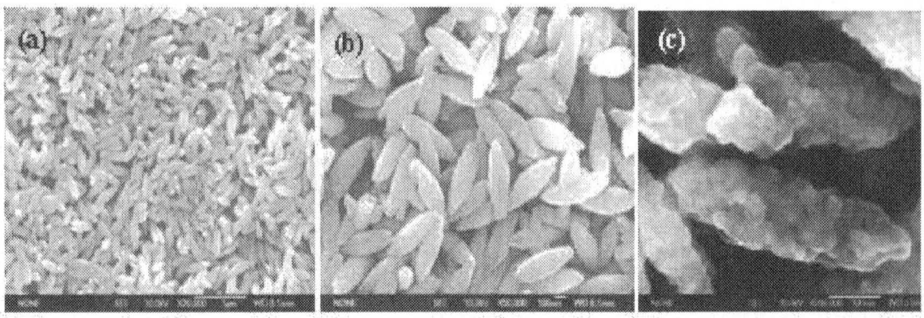

Fig. 10. SEM micrographs of $SrCO_3$ prepared using $(NH_4)_2CO_3$ and $Sr(NO_3)_2$ by microwave heating at 90 °C for 5 min in ethylene glycol. Reproduced with permission from J. Nanosci. Nanotechnol. 2007, 7, 4552. Copyright 2007 *ASP*.

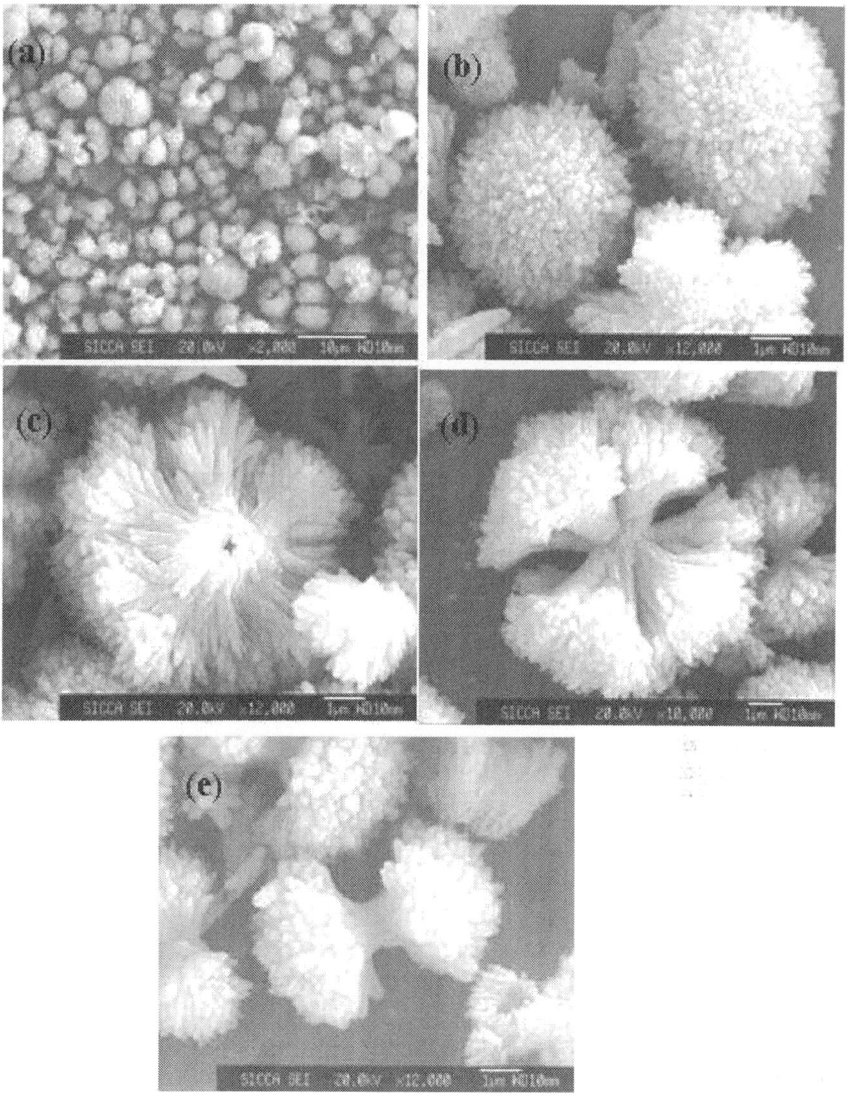

Fig. 11. SEM micrographs of $SrCO_3$ prepared by microwave heating an aqueous solution of $(NH_4)_2CO_3$ and $Sr(NO_3)_2$ at 90 °C for 5 min. (a) at a low magnification, (b) the top view of a typical flower-like morphology, (c) the bottom view of a typical flower-like morphology, (d) fully assembled flower-like morphology, (e) a typical bundle-like morphology. Reproduced with permission from J. Nanosci. Nanotechnol. **2007**, *7*, 4552. Copyright **2007** *ASP*.

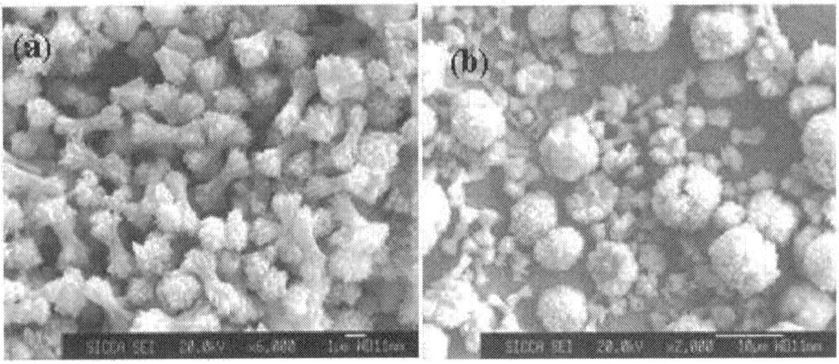

Fig. 12. SEM micrographs of $SrCO_3$ prepared by microwave heating an aqueous solution of $(NH_4)_2CO_3$ and $Sr(NO_3)_2$ at 90 °C. (a) for 30 s, and (b) for 1 min. Reproduced with permission from J. Nanosc. Nanotechn. **2007**, *7*, 4552. Copyright **2007** *ASP*.

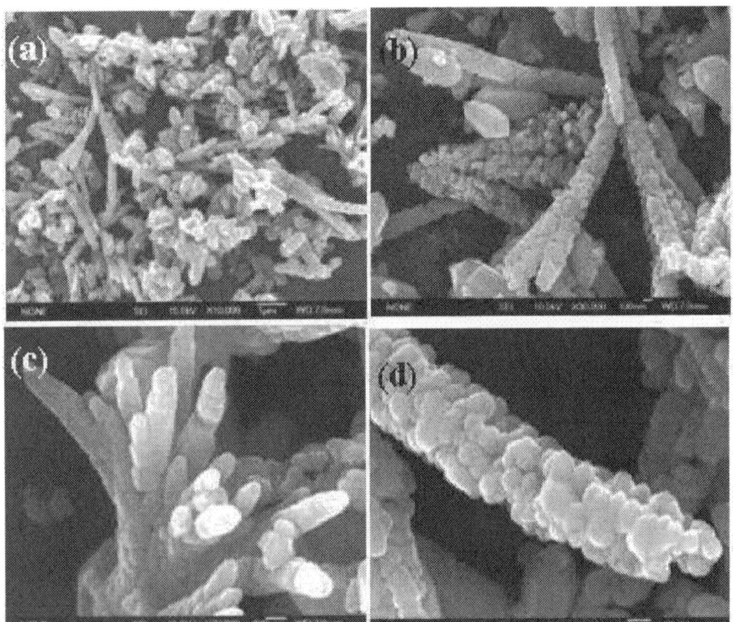

Fig. 13. SEM micrographs of $SrCO_3$ prepared by microwave heating an aqueous solution of $(NH_4)_2CO_3$, $Sr(NO_3)_2$ and EDA at 90 °C for 20 min. (a) at a lower magnification, (b) at a higher magnification, (c) the top view of the branch-like morphology, (d) a typical single branch assembled from nanoparticles. Reproduced with permission from Mater. Lett. **2008**, *62*, 2512. Copyright **2008** *Elsevier*.

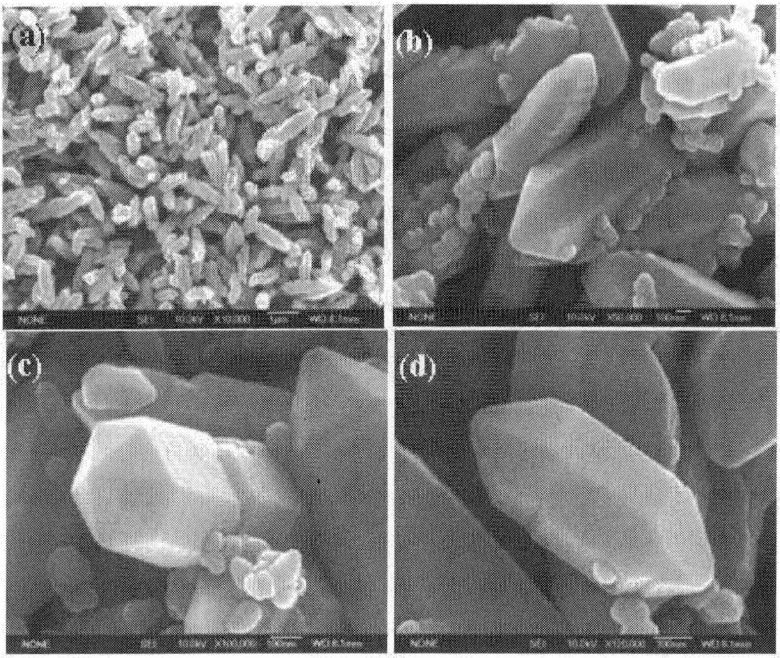

Fig. 14. SEM micrographs of $SrCO_3$ prepared by microwave heating an aqueous solution of $(NH_4)_2CO_3$, $Sr(NO_3)_2$ and ethylenediamine at 90 °C for 5 min. (a) at a lower magnification, (b) at a higher magnification, (c) the top view of the hexagonal cone, (d) a typical single hexagonal cone. Reproduced with permission from Mater. Lett. **2008**, *62*, 2512. Copyright **2008** *Elsevier*.

Ethylenediamine is a bidentate ligand and has strong coordination ability. In the presence of ethylenediamine, the complex of $Sr(en)_2^{2+}$ formed due to the strong coordination ability of ethylenediamine, then dissolved Sr^{2+} and CO_3^{2-} species would spontaneously form the $SrCO_3$ nuclei at room temperature because of small solubility product of $SrCO_3$ (at 25 °C, $K_{sp}=1.1\times10^{-10}$). Then the $SrCO_3$ nuclei grew to form nanocrystals. The microwave heating leads to a high heating rate and a rapid increase in temperature during the nucleation process, which is important for fast nucleation and growth of crystals. The rapidly changing electric field of the microwave reactor induced the oriented self-assembly of $SrCO_3$ nanocrystals. The self-assembly of nanocrystals depends on the interparticle interactions, crystal size distribution and shape. The microwave heating favored the formation of nanoparticles with a narrow size distribution. Ethylenediamine molecules also acted as the capping ligands that selectively adsorbed onto the surfaces of nanocrystals, leading to the oriented self-assembly of $SrCO_3$ nanocrystals to form branch-like morphology.

Barium chromate ($BaCrO_4$, also called hshemite) is often used as an oxidizing agent, as a catalyst for enhancing vapor-phase oxidation reactions (Economy et al., 1965) and as a highly efficient photocatalyst with a response to visible light irradiation (Yin et al., 2003). $BaCrO_4$ with various morphologies (Ma et al., 2009) such as X-shaped, shuttle, rhombus was produced by using poly(ethylene oxide)-poly(propylene oxide)-poly(ethylene oxide) (P123) as a structure directing agent at room temperature.

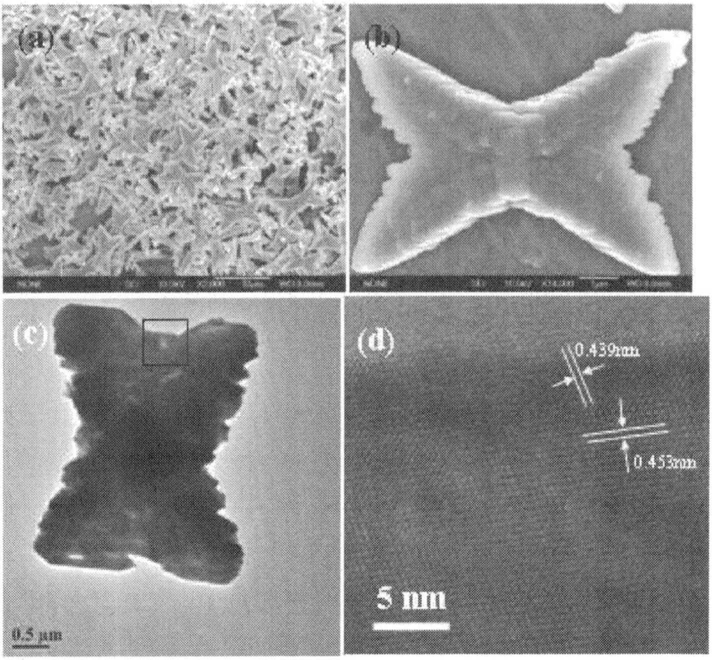

Fig. 15. (a) XRD pattern; (b) and (c) SEM micrographs; and (d) TEM micrograph of the typical $BaCrO_4$ sample. The HRTEM image of the individual X-shaped structure shown in (d) is given in (e). Reproduced with permission from Mater. Res. Bull., **2009**, *44*, 288. Copyright **2009** *Elsevier*.

The typical sample prepared from the solution containing $Ba(NO_3)_2$, K_2CrO_4, NaOH and P123 for 12 h. The reflection peaks can be indexed to a single phase of $BaCrO_4$ with an orthorhombic structure (JCPDS 35-0642). The morphology of the product was investigated by SEM, as shown in Fig. 15b and c, indicating that the sample consisted of X-shaped structures (majority) and some flower-like assembly (minority). Fig. 15c shows an individual X-shaped $BaCrO_4$ structure with four branches. Sawtooth-like edge and clear growth steps can be seen from Fig. 15c. The morphology was further investigated by TEM. Fig. 15d shows the typical individual structure. The corresponding SAED pattern of an individual X-shaped $BaCrO_4$ structure indicates the single-crystalline structure of the $BaCrO_4$. Fig. 15e shows the corresponding HR-TEM micrograph of an individual X-shaped $BaCrO_4$ structure. The periodic fringe spacings of ~4.53 and 4.39 Å correspond to the d-spacing of (200) and (011) planes, respectively. This result is in accord with the SAED result.

In our experiment, the sample underwent the ripening process. In order to investigate the effect of time on the morphology of $BaCrO_4$, the samples were fabricated for different times. When the time was only 5 min (Fig. 16a), the shuttle-like morphology with relatively uniform sizes was obtained, indicating rapid nucleation and growth process. Sawtooth-like edge and clear growth steps can be seen from the insets of Fig. 16a. When the time was prolonged to 3 h, the similar morphology was observed (Fig. 16b). The second nucleation

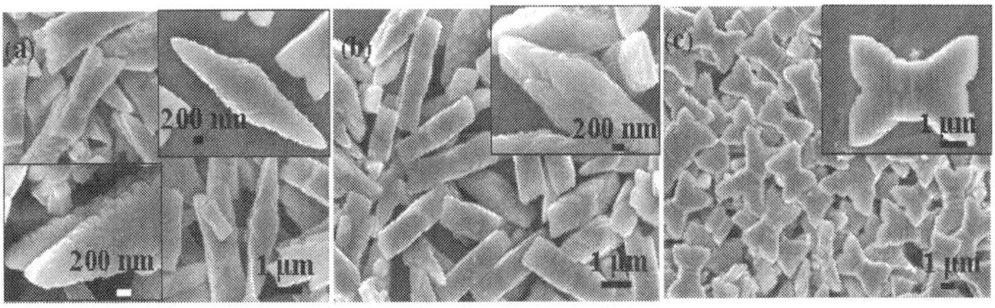

Fig. 16. SEM micrographs of $BaCrO_4$ crystals prepared for different time. (a) 5 min; (b) 3 h; and (c) 6 h. Reproduced with permission from Mater. Res. Bull., **2009**, *44*, 288. Copyright **2009** *Elsevier.*

was observed from the inset of Fig. 16b. When the time was increased to 6 h, the X-shaped structures with four branches with relatively uniform sizes (the lengths were about 2.4 μm) were obtained. From Fig. 16a-c and Fig. 15b, one can clearly see the morphological change process of $BaCrO_4$ with increasing time. The degree of split and the size of X-shaped structures increased with increasing time. The growth mechanism of $BaCrO_4$ may follow the well-known Ostwald ripening process, in which the larger particles grow at the expense of the smaller ones (Sugimoto, 1987).

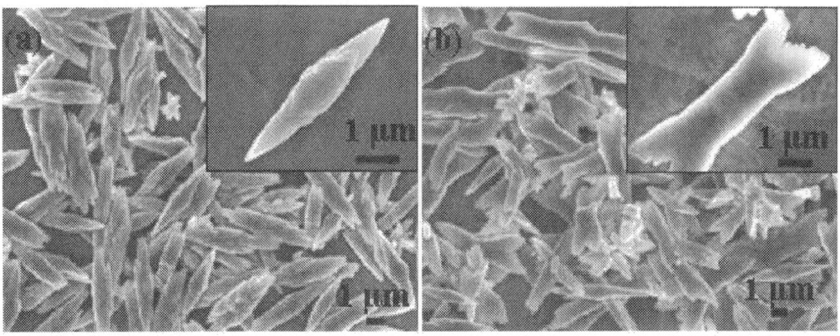

Fig. 17. SEM micrographs of $BaCrO_4$ crystals prepared using different P123 concentration. (a) [P123] = 2.9 g L^{-1} and (b) [P123] = 5.8 g L^{-1}. The insets of (a) and (b) show the individual $BaCrO_4$ crystals. Reproduced with permission from Mater. Res. Bull., **2009**, *44*, 288. Copyright **2009** *Elsevier.*

The effect of P123 concentration on the morphology of $BaCrO_4$ was investigated. When the concentration of P123 was increased from 0.58 to 2.9 g L^{-1} and the other conditions were kept the same, the different morphology was obtained (Fig. 17a) compared with Fig. 15b. The shuttle-like morphology was observed. When the concentration of P123 was increased to 5.8 g L^{-1}, the size and the morphology were not uniform (Fig. 17b). Therefore, the appropriate concentration of P123 is important for preparing uniform X-shaped morphology of $BaCrO_4$. In the absence of P123, the butterfly-like morphology was obtained (Fig. 18a). In the absence of both P123 and NaOH, the cross-like branches were observed (Fig. 18b). The insets of (a) and (b) show the individual $BaCrO_4$ structures. It is well known that CrO_4^{2-} ions exist in a basic solution, $Cr_2O_7^{2-}$ ions exist in an acid solution, and CrO_4^{2-} and $Cr_2O_7^{2-}$ can transform to each other in the aqueous solution. So the addition of NaOH favors the synthesis of $BaCrO_4$.

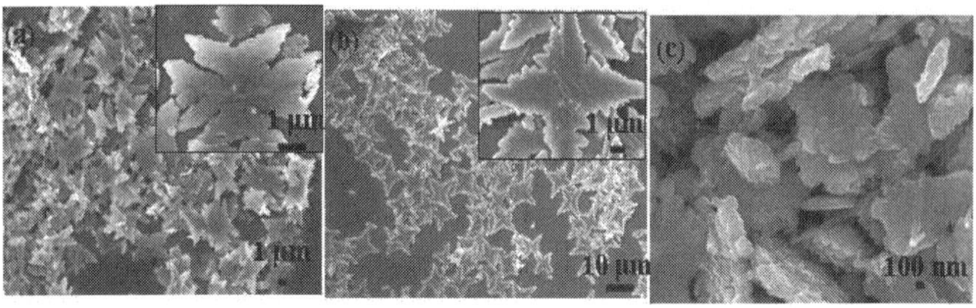

Fig. 18. SEM micrographs of $BaCrO_4$ structures. (a) in the absence of P123; (b) in the absence of P123 and NaOH; (c) 15 mL 0.58 g L^{-1} P123, $Ba(NO_3)_2$ concentration increased from 0.05 to 0.20 mol L^{-1} (0.5 mL), 1 mL 0.50 mol L^{-1} NaOH. Reproduced with permission from Mater. Res. Bull., **2009**, *44*, 288. Copyright **2009** *Elsevier.*

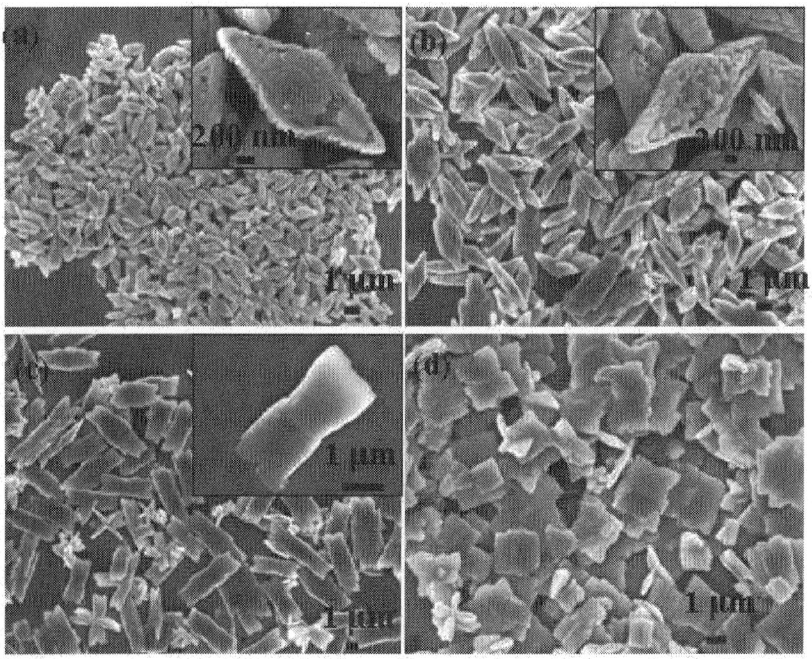

Fig. 19. (a)-(c) SEM micrographs of $BaCrO_4$ crystals prepared in the presence of both P123 and CTAB. (a) [P123] = 0.580 g L^{-1}, 6 h; (b) [P123] = 0.580 g L^{-1}, 12 h; (c) [P123] = 5.80 g L^{-1}, 12 h. (d) SEM micrograph of $BaCrO_4$ crystals prepared in the presence of CTAB. The insets of (a), (b), and (c) show the individual $BaCrO_4$ crystal. Reproduced with permission from Mater. Res. Bull., **2009**, *44*, 288. Copyright **2009** *Elsevier.*

When increasing the concentration of Ba^{2+} from 0.05 mol L^{-1} to 0.20 mol L^{-1}, the flakes consisted of particles were observed (Fig. 18c). When the high concentration of Ba^{2+} was used, the nucleation of $BaCrO_4$ was fast and the growth was restricted. So the particles were obtained. These results indicate that the morphology of $BaCrO_4$ is sensitive to the experimental conditions.

The combination effect of P123 and CTAB on the morphology of $BaCrO_4$ was investigated (Fig.19). When both P123 and CTAB were used, the rhombus-like structures consisted of particles were observed and porous structures were seen on the surface. The sizes of rhombus-like structures increased with increasing time. However, when the concentration of P123 was increased from 0.58 to 5.80 mol L^{-1}, different morphology was observed (Fig. 19c). When only CTAB was used without P123, the sheet-like morphology was obtained (Fig. 19d).

Various factors including inorganic anions, organic additives and solvents have effects on the morphologies of crystals. The specific adsorption of the additive to particular faces inhibits the growth of these faces by lowering their surface energy, induced the anisotropic

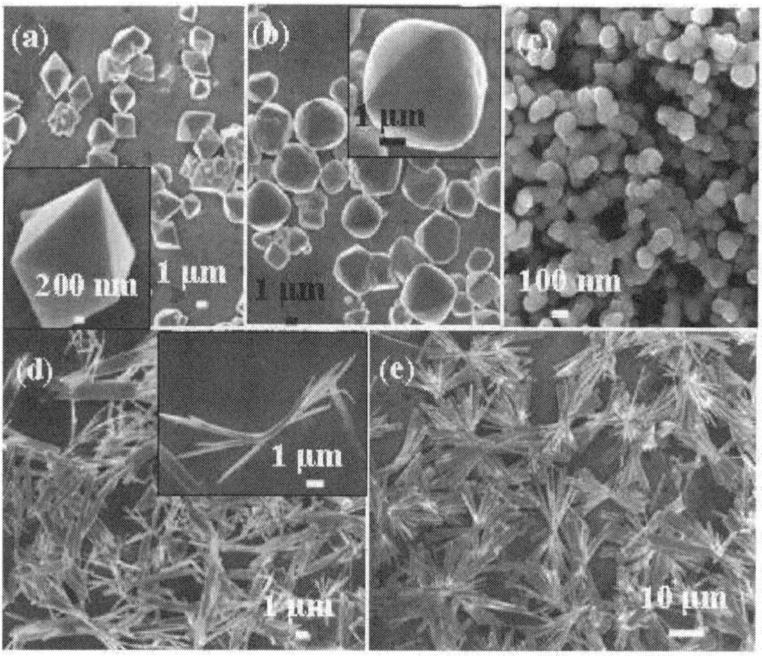

Fig. 20. (a)-(c) SEM micrographs of $BaWO_4$ crystals prepared from the solution of 15 mL P123, 0.5 mL 0.05 mol L^{-1} $Ba(NO_3)_2$, 1 mL 0.50 mol L^{-1} NaOH, and 0.5 mL 0.05 mol L^{-1} Na_2WO_4 for 12 h. (a) [P123]= 0.580 g L^{-1}; (b) [P123]= 5.80 g L^{-1}; (c) in the absence of P123 and NaOH. (d) and (e) SEM micrographs of Pb_2CrO_5 crystals prepared from the solution of 15 mL 0.580 g L^{-1} P123, 0.5 mL 0.05 mol L^{-1} $Pb(NO_3)_2$, 1 mL 0.50 mol L^{-1} NaOH, and 0.5 mL 0.05 mol L^{-1} Na_2CrO_4.: (d) 6 h; (e) 12 h. The insets of (a), (b) and (d) show the individual crystal. Reproduced with permission from Mater. Res. Bull., **2009**, *44*, 288. Copyright **2009** *Elsevier.*

growth of the crystals, and influenced the crystal morphology. Due to the electrostatic interaction with Ba^{2+} ions, the negatively charged of polymer polar groups acted as active sites for the nucleation of $BaCrO_4$. Yu et al. (2003) reported that some faces of the $BaCrO_4$ crystal could adsorb negatively charged groups such as $-PO_3H_2$, -COOH of polymer by electrostatic attraction and block these faces from further growth. Some interesting morphologies prepared using both polymer and surfactant as crystallization templates were reported (Shi et al., 2003; Wei et al., 2004a,b).

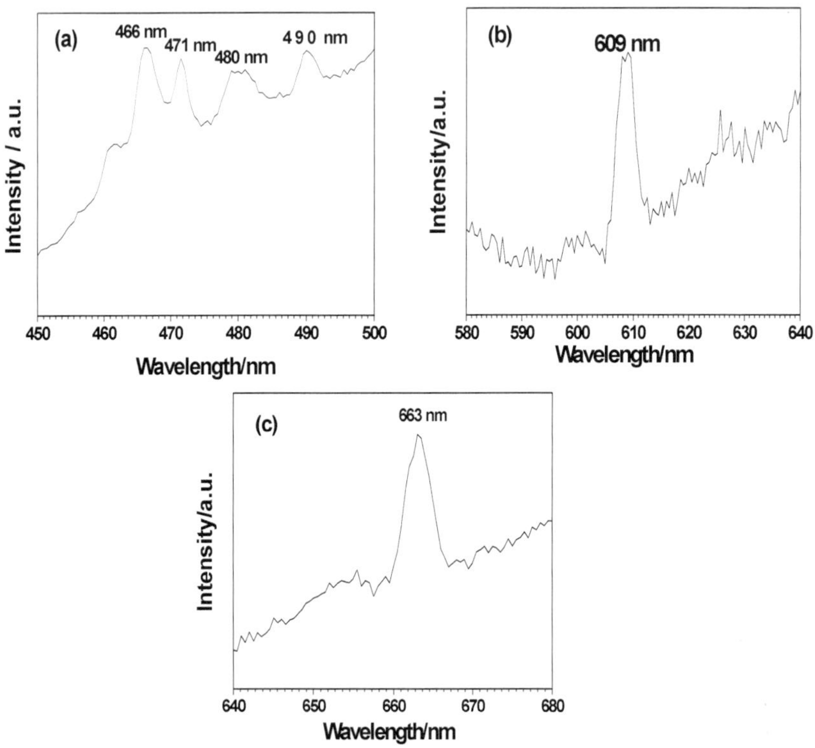

Fig. 21. PL spectra of the $BaCrO_4$ sample as shown in Fig. 15: (a) λ_{ex} = 276 nm; (b) λ_{ex} = 454 nm; (c) λ_{ex} = 488 nm. Reproduced with permission from Mater. Res. Bull., **2009**, *44*, 288. Copyright **2009** *Elsevier.*

$BaWO_4$ and Pb_2CrO_5 were slao fabricated using this synthetic route, and the corresponding results were displayed in Fig.6. The $BaWO_4$ sample consisted of octahedral crystals (Fig. 20a). The XRD pattern shows that the sample consisted of a single phase of crystalline tetragonal sheelite type $BaWO_4$ (JCPDS 43-0646). When the concentration of P123 was increased from 0.580 to 5.80 mol L^{-1}, the polyhedrons were observed (Fig. 20b). In the absence of P123 and NaOH, $BaWO_4$ particles were obtained (Fig. 20c), which is different from the morphologies in Fig. 20a and b. Fig. 20d shows the SEM micrograph of the Pb_2CrO_5 sample synthesized for 6 h, the long flakes with the split at two ends were observed. The inset of Fig. 6d displays the detailed structure. When the time was increased to 12 h, the bundles of nanoflakes were obtained (Fig. 20e). The XRD pattern shows that the sample consisted of a single phase of crystalline monoclinic Pb_2CrO_5 (JCPDS 29-0768).

Recently, the diverse luminescent spectra of $BaCrO_4$ were obtained when $BaCrO_4$ (Yan et al., 2006) was excited by 276, 454 and 488 nm, respectively. The PL spectra of our $BaCrO_4$ sample were obtained using the same excitation wavelengths. When excited at 276 nm, four weak emission band peaks were observed at 466, 471, 480, and 490 nm (Fig.21a). The emission band peak was not observed in the range of 300-450 nm. When excited at 454 and 488 nm, the $BaCrO_4$ sample had the strong emission band peak at 609 and 663 nm (Fig. 21b and c), respectively. Using the same excitation wavelength, Yan et al. (2006) observed the broad emission band peaks appeared at 607 and 640 nm, respectively. This phenomenon indicated that the $BaCrO_4$ sample had the diverse luminescent properties and potential application in electronic devices. Blasse (1980) proposed that the isoelectronic system CrO_4^{2-} was nonluminescent because of rapid radiationless deactivation. The metastable triplet state of the chromate ion may have an effect on the luminescent properties of $BaCrO_4$ (Dalhoeven et al., 1980; Miller & Tinti,1986; Speket al., 1996). The intrinsic mechanism still needs to be investigated because of few reports about luminescent properties of $BaCrO_4$ sample.

4. Morphology, structure, and function biomineral synthesis of other nanomaterials

Biomineral synthesis includes morphology, structure, and function biomineral synthesis. It is well known that the structure determines property and the morphology is the external display of structure. In chemistry, biomimetic synthesis is a man-made chemical synthesis inspired by biochemical processes. Here, we intend to review recent progress in biomineral synthesis of other nanomaterials in this section.

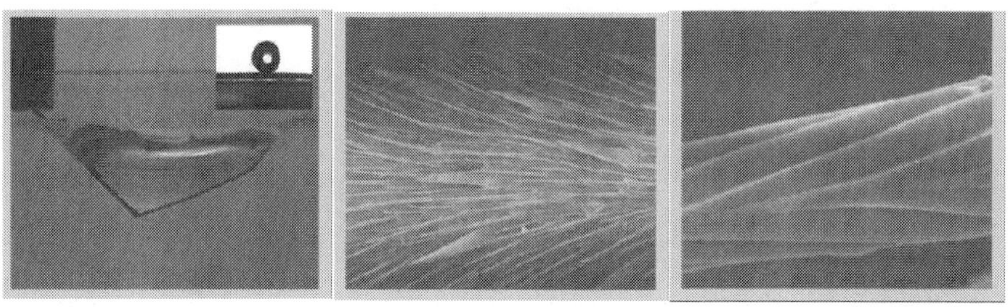

Fig. 22. The non-wetting leg of a water strider. **a,** Typical side view of a maximal-depth dimple (4.38±0.02 mm) just before the leg pierces the water surface. Inset, water droplet on a leg; this makes a contact angle of 167.6±4.4°. **b, c,** Scanning electron microscope images of a leg showing numerous oriented spindly microsetae (**b**) and the fine nanoscale grooved structures on a seta (**c**). Scale bars: **b,** 20 μm; **c,** 200 nm. Reproduced with permission from Nature, **2004**, *432*, 36. Copyright **2004** *Nature Publishing Group.*

Since the discovery of carbon nanotubes in 1991 (Iijima, 1991), carbon and carbon-based nanocomposites have been receiving more attention due to its unique properties such as mechanical properties, high thermal stability, electrical properties, high-temperature and high-pressure stability and resists attacks from acids, bases, and solvents, and promising potential applications in electronic conductors (White & Todorov, 1998), microelectrode (Teo et al., 2005), field emission transistors (Keren et al., 2003), hydrogen storage (Lin, 2000). carbon nanotubes are a excellent candidate in biomineral synthesis field.

Many biological surfaces in both the plant and animal kingdom possess unusual structural features at the micro- and nanometre-scale that control their interaction with water and hence wettability. Some paints and roof tiles have been engineered to be self-cleaning by copying the mechanism from the Nelumbo lotus. Jiang et al. reveal the mechanism of standing effortlessly and moving quickly on water of water striders in 2004 (Gao & Jiang, 2004), which has unique hierarchical micro- and nanostructuring on the leg's surface (Fig. 22). This discovery favors in the design of miniature aquatic devices and non-wetting materials. They also discover the micro- and nanoscale hierarchical structures on the surface of a lotus leaf (branch-like nanostructures on top of the micropapillae), which can induce super-hydrophobic surfaces with large contact angle and small sliding angle (Fig. 23a,b) (Zhai et al., 2002) and the micro- and nanostructures of a rice leaf, which are arranged in

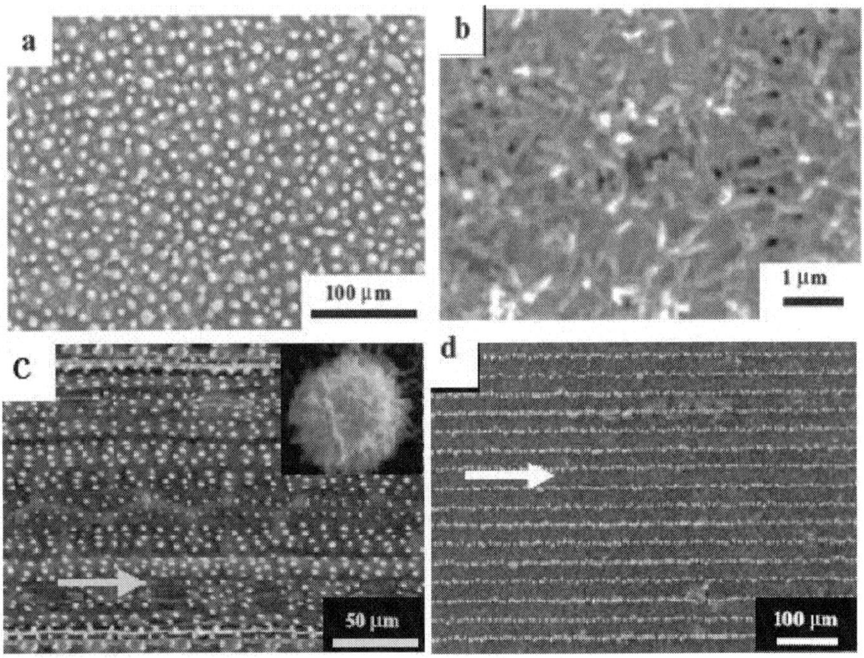

Fig. 23. a)Large-area SEM image of the surface of a lotus leaf (*Nelumbo nucifera*). Every epidermal cell forms a papilla and has a dense layer of epicuticular waxes superimposed on it. b) SEM image of the lower surface of the lotus leaf. c) Large-area SEM image of the surface of a rice leaf (*Oryza sativa*) with different magnifications. d) SEM image of the top view of a rice-like ACNT film. Reproduced with permission from Physics, **2002**, *31*, 483 and Adv. Mater., **2002**, *14*, 1857. Copyright **2002** *Elsevier and VCH.*

one-dimensional order parallel to the leaf edge with sliding angle 3-5° and randomly in the other directions with sliding angle 9-15° (Fig. 23c). Based on the finding, they biomineral synthesized the rice-like aligned carbon nanotube films with the similar micro- and nanostructures with super-hydrophobic nanochannels (Fig. 23d) (Feng et al., 2002). Aligned structure of carbon nanotube films with fairly uniform length of (3 μm) and external diameter (60 nm) and super-amphiphobic properties was biomineral synthesized by high temperature pyrolysis method using phthalocyanine complexes as raw materials (Li et al., 2001). The experimental results show that the untreated aligned carbon nanotube films are super-hydrophobic and super-lipophilic, fluoride membrane surface modification of carbon nanotubes are both hydrophobic and lipophobic properties, indicating that the presence of nanostructure led to the super-amphiphobic surface. Moreover, they designed artificial fibres that mimic the structural features of silk and exhibit its directional water-collecting ability, inspired by the finding that the water-collecting ability of the capture silk of the cribellate spider *Uloborus walckenaerius* is the result of a unique fibre structure that forms after wetting, with the 'wet-rebuilt' fibres characterized by periodic spindle-knots made of random nanofibrils and separated by joints made of aligned nanofibrils (Zheng et al., 2010).

It is well known that the ability of gecko lizards to adhere to a vertical solid surface is due to their remarkable feet with aligned microscopic elastic hairs. Qu et al. (2008) biomineral

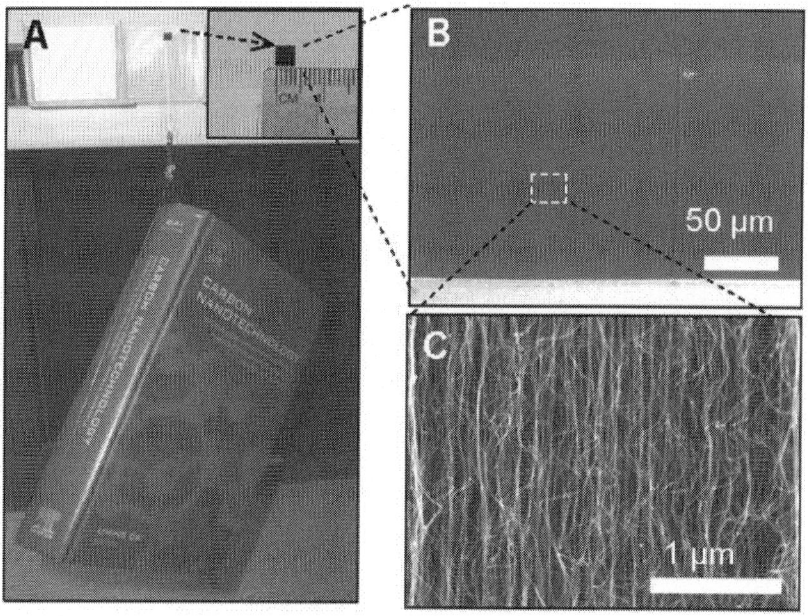

Fig. 24. (A) A book of 1480 g in weight suspended from a glass surface with use of VA-MWNTs supported on a silicon wafer. The top right squared area shows the VA-MWNT array film, 4 mm by 4 mm. (B and C) SEM images of the VA-MWNT film under different magnifications. Reproduced with permission from *Science*. **2008**, *322*, 238. Copyright **2008** *AAAS*.

synthesized the gecko-foot-mimetic dry adhesives with macroscopic adhesive forces of ~100 newtons per square centimeter using carbon nanotube arrays by simulating the walking of a living gecko (Fig. 24).

Bioinspired synthesis and self-assembly of advanced inorganic materials is fascinating field. Yu and co-workers used biomimetic synthesis method, in which the mineralization of inorganic materials was carried out in a glass bottle, which was put into a closed dessicator at room temperature, similar to that described by Addadi and co-workers (1996).

Yu et al (2005). reported the biomimetic synthesis of helices alignment achiral $BaCO_3$ nanocrystals in the presence of double hydrophilic block copolymers by a racemic polymer controlled biomineralization processes through selective adsorption on the (110) face of nanocrystals (Fig. 25). The results show that the spontaneous formation of spiral structure can be fabricated by directed tectonic assembly of inorganic particles and a new mechanism of the formation of spiral structure was proposed, that due to non-homogeneous polymer adsorption, making new modes of spontaneous symmetry breaking on the mesoscale, generating chiral contributions in the mutual interaction potentials of the building blocks. Moreover, facile biomimetic method is reported for the synthesis of novel $BaCO_3$ nanofibres with double-stranded and cylindrical helical morphologies (Zhu et al., 2009) *via* a phosphonated block co-polymer-controlled mineralization process.

Well-defined concaved cuboctahedral superstructures of copper sulfide (Wu et al., 2006) were large scale synthesized by a solvothermal reaction in ethylene glycol (Fig. 26). Each caved cuboctahedron is apparently "caved" with 14 highly symmetric cavities and is constructed by four identical hexagonal flakes while sharing the 24 edges in a dymaxion way. The results demonstrate that the branching growth process in solution can be precisely manipulated for the controlled growth of amazingly complex crystalline structures with high geometrical symmetry, which is not reflected in the primary crystal symmetry. This complex superstructure is similar to the image by M. C. Escher (1948).

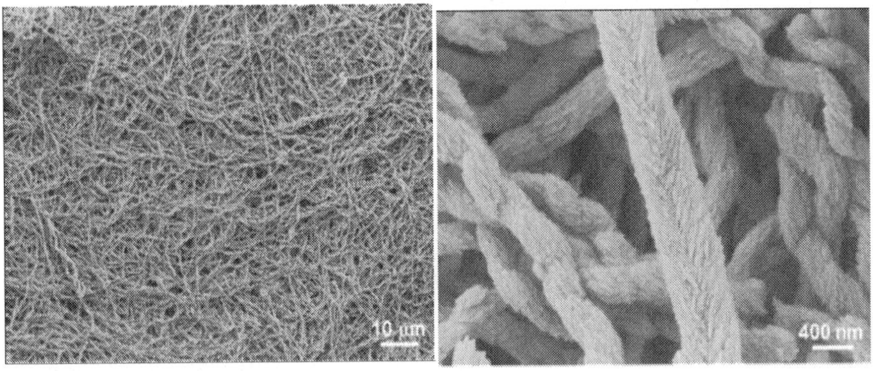

Fig. 25. Helical nanoparticle superstructures. a, The helical fi bres formed at room temperature with PEG-b-DHPOBAEE, 1 gL-1, starting pH=4, [$BaCl_2$] = 10 mM. **b**, Detailed surface structure. Reproduced with permission from *Nature Materials* **2005**, *5*, 51. Copyright **2005** *Nature Publishing Group*.

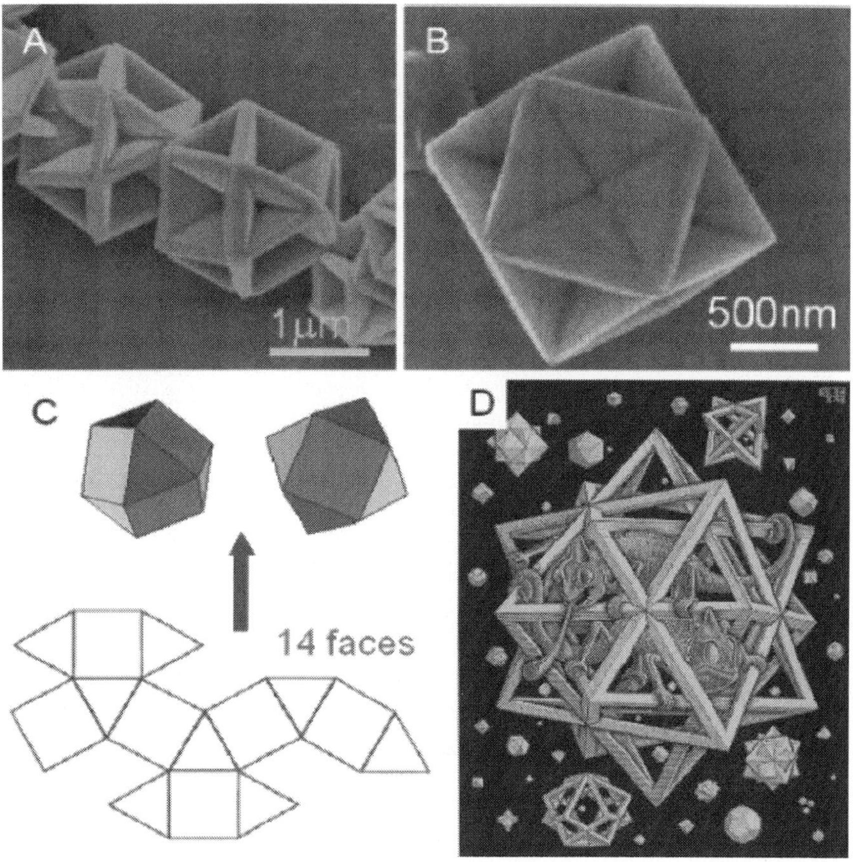

Fig. 26. (A and B) SEM images of the typical caved cuboctahedral crystals, synthesized by the solvothermal process at 140 °C for 24 h. (C) Schematic illustration of a cuboctahedron with 14 faces (six squares and eight triangles), composing the structure by sharing the identical 24 edges in a dymaxion way. (D) Cuboctahedron appearing as one of the polyhedral "stars" in M. C. Escher's 1948 wood engraving *Stars*. Reproduced with permission from Chem. Mater. **2006**, *18*, 3599. Copyright **2006** *ACS*.

The unique necklace-like Cu@cross-linked poly-(vinyl alcohol) (PVA) microcables (Zhan et al., 2008) that have strict wire-bead forms were biomimetic synthesized using a mixture of CuCl and $CuCl_2{\cdot}2H_2O$ by hydrothermal method at lower pH values (Fig. 27). One-dimensional magnetic Ni-Co alloy microwires (Hu & Yu, 2008) with different microstructures and differently shaped building blocks including spherical particles, multilayer stacked alloy plates, and alloy flowers, have been synthesized by an external magnetic field-assisted solvothermal reaction of mixtures of cobalt(II) chloride and nickel(II) chloride in 1, 2-propanediol with different NaOH concentrations (Fig. 28).

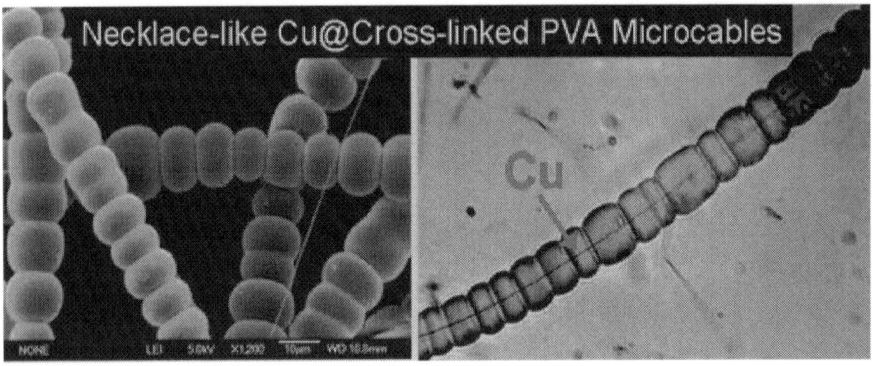

Fig. 27. SEM images of the necklace-like microcables with different magnifications. Reproduced with permission from J. Am. Chem. Soc. **2008**, *130*, 5650. Copyright **2008** *ACS*.

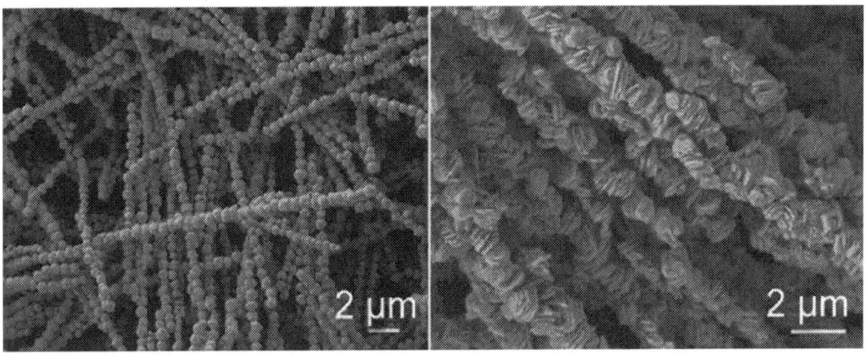

Fig. 28. SEM images of the one-dimensional assembly of Ni_xCo_{1-x} alloy microparticles. Reproduced with permission from Nano Research **2008**, *1*, 303. Copyright **2008** *springer*.

The calcite pancakes with controlled surface structures (Chen et al., 2005) was fabricated by double-hydrophilic block copolymer-directed self-assembly using the macrocycle-coupled block copolymer,poly(ethylene glycol)-b-poly (1,4,7,10,13,16-hexaazacyclooctadecan ethylene imine), macrocycle (PEG-B-hexacyclen) as a crystal modifier (Fig. 29a). Highly monodisperse $CaCO_3$ (vaterite) microspheres (Guo et al., 2006) were prepared by a slow gas-liquid diffusion reaction with an artificial peptide-type block copolymer, PEG(110)-b-pGlu(6), as a crystal-growth modifier in a mixture of solvents by using a suitable volume ratio of N,N-dimethylformamide/nonionic water and by taking advantage of the synergistic effects of the block copolymer and the solvent mixture (Fig. 29b,c). The results demonstrate that the solvent mixture plays a key role in controlling the growth, polymorphism, and shape of the $CaCO_3$ mineral. Polymorph discrimination of $CaCO_3$ mineral in an ethanol/water solution: Formation of complex vaterite superstructures and aragonite rods (Fig. 29d-f) (Chen et al., 2006).

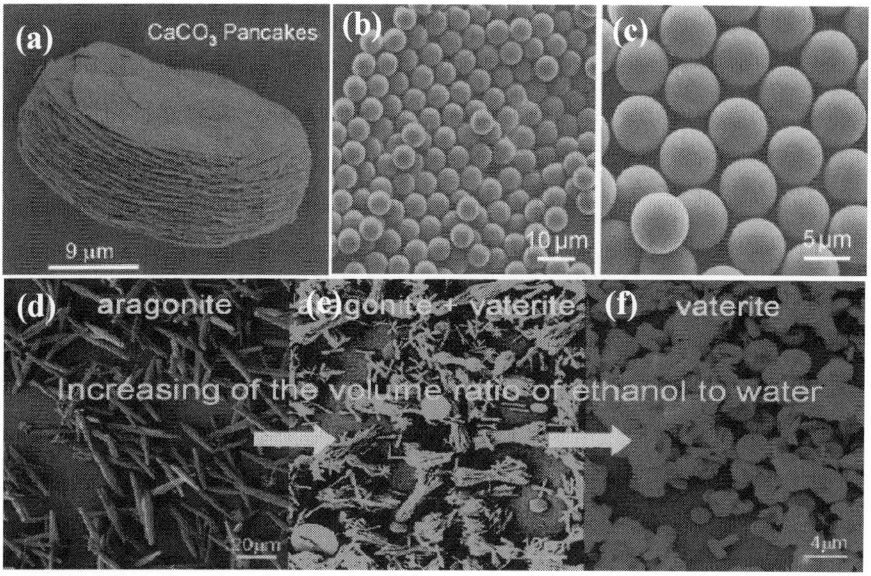

Fig. 29. SEM images of the $CaCO_3$: (a) calcite pancakes; (b,c) monodisperse $CaCO_3$ (vaterite) microspheres; (d-f) vaterite superstructures and aragonite rods. Reproduced with permission from Adv. Mater. **2005**, *17*, 1461, Angew. Chem. Int. Ed. **2006**, *45*, 3977, and Chem. Mater. **2006**, 18, 115. Copyright **2010** *ACS* and *VCH*.

5. Conclusion

In recent years, rapid progress has been made in the research of biomineralization and biomimetic synthesis. The effect research of bimolecular on the structure of biomaterials has great scientific significance and widely applications. However, the present research was still at the initial stage. In future, the follow problems should be explored. For example, the relationship of properties and microstructure in biominerals; the intrinsic mechanism of biomineralization; the experimental examples for better understanding of the molecular recognition mechanism; how to simulate the biomineralization and realize biomimetic synthesis?

6. Acknowledgments

Financial support from the National Natural Science Foundation of China (31070511) China Postdoctoral Science Special Foundation (20100359), and Major State Basic Research Development Program of China (973 Program) (No.2010CB732204) is gratefully acknowledged.

7. References

Banfield, J. F.; Welch, S. A.; Zhang, H. Z.; Ebert, T. T. & Penn, R. L. (2000). *Science* 289,751-54.

Bastow, T. J. (2002). *Chem. Phys. Lett.* 354, 156.

Blasse, G. (1980). *Struct. Bonding*, 42, 1.

Bohner, M. (2004). New hydraulic cements based on a-tricalcium phosphate-calcium sulfate dihydrate mixtures. *Biomaterials*, 25, 741-9.

Boskey, A. L.; Young, M. F.; Kilts, T. &Verdelis, K. (2005). Variation in mineral properties in normal and mutant bones and teeth. *Cells Tissues Organs*, 181, 144-53.

Cameron, H. U.; Macnab, I. & Pilliar, R. M. (1977). Evaluation of a biodegradable ceramic. *J. Biomed. Mater. Res.*, 11, 179-86.

Chen, S. F.; Yu, S. H.; Jiang, J.; Li, F. Q. & Liu, Y. K. (2006). Polymorph discrimination of $CaCO_3$ mineral in an ethanol/water solution: Formation of complex vaterite superstructures and aragonite rods. *Chem. Mater., 18*, 115-122.

Chen, S. F.; Yu, S. H.; Wang, T. X.; Jiang, J.; Cölfen, H.; Hu, B. & Yu, B. (2005). Polymer directed formation of unusual $CaCO_3$ pancakes with controlled surface structures. *Adv. Mater., 17*, 1461-1465.

Cheng, X. K.; He, Q. J.; Li, J. Q.; Huang, Z. L. & Chi, R. A. (2009). Control of pore size of the bubble-template porous carbonated hydroxyapatite microsphere by the adjustable pressure. *Crystal Growth & Design*, 9, 2770-5.

Chi, C. W. (2010). US7687098.

Chow, L. C. & Sun, L. M. (2010). US7670579.

Cortes, D. A.; Medina, A.; Escobedo, J. C.; Escobedo, S. & Lopez, M. A. (2004). Effect of wollastonite ceramics and bioactive glass on the formation of a bonelike apatite layer on a cobalt base alloy. *J. Biomed. Mater. Res.* A 70A, 341-6.

Cotton, F. A.; Wilkinson, G.; Murillo, C. A. & Bochmann, M. (1999). *Adv. Inorganic Chem. 6th ed.*; Wiley: New York.

Cui, X. J.; Yu, S. H.; Li, L. L.; Biao, L.; Li, H. B.; Mo, M. S. & Liu, X. M. (2004). *Chem. Eur. J.*, 10, 218-23.

Dadyburjor, D. B. & Ruckenstein, E. (1977). *J. Cryst. Growth*, 40, 279.

Dalhoeven, G. A. M. & Blasse, G. (1980). *Chem. Phys. Lett.*, 76, 27-29.

Ding, S. J. (2009). US2009198345.

Dorozhkin, S. V. (2007). Calcium orthophosphates. *J. Mater. Sci.*, 42, 1061-95.

Economy, J.; Meloon Jr., D. T. & Ostrozynski, R. L. (1965). *J. Catal.* 4, 446.

Erdemoğlu, M. & Canbazoğlu, M. (1998). *Hydrometallurgy* 49, 135.

Escher, M. C. *Stars* wood engraving, 1948; http://www.mcescher.com/Gallery/back-bmp/LW359.jpg.

Feng, L.; Li, S. H.; Li, Y. S.; Li, H. J.; Zhang, L. J.; Zhai, J.; Song, Y. L.; Liu,B. Q.; Jiang, L.; & Zhu. D. B. (2002). Super-hydrophobic Surfaces: From Natural to Artificial. *Adv. Mater.*, 14, 1857

Fujii, S.; Okada, M.; Sawa, H.; Furuzono, T. & Nakamura, Y. (2009). Hydroxyapatite nanoparticles as particulate emulsifier: fabrication of hydroxyapatite-coated biodegradable microspheres. *Langmuir* 25, 9759-66.

Furuzono, T.; Kisida, A.; Tanaka, J. & Matsuda, A. (2009). US7473731.

Gao, F.; Lu, Q. Y.; Xie, S. H. & Zhao, D. Y. (2002). *Adv. Mater.* 14,1537-40.

Gao, X. F. & Jiang, L. (2004). Striking water repellence by water striders' legs. *Nature*, 432,36

Garcia-Sanz, F. J.; Mayor, M. B.; Arias, J. L.; Pou, J.; Leon, B. & Perez-Amor, M. (1997). Hydroxyapatite coatings: a comparative study between plasma-spray and pulsed laser deposition techniques. *J. Mater. Sci. Mater. Med.*, 8, 861-5.

Getter, L.; Bhaskar, S. N.; Cutright, D. E.; Perez, B.; Brady, J. M.; Driskell, T. D. & O'Hara, M. J. (1972). Three biodegradable calcium phosphate slurry implants in bone. *J. Oral. Surg.*, 30, 263-8.

Gindl, W. & Keckes, J. (2004). Tensile properties of cellulose acetate butyrate composites reinforced with bacterial cellulose. *Comp. Sci. Techn.*, 64, 2407-13.

Godber, J. & Leite, L. (2009). US7468172.

Griffiths, J. (1985). *Ind. Miner.* 218, 21.

Groot, D. & Mitchell, J. C. (1981). Oro-pharyngeal mucosal reaction to fenoterol. *Contact Dermatitis*, 7, 48.

Gross, K. A; Berndt, C. C. & Iacono, V. J. (1998). Variability of hydroxyapatite-coated dental implants. *Int. J. Oral. Maxillofac Implants*, 13, 601-610.

Gross, K. A.; Ray, N. & Rokkum, M. (2002). The contribution of coating microstructure to degradation and particle release in hydroxyapatite coated prostheses. *J, Biomed, Mater, Res.*, 63, 106-14.

Guo, X. H.; Yu, S. H. & Cai, G. B. (2006). A New controlled crystallization approach in a mixed solution using an artificial peptide type block copolymer as a crystal modifier: highly monodisperse $CaCO_3$ microspheres and morphology control. *Angew. Chem. Int. Ed., 45*, 3977-3981.

Gutmann, B. & Chalup, A. (2000). *Am. Ceram. Soc. Bull.* 79, 63.

Hing, K. A. (2004). Bone repair in the twenty-first century: biology, chemistry or engineering. *Philos. Trans. R. Soc. A* 362, 2821-50.

Hu,M. J.; Lin, B. & Yu, S. H. (2008). Magnetic-Field Induced Solvothermal Synthesis of Uniform One-Dimensional Assembly of Ni_xCo_{1-x} Alloy Microparticles. *Nano Research,1*, 303-312.

Iguchi, M.; Yamanaka, S. & Budhiono, A. (2000). Bacterial cellulose-a masterpiece of nature's arts. *J. Mater. Sci.*, 35, 261-70.

Iijima S. (1991). Helical microtubules of grapgitic carbon, *Nature*, 354, 56.

Islas-Blancas, M. E.; Cervantes, J. M.; Vargas-Coronado, R.; Cauich-Rodriguez, J. V.; Vera-Graziano, R. & Martinez-Richa, A. (2001). Characterization of bone cements prepared with functionalized methacrylates and hydroxyapatite. *J. Biomater. Sci. Polym. Ed.*, 12, 893-910.

Jain, S. K.; Awasthi, A. M.; Jain, N. K. & Agrawal, G. P. (2005). Calcium silicate based microspheres of repaglinide for gastroretentive floating drug delivery: preparation and in vitro characterization. *J. Control Release* 107, 300-9.

Kanakis, J.; Chrissanthopoulos, A.; Tzanetos, N. P.; Kallitsis, J. K. & Dalas, E. (2006). Crystallization of hydroxyapatite on oxadiazole-based homopolymers. *Cryst. Growth Des.* 6, 1547-52.

Kano, S.; Yamazaki, A.; Otsuka, R.; Ohgaki, M.; Akao, M. & Aoki, H. (1994). Application of hydroxyapatite-sol as drug carrier. *Biomed. Mater. Eng.*, 4, 283-90.

Keren, K.; Berman, R. S.; et al. (2003). DNA-templated carbon nanotube field-effect transistor, *Science*, 302, 1380.

Kim, H. W.; Lee, H. H.; Knowles, J. C. (2006). Electrospinning biomedical nanocomposite fibers of hydroxyapaite/poly(lactic acid) for bone regeneration. *J. Biomed. Mater. Res. Part A*, 79A, 643-9.

Kim, H. W.; Knowles, J. C. & Kim, H. E. (2004). Hydroxyapatite/poly (epsilon-caprolactone) composite coatings on hydroxyapatite porous bone scaffold for drug delivery. *Biomaterials*, 25, 1279-87.

Kim, I. Y.; Sugino, A.; Kikuta, K. & Ohtsuki , C. (2009). Bioactive composites consisting of PEEK and calcium silicate powders. *J. Biomater. Applications* 24, 105-18.

Kithva, P.; Grondahl, L.; Martin, D. & Trau, M. (2010). Biomimetic synthesis and tensile properties of nanostructured high volume fraction hydroxyapatite and chitosan biocomposite films. *J. Mater. Chem.* 20, 381-9.

Koga, N.; Nakagoe, Y. Z. & Tanaka, H. (1998). *Thermochimica Acta*, 318, 239.

Kojima, Y.; Kawanobe, A.; Yasue, T. & Arai, Y. (1993). *J. Ceram. Soc. Japan* 101, 1145.

Kokubo, T.; Kawai, M.; Kawashita, M.; Yamamoto, K. & Nakamura, T. (2005). Fabrics of polymer fibers modified with calcium silicate for bone substitute. *Key Engineer. Mater.*, 284-286, 775-8.

Lacout, J. L.; Freche, M.; Goncalves, S. & Rodriguez, F. (2009). US6923989.

Lamer, V. K. & Dinegar, R. H. (1950). *J. Am. Chem. Soc.*, 72, 4847.

Landi, E.; Tampieri, A.; Celotti, G.; Vichi, L. & Sandri, M. (2004). Influence of synthesis and sintering parameters on the characteristics of carbonate apatite. *Biomaterials,* 25, 1763-70.

Lee, D. D.; Rey, C.; Aiolova, M. &Tofighi, A. (2009).US7517539.

Li,H. J.; Wang, X. B.; Song,Y. L.; Liu, Y. Q.; Li, Q. S.; Jiang, L. & Zhu. D. B. (2001). Super-"amphiphobic" aligned carbon nanotube films. *Angew.Chem.Int.Ed.*, 40, 1743.

Li, H. Y. & Chang, J. (2005). Preparation, characterization and in vitro release of gentamicin from PHBV/wollastonite composite microspheres. *J. Controlled Release* 107, 463.

Li, H. Y. & Chang, J. (2005). Preparation, characterization and in vitro release of gentamicin from PHBV/wollastonite composite microspheres. *J. Control Release* 107, 463-73.

Lin, J. Y. (2000). Hydrogen storage in nanotubes, *Science*, 287, 1929.

Liu, J. K.; Wu, Q. S. & Ding, Y. P. (2005). Self-assembled synthesis and fluorescent modification of hydroxyapatite nanoribbons spherulites. *Eur. J. Inorg. Chem.*, 4145-9.

Lima, R. S.; Khor, K. A.; Li, H.; Cheang, P. & Marple, B. R. (2005). HVOF spraying of nanostructured hydroxyapatite for biomedical applications. *Mater. Sci. Engin. A-Struct. Mater. Prop.s Microstr. Proc.*, 396, 181-7.

Li, Q.; Ding, Y.; Li, F. Q.; Xie, B. & Qian, Y. T. (2002). *J. Cryst .Growth 236*, 357.

Li, S. M.; Jia, N.; Zhu, J. F.; Ma, M. G. & Sun, R. C. (2010). Synthesis of cellulose-calcium silicate nanocomposites in ethanol/water mixed solvents and their characterization. *Carbohydr. Polym.* 80, 270-5.

Li, T. & Feng, Y. Q. (2009). Biomimetic fabrication of hydroxyapatite-coated zirconia-magnesia composite and its application in the separation of proteins. *Talanta.* 80, 889-94.

Li, T. T., Lee, J. , Kobayashi, T. & Aoki, H. (1992). Hydroxyapatite coating by dipping method, and bone bonding strength. *J. Mater. Sci.: Mater. in Medic.* 7, 355-7.

Li, Y. D.; Wang, J. W.; Deng, Z. X.; Wu, Y. Y.; Sun, X. M. & Yu, D. P. (2001). *J. Am. Chem. Soc.* 123, 9904-05.

Lu, X. & Leng, Y. (2005). Theoretical analysis of calcium phosphate precipitation in simulated body fluid. *Biomaterials* 26, 1097-108.

Ma, M. G. & Zhu, J. F. (2009). Solvothermal synthesis and characterization of hierarchically nanostructured hydroxyapatite hollow spheres. *Eur. J. Inorg. Chem.*, 5522-6.

Ma, M. G. & Zhu, J. F. (2010). Recent progress on fabrication of calcium-based inorganic biodegradable nanomaterials. *Recent Patents on Nanotechnology*, 4, 164-70.

Ma, M. G.; Zhu, J. F.; Jia, N.; Li, S. M.; Sun, R. C.; Cao, S. W. & Chen, F. (2010). Rapid microwave-assisted synthesis and characterization of cellulose-hydroxyapatite nanocomposites in *N,N*-dimethylacetamide solvent. *Carbohydr. Res.*, 345, 1046-50.

Ma, M. G.; Zhu, Y. J. & Chang, J. (2008). Solvothermal preparation of hydroxyapatite microtubes in water-*N,N*-dimethylformamide mixed solvents. *Mater. Lett.*, 62, 1642-5.

Ma, M. G.; Zhu, Y. J.; Cheng, G. F. & Huang, Y. H. (2008). Fabrication and characterization of $BaCO_3$ nanostructure. *Materials Letters*, 62, 3110-3113.

Ma, M. G.; Zhu, Y. J.; Zhu, J. F. & Xu, Z. L. (2007). A simple route to synthesis of $BaCO_3$ nanostructures in water/ethylene glycol mixed solvents. *Materials Letters*, 61, 5133-5136.

Ma, M. G.; Zhu, Y. J.; Zhu, J. F. & Cheng, G. F. (2006). Microwave-assisted fabrication and characterization of $BaCO_3$ nanorods, *Chemistry Letters* 35, 10, 1138-1139.

Ma, M. G.; Zhu, Y. J. & Li , S. H. (2009). A simple route to synthesis of $BaCrO_4$ microstructures at room temperature, *Materials Research Bulletin*, 44(2), 288-293.

Ma, M. G.; Jiang, J. X. & Sun, R. C. (2010). Microwave-assisted controlled synthesis of $CaCO_3$ with various biomimetic morphologies using basic additives in polyol. *Advanced Materials Research*, 92, 139-145.

Ma, M. G. & Zhu, Y. J. (2008). Microwave synthesis of $SrCO_3$ one-dimensional nanostructures assembled from nanocrystals using ethylenediamine additive. *Materials Letters*, 62, 2512-2515.

Ma, M. G. & Zhu, Y. J. (2007). A simple route to synthesis of $SrCO_3$ with olive-like and flower-like morphologies, *Journal of Nanoscience and Nanotechnology*, 7, 4552-4556.

Ma, M. Y.; Zhu, Y. J.; Li, L. & Cao, S. W. (2008). Nanostructured porous hollow ellipsoidal capsules of hydroxyapatite and calcium silicate: preparation and application in drug delivery. *J. Mater. Chem.*, 18, 2722-7.

Marqusee, J. A. & Ross, J. (1983). *J. Chem. Phys.* 79, 373.

Matsumoto, T. &Nakasu, M. (2010). US7687138.

Matsuoka, H.; Akiyama, H.; Okada, Y.; Ito, H.; Shigeno, C.; Konishi, J.; Kokubo, T. & Nakamura, T. (1999). In vitro analysis of the stimulation of bone formation by highly bioactive apatite- and wollastonite-containing glass-ceramic: released calcium ions promote osteogenic differentiation in osteoblastic ROS17/2.8 cells. *J. Biomed. Mater. Res.*, 47, 176-88.

McGrath, K. M. (2001),*Adv. Mater.* 13, 989.

McKee, M. D.; Wild, L. M.; Schemitsch, E H. & Waddell, J. P. (2002). The use of an antibiotic-impregnated, osteoconductive, bioabsorbable bone substitute in the treatment of infected long bone defects: early results of a prospective trial. *J. Orthop. Trauma*, 16, 622-7.

Miller, R. M. & Tinti, D. S. (1986). *J. Lumin.*, 36, 143-147.

Mirtchi, A. A.; Lemaitre, J. & Munting, E. (1990). *Calcium phosphate* cements: *study of* the alfa-*tricalcium* phosphate-dicalcium phosphate-calcite *cements, Biomaterials*, 11: 83-8.

Moheno, P. & Pfleiderer, W. (2010). US7662820.

Muller-Mai, C. M.; Voigt, C. & Gross, U. (1990). Incorporation and degradation of hydroxyapatite implants of different surface roughness and surface structure in bone. *Scanning Microsc*, 4, 613-22.

Nagano, M.; Nakamura, T.; Kokubo, T.; Tanahashi, M. & Ogawa, M. (1996). Differences of bone bonding ability and degradation behaviour in vivo between amorphous calcium phosphate and highly crystalline hydroxyapatite coating. *Biomaterials*, 17, 1771-7.

Nilsson, M.; Fernandez, E.; Sarda, S.; Lidgren, L. & Planell, J. A. (2002). Characterization of a novel calcium phosphate/sulphate bone cement. *J. Biomed. Mater. Res.* 61, 600-7.

Oktar, F. N.; Kesenci, K. & Piskin, E. (1999). Characterization of processed tooth hydroxyapatite for potential biomedical implant applications. *Artif Cells Blood Substit Immobil Biotechnol.* 27, 367-79.

Oyane, A.; Kawashita, M.; Nakanishi, K.; Kokubo, T.; Minoda, M.; Miyamoto, T. & Nakamura, T. (2003). *Bonelike apatite formation* on *ethylene*-vinyl alcohol copolymer modified with silane coupling agent and calcium silicate solutions. *Biomaterials* 24, 1729-35.

Owusu, G. & Litz, J. E. (2000). *Hydrometallurgy* 57, 23.

Pacholski, C.; Kornowski, A. & Weller, H. (2002). *Angew. Chem. Int. Ed.* 41, 1188-91.

Penn, R. L. & Banfield, J. F. (1999). *Geochimica et Cosmochimica Acta* 63,1549-57.

Qu, L. T.; Dai, L. M.; Stone, M.; Xia, Z. H. & Wang, Z. L. (2008). Carbon Nanotube Arrays with Strong Shear Binding-On and Easy Normal Lifting-Off. *Science.*, 322, 238.

Rauschmann, M. A.; Wichelhaus, T. A.; Stirnal, V.; Dingeldein, E.;, Zichner, L.; Schnettler, R. & Alt, V. (2005). Nanocrystalline hydroxyapatite and calcium sulphate as biodegradable composite carrier material for local delivery of antibiotics in bone infections. *Biomaterials*, 26, 2677-84.

Riihonen, R.; Nielsen, S.; Vaananen, H. K.; Laitala-Leinonen, T. & Kwon, T. H. (2010). Degradation of hydroxyapatite in vivo and in vitro requires osteoclastic sodium-bicarbonate co-transporter NBCn1. *Matrix Biology*, 29, 287-94.

Rodríguez-Lorenzo, L. M. ; García-Carrodeguas, R.; Rodríguez, M. A.; DeAza, S.; Jime´nez, J.; López-Bravo, A.; Fernandez, M. & Román, J. S. (2009). Synthesis, characterization, bioactivity and biocompatibility of nanostructured materials based on the wollastonite-poly (ethylmethacrylate-co-vinylpyrrolidone) system. *J. Biomed.Mater. Res. A* 88, 53-64.

Rudin, V. N.; Komarov, V. F.; Melikhov, I. V.; Minaev, V. V.; Orlov, A. Y. & Bozhevolnov, V.E. (2009). US7169372.

Sakai, H.; Ito, E.; Cai, R. X.; Yoshioka, T.; Kubota, Y.; Hashimoto, K. & Fujishima, A. (1994). Intracellular Ca^{2+} concentration change of T24 cell under irradiation in the presence of TiO_2 ultrafine particles. *Biochim. Biophys. Acta* 1201, 259-65

Sato, S.; Koshino, T. & Saito, T. (1998). Osteogenic response of rabbit tibia to hydroxyapatite particle-plaster of paris mixture. *Biomaterials*, 19, 1895-900.

Shi, H.; Qi, L. M.; Ma, J. & Cheng, H. (2003). *J. Am. Chem. Soc.* 125, 3450.

Shi, J. J.; Li, J. J.; Zhu, Y. F.; Wei, F. & Zhang, X. R. (2002). *Anal. Chim. Acta* 466, 69.

Shoda, M. & Sugano Y. (2005). Recent advances in bacterial cellulose production. *Biotechnol. Bioproc. Engin.*, 10, 1-8.

Shum, H. C.; Bandyopadhyay, A.; Bose, S. & Weitz, D. A. (2009). Double emulsion droplets as microreactors for synthesis of mesoporous hydroxyapatite. *Chem. Mater.*, 21, 5548-55.

Sotome, S.; Uemura, T.; Tanaka, J.; Kikuchi, M.; Shinomiya, K. & Tateishi, T. (2009). US7494664.

Spek, A. L.; Duisenberg,A. J. M.; Coremans,C. J. M. & der Waals, J. H. (1996). *J. Lumin.*, 69, 319-323.

Suchanek, W. L.; Shuk, P.; Byrappa, K.; Riman, R. E.; TenHuisen, K. S. & Janas, V. F. (2002). Mechanochemical hydrothermal synthesis of carbonated apatite powders at room temperature. *Biomaterials*, 23, 699-710.

Sugihara, H.; Anan, T.; Adachi, K.; Baba, A.; Egashira, N. & Nishiguchi, H. (1997). *J. Ceram. Soc. Japan* 105, 886-90.

Sugimoto, S. (1978). *J. Colloid Interface Sci.* 63, 16.

Sugimoto, T. (1987). *Adv. Colloid Interface Sci.* 28, 65.

Sun, R. X.; Lu, Y. P. & Chen, K. Z. (2009). Preparation and characterization of hollow hydroxyapatite microspheres by spray drying method. *Mater. Sci. Eng. C* 29, 1088-92.

Tarasevich, B. J.; Chusuei, C. C. & Allara, D. L. (2003). Nucleation and growth of calcium phosphate from physiological solutions onto self-assembled templates by a solution-formed nucleus mechanism. *J. Phys. Chem. B* 107, 10367-77.

Teo, K. B. K.; Minoux, E.; et al. (2005). Microwave devices- Carbon nanotubes as cold cathodes, *Nature*, 437, 968.

Thian, E. S.; Huang, J.; Vickers, M. E.; Best, S. M.; Barber, Z. H. & Bonfield, W. (2006). Silicon-substituted hydroxyapatite (SiHA): A novel calcium phosphate coating for biomedical applications. *J. Mater. Sci.*, 41, 709-17.

Tofighi, A. N. & Rey, C. (2010). US7686239.

Venugopal, A. & Scurrell, M. S. (2003). Hydroxyapatite as a novel support for gold and ruthenium catalysts - Behaviour in the water gas shift reaction. *Appl. Catalys. A-General*, 245, 137-47.

Wahl, D. A. & Czernuszka, J. T. (2006). Collagen-hydroxyapatite composites for hard tissue repair. *Europ. Cells Mater.*, 11, 43-56.

Wang, X.; Zhuang, J.; Peng, Q. & Li Y. D. (2006). Liquid-solid-solution synthesis of biomedical hydroxyapatite nanorods. *Adv. Mater.*, 18, 2031-4.

Wang, H. B.; Lee, J. K.; Moursi, A. & Lannutti, J. J. (2003). Ca/P ratio effects on the degradation of hydroxyapatite in vitro. *J. Biomedical Mater. Res. Part A*, 67A, 599-608.

Wang, K. W.; Zhou, L. Z.; Sun, Y.; Wu, G. J.; Gu, H. C.; Duan, Y. R.; Chen, F. & Zhu, Y. J. (2010). Calcium phosphate/PLGA-mPEG hybrid porous nanospheres: A promising vector with ultrahigh gene loading and transfection efficiency. *J. Mater. Chem.*, 20, 1161-6.

Wang, L. F.; Sondi, I. & Matijevic. E. (1999). *J. Colloid Interf. Sci.* 218, 545.

Wang, W. W. & Zhu, Y. (2005). *J. Crystal Growth & Design*, 5, 505-507.

Wei, H.; Shen, Q.; Zhao, Y.; Wang, D. & Xu, D. (2004a). *J. Cryst. Growth*, 260, 511.

Wei, H.; Shen, Q.; Zhao, Y.; Wang, D. & Xu, D. (2004b). *J. Cryst. Growth*, 260, 545.

Wei, J.; Chen, F. P.; Shin, J. W.; Hong, H.; Dai, C. L.; Su, J. C. & Liu, C. S. (2009). Preparation and characterization of bioactive mesoporous wollastonite -polycaprolactone composite scaffold. *Biomaterials*, 30, 1080-8.

Wei, J.; Heo, S. J.; Li, C. S.; Kim, D. H.; Kim, S. E.; Hyun, Y. T.; Shin, J. W. & Shin, J. W. (2009). Preparation and characterization of bioactive calcium silicate and poly(epsilon-caprolactone) nanocomposite for bone tissue regeneration. *J. Biomed. Mater.Res. Part A* 90A, 702-12.

Weiner, S.; Albeck, S. & Addadi, L. (1996). *Chem.Eur.J.*, 2, 278.

Wen, C. L.; Guan, S. K.; Peng, L.; Ren, C. X.; Wang, X. & Hu, Z. H. (2009). Characterization and degradation behavior of AZ31 alloy surface modified by bone-like hydroxyapatite for implant applications. *Appl. Surf. Sci.,* 255, 6433-8.

Wenisch, S.; Stahl, J. P.; Horas, U.; Heiss, C.; Kilian, O.; Trinkaus, K.; Hild, A. & Schnettler, R. (2003). In vivo mechanisms of hydroxyapatite ceramic degradation by osteoclasts: Fine structural microscopy. *J. Biomedical Mater. Res. Part A* 67A, 713-718.

White, C. T. & Todorov, T. N. (1998). Carbon nanotubes as long ballistic conductors, Nature, 393,240.

Wu, J.; Zhu, Y. J.; Cao, S. W. & Chen, F. (2009). Hierachically nanostructured mesoporous spheres of calcium silicate hydrate: surfactant-free sonochemical synthesis and drug-delivery system with ultrahigh drug-loading capacity. *Adv. Mater.,* 22, 749-53.

Wu, C. Y.; Yu, S. H.; Antonietti, M. (2006). Complex concaved cuboctahedrons of copper sulfide crystals with highly geometrical symmetry created by a solution process. *Chem. Mater., 18,* 3599-3601.

Wu, H. C.; Wang, T. W.; Bohn, M. C.; Lin, F. H. & Spector M. (2010). Novel magnetic hydroxyapatite nanoparticles as non-viral vectors for the glial cell line-derived neurotrophic factor gene. *Adv. Funct. Mater.,* 20, 67-77.

Yamaguchi, K.; Hirano, T.; Yoshida, G. & Iwasaki, K. (1995). Degradation-resistant character of synthetic hydroxyapatite blocks filled in bone defects. *Biomaterials,* 16, 983-5.

Yan, Y.; Wu, Q. S.; Li, L. & Ding, Y. P. (2006). *Crystal Growth & Design* 6, 769-773

Yasukawa, A.; Yokoyama, T.; Kandori, K. & Ishikawa, T. (2004). Ion-exchange property and mechanism of magnesium-calcium hydroxyapatite solid solutions. *Colloids Surf. A-Physicochem. Engin. Aspects.* 238, 133-9.

Yaszemski, M.; Currier, B. L.; Jabbari, E. & Lu, L. (2010). US7642300.

Yin, J.; Zou, Z. & Ye, J. (2003). *Chem. Phys. Lett.* 378, 24-28.

Yu, S. H.; Colfen, H. & Antonietti, M. (2003). *Adv.Mater.* 15, 133.

Yu, S. H.; Cölfen, H.; Tauer, K. & Antonietti, M. (2005). Tectonic arrangement of $BaCO_3$ nanocrystals into helices induced by a racemic block copolymer. *Nature Materials 5,* 51-55.

Yuan, Y.; Liu, C. S.; Qjan, J. C.; Wang, J. & Zhang, Y. (2010). Size-mediated cytotoxicity and apoptosis of hydroxyapatite nanoparticles in human hepatoma HepG2 cells. *Biomaterials,* 31, 730-40.

Zeller, A. F. (1981). *Chem. Tech.* 19, 762.

Zhai, J.; Li, H.J.; Li,Y.S.; Li, S.H. & Jiang, L. (2002). *Physics,* 31, 483.

Zhan, J. H.; Lin, H. P. & Mou, C. Y. (2003). *Adv. Mater.* 15, 621-23.

Zhan, Y. J. & Yu, S. H. (2008). Necklace-Like Cu@cross-linked poly(vinyl alcohol) (PVA) core-shell Microncables, *J. Am. Chem. Soc., 130,* 5650-5651.

Zhang, Z. J.; Sun, J. M.; Cao, H. F.; Zhang, X. Y.; Wang, Y. W. & Yao, Q. (2009). CN101591023.

Zheng, Y. M.; Bai, H.; Huang, Z. B.; Tian, X. L.; Nie, F . Q.; Zhao, Y.; Zhai , J. & Jiang, L. (2010). Directional water collection on wetted spider silk. *Nature* 463, 640-643.

Zhu, J. H.; Yu, S. H.; Xu, A. W. & Cölfen, H. (2009). Biomimetic mineralization of double-stranded and cylindrical helical $BaCO_3$ nanofibres, *Chem. Commun.* 1106-1108.

3

The Biomimetic Mineralization Closer to a Real Biomineralization

Binbin Hu, Zhonghui Xue and Zuliang Du
Key Lab for Special Functional Materials of Ministry of Education, Henan University, 475004 Kaifeng, P. R. China

1. Introduction

In view of the huge timeframe Nature has to optimize and perfect functional materials to survive during the evolution and natural selection, as a result, biominerals, the organic-inorganic hybrid materials are formed through biomineralzation, one of the most important processes for the organisms to produce for a variety of purposes, including mechanical support, navigation, protection, and defense (Lowenstam & Weiner, 1989; Stupp, et al., 1993; Weiner & Addadi, 2003). These biomaterials are generally molded into specifically designed devices with fascinating properties of superior materials properties and environmentally friendly synthesis and biocompatibility (Xu, et al., 2007) , in which the structure, size, shape, orientation, texture, and assembly of the constituents are precisely controlled over several hierarchy levels. Therefore, the understanding and ultimately mimicking of the processes involved in biomineralization may provide new approaches to the fabrication of specialized organic-inorganic hybrid materials, in other words, nature provides a perfect model for people to design and fabricate novel materials with special structures and functions through the biomimetic mineralization method (Mann, 2000).
Based on these ideas a rapidly developing research field has evolved, which can be summarized as bioinspired or biomimetic materials chemistry (Mann, 1995; Cölfen & Yu, 2005), is meanwhile already an important branch in the broad area of biomimetics (Mann, et al., 1993; Davis, et al., 2001; Cölfen, 2003; Meldrum, 2003; Yu & Cölfen, 2004). As the research is continuously developed, the main aim to mimic the syntheses of these biominerals, is not only to emulate a particular biological architecture or system, but also to abstract the guiding principles and ideas and use such knowledge for the preparation of new synthetic materials and devices (Dujardin & Mann, 2002). During the past decades, exploration as well as application of these bio-inspired synthesis strategies has resulted in the generation of complex materials with specific size, shape, orientation, composition, and hierarchical organization (Archibald & Mann, 1993; Antonietti & Göltner, 1997; Yang, et al., 1997; Li, et al., 1999; Estroff & Hamilton, 2001; Jones & Rao, 2002; Cölfen & Mann, 2003; Dabbs & Aksay, 2003; Aizenberg, 2004). The human efforts in the fields of chemistry and materials science have led to the development of a complementary set of inorganic and hybrid materials with special characteristics. However, by mimicking the design and synthesis of, e.g., biomaterials, to date no synthetic materials have evolved that show properties which are superior to those found in their natural counterparts (Sommerdijk & With, 2008). It is

evident that the understanding and ultimately the mimicking of the processes involved in biomineralization has been a motivation for humans to copy Nature and to adapt ideas from Nature to achieve functional, aesthetic, and societal value (Mann, 2000; Xu, et al., 2007), and it still has a long way to go. A proper biomimetic system closer to a real environment and process of biomineralization is necessary to both understand the mechanism of biomineralization and instruct materials synthesis using biomimetic mineralization approaches (Towe, 1990).

Many methods have been established to study and mimic the biomineralization process with the aim to synthesize superstructures that mimic natural biominerals and to gain an insight into the biomineralization mechanism. Among these approaches, as shown in Fig. 1, organic Langmuir monolayer (b) has an obvious structural feature of approximation to half of the bilayer structure of a biomembrane (a), as a result, organic Langmuir monolayer has been often used as a convenient model to approach the two-dimensional structure of biomembrane (Stine, 1994; Gzyl-Malcher & Paluch, 2008). For this, Langmuir monolayer usually can serve as an ideal model system for simulating and studying biomacromolecules and biomacromolecule-controlled mineralization at the air-water interface. Therefore, it has been widely used as the organic templates in the research of biomimetic mineralization to guide the growth of inorganic crystals with special structural features and to better understand the interface nature of organic-mineral interface and what occurs at the interface between organic molecules and inorganic materials (Mann, et al., 1988; Heywood & Mann, 1992; Heywood, 1992; Mann, et al., 1993; Heywood & Mann, 1994; Mann & Ozin, 1996; Mann, 2001; Zhang, et al., 2004; Amos, et al., 2007; Popescu, et al., 2007; Pichon, et al., 2008).

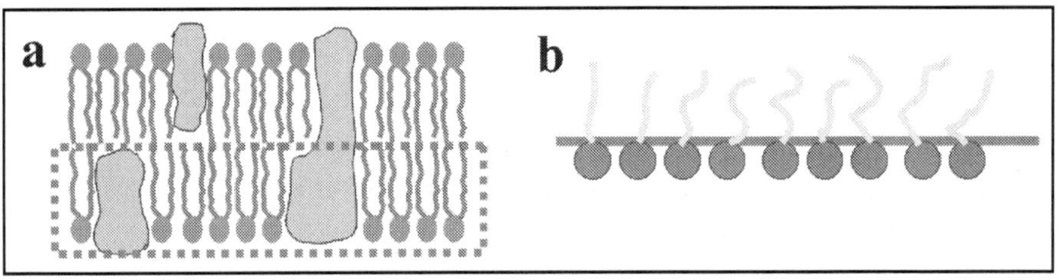

Fig. 1. The schematic diagrams of a biomembrane (a) and a Langmuir monolayer (b).

There has been so much biomimetic mineralization research in the past several decades using many kinds of Langmuir monolayer template system, such as small organic molecules, polymers, cells of organisms and so on. However, the proteins, the most important and the most frequently presented matrix in the biomineralization process of organisms, have not been researched enough in the biomimetic mineralization in a manner of Langmuir monolayer.

On the other hand, in the usual research of biomimetic mineralization, the regulation of organic Langmuir monolayer on the nucleation and growth of inorganic materials has been researched extensively as the important foundation of biomimetic synthesis. However, as an equally important factor for the special structural features of the biominerals in the real environment and process of biomineralization, the kinetic control of inorganic crystals growth in the biomimetic mineralization system has not gotten due diligence.

Fortunately, these two problems have attracted more and more attention in the recent years. The protein Langmuir monolayer and the kinetic control factor has been gradually introduced into the systems in order to make the biomimetic mineralization much closer to a real environment and process of biomineralization, which on the one hand provides a perfect model for biomineralization research; on the other hand, more opportunities to get inorganic materials with special structural features can also be obtained through introducing more conditions of controlling on the basis of a usual organic template system, providing an effective experimental method for controllable fabrication of functional materials. So in this chapter, particular emphasis is placed on what has been accomplished in the research on both the biomimetic mineralization of calcium carbonate under a protein, especially bovine serum albumin (BSA) Langmuir monolayer and the novel biomimetic interface system named dual-template approach in which the inorganic materials are grown under a Langmuir monolayer in the presence of kinetic control generated from ammonia diffusion.

2. Biomineralization and biomimetic mineralization of calcium carbonate under a protein Langmuir monolayer

2.1 Biomineralization and biominerals

Biomineralization is the process by which living organisms secrete inorganic minerals in an organized fashion with exceptional physical properties, by virtue of finely controlled microstructure, morphology, and hierarchical organization of the minerals and accompanying organic material (DiMasi, et al., 2003; Xu, et al., 2007). It is already a rather old process in the development of life, which was adapted by living beings probably at the end of the Precambrian more than 500 million years ago (Wood, et al., 2002). There are more than 60 biologically formed minerals identified, examples include iron and gold deposits in bacteria and other unicellular organisms, silicates in algae and diatoms, carbonates in diatoms and nonvertebrates, and calcium phosphates and carbonates in vertebrates (Boskey, 2003).

Biominerals formed through biomineralization process are highly optimized materials with remarkable structural features and functional properties, which attracted a lot of recent attention. Fig. 2 shows three kinds of typical biominerals: combination coccosphere (a), the silica wall of the marine benthic diatom Amphora coffeaeformis (b), and a part of the skeleton of a brittlestar Ophiocoma wendtii (c). Obviously, the abilities to design and construct those inorganic materials with specified atomic structure, size, shape, orientation, and number of defects and to integrate these architectures into functioning devices is an important foundation for the survival of the organisms. These inorganic biominerals provide a wonderful and peerless foundation for advances in technologies that rely on the devices' electrical, optical, magnetic, and chemical outputs. Their formation and impressive properties have inspired chemists to take a biomimetic approach to the synthesis of materials. However, assembly methods that allow simultaneous control of these features at lengths from the nanometer scale to the macroscale is still extremely difficult to replicate synthetically for scientists and engineers. The ability to build architectures with such control would consequentially bring many new areas of technology—some already enumerated in the literature and others the outcomes of unanticipated surprises that are the direct consequences of the precision in assembly (Davis, 2004).

If there were constructors that could sequester inorganic ions from water, accumulate and concentrate them to produce architectures controlled over length scales from nanometers to tens of centimeters, and do all of this in a matter of hours at ambient temperatures (Davis,

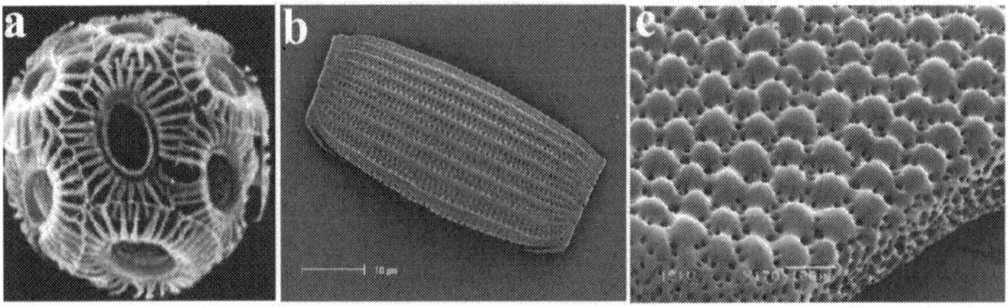

Fig. 2. Selection of biomineral structures. Each of them performs a specific function. a: Coccoliths calcite plates on the exterior of a single celled coccolithophorid alga, Emiliania huxleyi. Coccoliths are thought to provide protection against grazing, improve buoyancy, and scatter light to protect against damage from intense UV as well as improving light capture for species at depth (Cusack & Freer, 2008) (from Ref (Young, et al., 1999) with permission). b: Intricate walls. Scanning electron micrograph of the silica wall of the marine benthic diatom Amphora coffeaeformis. Note the ornate structure, patterning, and porosity of the silica wall (from Ref (Wetherbee, 2002) with permission of professor Richard Wetherbee). c: Scanning electron micrograph (SEM) of a part of the skeleton of a brittlestar Ophiocoma wendtii (Ophioroidea, Echinodermata). The entire structure (the mesh and the array of microlenses) is composed of a single calcite crystal used by the organism for mechanical and optical functions (Aizenberg, et al., 2001) (from Ref (Aizenberg, et al., 2003). (Reprinted with permission from AAAS).

2004), obviously, they will present an excellent model and bring a bright future for material science. In fact, such constructors are not inventions of science fiction novels but rather unicellular microalgae called diatoms with highly sculpted walls of silica. Because living cells must constantly interact with their environment, the diatom walls have myriad openings (such as pores and slits) that facilitate such exchanges (Aizenberg, Muller et al., 2003). The intricate patterns and symmetries (Fig. 2b) are species-specific and genetically determined (Pickett-Heaps, et al., 1990). And Kröger et al. (Kröger, Lorenz et al., 2002) have also found that silaffins have been implicated in the biogenesis of diatom biosilica and are crucial for the formation of these diatom walls. It is also found by Aizenberg et al. (Aizenberg, et al.,, 2001) that certain single calcite crystals (Fig. 2c) used by brittlestars for skeletal construction (Wainwright, et al., 1976; Lowenstam & Weiner, 1989) are also a component of specialized photosensory organs, conceivably with the function of a compound eye. The analysis of arm ossicles in Ophiocoma (Hendler & Byrne, 1987) shows that in light-sensitive species, the periphery of the labyrinthic calcitic skeleton extends into a regular array of spherical microstructures that have a characteristic double-lens design to minimize spherical aberration and birefringence and to detect light from a particular direction. The optical performance is further optimized by phototropic chromatophores that regulate the dose of illumination reaching the receptors. These structures represent an excellent and astonishing example of a multifunctional biomaterial with both mechanical and optical functions (Aizenberg, et al., 2001). It illustrates a remarkable example of organisms, through the process of evolution, to optimize one material for several functions, and provides new ideas for the fabrication of smart materials (Mann & Ozin, 1996; Belcher, et al., 1998).

Biological materials constitute most of the body of plants and animals around us. They allow cells to function, eyes to capture and interpret light, plants to stand up to the light and animals to move or fly. This multitude of solutions has always inspired mankind to make materials and devices, which simplify many of our day-to-day functions (Fratzl, 2007). However, the design strategies of biominerals are not immediately applicable to the design of new engineering materials, since there are some remarkable differences between the strategies common in engineering and those used by nature (Fratzl, 2007). Firstly, the range of choice of elements in natural materials is much less than that in manmade materials. Natural materials consist of relatively few constituent elements that are used to synthesize a variety of polymers and minerals, but human use many more elements. Secondly, manmade materials usually require high temperatures for fabrication but biological organisms have no access to them. For example, the diatom silica walls and single calcite crystals of skeleton of brittlestar with high degree of complexity and hierarchical structures are just achieved under mild physiological conditions. Meanwhile, nature grows both the material and the whole organism using the principles of biologically controlled self-assembly according to a recipe stored in the genes, rather than being fabricated according to an exact design, which is usually the basic principle for manmade materials (Fratzl, 2007). Therefore, the improved understanding of biomineralization process will unambiguously lead to the creation of better technologies (Davis, 2004). For example, some structures produced by biomineralization have superior properties to those of man-made counterparts. Nacre, the mother-of-pearl layer found on the inner surface of shells, has fracture toughness approximately 3000 times that of the synthetic analogue aragonite (Zaremba, et al., 1996). Nacre is composed of thin (circa 30 nm) layers of a protein-polysaccharide intercalated between 0.5-μm-thick layers of aragonite tablets. The weak interface between the organic and inorganic layers is thought to dissipate the energy of crack propagation and thus strengthen the composite structure. Recently, Much et al. (Munch, et al., 2008) emulate Nature's toughening mechanism through the combination of two ordinary compounds, alumina oxide and polymethylmethacrylate, into ice-template structures whose toughness can be over 300 times that of their constituents. This sophisticated architecture provides clues as to how man-made structures can be improved. It should be mentioned that biological structures are a constant source of inspiration for solving a variety of technical challenges in materials science (Jeronimidis & Atkins, 1995). Careful investigation of a biological system serving as the model is necessary for biomimetic materials research, as the elementary step, the design and construction of biomimetic mineralization system closer to native biomineralization process is a promise and important way to understand basic mechanism of biomineralization and get man-made materials with structural and functional features closer to the biominerals.

2.2 Biomimetic mineralization of calcium carbonate under a bovine serum albumin (BSA) Langmuir monolayer

The basic building blocks available to evolution when deciding skeletal structure are just Ca^{2+} and HCO_3^- or HPO_4^{2-}, this dichotomy is resolved when vertebrates evolve utilizing phosphate and (most) invertebrates evolve utilizing carbonate (Cusack & Freer, 2008). However, Nature has created a staggering diversity of perfect structures in the carbonate zone and continuing evolutionary masterpieces in the vertebrates using so limited fundamental building blocks. The secret to this diversity is the inclusion of organic materials, such as protein, carbohydrate and lipid as the thread to stitch together complicated structures from a simple cloth through biomineralization process (Cusack & Freer, 2008). Just as mentioned above, the success of diatoms in processing silica results from specific interactions at the organic-inorganic interface, between highly modified peptides called silaffins and silica (Kröger, et al., 2002). It is the variety of biomineral ultrastructures and chemical compositions, in combination with the organic components that ultimately determines the physical and material properties of these biocomposites, facilitating the specific functions (Cusack & Freer, 2008).

In pursuit of comparable synthetic materials, the processes by which minerals nucleate from solution in the presence of organic species have been under intense study in recent years, because it is clear that the organic matter controls and defines the end product in biomineralization (DiMasi, et al., 2003). One of the most challenging scientific problems is to gain greater insight into the molecular interactions occurring at the interface between the inorganic mineral and the macromolecular organic matrix. Many studies have been devoted to the putative mechanisms underlying the formation of highly organized mineral structures in molluscs and similar organisms. Due to the various experimental difficulties of observing crystal growth in living molluscs, scientists have sought out suitable model systems for mimicking biomineralization processes to reflect the mineral/matrix interactions active at the atomic or molecular level of structural complexity (Fricke & Volkmer, 2007). Seminal contributions were made by Mann and Heywood, who studied the controlled nucleation and crystallization of $CaCO_3$ under Langmuir monolayers of stearic acid (Mann, et al., 1988), which should be considered as extremely important work, as it placed the use of Langmuir monolayer studies, a technique well established in the field of physical chemistry in past century, now in the context of biomineralization. Importantly, the work noted that partially compressed Langmuir monolayers were optimal in inducing crystal formation, which was related to the possibility that the stearate molecules would adopt a Ca-induced local ordering resulting in a configuration tailored for nucleation of these crystals. This paper clearly is the onset for a large number of papers using Langmuir monolayers to study the nucleation of calcium carbonate and other minerals (Sommerdijk & With, 2008). As a general advantage, the biomimetic mineralization system using Langmuir monolayer as organic template allows for creating conveniently a smooth and clean interface and for depositing a measured quantity of amphiphilic molecules in a highly controlled way, the average area per molecule can be easily adjusted by a movable barrier, and the surface pressure is monitored by a pressure sensor. In many cases it is straight-forward to obtain a first approximation model to half of the bilayer structure of a biomembrane. All of these features make it possible to research precisely the structural relation between the organic matrixes and inorganic crystals. $CaCO_3$ is not only one of the most abundant biominerals, but also the mineral of choice for fundamental studies on template-mineral interactions due to its sensitivity to template effect (Dey, et al., 2010). Therefore, the model system of crystallization of calcium carbonate underneath Langmuir monolayer is often regarded as a straight-forward experimental approach toward biomimetic mineralization (Fricke & Volkmer, 2007).

Although the mechanisms by which organisms generate mineral crystals are not well understood, there is widespread belief that proteins play important roles. Thus, biomineralization can be seen as an interfacial phenomenon in which (usually extracellular) proteins interact with nascent crystals in order to control their growth (Hunter, et al. 2010), and Calcium carbonate grown under a Langmuir monolayer of protein should be a perfect model closer to a real biomineralization to get more insight on the mechanisms of biomineralization. As mentioned above, as one of the most important substances in the organisms, proteins are often implicated in the biomineralization. Proteins both collect and transport raw materials, and consistently and uniformly self- and co-assemble subunits into short- and long-range-ordered nuclei and substrates (Lowenstam & Weiner, 1989; Sarikaya, et al., 2003). Whether in controlling tissue formation, biological functions or physical performance, proteins are an indispensable part of biological structures and systems. A simple conclusion is that next-generation biomimetic systems should include proteins in synthesis, assembly or function (Bayley & Cremer, 2001; Sarikaya, et al., 2003). And proteins have widely been used for preparation of inorganic materials by biomimetic method. Comprehensive reviews on the synthesis of inorganic nanomaterials mediated by proteins assemblies (Behrens, 2008) and peptides (Chen & Rosi, 2010) have been given by Behrens and Chen et al., respectively. On the other hand, it is also important and necessary that proteins are introduced in the mineralization mimic and biomimetic syntheses research in appropriate manner closer to the real biomineralization process because of the special features of proteins, e.g., the large diversity of natural and synthetic proteins and their adjustability provide high probability that proteins recognize, interact with, and direct the formation of many inorganic materials. More importantly, the motivation and advantage using protein Langmuir monolayer as organic template for biomimetic mineralization is that it is easy to realize the structural changes of the protein molecules by simply controlling the surface pressure, which provides a great convenience for researching the influence of structural changes of protein molecules on the structural formation of biominerals.

Bovine serum albumin (BSA) is a popular candidate for biomimetic studies because some of the sequence characteristics is native to biomineralization proteins, at the same time, it is in readily available and inexpensive (Dickerson, et al., 2008). Xue et al. (Xue, et al. 2009) researched the templated crystallization of calcium carbonate nanoparticles beneath the Langmuir monolayer of bovine serum albumin (BSA). Through researching the area-time curve of BSA Langmuir monolayer on the supersaturated $Ca(HCO_3)_2$ solution subphase, they found that it takes about 18 min for the BSA Langmuir monolayer to be compressed to a surface pressure of 15 mN m^{-1}, and the area between the two barriers decreases as much as 26% during keeping the surface pressure at 15 mN m^{-1} for 1 h, which means the area per molecule has a 26% decrease during the crystallization of calcium carbonate. Such a decrease is closely related to the structural flexibility of the BSA Langmuir monolayer. The interaction between the BSA molecules and the Ca^{2+} ions in the subphase solution can affect the structure self-regulation of the BSA monolayer along with the formation of the inorganic crystal. Simultaneously, the structure self-regulation of the BSA monolayer affects in turn the formation of the inorganic crystal as well. The formation of the $CaCO_3$ crystals beneath the BSA Langmuir monolayer can be thought as a mutual-correlating, influencing, and adjusting process, where the key worth of special emphasis is that the structural flexibility of the BSA Langmuir monolayer helps to provide enough room for the $CaCO_3$ crystals to modulate and self-regulate their structure. BSA molecule contains charged amino acids such as 41 aspartic acids, 58 glutamic acids, and 60 lysine arrayed along certain directions at the interface between the BSA Langmuir monolayer and subphase solution. In addition to the putative BSA cation-binding by Asx residues, the presence of Lys and Arg residues may provide active sites for interaction with carbonate counterion. These acidic and basic residues, in conjunction with Ser and Glx residues, also provide active sites for hydrogen-bonding with water, and the presence of Gly residues generate considerable flexibility along the protein backbone (Xue, et al., 2009). The BSA molecules usually tend to have α-helix conformation when being spread onto the air/water interface. The Ca^{2+} ions in (104) plane has the similar structure of orthogonal repeat units to the α-helix conformation, which provides convenience for their structural regulation to grow along the (104) plane, while the template and structural adaptability play a key role in the oriented crystallization of $CaCO_3$ (Xue, et al., 2009). In the experiments, the transformation of calcium carbonate from unstable amorphous calcium carbonate (ACC) phase to stable calcite crystals was also observed, indicating a multistep crystallization process found in other biomimetic mineralization of calcium carbonate crystals (Xu, et al., 1998; Pouget, et al., 2009).

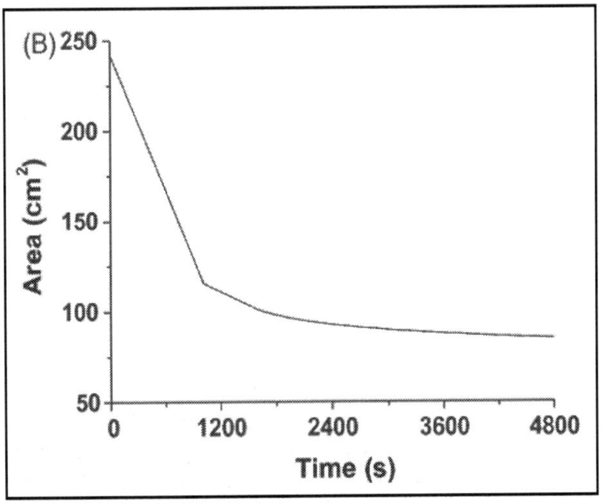

Fig. 3. The area–time curve of BSA Langmuir monolayer compressed and kept for 60 min on calcium bicarbonate solution subphase (from (Xue, et al., 2009) with permission).

Aside from the BSA Langmuir monolayer, some factors such as pH, temperature, and supersaturation degree also play key roles in controlling the growth and morphologies of $CaCO_3$ crystals. As one of the thermodynamic driving forces, the supersaturation degree is the most decisive parameter for crystallization process and has a different subphase concentrations. The influence of different subphase concentrations on the growth process and morphology evolution of calcium carbonate crystals under a BSA Langmuir monolayer was investigated (Xue, et al. 2009). The morphologies of the $CaCO_3$ crystals grown under the BSA Langmuir monolayer experienced a great evolution from disk-like calcite particles with an average diameter of 0.75 μm at a subphase concentration of 2.5 mM (Fig. 4a, b), to bowknot-like calcite particles formed at 5.0 mM (Fig. 4c, d), and to hexagonal-shaped morphology with a size of 16–18 μm at 7.5 mM (Fig. 4e, f). The result shows that the concentration is a key factor for the structural control in the biomimetic mineralization systems. Certainly, further work is needed to reveal the role of the BSA Langmuir monolayer and subphase concentration in the nucleation and growth process of calcium carbonate in more details (Xue, et al., 2009).

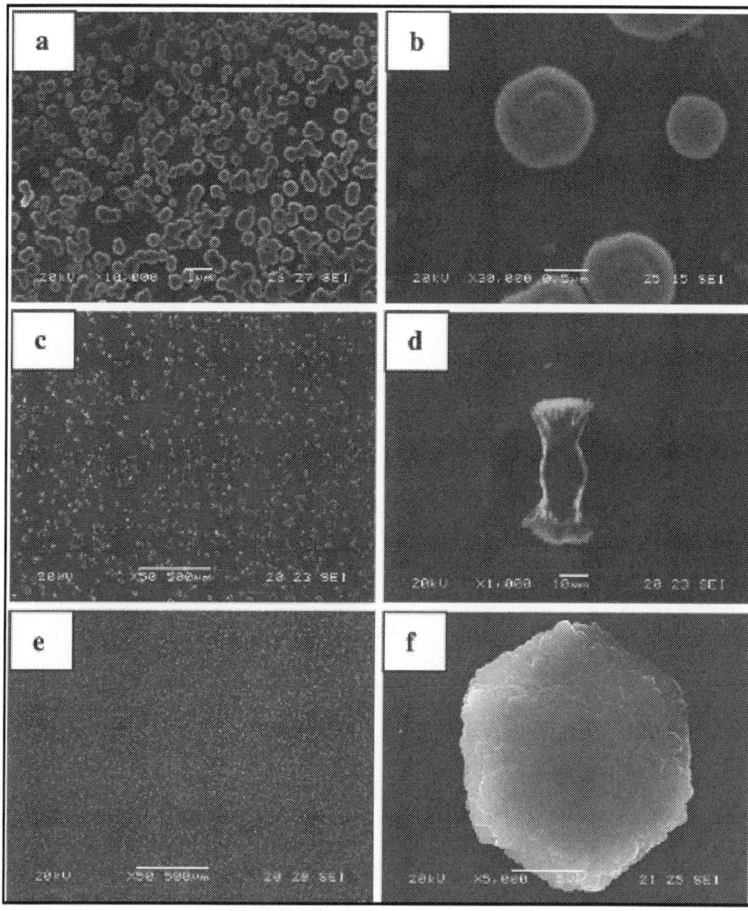

Fig. 4. SEM images of calcium carbonate formed at different subphase concentrations: (a and b) 2.5 mM, (c and d) 5.0 mM, (e and h) 7.5 mM from ref (Xue, et al., 2009) with permission.

3. Biomimetic mineralization in the presence of kinetic control from ammonia diffusion

Biomimetic synthesis inspired from biomineralization has recently been attracting more and more attention as a green and environment-friendly method, developing to be a multi-disciplinary hot spot. In the usual research of biomimetic mineralization, the regulation of organic Langmuir monolayer on the nucleation and growth of inorganic materials is considered and researched as the important foundation of biomimetic synthesis. However, as an equally important factor for the special structural features of the biominerals in a real biomineralization, the kinetic control of inorganic crystals growth has not gotten enough attention.

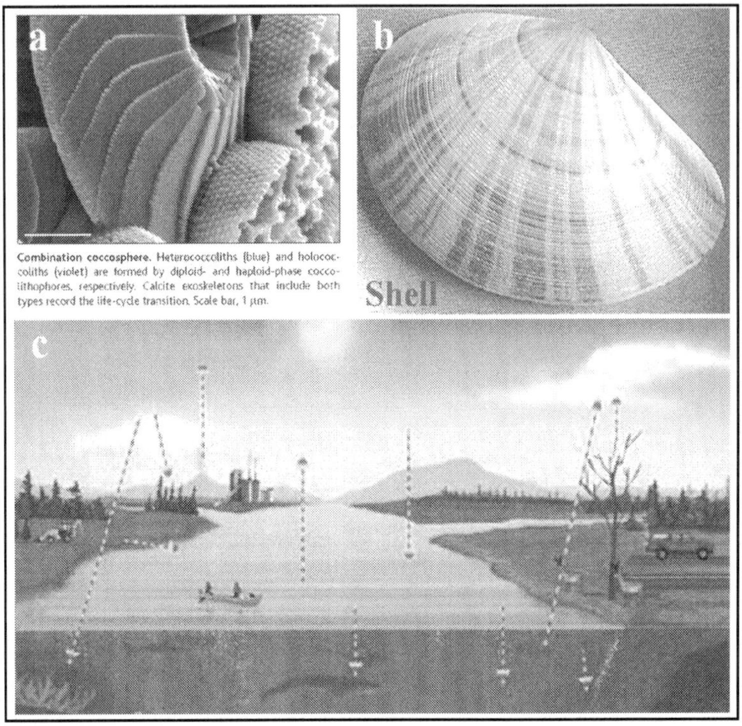
a
Combination coccosphere. Heterococcoliths (blue) and holococ-
coliths (violet) are formed by diploid- and haploid-phase cocco-
lithophores, respectively. Calcite exoskeletons that include both
types record the life-cycle transition. Scale bar, 1 μm.
b
Shell
c

Fig. 5. Calcite of coccosphere (a) (from (Davis, 2004) with permission), shell (b), schematic circle diagram of carbon dioxide in nature (c).

In fact, the growth of natural inorganic biominerals is also regulated by the kinetic control except of the regulation of organic matrix that is emphasized in the usual biomineralization and biomimetic research. As shown in Fig. 5, both the calcite of coccosphere (a) (Davis, 2004) and shell (b) show perfect structural features. What's the most important, they both present specific properties, e.g., nacre, the mother-of-pearl layer found on the inner surface of shells, has fracture toughness approximately 3000 times that of the synthetic analogue aragonite, and such a mechanical capacity results from the organic components and its special formation (Zaremba, et al., 1996). While the special formation results from the kinetic control as well as the genetic regulation and the participation of organic components. Fig. 5c is a schematic circle diagram of carbon dioxide in nature. Statistics show that the carbon dioxide concentration in the atmosphere is much less than that of human emissions and a large part of carbon dioxide is absorbed by the oceans (Ridgwell, et al., 2003). Carbonic anhydrase exists in the body of many sea creatures can catalyze the transformation reaction between carbon dioxide and hydrogen carbonate. Under the nucleation and growth control of the organic matrix, the calcium ions in the body combine with the hydrogen carbonates and finally form those biominerals with sophisticated architecture and special properties. In such a process, the slow catalysis of transformation from carbon dioxide to hydrogen carbonate plays a key role on the structures of inorganic crystals. Obviously, the environment and the speed of such a process have important influence on the formation and growth of inorganic biominerals. Clams, oysters and some other microbes are through this process for synthesis of shells and other hard minerals.

These natural examples indicate that the kinetic control plays an important role on the formation of special morphological and structural features for these biominerals. Therefore, more attention should be paid to the kinetic control factors in the biomimetic mineralization research. If a kinetic control can be introduced into the biomimetic growth system on the basis of regulation effect of organic template through designing novel and suitable biomimetic interface system, one hand, the biomimetic synthesis can be much closer to a real biomineralization environment, providing a perfect model for biomineralization mimic research; on the other hand, more opportunities to get inorganic materials with special structural features can also be obtained through introducing more conditions of controlling on the basis of a usual organic template system, providing an effective experimental method for controllable fabrication of functional materials. So it is meaningful for both understanding biomineralization phenomena and instructing biomimetic synthesis of inorganic functional materials.

Nanocrystalline TiO_2 (Sumerel, et al., 2003) and Ga_2O_3 (Kisailus, et al., 2005) were fabricated using a biomimetic synthesis method where silicatein, a catalytically active, structure-directing enzyme (Morse, 1999), was used as a catalyst and template for the hydrolysis and subsequent polycondensation of water stable molecular complexes of titanium and gallium to form nanocrystalline TiO_2 (Sumerel, et al., 2003) and Ga_2O_3 (Kisailus, et al., 2005), respectively. Ferroelectric $BaTiO_3$ nanocrystals were also synthesized by using an assembly of bola-amphiphile peptide, a linear type of peptide monomer with two amide head groups connected by a hydrocarbon tail group (Nuraje, et al., 2006). When a solution of the peptide monomers was added to the $BaTi(O_2CC_7H_{15})[OCH(CH_3)_2]_5$ precursor, ring-shaped peptide assemblies and tetragonal $BaTiO_3$ crystals were formed. During this process, the peptides were self-assembled into nanorings simultaneously as the precursor was hydrolyzed inside the cavity of the assembly. As the cavity size of the nanorings was a function of the pH value, the diameter of the particles could be varied from 6 to 12 nm. The surface chemical structure as well as the confinement effect of the peptide nanorings was likely to induce the unusual crystallization of the tetragonal $BaTiO_3$ nanoparticles (Nuraje, et al., 2006). By using the similar method, β-Ga_2O_3 semiconductor crystals that are known to be kinetically unfavoured to grow under ambient conditions, were successfully synthesized (Lee, et al. 2007). Where, the peptide assembly captured primary GaOOH particles, mineralized them into β-Ga_2O_3 crystals by its catalytic functions, and then fused them to grow monodisperse, single-crystalline, 50 nm particles in the cavity of the peptide assembly. It was suggested that the carboxyl groups of the peptide which were hydrogen-bonded with neighbouring amines catalyzed the hydrolysis of the gallium precursor (Behrens, 2008). Inspired by that some protein filaments shown in vitro to catalyze the hydrolysis and structurally direct the polycondensation of metal oxides at neutral pH and low temperature, Kisailus et al. (Kisailus, et al., 2006) designed and fabricated a bifunctional self-assembled monolayer surfaces containing the essential catalytic and templating elements by using alkane thiols microcontact-printed on gold substrates. The interface between chemically distinct self-assembled monolayer domains provided the necessary juxtaposition of nucleophilic (hydroxyl) and hydrogen-bonding (imidazole) agents to catalyze the hydrolysis of a gallium oxide precursor and template the condensed product to form GaOOH and the defect spinel, γ-Ga_2O_3. These methods use the similar principles borrowed from biomimetic synthesis routes (Sumerel, et al., 2003; Kisailus, et al., 2005; Schwenzer, et al., 2006): 1) slow catalysis of synthesis from molecular precursors provides the opportunity for kinetic control; and 2) crystal growth is vectorially regulated by a template, operating in concert with kinetic control to provide spatial and temporal control of crystal polymorph, orientation and morphology. And the results indicate that the kinetic control can provide an opportunity to get the materials with special structural features.

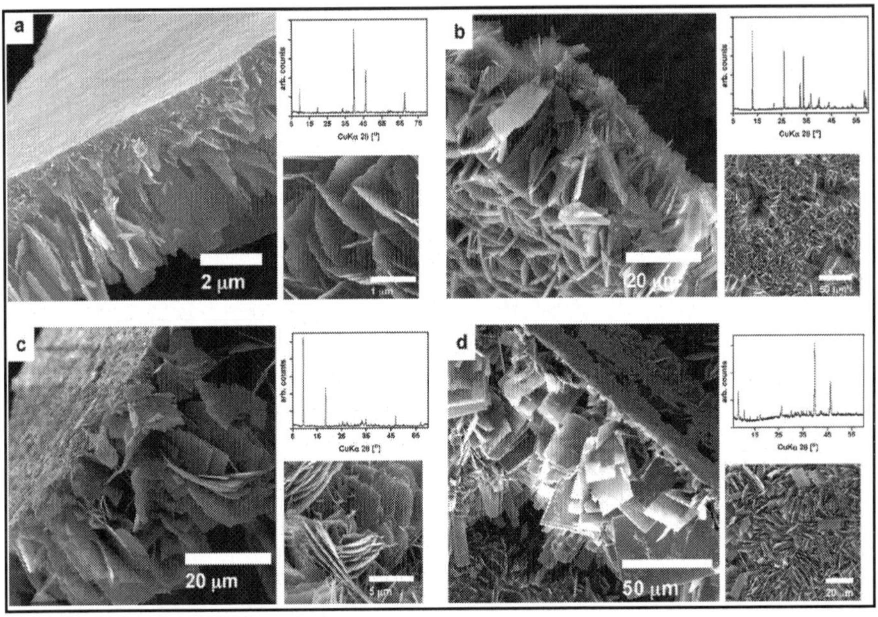

Fig. 6. Morphological and crystallographic characterization of metal hydroxide and phosphate thin films. Scanning electron microscopy (SEM; side- and bottom-view) images and XRD patterns of (a) $Co_5(OH)_8(NO_3)_2 \cdot 2H_2O$ (hydrotalcite-like structure), (b) $Cu_2(OH)_3(NO_3)$ (rouaite structure), (c) $Zn_5(OH)_8(NO_3)_2 \cdot 2H_2O$ (hydrotalcite-like structure) and (d) $Mn_3(PO_4)_2 \cdot 7H_2O$ (switzerite structure). Peaks at 39.7° and 46.2° in the XRD spectra of (a) and (d) result from the Pt holder of the instrument (from ref (Schwenzer, et al., 2006) *Reproduced by permission of The Royal Society of Chemistry*).

However, Morse et al. (Schwenzer, et al., 2006) believe that protein filaments that catalyzed and templated synthesis of nanocrystalline TiO_2 (Sumerel, et al. 2003) and Ga_2O_3 (Kisailus, et al. 2005) will incorporate the carbon impurities and degrade the performance of the materials for device applications that require high purity materials. In order to prevent the carbon impurities originating from the use of organic template, at the same time to capture the advantage of the slow catalysis and anisotropic, vectorial control of biocatalytic crystal growth, they developed a low-temperature, solution-based method employing the slow diffusion of ammonia vapor as a catalyst or hydrolysis of metal-containing molecular precursors. The diffusion through a solution of molecular precursor can establish spatially and temporally regulated gradient of the catalyst, while the vapor–liquid interface serves as a nucleation template. The resulting vectorially controlled combination of the molecular precursor and hydrolysis catalyst at room temperature yields a nanostructured thin film at the vapor–liquid interface. The diffusion of the basic catalyst (ammonia) into the aqueous solution creates a pH gradient that determines the morphology of the growing film, resulting in a unique structure of the film. Nanostructured $Co_5(OH)_8Cl_2 \cdot 3H_2O$, $Co_5(OH)_8(NO_3)_2 \cdot 2H_2O$, $Co_5(OH)_8SO_4 \cdot 2H_2O$, $Cu_2(OH)_3(NO_3)$, $Zn_5(OH)_8(NO_3)_2 \cdot 2H_2O$, $Mn_3(PO_4)_2 \cdot 7H_2O$ (Schwenzer, Roth et al., 2006) and ZnO (Kisailus, et al., 2006) thin films were prepared by this kinetically controlled vapor-diffusion method as shown in Fig. 6.

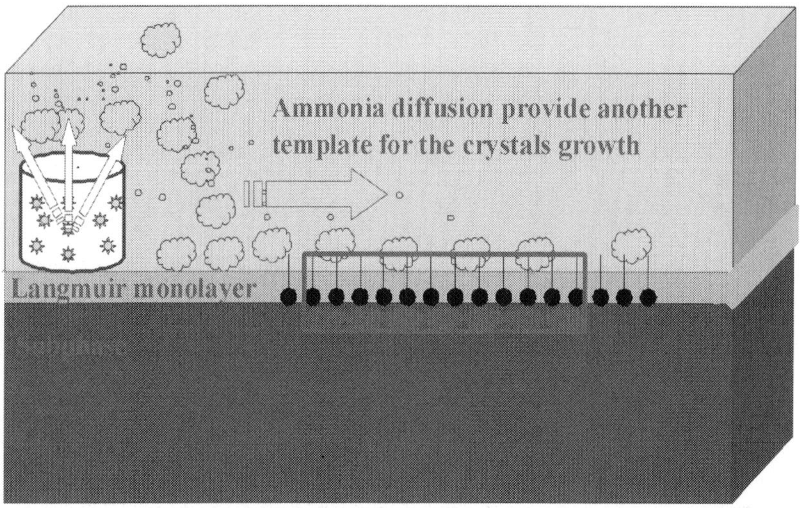

Fig. 7. Schematic diagram of the dual-template approach. A Langmuir monolayer is used as organic template; and the kinetic control of the hydrolysis degree of the molecular precursor, the species and concentration ratio of the cations and anions at the vapor-liquid interface is also realized through the pH value gradient, concentration gradient of reactants, and surface tension gradient generated from the vapor-diffusion and decided by the mode and the rate of ammonia diffusion, which directly influences the nucleation rate and crystal growth mode. The vapor-liquid interface generated from ammonia diffusion provides template information for the crystal growth, which is used as a kinetic template, and the system is named as dual-template approach. Obviously, it is much closer to a real biomineralization process.

Although hydrogen sulfide gas is widely used to fabricate PbS (Wang, et al., 1987; Zhao, et al., 1992; Zhu, et al., 1992; Tassoni & Schrock, 1994; Yang & Fendler, 1995; Mukherjee, et al., 1997; Shenton, et al., 1999; Ni, et al., 2004; Lu, et al., 2005) and CdS (Lianos & Thomas, 1987; Wang & Mahler, 1987; Facci, et al., 1994; Cui, et al., 2005; Lu, et al., 2005) nanoparticles, it only served as a gas reactant, which is completely different from the concept that ammonia used as a catalyst dissolves in an aqueous metal salt solution to initiate hydrolysis. It should be noted that Morse et al., (Schwenzer, et al., 2006) for the first time, put forward the concept that the vapor-liquid interface generated by the vapor-diffusion of catalyst (ammonia) can work as the nucleation template (Hu, et al., 2009). However, as shown in Fig. 6, the morphologies of the thin films obtained by the vapor-liquid interface template method are not very uniform, furthermore, their crystallographic orientation is random, the reason of which is the absence of organic matrix templates in synthetic conditions. Additionally, as mentioned above, it has been proved that Langmuir monolayers as organic matrix templates can play a key role in controlling morphology and crystallinity of the products in many biomimetic processes (Mann, et al., 1988; Heywood & Mann, 1992; Mann, et al., 1993; Yang, et al., 1995; Estroff & Hamilton, 2001; DiMasi, et al., 2002; With, 2008). Considering the nucleation effect of the vapor-liquid interface template and the matrix role of the organic template, we think that the combination of both templates will construct uniform morphological and well-oriented thin films at ambient temperature. With this consideration in mind, we developed a combination strategy of the vapor-liquid interface nucleation template and the organic matrix template, which was named as dual-template approach, and the schematic diagram is shown in Fig. 7 (Hu, et al., 2009). The experimental results proved that this dual-template approach was rather effective in the preparations of uniform morphological and well-oriented thin films of pure or doped metal hydroxide nitrates. The most important characteristic of our developed dual-template approach is the synergetic effect of the vapor-liquid interface nucleation template and the organic matrix template.

Firstly, the effect of organic matrix template in the dual-template system on the crystals growth is investigated. Fig. 8a shows the TEM image of crystals formed under a BSA Langmuir monolayer template at the surface pressure of 15 mN m^{-1} for 2 h. Individual nanosheets crystals can be observed in Fig. 8a, large area nanosheets are uniformly distributed on the substrate and some crystals stand while some lie, which is further confirmed by SEM images (Fig. 8d-8e). Their lengths and widths are ca. 2−4 μm and ca. 200−300 nm, respectively. The pattern of selected area electron diffraction (SAED) (Fig. 8b), recorded at the rectangular area shown in Fig. 8a, shows 6-fold symmetry and confirms that nanosheets are highly ordered single crystal structure. A high-resolution TEM image (HR-TEM) shown in Fig. 8c presents good crystallinity, and clear well-defined lattice fingers are in good agreement with the SAED pattern taken at the same area shown in Fig. 8b (Hu, et al., 2009).

It is remarkable that an interesting phenomenon in the recent publication, Casse et al. (Casse, et al., 2008) has found that even a rather flexible matrix like the block copolymers film at the vapor-liquid interface not only leads to uniform particles with identical particle sizes, but also can act as a tool for the 2D arrangement of the resulting particles in a near-crystalline order in a distorted hexagonal lattice. Regulating mineralization on the atomic (crystal phase) and the nanoscopic (particle size and shape) scale in the reported work is often encountered in the case that inorganic crystals are mineralized under organic matrix templates. Those mineralized inorganic crystals usually adopt a preferred orientation along a specific plane, even a single crystal structure at the atomic scale, meanwhile, display a uniform particle size and shape at the nanoscopic scale, just as the results shown in Fig. 8. However, it is seldom observed for the 2D arrangement of the resulting particles in a near-crystalline order. The main reason for the phenomenon is perhaps due to a special stage of balance between the nucleation and the growth of calcium phosphate at a very low concentration and a suitable pH value of the subphase, such conditions make the nucleation and growth process of minerals well-defined. In our recent work, we have also found that our dual template approach can lead to a 2D aggregation of crystals with a special fractal structure. In a word, these works give an implication that the organic matrix templates can realize an effective control for the mineralization of inorganic crystals, which provides us a good model for biological mineralization and an opportunity to obtain a series of inorganic materials with special structural features.

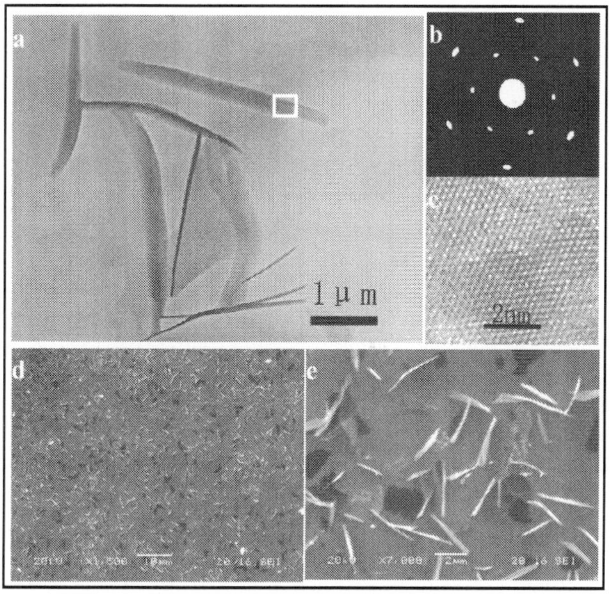

Fig. 8. TEM image (a), SAED pattern (b), HR-TEM image (c), and SEM images (d and e) of the nanosheets grown under the BSA Langmuir monolayer for 2 h at surface pressure of 15 mN m−1. The scale bars in a: 1μm, c: 2 nm, d: 10 μm and d: 2 μm (from ref (Hu, et al., 2009) *Reproduced by permission of The Royal Society of Chemistry*).

However, when the vapour-liquid interface template generated by the kinetically controlled vapor-diffusion of ammonia exists together with the organic matrix template on the surface of the subphase, it is notably different from the situation when only organic matrix template is present. The TEM images of $Zn_5(OH)_8(NO_3)_2 \cdot 2H_2O$ films formed at 2 h under a BSA Langmuir monolayer at surface pressure of 15 mN m^{-1} in the presence of ammonia diffusion are shown in Fig. 9. Compared with Fig. 8, Fig. 9 shows a continuous film other than the individual nanosheets in the presence of ammonia. It is obvious that the vapor-liquid interface template generated by the kinetically controlled vapor-diffusion of ammonia plays a key role in the formation of the thin films. The diffusion through a solution of molecular precursor $[Zn(NO_3)_2 \cdot 6H_2O]$ establishes a spatially and temporally regulated gradient of the catalyst (ammonia), to control the supersaturation of $Zn_5(OH)_8(NO_3)_2 \cdot 2H_2O$ through the formation of complexes (Kisailus, et al., 2006), while the vapor–liquid interface serves as the nucleation template (Schwenzer, et al., 2006; Hu, et al., 2009). Such a template as assistant of the BSA organic template directs crystal growth where there are no nanosheets induced by BSA Langmuir monolayer (like the blank areas in Fig. 8a). The co-operation effect between the vapor-liquid interface template and the organic template directs the growing materials to adopt a continuous film morphology, in contrast, the competition effect between the two templates leads to the morphological differences between nanosheets in the films and those as shown in Fig. 8a. The inset in Fig. 9b is the ED pattern of films, indicating a polycrystallinity structure. In comparison with Fig. 8 and Fig. 9, it is easy to see that the organic template favors to the formation of individual single-crystal nanosheets whereas the dual template is propitious to the construction of continuous polycrystalline films, but there exist still some single-crystal domains in polycrystalline films. This observation confirms that co-operation and competition (synergetic effect) of the dual template at the interface lead to the structure containing single-crystal domains in the polycrystalline films (Hu, et al., 2009).

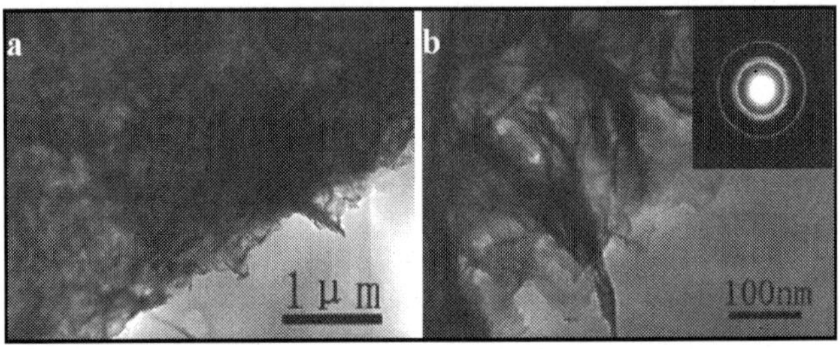

Fig. 9. TEM images of $Zn_5(OH)_8(NO_3)_2 \cdot 2H_2O$ thin films formed at 2 h in the presence of dual template. The scale bars are 1 μm in a, 100 nm in b. The insets in b, is the corresponding ED pattern (from ref (Hu, et al., 2009) *Reproduced by permission of The Royal Society of Chemistry*).

Through changing the composition of subphase solutions, $Co_5(OH)_8(NO_3)_2 \cdot 2H_2O$, and Co-doped $Zn_5(OH)_8(NO_3)_2 \cdot 2H_2O$ thin films were also successfully prepared using such a method, indicating the dual-template biomimetic mineralization system can be a promise method for preparing many other kinds inorganic thin films. The Fig. 10 and Fig. 11 are the SEM images and XRD patterns of the thin films, respectively. Obviously, the products shows a much more uniform morphology than that of ref (Kisailus, et al., 2006; Schwenzer, et al., 2006) and a preferred orientation along (200) plane.

The uniform surface morphologies and the preferred orientation along (200) plane of the films are ascribed to the special structural features of the materials and the synergetic effect of the dual template in the novel biomimetic system. As for $Zn_5(OH)_8(NO_3)_2 \cdot 2H_2O$, as we know, it consists of layered sheets with octahedrally coordinated Zn^{2+} ions in the brucite layer, one quarter of which are replaced by two tetrahedrally coordinated Zn^{2+} ions located above and below the plane of the octahedrally coordinated Zn^{2+} ions (Stählin & Oswald, 1970; Biswick, et al., 2007). The nitrates anions are located between the sheets and do not directly coordinate to the zinc atoms. There are only zinc atoms in the (200) plane, which indicates that the (200) plane is a polar plane. When BSA molecules are spreaded on the surface of $Zn(NO_3)_2$ solution, the Zn^{2+} are strongly attracted by the negative charge of BSA Langmuir monolayers through electrostatic interactions, therefore, the nucleation along the (200) plane is facilitated because of the strong polarity of (200) plane. Furthermore, it has been proposed that structural flexibility in the organic monolayer plays an important role in the orientation growth of inorganic crystals (Cooper, et al., 1998). A cooperative interaction between the organic templates and inorganic phases leads to local re-arrangement of the Langmuir films during the nucleation stage. Here, the interactions between the BSA molecules and Zn^{2+} ions in the subphase solution make the monolayer self-regulate its structure during the formation of the inorganic crystals; meanwhile, the formation of inorganic crystals is also influenced by the self-regulation of the monolayer, which should be a synergetic process of adapting each other and adjusting each other. What's the most important is that the structural flexibility of BSA monolayer provides a probability for the regulating and adjusting. All of those factors above lead to the decrease of the interfacial energy and improve the preferred orientation along the (200) plane. As for $Co_5(OH)_8(NO_3)_2{\cdot}2H_2O$ and Co-doped $Zn_5(OH)_8(NO_3)_2{\cdot}2H_2O$, a similar situation takes place.

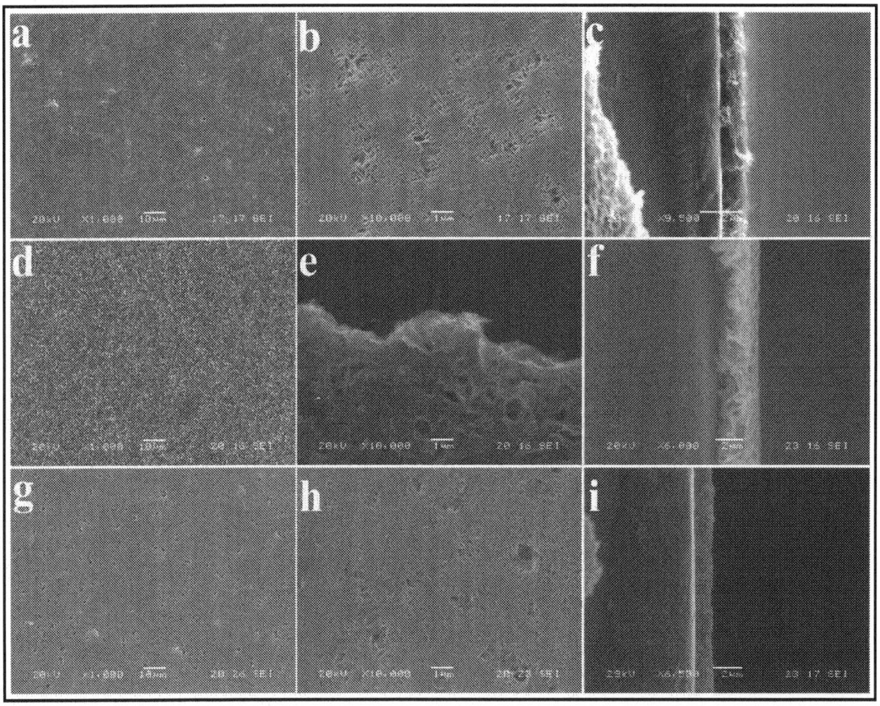

Fig. 10. SEM images of the films obtained at 2 h in the presence of dual template: top view in different magnification of $Zn_5(OH)_8(NO_3)_2{\cdot}2H_2O$ (a and b), $Co_5(OH)_8(NO_3)_2{\cdot}2H_2O$ (d and e), and Co-doped $Zn_5(OH)_8(NO_3)_2{\cdot}2H_2O$ thin films (g and h); side view of $Zn_5(OH)_8(NO_3)_2{\cdot}2H_2O$ (c), $Co_5(OH)_8(NO_3)_2{\cdot}2H_2O$ (f), and Co-doped $Zn_5(OH)_8(NO_3)_2{\cdot}2H_2O$ thin films (i). Scale bars are 10 μm in a, d, g; 1 μm in b, e, h; and 2 μm in c, f, I, respectively (from ref (Hu, et al., 2009) *Reproduced by permission of The Royal Society of Chemistry*).

In a word, such a dual-template approach make the usual biomimetic mineralization system only using Langmuir monolayer as organic template closer to a real biomineralization process, which captures the advantages of both the vapor-liquid interface generated by the vapor-diffusion of catalyst (ammonia) served as the other nucleation template providing a kinetic control and the crystal growth regulated by the organic matrix template providing control of crystal structures and morphologies (Sumerel, et al., 2003; Hosono, et al., 2005; Kisailus, et al., 2005). The regulation effect of Langmuir monolayer on the crystal growth was realized in the novel interface system, meanwhile, the kinetic control of materials was also realized through the pH value gradient, concentration gradient of reactants, and surface tension gradients generated from the vapor-diffusion. The novel biomimetic interface system unambiguously influenced the growth mode and habit of inorganic crystals, being a promise method for realizing structural controllable fabrication of inorganic functional materials at room temperature.

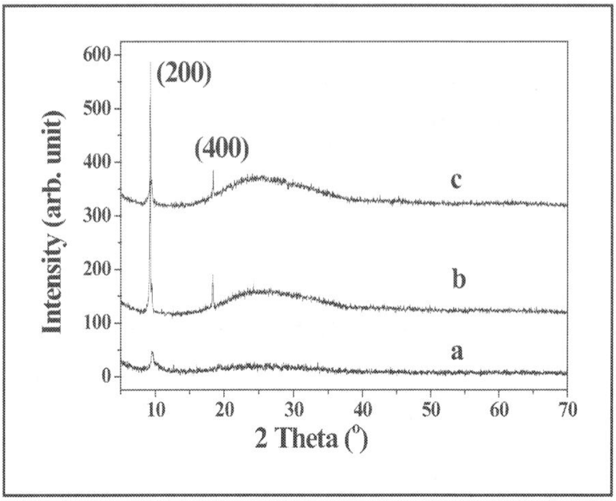

Fig. 11. XRD patterns of the films formed under BSA Langmuir monolayer at surface pressure of 15 mN m^{-1} at 2 h on the surfaces of 0.03 M Co^{2+} solution (a), 0.03 M Zn^{2+} solution (b) and 0.03 M Zn^{2+}/Co^{2+} mixed solution (c) in the presence of ammonia diffusion (from ref (Hu, et al., 2009) *Reproduced by permission of The Royal Society of Chemistry*).

4. Conclusion

How do mussels form their shells? Why is a sea-urchin spine so mechanically stable? Can we grow teeth in the test-tube? Why is bone hard as well elastic? These questions are still mainly unresolved (Becker, et al., 2003). Biomineralization processes can form biominerals with delicate structures and various functions, attracting peoples to strive to understand molecular mechanisms of the assembly of inorganic materials. Obviously, the elucidation of the mechanisms for the formation of these composite materials will lead to new strategies for assembling other inorganic-organic composites and bring a bright future for materials science (Bensaude-Vincent, et al., 2002). Although many researches of biomineralization mimic and biomimetic mineralization have been carried out from disciplinary of biology, chemistry, crystallography and materials science, our understanding on the essence of biomineralization is still very limited.

It is well known that biomineralization takes place at a biomembrane interface, so an appropriate mimic model of biomembrane is indispensable for exploring the secret in Nature. As an approximation to half of the bilayer structure of a biomembrane, organic Langmuir monolayers can usually serve as a convenient model to approach the two-dimensional structure of biomembranes through easy control, and therefore, Langmuir monolayer is an ideal model interface for biomimetic mineralization and has been widely used as the organic templates in the research of biomimetic mineralization to guide the growth of inorganic crystals with special structure, size, and morphology. Meanwhile, although the mechanisms by which organisms generate mineral crystals are not well understood, there is widespread belief that proteins play important roles. So proteins should be paid more attention in the biomimetic mineralization research, especially in a manner of Langmuir monolayer. The large diversity of natural and synthetic proteins and their adjustability provide high probability that proteins recognize, interact with, and direct the formation of many inorganic materials. At the same time, it is easy to realize the structural changes of the protein molecules by simply controlling the surface pressure of a protein Langmuir monolayer, which provides a great convenience for researching the influence of structural changes of protein molecules on the structural formation of biominerals. As an equally important factor for the special structural features of the biominerals in the real biomineralization, the kinetic control of inorganic crystals growth in the biomimetic mineralization system has not gotten due diligence. The kinetic control of the hydrolysis degree of molecular precursor, the species and concentration ratio of the cations and anions at the vapor-liquid interface is also realized through the pH value gradient, concentration gradient of reactants, and surface tension gradient generated from ammonia diffusion. So, the dual-template interface system introducing the kinetic control generated from ammonia diffusion into a usual biomimetic mineralization interface of only a protein Langmuir monolayer should be a preliminary ideal biomimetic mineralization interface system, it is still faraway from but much closer to a real biomineralization process.

If one day we want to be able to manufacture materials with hierarchical structures similar to those of nature, learning from a real biomineralization process is important and necessary. The design and construction of biomimetic mineralization system closer to the real environment and process of biomineralization should be undoubtedly a promise way, which on the one hand provides a perfect model for biomineralization research; on the other hand, more opportunities to get inorganic materials with special structural features can also be obtained through introducing more conditions of controlling, providing an effective experimental method for controllable fabrication of functional materials. It is meaningful for both deepening the understanding on the mechanism of biomineralization and promoting the ability of fabricating materials using biomimetic mineralization approach.

5. Acknowledgments

The authors are grateful to National Natural Science Foundation of China (No. 20371015, 20903034 and 10874040), State Key Basic Research "973" Plan of China (No. 2002CCC02700 and 2007CB616911), the Program for New Century Excellent Talents in University of China (No. NCET-04-0653), and the Cultivation Fund of the Key Scientific and Technical Innovation Project, Ministry of Education of China (No. 708062) for financial support. The corresponding author: professor Zuliang Du, E-mail: zld@henu.edu.cn.

6. References

Aizenberg, J. (2004). "Crystallization in patterns: a bio-inspired approach." *Advanced Materials,* 16. 15. 1295-1302, 0935-9648

Aizenberg, J.; Muller, D. et al. (2003). "Direct fabrication of large micropatterned single crystals." *Science,* 299. 5610. 1205-1208, 0036-8075

Aizenberg, J.; Tkachenko, A. et al. (2001). "Calcitic microlenses as part of the photoreceptor system in brittlestars." *Nature,* 412. 6849. 819-822, 0028-0836

Amos, F.; Sharbaugh, D. et al. (2007). "Formation of single-crystalline aragonite tablets/films via an amorphous precursor." *Langmuir,* 23. 4. 1988-1994, 0743-7463

Antonietti, M. & Göltner, C. (1997). "Superstructures of functional colloids: chemistry on the nanometer scale." *Angewandte Chemie International Edition in English,* 36. 9. 910-928, 1433-7851

Archibald, D. & Mann S. (1993). "Template mineralization of self-assembled anisotropic lipid microstructures." *Nature,* 364. 6436. 430-433, 0028-0836

Bayley, H. & Cremer, P. (2001). "Stochastic sensors inspired by biology." *Nature,* 413. 6852. 226-230, 0028-0836

Becker, A.; Becker, W. et al. (2003). "In-vitro Crystallization of Calcium Carbonate in the Presence of Biological Additives - Comparison of the Ammonium Carbonate Method with Double-Diffusion Techniques." *Zeitschrift Fur Anorganische Und Allgemeine Chemie,* 629. 2305-2311, 0044-2313

Behrens, S. (2008). "Synthesis of inorganic nanomaterials mediated by protein assemblies." *Journal of Materials Chemistry,* 18. 32. 3788-3798, 0959-9428

Belcher, A.; Hansma, P. et al. (1998). "First steps in harnessing the potential of biomineralization as a route to new high-performance composite materials." *Acta materialia,* 46. 3. 733-736, 1359-6454

Bensaude-Vincent, B.; Arribart, H. et al. (2002). "Chemists and the school of nature." *New journal of chemistry,* 26. 1. 1-5, 1144-0546

Biswick, T.; Jones, W. et al. (2007). "The role of anhydrous zinc nitrate in the thermal decomposition of the zinc hydroxy nitrates $Zn_5(OH)_8(NO_3)_2 \cdot 2H_2O$ and $ZnOHNO_3 \cdot H_2O$." *Journal of Solid State Chemistry,* 180. 1171-1179, 0022-4596

Boskey, A. L. (2003). "Biomineralization: An Overview." *Connective Tissue Research,* 44. 1. 5-9, 0300-8207

Casse, O.; Colombani, O. et al. (2008). "Calcium phosphate mineralization beneath monolayers of poly (n-butylacrylate) - block - poly (acrylic acid) block copolymers." *Faraday Discussions,* 139. 179-197, 1364-5498

Chen, C. & Rosi, N. L. (2010). "Peptide-Based Methods for the Preparation of Nanostructred Inorganic Materials." *Angewandte Chemie International Edition,* 49. 1924-1942, 1433-7851

Cölfen, H. (2003). "Precipitation of carbonates: recent progress in controlled production of complex shapes." *Current Opinion in Colloid & Interface Science,* 8. 1. 23-31, 1359-0294

Cölfen, H. & Mann S. (2003). "Higher-order organization by mesoscale self-assembly and transformation of hybrid nanostructures." *Angewandte Chemie International Edition,* 42. 21. 2350-2365, 1433-7851

Cölfen, H. & Yu S. (2005). "Biomimetic mineralization/synthesis of mesoscale order in hybrid inorganic-organic materials via nanoparticle self-assembly." *MRS Bulletin,* 30. 727-735, 0883-7694

Cooper, S.; Sessions, R. et al. (1998). "A new mechanism for nucleation beneath monolayer films?" *Journal of the Amecrican Chemical Society,* 120. 9. 2090-2098, 0002-7863

Cui, T.; Zhang, J. et al. (2005). "CdS-nanoparticle/polymer composite shells grown on silica nanospheres by atom-transfer radical polymerization." *Advanced Functional Materials,* 15. 3. 481-486, 1616-301X

Cusack, M. & Freer A. (2008). "Biomineralization: elemental and organic influence in carbonate systems." *Chemical reviews,* 108. 11. 4433-4454, 0009-2665
Dabbs, D. & Aksay I. (2003). "Self-assembled ceramics produced by complex-fluid templation." *Annual Review of Physical Chemistry,* 51. 601-622, 0066-426X
Davis, M. (2004). "How Life Makes Hard Stuff." *Science,* 305. 5683. 480-480, 0036-8075
Davis, S.; Breulmann, M. et al. (2001). "Template-directed assembly using nanoparticle building blocks: A nanotectonic approach to organized materials." *Cheimistry of Materials,* 13. 10. 3218-3226, 0897-4756
Dey, A.; With, G. et al. (2010). "In situ techniques in biomimetic mineralization studies of calcium carbonate." *Chemical Society reviews,* 39. 2. 397-409, 0306-0012
Dickerson, M.; Sandhage, K. et al. (2008). "Protein-and peptide-directed syntheses of inorganic materials." *Chemical reviews,* 108. 11. 4935-4978, 0009-2665
DiMasi, E.; Olszta, M. et al. (2003). "When is template directed mineralization really template directed?" *CrystEngComm,* 5. 61. 346-350, 1466-8033
DiMasi, E.; Patel, V. et al. (2002). "Polymer-controlled growth rate of an amorphous mineral film nucleated at a fatty acid monolayer." *Langmuir,* 18. 23. 8902-8909, 0743-7463
Dujardin, E. & Mann S. (2002). "Bio-inspired materials chemistry." *Advanced Materials,* 14. 11. 775-788, 0935-9648
Estroff, L. & Hamilton A. (2001). "At the interface of organic and inorganic chemistry: Bioinspired synthesis of composite materials." *Cheimistry of Materials,* 13. 10. 3227-3235, 0897-4756
Facci, P.; Erokhin, V. et al. (1994). "Formation of ultrathin semiconductor films by CdS nanostructure aggregation." *The Journal of Physical Chemistry,* 98. 50. 13323-13327, 0022-3654
Fratzl, P. (2007). "Biomimetic materials research: what can we really learn from nature's structural materials?" *Journal of the Royal Society Interface,* 4. 15. 637, 1742-5689
Fricke, M. & Volkmer D. (2007). "Crystallization of Calcium Carbonate Beneath Insoluble Monolayers: Suitable Models of Mineral-Matrix Interactions in Biomineralization?" *Topics in Current Chenistry,* 270, 1-41, 0340-1022
Gzyl-Malcher, B. & Paluch M. (2008). "Studies of lipid interactions in mixed Langmuir monolayers." *Thin Solid Films,* 516. 24. 8865-8872, 0040-6090
Hendler, G. & Byrne M. (1987). "Fine structure of the dorsal arm plate of Ophiocoma wendti: evidence for a photoreceptor system (Echinodermata, Ophiuroidea)." *Zoomorphology,* 107. 5. 261-272, 0720-213X
Heywood, B. & Mann S. (1992). "Template-directed inorganic crystallization: oriented nucleation of barium sulfate under Langmuir monolayers of an aliphatic long chain phosphonate." *Langmuir,* 8. 5. 1492-1498, 0743-7463
Heywood, B. & Mann S. (1994). "Molecular construction of oriented inorganic materials: controlled nucleation of calcite and aragonite under compressed langmuir monolayers." *Cheimistry of Materials,* 6. 3. 311-318, 0897-4756
Heywood, B. R. & Mann, S. (1992). "Organic Template-Directed Inorganic Crystallization: Oriented Nucleation of $BaSO_4$ under Compressed Langmuir Monolayers." *Journal of the Amecrican Chemical Society,* 114. 4681-4686, 0002-7863
Hosono, E.; Fujihara, S. et al. (2005). "Superhydrophobic perpendicular nanopin film by the bottom-up process." *Journal of the Amecrican Chemical Society,* 127. 39. 13458-13459, 0002-7863

Hu, B.; Xue, Z. et al. (2009). "Biomimetic syntheses of pure or doped metal hydroxide nitrate thin films by a dual-template approach." *Journal of Materials Chemistry,* 19. 16. 2373-2379, 0959-9428

Hunter, G. K.; Young, J. O. et al. (2010) "The Flexible Polyelectrolyte Hypothesis of Protein-Biomineral Interaction." *Langmuir,* DOI: 10.1021/la100401r, 0743-7463

Jeronimidis, G. & Atkins A. (1995). "Mechanics of biological materials and structures: Nature's lessons for the engineer." *Proceedings of the Institution of Mechanical Engineers. Part C. Mechanical engineering science,* 209. 4. 221-235, 0263-7154

Jones, W. & Rao C. (2002). *Supramolecular organization and materials design.* Cambridge Univ Press, ISBN-13: 9780521662406, Cambridge

Kisailus, D.; Choi, J. et al. (2005). "Enzymatic synthesis and nanostructural control of gallium oxide at low temperature." *Advanced Materials,* 17. 3. 314-318, 0935-9648

Kisailus, D.; Schwenzer, B. et al. (2006). "Kinetically controlled catalytic formation of zinc oxide thin films at low temperature." *Journal of the Amecrican Chemical Society,* 128. 31. 10276-10280, 0002-7863

Kisailus, D.; Truong, Q. et al. (2006). Self-assembled bifunctional surface mimics an enzymatic and templating protein for the synthesis of a metal oxide semiconductor, *Proceedings of the National Academy of Sciences of the United States of America,* 103. 15. 5652-5657, 0027-8424

Kröger, N.; Lorenz, S. et al. (2002). "Self-assembly of highly phosphorylated silaffins and their function in biosilica morphogenesis." *Science,* 298. 5593. 584-586, 0036-8075

Lee, S.; Gao, X. et al. (2007). "Biomimetic and Aggregation-Driven Crystallization Route for Room-Temperature Material Synthesis: Growth of β-Ga_2O_3 Nanoparticles on Peptide Assemblies as Nanoreactors." *Journal of the Amecrican Chemical Society,* 129. 10. 2954-2958, 0002-7863

Li, M.; Schnablegger, H. et al. (1999). "Coupled synthesis and self-assembly of nanoparticles to give structures with controlled organization." *Physical Review Letters,* 82. 1345-1349, 0031-9007

Lianos, P. & Thomas J. (1987). "Small CdS particles in inverted micelles." *Journal of Colloid and Interface Science,* 117. 2. 505-512, 0021-9797

Lowenstam, H. & Weiner S. (1989). *On biomineralization.* Oxford University Press, ISBN 0195049772, New York

Lu, X.; Zhao, Y. et al. (2005). "Fabrication of PbS nanoparticles in polymer-fiber matrices by electrospinning." *Advanced Materials,* 17. 20. 2485-2488, 0935-9648

Lu, X.; Zhao, Y. et al. (2005). "Fabrication of CdS nanorods in PVP fiber matrices by electrospinning." *Macromolecular Rapid Communications,* 26. 16. 1325-1329, 1022-1336

Mann, S. (1995). "*Biomimetic materials chemistry.* " John Wiley & Sons. Inc., ISBN 1-56081-669-4, New York

Mann, S. (2000). "The chemistry of form." *Angewandte Chemie International Edition,* 39. 19. 3392-3406, 1433-7851

Mann, S. (2001). "*Biomineralization: principles and concepts in bioinorganic materials chemistry.*" Oxford University Press, ISBN 0198508824, Oxford

Mann, S.; Archibald, D. et al. (1993). "Crystallization at inorganic-organic interfaces: biominerals and biomimetic synthesis." *Science,* 261. 5126. 1286-1292, 0036-8075

Mann, S.; Heywood, B. et al. (1988). "Controlled crystallization of $CaCO_3$ under stearic acid monolayers." *Nature,* 332. 119-124, 0028-0836

Mann, S. & Ozin G. (1996). "Synthesis of inorganic materials with complex form." *Nature,* 382. 6589. 313-318, 0028-0836

Morse, D. (1999). "Silicon biotechnology: harnessing biological silica production to construct new materials." *Trends in Biotechnology,* 17. 6. 230-232, 0167-7799

Mukherjee, M.; Datta, A. et al. (1997). "Growth of nanocrystalline PbS within a glass." *Journal of Materials Research,* 12. 10. 2507-2510, 0884-2914

Munch, E.; Launey, M. et al. (2008). "Tough, bio-inspired hybrid materials." *Science,* 322. 5907. 1516-1520, 0036-8075

Ni, Y.; Liu, H. et al. (2004). "PbS crystals with clover-like structure: Preparation, characterization, optical properties and influencing factors." *Crystal Research and Technology,* 39. 3. 200-206, 0232-1300

Nuraje, N.; Su, K. et al. (2006). "Room temperature synthesis of ferroelectric barium titanate nanoparticles using peptide nanorings as templates." *Advanced Materials,* 18. 6. 807-811, 0935-9648

Pichon, B.; Bomans, P. et al. (2008). "A quasi-time-resolved CryoTEM study of the nucleation of $CaCO_3$ under langmuir monolayers." *Journal of the Amecrican Chemical Society,* 130. 12. 4034-4040, 0002-7863

Pickett-Heaps, J.; Schmid, A. et al. (1990). "The cell biology of diatom valve formation." in *Progress in Phycological Research 7* (Round, F. E. & Chapman, D. J. eds) pp.1- 168, Biopress Ltd., Bristol, UK

Popescu, D.; Smulders, M. et al. (2007). "Template adaptability is key in the oriented crystallization of $CaCO_3$." *Journal of the Amecrican Chemical Society,* 129. 45. 14058-14067, 0002-7863

Pouget, E.; Bomans, P. et al. (2009). "The Initial Stages of Template-Controlled $CaCO_3$ Formation Revealed b Cyro-TEM." *Science,* 323. 1455-1458, 0036-8075

Ridgwell, A. J.; Kennedy, M. J. & Caldeira K. (2003). "Carbonate Deposition, Climate Stability, and Neoproterozoic Ice Ages." *Science,* 302. 859-862, 0036-8075

Sarikaya, M.; Tamerler, C. et al. (2003). "Molecular biomimetics: nanotechnology through biology." *Nature materials,* 2. 9. 577-585, 1476-1122

Stählin, W. & Oswald, H. R. (1970). "The crystal structure of zinc hydroxide nitrate, $Zn_5(OH)_8(NO_3)_2 \cdot 2H_2O$." *Acta Crystallographica Section B,* 26. 6. 860-863, 0108-7681

Schwenzer, B.; Roth, K. M. et al. (2006). "Kinetically controlled vapor-diffusion synthesis of novel nanostructured metal hydroxide and phosphate films using no organic reagents." *Journal of Materials Chemistry,* 16. 401-407, 0959-9428

Shenton, W.; Douglas, T. et al. (1999). "Inorganic-organic nanotube composites from template mineralization of tobacco mosaic virus." *Advanced Materials,* 11. 3. 253-256, 0935-9648

Sommerdijk, N. A. J. M. & With G. (2008). "Biomimetic $CaCO_3$ mineralization using designer molecules and interfaces." *Chemical reviews,* 108. 11. 4499-4550, 0009-2665

Stine, K. (1994). "Investigations of monolayers by fluorescence microscopy." *Microscopy research and technique,* 27. 5. 439-450, 1059-910X

Stupp, S.; Mejicano, G. et al. (1993). "Organoapatites: materials for artificial bone. II. Hardening reactions and properties." *Journal of biomedical materials research,* 27. 3. 289-299, 1549-3296

Sumerel, J.; Yang, W. et al. (2003). "Biocatalytically templated synthesis of titanium dioxide." *Chemistry of Materials,* 15. 25. 4804-4809, 0897-4756

Tassoni, R. & Schrock R. (1994). "Synthesis of PbS nanoclusters within microphase-separated diblock copolymer films." *Chemistry of Materials,* 6. 6. 744-749, 0897-4756

Towe, K. M. (1990). "Overviews of Biomineralization." *Paleobiology,* 16. 4. 521-526, 0094-8373

Wainwright, S.; Biggs, W. et al. (1976). "*Mechanical Design in Organisms.*" Princeton University Press, ISBN 0-691-08306-1, Princeton, NJ

Wang, Y. & Mahler W. (1987). "Degenerate four-wave mixing of CdS/polymer composite." *Optics Communications,* 61. 3. 233-236, 0030-4018

Wang, Y.; Suna, A. et al. (1987). "PbS in polymers. From molecules to bulk solidsa." *Journal of Chemical Physics,* 87. 12. 7315-7322, 0021-9606

Weiner, S. & Addadi, L. (2002). "At the Cutting Edge." *Science,* 298. 375-376, 0036-8075

Wetherbee, R. (2002). "The diatom glasshouse." *Science,* 298. 5593. 547-547, 0036-8075

Wood, R.; Grotzinger, J. et al. (2002). "Proterozoic modular biomineralized metazoan from the Nama Group, Namibia." *Science,* 296. 5577. 2383-2386, 0036-8075

Xu, A.; Ma, Y. et al. (2007). "Biomimetic mineralization." *Journal of Materials Chemistry,* 17. 5. 415-449, 0959-9428

Xu, G.; Yao, N. et al. (1998). "Biomimetic Synthesis of Macroscopic-Scale Calcium Carbonate Thin Films. Evidence for a Multistep Assembly Process." *Journal of the Amecrican Chemical Society,* 120. 46. 11977-11985, 0002-7863

Xue, Z. H.; Dai, S. X. et al. (2009). "Effect of Langmuir monolayer of bovine serum albumin protein on the morphology of calcium carbonate." *Materials Science and Engineering: C,* 29. 6. 1998-2002, 0928-4931

Xue, Z.; Hu, B. et al. (2009). "Effect of the interaction between bovine serum albumin Langmuir monolayer and calcite on the crystallization of $CaCO_3$ nanoparticles." *Materials Chemistry and Physics,* 114. 1. 47-52, 0254-0584

Yang, H.; Coombs, N. et al. (1997). "Morphogenesis of shapes and surface patterns in mesoporous silica." *Nature,* 386. 692-695, 0028-0836

Yang, J. & Fendler J. (1995). "Morphology control of PbS nanocrystallites, epitaxially grown under mixed monolayers." *The Journal of Physical Chemistry,* 99. 15. 5505-5511, 0022-3654

Yang, J.; Meldrum, F. et al. (1995). "Epitaxial growth of size-quantized cadmium sulfide crystals under arachidic acid monolayers." *The Journal of Physical Chemistry,* 99. 15. 5500-5504, 0022-3654

Young, J.; Davis, S. et al. (1999). "Coccolith ultrastructure and biomineralisation." *Journal of Structural Biology,* 126. 3. 195-215, 1047-8477

Yu, S. & Cölfen H. (2004). "Bio-inspired crystal morphogenesis by hydrophilic polymers." *Journal of Materials Chemistry,* 14. 14. 2124-2147, 0959-9428

Zaremba, C.; Belcher, A. et al. (1996). "Critical transitions in the biofabrication of abalone shells and flat pearls." *Chemistry of Materials,* 8. 3. 679-690, 0897-4756

Zhang, L.; Liu, H. et al. (2004). "Mineralization mechanism of calcium phosphates under three kinds of Langmuir monolayers." *Langmuir,* 20. 6. 2243-2249, 0743-7463

Zhao, X.; Yang, J. et al. (1992). "Epitaxial formation of lead sulfide crystals under arachidic acid monolayers." *The Journal of Physical Chemistry,* 96. 24. 9933-9939, 0022-3654

Zhu, R.; Min, G. et al. (1992). "Scanning tunneling microscopy and UV-visible spectroscopy studies of lead sulfide ultrafine particles synthesized in Langmuir-Blodgett films." *The Journal of Physical Chemistry,* 96. 21. 8210-8211, 0022-3654

4

The Biomimetic Approach to Design Apatites for Nanobiotechnological Applications

Norberto Roveri and Michele Iafisco
Alma Mater Studiorum, Università di Bologna
Italy

1. Introduction

Mimicking Nature and designing bioinspired materials represents a promising way to reach technological innovations in many interdisciplinary scientific fields, since biological materials exhibit a high degree of sophistication, hierarchical organisation, hybridisation, efficiency, resistance and adaptability. These properties, which biogenic materials have achieved through specific building principles selected by evolution, can only be partially possessed in man-made materials by present synthetic processes. For this reason Nature is a school for material scientists, in view of the fact that living organisms can produce different amazing high-performance materials (Sanchez et al., 2005).

Nature produces soft and hard materials exhibiting remarkable functional properties by controlling the hierarchical assembly of simple molecular building blocks from the nano- to the macro-scale. Biogenic materials are nucleated in defined nano–micro dimensioned sites inside the biological environments, in which chemistry can be spatially controlled (Mann et al., 1993; Weiner & Addadi 1997). The spatial delimitation is essential to biological mechanisms for controlling the size, shape and structural organisation of biomaterials. Recently, with the development of nanotechnology, this strategy employing natural material genesis has attracted a lot of attention in designing bioinspired materials such as polymeric micelles, nanoparticles, dendrimers and nanocrystals synthesised in nanoscale dimensions (Sarikaya et al., 2003; Tamerler & Sarikaya 2007; Vriezema et al., 2005).

One of the most exciting and economical rewarding research areas of materials science involves the applications of materials to health care, especially to reconstructive surgery. In the past, many implantations failed due to infections or a lack of knowledge about toxicity of the selected materials. In this case, the use of calcium phosphates, since they are the most important inorganic constituents of hard tissues in vertebrates, is valid due to their chemical similarity to the mineral component of mammalian bones and teeth. Thus, calcium phosphate based biomaterials are now used in many different applications throughout the body, covering all areas of the skeleton. These applications include dental implants, percutaneous devices and use in periodontal treatment, treatment of bone defects, fracture treatment, total joint replacement (bone augmentation), orthopaedics, cranio-maxillofacial reconstruction, otolaryngology and spinal surgery (Dorozhkin 2010).

In this chapter we will give details about the principal characteristics of bone, tooth and pathological calcifications where the calcium phosphates are present (section 2); the chemical-physical characteristics and the methods to synthesize biomimetic hydroxyapatites (section 3); and the main applications of these in the nanobiotechnology field (section 4).

2. Biogenic hydroxyapatite

In biological systems, calcium phosphates are the principal inorganic constituent of normal (bones, teeth, fish enameloid, deer antlers and some species of shells) and pathological (dental and urinary calculus and stones, atherosclerotic lesions) calcifications. Except for small portions of the inner ear, all hard tissue of the human body is made of calcium phosphates. Structurally, they occur mainly in the form of poorly crystallized non-stoichiometric F, Na, Mg and carbonate substituted hydroxyapatite [$Ca_{10}(PO_4)_6(OH)_2$] (HA) (Dorozhkin 2010). We will thus give details in this section about the principal characteristics of bone, tooth and pathological calcifications, highlighting the fact that the living organisms can produce different amazing high-performance materials.

2.1 Bone

Bones are rigid organs that form part of the endoskeleton of vertebrates. Their function is to move, support and protect the various organs of the body, produce red and white blood cells and store minerals (Loveridge 1999; Reddi 1994). Bones appear in a variety of shapes and have a complex internal and external structure, they are lightweight, yet strong and hard, in addition to satisfying their many other functions. One of the types of tissues that constitutes bone is the mineralized osseous tissue, also called bone tissue, that gives it rigidity and honeycomb-like three-dimensional structure (Cowles et al., 1998). Other types of tissue found in bones include marrow, endosteum and periosteum, nerves, blood vessels and cartilage (Tzaphlidou 2008). There are 206 bones in the adult body and about 300 bones in the infant body. Bone tissue consists of cells embedded in a fibrous, organic matrix, the osteoid, which is primarily constituted by type I collagen (90%) and 10% amorphous ground substance (primarily glycosaminoglycans and glycoproteins). Osteoid comprises approximately 50% of bone by volume and 25% by weight (Urist 2002).

Osteoblasts are mono-nucleate cells responsible for the secretion of osteoid and subsequent bone formation through the mineralization of the osteoid matrix. They strongly produce alkaline phosphatase, an enzyme that has a role in the mineralisation of bone, as well as many matrix proteins. When osteoblasts are trapped in the bone matrix, which they themselves produced, they become star-shaped cells named osteocytes, the most abundant cells found in bone (Wozney 1992).

Osteocytes are mature bone cells, networked to each other via long processes that occupy tiny canals called canaliculi, which are used for exchange of nutrients and waste. They are actively involved in the maintenance of bony matrix, through various mechanosensory mechanisms regulating the bone's response to stress. Bone is a dynamic tissue constantly being reshaped by osteoblasts, cells which build bone, and osteoclasts, cells which resorb it (Manolagas 2000).

Osteoclasts are multi-nucleated cells responsible for the resorption of bone through the removal of the bone's mineralized matrix. The removal process begins with the attachment of the osteoclast to the osteon (predominant structures found in compact bone); the osteoclast then induces an infolding of its cell membrane and secretes collagenase and other enzymes important in the resorption process, such as tartrate resistant acid phosphatase,

secreted against the mineral substrate. During childhood, bone formation exceeds resorption but, as the aging process occurs, resorption exceeds formation (Legeros & Craig 1993).
The characteristic rigidity and strength of bone derives from the presence of mineral salts, that permeate the organic matrix, formed by the osteoid mineralization, due to the secretion of vesicles containing alkaline phosphatase, by the osteoblasts (Boskey 2007). The mineral phase comprises approximately 50% of bone by volume and 75% by weight. The principal constituents of bone mineral are calcium phosphate, mainly carbonated hydroxyapatite, amorphous calcium phosphate and calcium carbonate, with lesser quantities of sodium, magnesium, silicon and fluoride (Palmer et al., 2008).
The whole architecture of bone is very complex: starting from the smallest constituting elements to the largest scales, the bone is not only organized in an anisotropic manner, but the arrangement of its constituting elements is hierarchical; this means that its structural units are organized at increasing size levels, and this feature confers unique properties to the whole bone structure. To better understand the complex bone architecture, several hierarchical models have been proposed. Weiner and Wagner have identified seven discrete levels of hierarchical organization in bone (Figure 1), which we describe here (Weiner & Wagner 1998). In their model, bone is considered as a family of materials with the mineralized collagen fibre as the primary building block for subsequent higher order architectures.

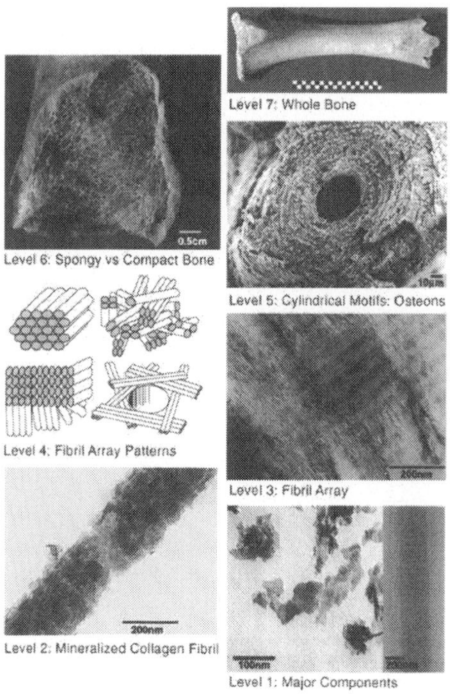

Fig. 1. Seven hierarchical levels of organization of the bone family of materials as proposed by Weiner and Wagner. Reproduced with permission from (Weiner & Wagner 1998).

The structure of bone differs greatly among the different locations in the skeleton, but the basic nanoscale structure consisting of mineralized collagen remains the same throughout. The first hierarchical level consists of the molecular components: water, HA, collagen and other proteins. The crystals of HA are plate-shaped and are among the smallest known biological crystals (Table 1).

Composition	Enamel	Dentin	Bone
Calcium [wt %][a]	36.5	35.1	34.8
Phosphorus (as P) [wt %][a]	17.7	16.9	15.2
Ca/P (molar ratio) [a]	1.63	1.61	1.71
Sodium [wt %][a]	0.5	0.6	0.9
Magnesium [wt %][a]	0.44	1.23	0.72
Potassium [wt %][a]	0.08	0.05	0.03
Carbonate (as CO_3^{2-}) [wt %][b]	3.5	5.6	7.4
Fluoride [wt %][a]	0.01	0.06	0.03
Chloride [wt %][a]	0.30	0.01	0.13
Pyrophosphate (as $P_2O_7^{4-}$) [wt %][b]	0.022	0.100	0.070
Total inorganic [wt %][b]	97	70	65
Total organic [wt %][b]	1.5	20	25
Water [wt %][b]	1.5	10	10
a axis [Å][c]	9.441	9.421	9.410
c axis [Å][c]	6.880	6.887	6.890
Crystallinity index, (HA=100)	70 – 75	33 - 37	33 - 37
Typical crystal sizes [nm]	100 × 50 × 50 μm	35 × 25 × 4	50 × 25 × 4
Ignition products (800 °C)	β-TCP + HA	β-TCP + HA	HA + CaO
Elasticity modulus (GPa)	80	15	0.34 - 13.8
Compressive strength (MPa)	10	100	150

Table 1. Comparative composition and structural parameters of inorganic phases of adult-human calcified tissues ([a]Ashed samples. [b]Unashed samples. [c]Lattice parameters: ± 0.003 Å).

Though the size of biological apatite crystals reported in the literature varies due to the different treatment methods and analysis techniques utilized, it is generally around the nanometric level, with values in the ranges of 30–50 nm (length), 15–30 nm (width) and 2–10 nm (thickness) (Fernandez-Moran & Engstrom 1957). In early studies, apatite needles were observed, but other studies suggest that platelets are the dominant morphology and that the apparent needles are most likely to be platelets viewed edge-on (Traub et al., 1989). Noncollagenous proteins (NCPs) are also present but make up 10% or less of the total protein content in the bone matrix. The specific functions of the NCPs are still not completely understood. In addition to influencing crystal nucleation and growth, NCPs also play roles in cell signalling and ion homeostasis (Feng et al., 2006).

The second level is formed by the mineralization of collagen fibrils. Tiny plate-like crystals of biological apatite in bone occur within the discrete spaces within the collagen fibrils and grow with specific crystalline orientation along the c-axes, which are roughly parallel to the long axes of the collagen fibrils (Termine et al., 1981). The HA growth is somehow limited by these small intercollagenous spaces, which are approximately 50 nm in length, 25 nm in width and 2-3 nm thick (Cui et al., 2007). The location of these crystals in the fibril was demonstrated in a study by Traub et al. that showed that mineralized collagen fibrils had the same banded pattern as negatively stained collagen fibrils (Traub et al., 1989). This indicated that mineral is concentrated in the hole zones of the fibril. It was proposed that these mineral platelets were arranged in parallel like a stack of cards within the interstices of the fibril. Olszta et al. concluded from electron diffraction studies that the mineral plates are not quite as ordered as previously assumed (Olszta et al., 2007). This imperfect arrangement of nearly parallel crystals has been supported by recent small-angle X-ray scattering (SAXS) and transmission electron microscopy (TEM) data from Burger et al. (Burger et al., 2008). The third level of hierarchy is composed of arrays of these mineralized collagen fibrils. These fibrils are rarely found isolated, but rather almost always associated as bundles or other arrangements, often aligned along their long axis. Type I collagen molecules are self-assembled into fibrils with a periodicity of 67 nm and with 40 nm gaps between the end and the head of their molecules, into which the apatite crystals are placed. A composite of these two constituents forms mineralized fibrils (Wahl & Czernuszka 2006; Bigi et al., 1991; Bigi et al., 1996; Bigi et al., 1997). The fourth level is the patterns of arrays that are formed. These include parallel arrays, woven arrangements, plywood like structures and radial arrays like those found in dentin. Cylindrical structures called osteons make up the fifth level. Osteons are formed with significant cellular activity and remodeling; osteoclasts resorb bone and form a tunnel and osteoblasts subsequently lay down lamellae in stacked layers until only a small channel (Haversian canal) is left behind. These channels serve as a conduit for nerves and blood supply to the bone cells. The sixth level of bone organization is the classification of osseous tissue as either spongy (trabecular or cancelous) or compact (cortical). Cancellous bone is extremely porous (75-95% porosity), providing space for marrow and blood vessels, but has much lower compressive strength. Cortical bone is the dense outer layer (5-10% porosity) that allows many of the support functions of bone (Fratzl et al., 2004). Therefore, the mechanical properties of cortical bone represent the benchmark for synthetic bone. The seventh level is simply the whole bone on the macroscopic scale, incorporating all of the lower levels of hierarchy.

2.2 Tooth

The mammalian body contains numerous mineralized tissues as reported in the previous paragraph, but the tissue with the most robust mechanical properties is enamel. Enamel is the hardest material formed by vertebrates and is the most highly mineralized skeletal tissue present in the body (Whittaker 1982). Mature enamel is composed of 95-97% carbonated HA by weight with less than 1% organic material. The high degree of mineralization makes enamel a fascinating model for understanding fundamental mineralization processes and processes that occur within an extracellular matrix.

It is distinct from bone in terms of architecture, pathology and the biological mechanisms mediating its formation. Understanding the biological formation of different mineralized structures could lead to innovative approaches toward engineering novel scaffolds and providing new therapeutics. Additionally, unlike other biomineralized tissues, such as bone and dentin, mature enamel is acellular and does not resorb or remodel. As a result, enamel regeneration cannot occur in vivo following failure and is therefore an attractive target for future biomimetic and therapeutic approaches. The mammalian tooth is made up of four distinct structures: enamel, dentin, pulp and cementum (Figure 2).

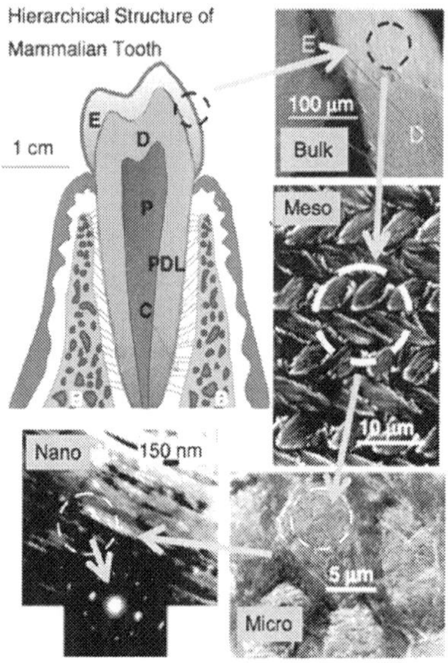

Fig. 2. Hierarchical architecture of mammalian enamel. Enamel (E) is the outermost layer at the crown of the tooth and resides above the dentin (D). The pulp (P) contains nerves and blood vessels, while the cementum (C) is the outermost layer of mineralized tissue surrounding the root of the tooth allowing the tooth to be anchored to the jawbone through the periodontal ligament (PDL). The bulk image depicts the E organ, the transition across the D-E junction, and the D below. On the mesoscale level, prismatic E consisting of weaving of rods (or prisms) that range from 3 to 5 µm in diameter can be visualized. Upon further magnification, the micrometer scale shows the composition of a single rod. The nanometer scale reveals a highly organized array of individual HA crystallites (approximately 30 nm thick, 60 nm wide, and several millimeters in length), which are preferentially aligned along the c-axis. Reproduced with permission from (Tamerler & Sarikaya 2008).

The pulp contains nerves, blood vessels, fibroblasts and lymphocytes, while the mineralized organs of the tooth include enamel, dentin and cementum (Tamerler & Sarikaya 2008). Enamel makes up the uppermost 1-2 mm of the tooth crown and contains a high mineral content, giving it a high modulus but also making it susceptible to cracking. Dentin lies below the enamel and is tougher, forming the bulk of the tooth and absorbing stresses from enamel, preventing its fracture (Arsenault & Robinson 1989). The composition of dentin is similar to that of bone. The cementum is the mineralized layer that surrounds the root of the tooth covering the dentin layer and some of the enamel layer. The cementum allows for the anchoring of the tooth to the alveolar bone (jawbone) through the periodontal ligament. The primary function of the tooth is for mastication of food; however, some species use them for attacking prey and for defence. It also faces the lifelong challenge of maintaining robust mechanical properties in a bacteria-filled environment.

The enamel and dentin tissues give rise to a tough, crack-tolerant and abrasion-resistant tissue through their unique architectures and mineral compositions. Enamel is highly patterned and consists of organized interweaving bundles of crystallites (called rods or prisms). It has a higher reported toughness than that of crystalline HA, indicating that the organization of the crystallites is essential for enamel function (White et al., 2001). Because of the high mineral content and minimal organic, enamel is brittle. Interestingly, the architecture of the enamel crystallites can deflect a propagating crack preventing it from reaching the dentin-enamel junction (DEJ), which also has been shown to resist delamination of the tissues despite their differences in composition (Imbeni et al., 2005). The mechanical properties of enamel, dentin and the DEJ are not completely understood and are a significant area of research. Understanding the properties of these tissues could serve to motivate further engineering of more robust dental materials as well as to inspire fabrication of nonbiological materials.

Similar to bone, enamel possesses a complex architecture, which can be broken into several hierarchical levels from the nanoscale to the macroscale (Paine et al., 2001). On the nanoscale, the protein-protein and protein-mineral interactions in the presence of supersaturated ions create a highly organized array of HA crystallites that grow preferentially along the c-axis (Wen et al., 2000). The sizes of these crystallites depend on the stage of the mineralization. The crystallites grow primarily in length during the secretory stage and continue to grow in width and thickness during the maturation stage. The assembly of amelogenin has been shown to be crucial for the proper development of enamel crystallites. Disruption of the assembly alters formation on the nanoscale, subsequently affecting larger length scales and giving rise to a diseased or malformed enamel phenotype.

On the mesoscale level, there are three main structural components: the rod, the interrod and the aprismatic enamel. The main component of enamel on the mesoscale includes rods, which are bundles of aligned crystallites that are "woven" into intricate architectures that are approximately 3-5 μm in diameter (Cui & Ge 2007).

The second structural component of the enamel matrix is the interrod (or interprismatic) enamel, which surrounds and packs between the rods. The difference between the rod and the interrod is the orientation of HA crystals; the rod contains aligned crystallites, whereas the mineral in the interrod is less ordered. These structures coalesce to form the tough tissue of enamel, which can withstand high forces and resist damage by crack deflection.

The third structure, aprismatic enamel, refers to the structures containing HA crystals that show no mesoscale or macroscale alignment. The macroscale architecture includes specific zones of enamel that have unique characteristics, which contribute to the whole tissue. The enamel adjacent to the DEJ exhibits a gradual transition from dentin to enamel. Aprismatic regions of enamel have been proposed to be primitive areas of the tooth serving as a toughening mechanism due to their flexible nature (Wang & Weiner 1998). Several authors have identified these aprismatic areas to be located adjacent to the DEJ and at the incisal surface of both deciduous and permanent human enamel (Kodaka et al., 1989). The Tomes' process, a unique structure present at the secretory pole of an enamel-forming cell, is responsible for aligned mineral formation in the prismatic enamel. The absence of this process may give rise to the aprismatic zone in the tooth.

2.3 Pathological calcifications

In the body of mammals, osteoblasts and odontoblasts fix ions of calcium and orthophosphate and then precipitate biological apatite onto an organic matrix. This is the process of physiological biomineralization that is restricted to the specific sites in skeletal tissues, including growth plate cartilage, bones and teeth. Unfortunately, owing to ageing, to various diseases and under certain pathological conditions, blood vessels and some internal organs are calcified as well (Daculsi et al., 1997). This process is called pathological calcification or ectopic mineralization and leads to a morbidity and a mortality. In general, any type of abnormal accumulation of calcium phosphates in wrong places is accounted for by a disruption of systemic defense mechanism against calcification (Kazama et al., 2006).
Unwanted depositions always lead to various diseases, for instance: soft tissue calcification (in damaged joints, blood vessels, dysfunctional areas in the brain, diseased organs, scleroderma, prostate stones) (Brancaccio & Cozzolino 2005), kidney and urinary stones (Achilles et al., 1995), dental pulp stones and dental calculus (Hayashizaki et al., 2008), salivary stones, gall stones, pineal gland calcification, atherosclerotic arteries and veins (Marra et al., 2006), coronary calcification, cardiac skeleton, damaged cardiac valves, calcification on artificial heart valves (Weissen-Plenz et al., 2008; Bigi et al., 1988), carpal tunnel, cataracts, malacoplakia, calcified menisci, dermatomyositis and other. All these cases are examples of a calcinosis, which might be described as a formation of calcium phosphate deposits in any soft tissue (Laird et al., 2006).
Contrary to the mineral phases of the normal calcifications (bone, dentin, enamel, cementum, antlers), which consist of only one type of calcium phosphate (namely, biological apatite), the mineral phases of abnormal and/or pathological calcifications are found to occur as single or mixed phases of other types of calcium phosphates and/or other phosphatic and non-phosphatic compounds, in addition to or in place of biological apatite (Wesson & Ward 2007). This happens because the solution pH is often relatively low in the places of pathological calcifications. However, in some cases, the chemical composition of an unwanted inorganic phase might depend on the age of the pathological calcification and its location (Legeros et al., 1988). It is interesting to note that the mineral phases of animal calculus (e.g., from dog) was found to consist of calcium carbonate and biological apatite, while human calculi do not contain calcium carbonate. Some findings suggested that the mechanisms and factors regulating the physiological biomineralization might be similar to those influencing the ectopic mineralization: both were initiated by various organics (i.e., membrane-enclosed particles released from the plasma membrane of mineralization-competent cells), that were present (Kirsch 2006).

3. Synthetic biomimetic hydroxyapatites

Biomimetism of synthetic calcium phosphates can be carried out at different levels, such as composition, structure, morphology, bulk and surface chemical-physical properties. Biomaterials can be turned into biomimetic imprinting all these characteristics in order not only to optimise their interaction with biological tissues, but also to mimic biogenic materials in their functionalities. Detailed information on calcium phosphates, their synthesis, structure, chemistry, other properties and biomedical application have been comprehensively reviewed recently (Dorozhkin 2010; LeGeros 2008).
In this section the chemical-physical characteristics and some methods to synthesize biomimetic calcium phosphates will be described.

3.1 Chemical-physical characteristics of nanocrystalline hydroxyapatites

The study of nanocrystalline calcium phosphate physical-chemical characteristics and, thereafter, the possibility to imitate bone mineral for the development of new advanced biomaterials is constantly growing. The possibility to synthesize in the laboratory synthetic biomimetic compounds makes it possible to consider these systems as a bone mineral "model", enabling to investigate on the one hand the interaction between bone-like apatite nanocrystals and the components of surrounding fluids (ions, proteins…) and, on the other hand, to follow surface interactions with drugs aimed at being delivered in vivo.

Among the peculiarities of these compounds, their plate-like morphology (elongated towards the *c*-axis) is one obvious specificity as compared to regular HA. Another difference is of course the mean crystallite size, of the order of 15-30 nm in length and ca. 6-9 nm in width. From a chemical point of view, the composition of nanocrystalline apatites also strongly differs from that of HA. Although it has been the object of much controversy during several decades in the middle of the 20th Century, the global chemical composition of biological apatites (or their synthetic analogues) can generally be described as:

$$Ca_{10-x}\ (PO_4)_{6-x}\ (HPO_4 \text{ or } CO_3)_x\ (OH \text{ or } \tfrac{1}{2}\, CO_3)_{2-x} \text{ with } 0 \leq x \leq 2$$

(except maybe for very immature nanocrystals which may depart from this generic formula). In particular, this expression underlines the presence of vacancies in both Ca and OH sites. For example, Legeros et al. (Legros et al., 1987) analyzed various cortical bone specimens, suggesting the following relatively homogeneous composition, unveiling high vacancy contents:

$$Ca_{8.3}\ (PO_4)_{4.3}\ (HPO_4 \text{ or } CO_3)_{1.7}\ (OH \text{ or } \tfrac{1}{2}\, CO_3)_{0.3}$$

Minor substitutions are also found in biological apatites involving for example monovalent cations (especially Na^+) in cationic sites. In this case, charge compensation mechanisms have to be taken into account.

It should however be kept in mind that such chemical formulas only enable to have a "global" insight on the nature and amount of ions present in the compound, but it does not reflect possible local variations that may be observed on the nanocrystals or in vivo within the osteons (Paschalis et al., 1996), linked to the local apatite crystal formation and, in vivo, to continuous bone remodelling.

The characterization of nanocrystalline apatites is a relatively arduous task due to their poor crystallinity and metastability. But despite the complexity of these systems, recent in-depth investigations have succeeded to reveal their particular surface features (and related reactivity in wet media) that may be exploited for the setup of new biomaterials, or for a better understanding of natural or pathological biomineralization phenomena. Recent advances in the characterization of apatite nanocrystals were obtained thanks to the use of spectroscopic techniques and, in particular, Fourier Transform Infrared (FT-IR) spectroscopy. FT-IR method is useful for drawing conclusions on the local chemical environment of phosphate, carbonate and hydroxide ions as well as water molecules in such systems. Detailed analyses of the phosphate groups by FT-IR have enabled to distinguish in nanocrystalline apatites the presence of additional bands that cannot be attributed to phosphate groups in a regular apatitic environment (Rey et al., 1990; Rey et al., 1989). These chemical environments have been referred to by Rey as "non-apatitic" environments.

Taking into account all the above data, nanocrystalline apatites (whether biological or their synthetic analogues prepared under close-to-physiological conditions) may thus most probably be described as the association of an apatitic core (often non stoichiometric) and a structured by fragile surface hydrated layer containing water molecules and rather labile ions (e.g. Ca^{2+}, HPO_4^{2-}, CO_3^{2-}...) (Drouet et al., 2009) occupying non-apatitic crystallographic sites (although in the case of biomimetic apatites the layer is directly exposed on the surface and not included in a "sandwich-like" structure between two "apatitic" layers). A schematic model for such nanocrystalline apatites is given in Figure 3 (Eichert et al., 2007).

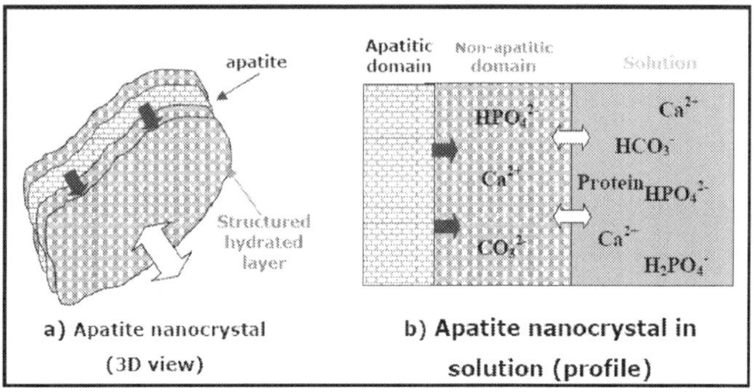

Fig. 3. Schematic modelling of a biomimetic apatite nanocrystal (a) and interaction with surrounding fluids (b) (from reference (Eichert et al., 2007)), with permission.

The presence of this hydrated surface layer (Sakhno et al., 2010) is thought to be responsible for most of the properties of biomimetic apatites and, in particular, their high surface reactivity in relation with surrounding fluids (which is probably directly linked to a high mobility of ionic species contained within this layer) may explain, from a physical-chemical viewpoint, the role of bone mineral in homeostasis in vivo. This layer indeed contains labile ions that can potentially be exchanged by other ions from the surrounding solution, or by small molecules, which may be exploited for couplings with proteins or drugs. It is interesting to remark that the typical non-apatitic features mentioned above tend to progressively disappear during the ageing of the nanocrystals in solution (Cazalbou et al., 2005; Drouet et al., 2009). This process is referred to as "maturation" and has been related to the progressive growth of apatite domains at the expense of the surface hydrated layer (Cazalbou et al., 2004).

This maturation process is thought to be linked to the metastability of such poorly-crystallized non stoichiometric apatites, which steadily evolve in solution towards stoichiometry and better crystallinity (Cazalbou et al., 2005; Cazalbou et al., 2004). This evolution can be for example witnessed by the decrease of the amount of non-apatitic HPO_4^{2-} ions upon ageing, or else by the decreased potentialities to undergo ion exchanges (Cazalbou et al., 2005). One illustration of such effects can be given for example by the decreased exchangeability of HPO_4^{2-} by CO_3^{2-} observed on carbonated apatites matured for incremented amounts of time. Additionally, beside this compositional evolution, some structural and microstructural features also tend to evolve such as the mean crystallite size which increases upon maturation. The control of synthesis parameters such as pH, temperature or maturation time can thus enable one to tailor the physical-chemical properties of biomimetic apatites (Drouet et al., 2009) and, in particular, their surface reactivity, so to mimic for example mature bone mineral or else newly-formed bone apatite.

3.2 Preparation of biomimetic hydroxyapatites

Many different methodologies have been proposed to prepare nanosized and/or nanocrystalline HAs (Schmidt 2000; Cushing et al., 2004; Wang et al., 2005; Mao et al., 2007). These are: wet chemical precipitation (Wang & Shaw 2007; Huang et al., 2004; Liou et al., 2004; Ganesan & Epple 2008; Zhang & Lu 2007), sol-gel synthesis (Sun et al., 2007; Chai & Ben-Nissan 1999; Ben-Nissan & Choi 2006; Choi & Ben-Nissan 2007), co-precipitation (Lopez-Macipe et al., 1998; Tas 2000), hydrothermal synthesis (Guo et al., 2007; Chaudhry et al., 2006), mechanochemical synthesis (Yeon et al., 2001), microwave processing (Siva Rama Krishna et al., 2007; Liu et al., 2005; Rameshbabu et al., 2005), vapour diffusion (Iafisco et al., 2010a), silica gel template (Iafisco et al., 2009a), emulsion-based syntheses (Phillips et al., 2003) and several other methods by which nanocrystals of various shapes and sizes can be obtained (Layrolle & Lebugle 1994; Ye et al., 2008). In general, the shape, size and specific surface area of the apatite nanocrystals appear to be very sensitive to both the reaction temperature and both the reactant addition rate. HAs with different stoichiometry and morphology have been prepared and the effects of varying powder synthesis conditions on stoichiometry, crystallinity and morphology, have been analysed. The effects of varying the concentration of the reagents, the reaction temperature, initial pH, ageing time and the atmosphere within the reaction vessel have also been studied (Koutsopoulos 2002). In order to optimise its specific biomedical applications, especially drug delivery function, the physical-chemical features that should be tailored in synthetic biomimetic HA are dimensions, porosity, morphology and surface properties (Roveri et al., 2008c; Tampieri et al., 2009). Biomimetic carbonate-hydroxyapatite nanocrystals have been synthesized by using the sitting drop vapour diffusion technique, for the first time by Iafisco et al. (Iafisco et al., 2010a). The method consists of diffusing vapours of an aqueous solution of NH_4HCO_3 through drops containing an aqueous mixture of $(CH_3COO)_2Ca$ and $(NH_4)_2HPO_4$ in order to increase slowly their pH. This synthesis has been performed in a crystallization mushroom, a glass device developed for protein and small molecules crystallization (Figure 4). The concentrations of the reagents, the final pH and the crystallization time have been optimized to produce pure carbonate-HA as a single phase. X-Ray diffraction, Fourier transformed infrared spectroscopy and transmission electron microscopy have been utilized to characterize the synthesized carbonated substituted HA crystals, which display nanometric dimensions, platelike morphology and low crystallinity degree, closely resembling the inorganic phase of bones, teeth and many pathological calcifications.

Porous HA biomimetic ceramics in simulating spongy bone morphology (porosity varying from a microporosity > 1 μm to a macroporosity ranging from 300 to 2000 μm) has been prepared using various technologies to control pore dimension, shape, distribution and interconnections. Pore sizes and pore morphology are directly related to bone formation, since they provide surface and space for cell adhesion and bone ingrowth. On the other hand, pore interconnection provides the way for cell distribution and migration, as well as it allows an efficient in vivo blood vessel formation suitable for sustaining bone tissue neo-formation and possibly remodelling. Namely, porous HA ceramics can be colonized by bone tissues (Mastrogiacomo et al., 2006; Karageorgiou & Kaplan 2005). Therefore, interconnecting macroporosity (pore size > 100 mm), which is defined by its capacity to be

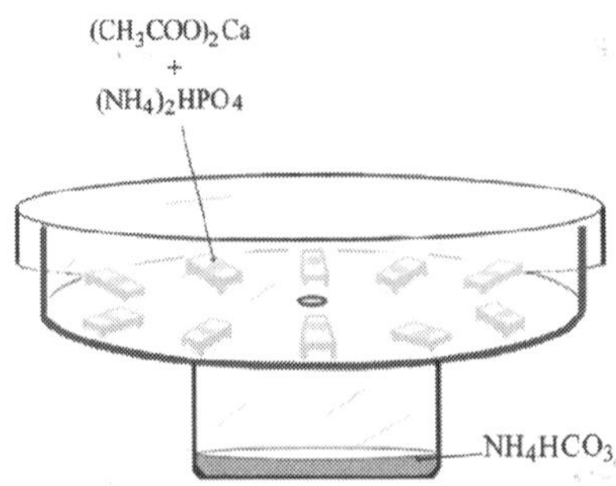

Fig. 4. Crystallization mushroom sketch. Carbonate-hydroxyapatite crystals were grown in sitting droplets on microbridges. $NH_3(g)$ and $CO_2(g)$ slowly diffused from the reservoir to the droplet through the small opening in the plate at bottom.

colonized by cells, is intentionally introduced in solid ceramics (Lu et al., 1999). Porous HA ceramics processed by high-temperature treatment present a significant reduction of bioreactivity and growth kinetics of new bone due to the lack of resorbability (Rodriguez-Lorenzo et al., 2001). However, the low resorbability of sintered HA-ceramics appears useful when they have to be implanted with a defined 3D form. Macroporosity is usually formed due to release of various volatile materials and, for that reason, incorporation of pore creating additives (porogens) is the most popular technique to create macroporosity. Among porogens additives we can mention paraffin, naphthalene, fluor, hydrogen peroxide, polyvinyl butyral, etc (Tancret et al., 2006; Walsh & Tanaka 2001; Chevalier et al., 2008). These additives are admixed to HA powders or slurries. After moulding, the organics burn away from the moulding body during sintering. This approach allows direct control of the pore characteristics, which are a function of the amount and properties of the volatile phase. Several other techniques, such as replication of polymer foams by impregnation, dual-phase mixing technique, freeze casting, strereolithography and foaming of gel-casting suspensions and transformation of porous calcium carbonate from biological origin (marine corals or echinoderms skeletons) into porous calcium phosphates by treatment with phosphate solutions under hydrothermal conditions have been applied to fabricate porous calcium phosphate ceramics (Gonzalez-McQuire et al., 2005; Liu 1997; Walsh et al., 2005; Charriere et al., 2003). By using the latter technique the interconnected porosity of the aragonitic or calcitic skeletons of corals or echinoderms is maintained after transformation to HA or mixtures of HA and other calcium phosphates (Araiza et al., 1999). The preparation methods of porous bioceramics has been recently reviewed by Sopiana et al. (Sopyan et al., 2007).

Many studies have demonstrated that HA ceramics can be used to deliver steroids, antibiotics, proteins, hormones, anticancer drugs. Porous ceramics closely mimicking spongy bone morphology have been synthesized by impregnation of cellulosic sponges with poorly crystalline HA water suspension (Figure 5) (Palazzo et al., 2005). These porous ceramics have been tested as controlled drug delivery bone grafts to evaluate the fundamental parameters that control release kinetics. A theoretical approach, based on the use of the Finite Element Method, was adopted to describe the ibuprofen-lysine and hydrocortisone Na-succinate release kinetics, comparing the numerical results with the experimental ones.

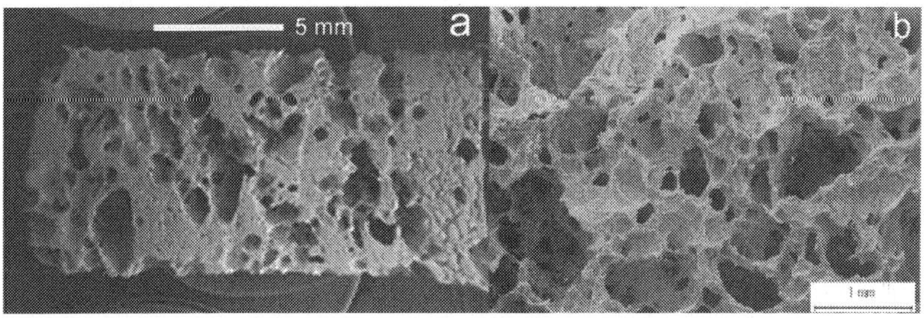

Fig. 5. Scanning electron microscopy image of porous hydroxyapatite

4. Applications of biomimetic hydroxyapatites

The main driving force behind the use of calcium phosphates as bone substitute materials is their chemical similarity to the mineral component of mammalian bones and teeth, as previously explained. As a result, in addition to being non-toxic, they are biocompatible, not recognized as foreign materials in the body and, most importantly, they exhibit bioactive behavior and integrate into living tissue by the same processes active in remodeling healthy bone. This leads to an intimate physical-chemical bond between the implants and bone, termed osteointegration (Puleo 2004). In fact, materials can interact with biomolecules as well as with living systems and these interactions can be used to develop new materials and technologies. In particular, surface interaction of proteins and peptides with calcium phosphates based biomaterial represents the first and pivotal event when materials are implanted within an organism and must integrate in the host tissues, affecting the accompanying biological responses, namely cell attachment and activation (Iafisco et al., 2008; Iafisco et al., 2010b; Palazzo et al., 2009). More to the point, calcium phosphates are also known to support osteoblast adhesion and proliferation (Hong et al., 2003; Sader et al., 2009). Even so, the major limitations to use calcium phosphates as load-bearing biomaterials are their mechanical properties; namely, they are brittle with a poor fatigue resistance (Dorozhkin 2009). The poor mechanical behavior is even more evident for highly porous ceramics and scaffolds because porosity greater than 100 μm is considered a requirement for proper vascularization and bone cell colonization (Sader et al., 2009). That is why, in biomedical applications, calcium phosphates are used primarily as fillers and coatings (de Groot 1993).

4.1 Scaffolds

Following the biomimetic approach, inspiring to Nature, natural wood templates have been selected as a starting point to obtain open-pore geometries with high surface area and microstructure allowing cell in-growth and reorganization and providing the necessary space for vascularisation (Li et al., 2006; Zimmerman et al., 2002). In fact, the alternation of fibre bundles and channel-like porous areas makes the wood an elective material to be used as template in starting the development of new bone substitute biomaterials by an ideal biomimetic hierarchic structure (Singh et al., 2003). Hydroxyapatite bone scaffolds characterized by highly organized hierarchical structures have been recently obtained by chemically transforming native woods through a sequence of thermal and hydrothermal processes. The whole chemical conversion has been carried out through five chemical steps from native wood to porous hydroxyapatite: i) pyrolysis of ligneous raw materials to produce carbon templates characterized by the natural complex anisotropic pore structure; ii) carburization process by vapour or liquid calcium permeation to yield calcium carbide; iii) oxidation process to transform calcium carbide into calcium oxide; iv) carbonation by hydrothermal process under CO_2 pressure for the further conversion into calcium carbonate; v) phosphatization process through hydrothermal treatment to achieve the final hydroxyapatite phase.

The five steps of the phase transformation process have been set up in order to achieve total phase conversion and purity maintaining the original native microstructure. An innovative biomimetic apatite hierarchically structured in parallel fastened hollow microtubules has been synthesized, structurally characterized and proposed as new inorganic biomorphic scaffold providing a biomimetic nanostructured surface for fascinating bone engineering applications (Tampieri et al., 2009). The SEM image reported in Figure 6A demonstrates that the structured anisotropy typical of the native woods was preserved on the macro-scale, exhibiting in the case of rattan pore sizes in the range 100–300 μm, revealing an ordered fastening of parallel micro-tubes 100-150 μm long and 15-30 μm wide with a hollow core of about 10-25 μm in diameter, organized like the cell morphology of the natural wood used as the starting template for its synthesis. SEM image reported in Figure 6B of the newly formed HA surface morphology shows typical needle-like nuclei grown on the surface, proving the concomitant occurrence of a dissolution/precipitation process at sub-micron level, in agreement with hypotheses previously reported. This surface nanostructured morphology of the unidirectional fastened hollow HA microtubules allows biological systems like cells to utilize biomorphic scaffolds on the micrometer level which are also biomimetic for composition and structure on the nanometer scale.

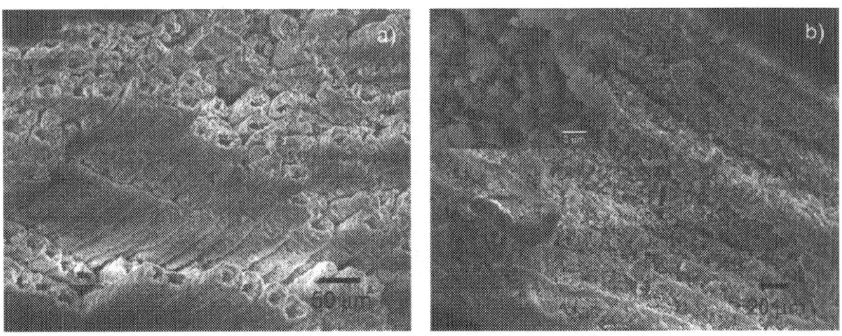

Fig. 6. Detailed SEM images of pine wood-derived hydroxyapatite: a) microstructure of wood-derived parallel fastened hydroxyapatite microtubes; b) typical needle-like HA nuclei grown on the micro-tube surface; inset in b shows an higher magnification of picture b. Reproduced with permission from (Tampieri et al., 2009).

4.2 Drug delivery

Over the past few decades, the rise of modern pharmaceutical technology and the amazing growth of the biotechnology industry have revolutionized the approach to drug delivery systems development. For most of the industry's existence, pharmaceuticals have primarily consisted of relatively simple, fast-acting chemical compounds that are dispensed orally (as solid pills and liquids) or injected. During the past three decades, however, complex formulations that control the rate and period of drug delivery (i.e., time-release medications) and that target specific areas of the body for treatment have become increasingly common. A controlled release drug delivery system should be able to achieve the following benefits: (i) maintenance of optimum therapeutic drug concentration in the blood with minimum fluctuation; (ii) predictable and reproducible release rates for extended duration; (iii) enhancement of activity duration for short half-life drugs; (iv) elimination of side effects, frequent dosing and wastage of drug; and (v) optimized therapy and improved patient compliance.

Hydroxyapatites and other calcium phosphates may find several applications in implant drug devices. In fact, as drug carriers, calcium phosphate nanoparticles have some advantageous properties. They are dissolved at low pH (around 4), e.g. in lysosomes after the cellular intake or in the environment of solid tumours, thereby releasing incorporated drugs or biomolecules (Roveri et al., 2008b; Epple et al., 2010). Their size can easily be controlled by stabilizing agents, such as polymers or nucleic acids. The nanoparticles can be made to fluoresce by the incorporation of lanthanide ions and they can also act as carriers for different drugs (Al-Kattan et al., 2010). For example, one of the most efficient ways to improve the bone forming ability of biomaterials is their association with bone morphogenetic proteins (Autefage et al., 2009). Thus the choice of the process used to prepare implantable bone biomaterials has an influence on the release of the associated bioactive molecules. Various techniques associating drugs with a calcium phosphate biomaterial have been reported: adsorption and impregnation allow the therapeutic agent to be incorporated at the surface of the biomaterial, whereas centrifugation and vacuum based-techniques enable it to enter into pores of biomaterials (Gautier et al., 2001; Gautier et al., 2000).

Generally bioactive molecules, such as growth factors, are incorporated in biomaterials by simple impregnation, followed by drying, and the type of bonding with the substrate and the release rate are often undetermined (Alam et al., 2001). It is suspected that such associations do not allow the chemical bonding of the growth factor to the biomaterial and thus the release rate is often difficult to control. For example, precipitation and clustering of the growth factor molecules may occur and the release is only determined by local dissolution and diffusion rules. The uncontrolled release of growth factors has, in some instances, been related to an accelerated resorption of bone tissue and of the implant (Autefage et al., 2009). Since growth factors agents can stimulate the degradation as well as the formation of bone (depending on their local concentrations), they could impair the osteoconductivity of the coated-implant surface (Liu et al., 2007).

Similarly, bisphosphonates molecules (BPs), by affecting bone remodeling, could also block the bone repair process: the drug at too high concentration could have detrimental effects on the fixation of the implant over longer periods of time. Zoledronate grafted to HA coating on titanium implants shows a dose-dependent effect on the inhibition of resorption activity according to the amount of zoledronate loaded (Peter et al., 2005). Local and slow administration of antineoplasic drug as methotraxate (MTX) is also useful to avoid systemic side effects and, because its time effect (the sensitivity of cells to this drug increases with time) is greater than dose effect (Lebugle et al., 2002).

Adsorption, on the contrary, leads to stable association and control of the amount of bioactive molecules contained in the solid implant and thus of the dose released. Generally, the release is rather low because most of the bioactive molecules adsorbed are irreversibly bound and they are not spontaneously released in a cell culture media (Errassif et al., 2010). They can only be displaced by mineral ions and/or soluble proteins with a stronger affinity for apatite surfaces but in a predicable manner, or by cell activity (Errassif et al., 2010). This characteristic has been observed for various growth factors like bone morphogenetic protein (BMP-2) or vascular endothelial growth factor (VEGF) (Midy et al., 2001; Boix et al., 2005), antiosteoporisis agents (Yoshinari et al., 2001; McLeod et al., 2006) and anticancer drugs as methotraxate and cisplatin (Barroug et al., 2004; Lebugle et al., 2002). It has been reported that slow release of MTX from calcium phosphate is not only due to the porosity like in most of the cases, but mainly due to the adsorption of MTX (Lebugle et al., 2002). A local release system of antibiotics could be used to prevent post-surgical infections favoring early osteointegration of prosthesis. Since some of the antibiotics containing carboxylic groups in their chemical structure, like cephalothin, were better adsorbed than others into calcium phosphate biomaterials, these molecules are slowly released from the carrier (Stigter et al., 2004). Moreover, the high binding capability of apatitic support for a wide range of therapeutic agents allows its surface functionalisation with linking agents, such as BPs molecules, to anchor biologically active molecules which can be released, breaking the linkage as a consequence of external stimuli or internal chemical factors, such as pH and ionic force variation due to physiological or pathological biological process. For example, some works have investigated the adsorption and "smart release" of antitumoral platinum complexes containing BPs onto apatitic nanocrystals as bone specific drug delivery devices to be used for the treatment of bone tumors upon local implantation (Iafisco et al., 2009b).

The adsorption and release of bioactive molecules are strongly affected not only by the chemical properties of the drug molecule, but also by the chemical and structural characteristics of the HA substrates. The adsorption and release of cisplatin, alendronate and di(ethylendiamineplatinum)medronate have been investigated using two biomimetic synthetic HA nanocrystal materials with either plate-shaped or needle-shaped morphologies and with different physical-chemical surface properties by Palazzo et al. (Palazzo et al., 2007). These bioactive molecules were chosen in order to compare the behaviour of metal based drugs to that of a classical organic drug (alendronate), evaluating the effect of the drug molecule overall charge in influencing the drug affinity for apatite nanocrystals with variable structural and chemical different properties. The HA surface area and surface charge (Ca/P ratio), as well as the charge on the adsorbed molecules and their mode of interaction with the HA surface, influence the adsorption and release kinetics of the three drugs investigated. The results demonstrated that HA nanocrystals and anti-tumour drugs can be selected in such a way that the bioactivity of the drug-HA conjugate could be tailored for specific therapeutic applications.

The adsorption of two different platinum complexes with cytotoxic activity, {ethylenediamineplatinum(II)-2-amino-1-hydroxyethane-1,1-diyl-bisphosphonate (A) and bis-{ethylenediamineplatinum(II)}medronate (B), on the synthesized biomimetic nanocrystals has been investigated by Iafisco et al. (Iafisco et al., 2009b). Both complexes contain a geminal bisphosphonate but, in addition, complex A contains a charged ammonium group (Figure 7).

This structural difference dramatically affects the affinity of A and B towards HA nanocrystals, complex A having a greater affinity for calcium phosphate nanocrystals. The release profiles of the platinum complexes from the HA nanoparticles follow an inverted

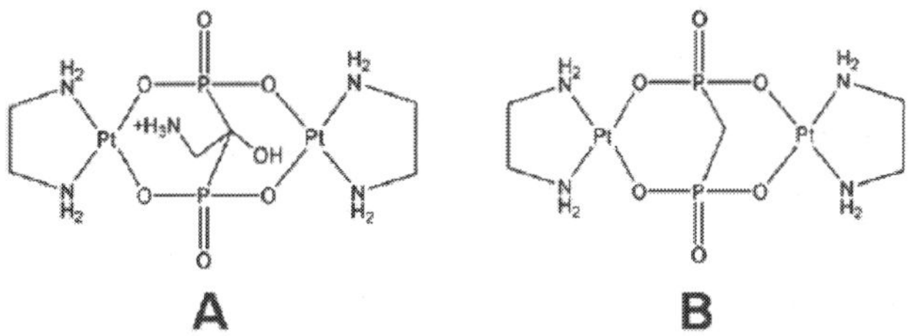

Fig. 7. Sketches of {ethylenediamineplatinum(II)}-2-amino-1-hydroxyethane-1,1-diyl-bisphosphonate (A) and bis-{ethylenediamineplatinum(II)}medronate (B).

trend (complex B > complex A) when compared with the adsorption process. Most probably the less effective desorption in the case of complex A could be due to the aminic group present on the bisphosphonate which remains anchored to the HA matrix, coordinating and holding some of the ethylenediamineplatinum (Pt(en)) residues. Unmodified and HA-adsorbed Pt complexes were tested for their cytotoxicity towards human cervix carcinoma cells (HeLa). The HA-loaded Pt complexes were more cytotoxic than the unmodified compounds A and B and their cytotoxicity was comparable to that of dichloridoethylenediamineplatinum [$PtCl_2$(en)] thus indicating a common active species. The above results demonstrate that HA nanocrystals and antitumor drugs can be conjugated in such a way to yield a smart bone filler delivery system, acting both as bone substitutes and as platinum drug releasing agents with the final goal of locally inhibiting the tumour re-growth and reducing the systemic toxicity. The one here described not only can ensure a prolonged release of active species but also improve the performance of the unmodified drug. Moreover, these results suggest the possibility of using the chemical-physical differences of HA nanocrystals, above all degree of crystallinity, crystal size and surface area, in order to strongly tailor the Pt complex release kinetics. Considering the biomimetic apatite nanocrystals functionalization effects, an attracting goal could be to obtain a drug delivery process characterized by a stimuli responsive kinetic. This aim induces to surface functionalize HA nanocrystals with different linking agents, such as bisphosphonates, to anchor biologically active molecules which can be released breaking the linkage as a consequence of external stimuli or internal chemical factors, such as pH and ionic force variation due to physiological or pathological biological process.

4.3 Preventive dentistry

The purpose of modern dentistry is the early prevention of tooth decay rather than invasive restorative therapy. However, despite tremendous efforts in promoting oral hygiene and fluoridation, the prevention and biomimetic treatment of early caries lesions are still challenges for dental research and public health, particularly for individuals with a high risk for developing caries, which is the most widespread oral disease. Recent studies indicate that nanotechnology might provide novel strategies in preventive dentistry, specifically in the control and management of bacterial biofilms or remineralization of submicrometre-sized tooth decay. Examples include liquids and pastes that contain nano-hydroxyapatites for biofilm management at the tooth surface, and products that contain nanomaterials for the remineralization of early submicrometre-sized enamel lesions (Hannig & Hannig 2010).

Initial carious lesions in the enamel caused by adherent biofilms yield a typical micromorphology with a pseudo-intact surface layer on top of the subsurface body of the lesion as a result of reprecipitating minerals. In contrast to caries lesions caused by acids from bacterial metabolism, enamel erosions are induced by frequent consumption of acidic foods and beverages, or by gastric juice (Figure 8). This direct and continuous surface demineralization is only slightly diminished by the pellicle present in eroded lacunae (Hannig et al., 2009).

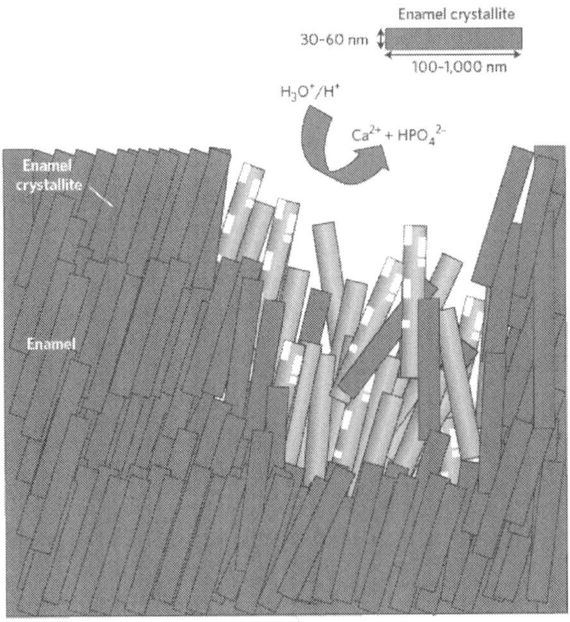

Fig. 8. Dental erosion caused by acidic beverages or food in the oral cavity. Low pH, (pH 1-4), destroys the enamel surface by partial and complete dissolution of the enamel crystallites, resulting in the release of Ca^{2+} and HPO_4^{2-} ions. This loosens the microstructure of the enamel and hydroxyapatite crystallites (pale blue) become demineralized, or are lost. Reproduced with permission from (Hannig & Hannig 2010).

A biomimetic approach for remineralization of initial submicrometre enamel erosions are based on nano-sized hydroxyapatite particles (Roveri et al., 2008a; Li et al., 2008). *In vitro* data indicate that repair at the enamel surface can be greatly improved if the dimensions of the apatite particles are adapted to the scale of the submicrometre- and nanosized defects caused by erosive demineralization of the natural apatite crystallites. HA with a size of 20 nm fits well with the dimensions of the nanodefects caused at the enamel surface during acidic erosion. These particles adsorb strongly to the etched enamel surface under *in vitro* conditions and, interestingly, retard further erosive demineralization (Li et al., 2008). Therefore, the use of well-sized nano-apatite particles could simultaneously repair and prevent initial enamel-erosive lesions.

In another approach, biomimetic carbonate HA nanoparticles that mimic the size of natural dentinal HA (20 nm) or enamel apatite (100 nm) were used to repair micrometre-sized tooth-surface defects *in vitro* (Roveri et al., 2008a; Roveri et al., 2009). Clusters of these nanocrystals have been incorporated into toothpastes or mouth-rinsing solutions to promote the repair of demineralised enamel or dentin surfaces by depositing apatite nanoparticles in the defects. Commercially available dental prophylactic products containing carbonate HA nanoparticles to fill microdefects at the etched enamel surface (for example, BioRepair from Coswell Laboratories, Italy and from Dr. Wolff, Germany) have been proved to be effective *in vitro* after a ten-minute application onto enamel or dentin surfaces (Roveri et al., 2009). Recently an *in vivo* study has been documented that a toothpaste containing zinc–carbonate HA nanocrystals significantly reduced dentinal hypersensitivity after 4 and 8 weeks, supporting its utility in clinical practice (Orsini et al., 2010).
Nano-hydroxyapatite toothpaste with either spheroidal or needle-like particles as an active component was shown to enhance the remineralization of etched enamel better than sodium fluoride solutions. However, the 5 - 10 day *in vitro* study had neglected the conditions of the oral cavity. In another *in vitro* study, nano-sized amorphous calcium carbonate particles that were applied twice a day for a period of 20 days promoted remineralization of artificial white-spot enamel lesions (Nakashima et al., 2009). Reconstitution and remineralization of dentin using nano-sized bioactive glass particles and beta-tricalcium phosphate was also tested *in vitro*, however, the mechanical properties of original dentin could not be reproduced (Shibata et al., 2008; Vollenweider et al., 2007). Owing to the complex organic and inorganic structure of the dentin, remineralizing dentin into a functional state remains one of the most difficult challenges in dental research (Bertassoni et al., 2009).

5. Conclusion

The biomimetism of biomaterials based hydroxyapatite could be carried out at different levels: composition, structure, morphology and surface reactivity. The aim of a researcher is to realise a biomaterial that is biomimetic in all these characteristics, in order not only to optimise the interaction of synthetic materials with biological materials but also, and more ambitiously, to mimic the biogenic materials in its functionality. This concept should be utilised in designing and preparing synthetic inorganic biomaterials in replacing hard and soft tissues. Nanotechnology has great potential in the biomimetism field to do just that: increase in efficacy by orders of magnitude. In fact, the nano-size of biological tissues building blocks is one of the bases of their self-organisational ability and one that needs to be replaced by synthetic materials in the synthesis of structured architectures with controlled organisation on a multiple-length scale.

6. Acknowledgements

We thank the University of Bologna, (funds for selected research topics) and the Inter University Consortium for Research on Chemistry of Metals in Biological Systems (C.I.R.C.M.S.B). This chapter book is in honour of Professor Alberto Ripamonti in the occurrence of the 80th birthday.

Declaration of interest

The authors state no conflict of interest and have received no payment in the preparation of this manuscript.

7. References

Achilles, W.; Jockel, U.; Schaper, A.; Burk, M. & Riedmiller, H. (1995). In-Vitro Formation of Urinary Stones - Generation of Spherulites of Calcium-Phosphate in Gel and Overgrowth with Calcium-Oxalate Using a New Flow Model of Crystallization. *Scanning Microscopy*, 9, 2, 577-586.

Al-Kattan, A.; Dufour, P.; Dexpert-Ghys, J. & Drouet, C. (2010). Preparation and Physicochemical Characteristics of Luminescent Apatite-Based Colloids. *Journal of Physical Chemistry C*, 114, 7, 2918-2924.

Alam, M. I.; Asahina, I.; Ohmamiuda, K.; Takahashi, K.; Yokota, S. & Enomoto, S. (2001). Evaluation of ceramics composed of different hydroxyapatite to tricalcium phosphate ratios as carriers for rhBMP-2. *Biomaterials*, 22, 12, 1643-51.

Araiza, M. A.; Gomez-Morales, J.; Clemente, R. R. & Castano, V. M. (1999). Conversion of the echinoderm Mellita eduardobarrosoi calcite skeleton into porous hydroxyapatite by treatment with phosphated boiling solutions. *Journal of Materials Synthesis and Processing*, 7, 4, 211-219.

Arsenault, A. L. & Robinson, B. W. (1989). The Dentino-Enamel Junction - a Structural and Microanalytical Study of Early Mineralization. *Calcified Tissue International*, 45, 2, 111-121.

Autefage, H.; Briand-Mesange, F.; Cazalbou, S.; Drouet, C.; Fourmy, D.; Goncalves, S.; Salles, J. P.; Combes, C.; Swider, P. & Rey, C. (2009). Adsorption and Release of BMP-2 on Nanocrystalline Apatite-Coated and Uncoated Hydroxyapatite/beta-Tricalcium Phosphate Porous Ceramics. *Journal of Biomedical Materials Research Part B-Applied Biomaterials*, 91B, 2, 706-715.

Barroug, A.; Kuhn, L. T.; Gerstenfeld, L. C. & Glimcher, M. J. (2004). Interactions of cisplatin with calcium phosphate nanoparticles: in vitro controlled adsorption and release. *J Orthop Res*, 22, 4, 703-8.

Ben-Nissan, B. & Choi, A. H. (2006). Sol-gel production of bioactive nanocoatings for medical applications. Part 1: an introduction. *Nanomedicine*, 1, 3, 311-319.

Bertassoni, L. E.; Habelitz, S.; Kinney, J. H.; Marshall, S. J. & Marshall, G. W. (2009). Biomechanical Perspective on the Remineralization of Dentin. *Caries Research*, 43, 1, 70-77.

Bigi, A.; Compostella, L.; Fichera, A. M.; Foresti, E.; Gazzano, M.; Ripamonti, A. & Roveri, N. (1988). Structural and chemical characterization of inorganic deposits in calcified human mitral valve. *J Inorg Biochem*, 34, 2, 75-82.

Bigi, A.; Gandolfi, M.; Koch, M. H. & Roveri, N. (1996). X-ray diffraction study of in vitro calcification of tendon collagen. *Biomaterials*, 17, 12, 1195-201.

Bigi, A.; Gandolfi, M.; Roveri, N. & Valdre, G. (1997). In vitro calcified tendon collagen: an atomic force and scanning electron microscopy investigation. *Biomaterials*, 18, 9, 657-65.

Bigi, A.; Ripamonti, A.; Cojazzi, G.; Pizzuto, G.; Roveri, N. & Koch, M. H. (1991). Structural analysis of turkey tendon collagen upon removal of the inorganic phase. *Int J Biol Macromol*, 13, 2, 110-4.

Boix, T.; Gomez-Morales, J.; Torrent-Burgues, J.; Monfort, A.; Puigdomenech, P. & Rodriguez-Clemente, R. (2005). Adsorption of recombinant human bone morphogenetic protein rhBMP-2m onto hydroxyapatite. *J Inorg Biochem*, 99, 5, 1043-50.

Boskey, A. L. (2007). Mineralization of bones and teeth. *Elements,* 3, 6, 385-391.

Brancaccio, D. & Cozzolino, M. (2005). The mechanism of calcium deposition in soft tissues. *Contrib Nephrol,* 149, 279-86.

Burger, C.; Zhou, H. W.; Wang, H.; Sics, I.; Hsiao, B. S.; Chu, B.; Graham, L. & Glimcher, M. J. (2008). Lateral packing of mineral crystals in bone collagen fibrils. *Biophysical Journal,* 95, 4, 1985-1992.

Cazalbou, S.; Combes, C.; Eichert, D.; Rey, C. & Glimcher, M. J. (2004). Poorly crystalline apatites: evolution and maturation in vitro and in vivo. *Journal of Bone and Mineral Metabolism,* 22, 4, 310-317.

Cazalbou, S.; Eichert, D.; Ranz, X.; Drouet, C.; Combes, C.; Harmand, M. F. & Rey, C. (2005). Ion exchanges in apatites for biomedical application. *Journal of Materials Science-Materials in Medicine,* 16, 5, 405-409.

Chai, C. S. & Ben-Nissan, B. (1999). Bioactive nanocrystalline sol-gel hydroxyapatite coatings. *Journal of Materials Science-Materials in Medicine,* 10, 8, 465-469.

Charriere, E.; Lemaitre, J. & Zysset, P. (2003). Hydroxyapatite cement scaffolds with controlled macroporosity: fabrication protocol and mechanical properties. *Biomaterials,* 24, 5, 809-817.

Chaudhry, A. A.; Haque, S.; Kellici, S.; Boldrin, P.; Rehman, I.; Fazal, A. K. & Darr, J. A. (2006). Instant nano-hydroxyapatite: a continuous and rapid hydrothermal synthesis. *Chemical Communications,* 21, 2286-2288.

Chevalier, E.; Chulia, D.; Pouget, C. & Viana, M. (2008). Fabrication of porous substrates: A review of processes using pore forming agents in the biomaterial field. *Journal of Pharmaceutical Sciences,* 97, 3, 1135-1154.

Choi, A. H. & Ben-Nissan, B. (2007). Sol-gel production of bioactive nanocoatings for medical applications. Part II: current research and development. *Nanomedicine,* 2, 1, 51-61.

Cowles, E. A.; DeRome, M. E.; Pastizzo, G.; Brailey, L. L. & Gronowicz, G. A. (1998). Mineralization and the expression of matrix proteins during in vivo bone development. *Calcified Tissue International,* 62, 1, 74-82.

Cui, F. Z. & Ge, J. (2007). New observations of the hierarchical structure of human enamel, from nanoscale to microscale. *Journal of Tissue Engineering and Regenerative Medicine,* 1, 3, 185-191.

Cui, F. Z.; Li, Y. & Ge, J. (2007). Self-assembly of mineralized collagen composites. *Materials Science & Engineering R-Reports,* 57, 1-6, 1-27.

Cushing, B. L.; Kolesnichenko, V. L. & O'Connor, C. J. (2004). Recent advances in the liquid-phase syntheses of inorganic nanoparticles. *Chemical Reviews,* 104, 9, 3893-3946.

Daculsi, G.; Bouler, J. M. & LeGeros, R. Z. (1997). Adaptive crystal formation in normal and pathological calcifications in synthetic calcium phosphate and related biomaterials. *International Review of Cytology - a Survey of Cell Biology, Vol 172,* 172, 129-191.

de Groot, K. (1993). Clinical applications of calcium phosphate biomaterials: A review. *Ceramics International,* 19, 5, 363-366.

Dorozhkin, S. V. (2009). Calcium orthophosphate-based biocomposites and hybrid biomaterials. *Journal of Materials Science,* 44, 9, 2343-2387.

Dorozhkin, S. V. (2010). Bioceramics of calcium orthophosphates. *Biomaterials,* 31, 7, 1465-85.

Drouet, C.; Bosc, F.; Banu, M.; Largeot, C.; Combes, C.; Dechambre, G.; Estournes, C.; Raimbeaux, G. & Rey, C. (2009). Nanocrystalline apatites: From powders to biomaterials. *Powder Technology,* 190, 1-2, 118-122.

Eichert, C.; Drouet, C.; Sfihi, H.; Rey, C. & Combes, C. (2007). Nanocrystalline apatite-based biomaterials: synthesis, processing and characterization. In *Biomaterials Research Advances,* ed. J. Kendall, 93-143. Nova Science Publishers.

Epple, M.; Ganesan, K.; Heumann, R.; Klesing, J.; Kovtun, A.; Neumann, S. & Sokolova, V. (2010). Application of calcium phosphate nanoparticles in biomedicine. *Journal of Materials Chemistry,* 20, 1, 18-23.

Errassif, F.; Menbaoui, A.; Autefage, H.; Benaziz, L.; Ouizat, S.; Santran, V.; Sarda, S.; Lebugle, A.; Combes, C.; Barroug, A.; Sfihi, H. & Rey, C. 2010. Adsorption on Apatitic Calcium Phosphates: Applications to Drug Delivery In *Advances in Bioceramics and Biotechnologies,* eds. R. Narayan, M. Singh & J. McKittrick. Wiley-VCH Verlag GmbH & Co. KGaA

Feng, J. Q.; Ward, L. M.; Liu, S.; Lu, Y.; Xie, Y.; Yuan, B.; Yu, X.; Rauch, F.; Davis, S. I.; Zhang, S.; Rios, H.; Drezner, M. K.; Quarles, L. D.; Bonewald, L. F. & White, K. E. (2006). Loss of DMP1 causes rickets and osteomalacia and identifies a role for osteocytes in mineral metabolism. *Nat Genet,* 38, 11, 1310-5.

Fernandez-Moran, H. & Engstrom, A. (1957). Electron microscopy and x-ray diffraction of bone. *Biochim Biophys Acta,* 23, 2, 260-4.

Fratzl, P.; Gupta, H. S.; Paschalis, E. P. & Roschger, P. (2004). Structure and mechanical quality of the collagen-mineral nano-composite in bone. *Journal of Materials Chemistry,* 14, 14, 2115-2123.

Ganesan, K. & Epple, M. (2008). Calcium phosphate nanoparticles as nuclei for the preparation of colloidal calcium phytate. *New Journal of Chemistry,* 32, 8, 1326-1330.

Gautier, H.; Daculsi, G. & Merle, C. (2001). Association of vancomycin and calcium phosphate by dynamic compaction: in vitro characterization and microbiological activity. *Biomaterials,* 22, 18, 2481-7.

Gautier, H.; Merle, C.; Auget, J. L. & Daculsi, G. (2000). Isostatic compression, a new process for incorporating vancomycin into biphasic calcium phosphate: comparison with a classical method. *Biomaterials,* 21, 3, 243-249.

Gonzalez-McQuire, R.; Green, D.; Walsh, D.; Hall, S.; Chane-Ching, J. Y.; Oreffo, R. O. C. & Mann, S. (2005). Fabrication of hydroxyapatite sponges by dextran sulphate/amino acid templating. *Biomaterials,* 26, 33, 6652-6656.

Guo, X.; Gough, J. E.; Xiao, P.; Liu, J. & Shen, Z. (2007). Fabrication of nanostructured hydroxyapatite and analysis of human osteoblastic cellular response. *J Biomed Mater Res A,* 82, 4, 1022-32.

Hannig, C.; Berndt, D.; Hoth-Hannig, W. & Hannig, M. (2009). The effect of acidic beverages on the ultrastructure of the acquired pellicle--an in situ study. *Arch Oral Biol,* 54, 6, 518-26.

Hannig, M. & Hannig, C. (2010). Nanomaterials in preventive dentistry. *Nature Nanotechnology,* 5, 8, 565-569.

Hayashizaki, J.; Ban, S.; Nakagaki, H.; Okumura, A.; Yoshii, S. & Robinson, C. (2008). Site specific mineral composition and microstructure of human supra-gingival dental calculus. *Archives of Oral Biology,* 53, 2, 168-174.

Hong, J.-Y.; Kim, Y. J.; Lee, H.-W.; Lee, W.-K.; Ko, J. S. & Kim, H.-M. (2003). Osteoblastic cell response to thin film of poorly crystalline calcium phosphate apatite formed at low temperatures. *Biomaterials*, 24, 18, 2977-2984.

Huang, J.; Best, S. M.; Bonfield, W.; Brooks, R. A.; Rushton, N.; Jayasinghe, S. N. & Edirisinghe, M. J. (2004). In vitro assessment of the biological response to nano-sized hydroxyapatite. *Journal of Materials Science-Materials in Medicine*, 15, 4, 441-445.

Iafisco, M.; Marchetti, M.; Morales, J. G.; Hernandez-Hernandez, M. A.; Ruiz, J. M. G. & Roveri, N. (2009a). Silica Gel Template for Calcium Phosphates Crystallization. *Crystal Growth & Design*, 9, 11, 4912-4921.

Iafisco, M.; Morales, J. G.; Hernandez-Hernandez, M. A.; Garcia-Ruiz, J. M. & Roveri, N. (2010a). Biomimetic Carbonate-Hydroxyapatite Nanocrystals Prepared by Vapor Diffusion. *Advanced Engineering Materials*, 12, 7, B218-B223.

Iafisco, M.; Palazzo, B.; Falini, G.; Di Foggia, M.; Bonora, S.; Nicolis, S.; Casella, L. & Roveri, N. (2008). Adsorption and conformational change of myoglobin on biomimetic hydroxyapatite nanocrystals functionalized with alendronate. *Langmuir*, 24, 9, 4924-4930.

Iafisco, M.; Palazzo, B.; Marchetti, M.; Margiotta, N.; Ostuni, R.; Natile, G.; Morpurgo, M.; Gandin, V.; Marzano, C. & Roveri, N. (2009b). Smart delivery of antitumoral platinum complexes from biomimetic hydroxyapatite nanocrystals. *Journal of Materials Chemistry*, 19, 44, 8385-8392.

Iafisco, M.; Sabatino, P.; Lesci, I. G.; Prat, M.; Rimondini, L. & Roveri, N. (2010b). Conformational modifications of serum albumins adsorbed on different kinds of biomimetic hydroxyapatite nanocrystals. *Colloids Surf B Biointerfaces*, 81, 1, 274-84.

Imbeni, V.; Kruzic, J. J.; Marshall, G. W.; Marshall, S. J. & Ritchie, R. O. (2005). The dentin-enamel junction and the fracture of human teeth. *Nature Materials*, 4, 3, 229-232.

Karageorgiou, V. & Kaplan, D. (2005). Porosity of 3D biomaterial scaffolds and osteogenesis. *Biomaterials*, 26, 27, 5474-91.

Kazama, J. J.; Amizuka, N. & Fukagawa, M. (2006). Ectopic calcification as abnormal biomineralization. *Therapeutic Apheresis and Dialysis*, 10, S34-S38.

Kirsch, T. (2006). Determinants of pathological mineralization. *Curr Opin Rheumatol*, 18, 2, 174-80.

Kodaka, T.; Nakajima, F. & Higashi, S. (1989). Structure of the So-Called Prismless Enamel in Human Deciduous Teeth. *Caries Research*, 23, 5, 290-296.

Koutsopoulos, S. (2002). Synthesis and characterization of hydroxyapatite crystals: a review study on the analytical methods. *J Biomed Mater Res*, 62, 4, 600-12.

Laird, D. F.; Mucalo, M. R. & Yokogawa, Y. (2006). Growth of calcium hydroxyapatite (Ca-HAp) on cholesterol and cholestanol crystals from a simulated body fluid: A possible insight into the pathological calcifications associated with atherosclerosis. *Journal of Colloid and Interface Science*, 295, 2, 348-363.

Layrolle, P. & Lebugle, A. (1994). Characterization and Reactivity of Nanosized Calcium Phosphates Prepared in Anhydrous Ethanol. *Chemistry of Materials*, 6, 11, 1996-2004.

Lebugle, A.; Rodrigues, A.; Bonnevialle, P.; Voigt, J. J.; Canal, P. & Rodriguez, F. (2002). Study of implantable calcium phosphate systems for the slow release of methotrexate. *Biomaterials*, 23, 16, 3517-22.

LeGeros, R. Z. (2008). Calcium Phosphate-Based Osteoinductive Materials. *Chemical Reviews,* 108, 11, 4742-4753.

Legeros, R. Z. & Craig, R. G. (1993). Strategies to Affect Bone Remodeling - Osteointegration. *Journal of Bone and Mineral Research,* 8, S583-S596.

Legeros, R. Z.; Orly, I.; Legeros, J. P.; Gomez, C.; Kazimiroff, J.; Tarpley, T. & Kerebel, B. (1988). Scanning Electron-Microscopy and Electron-Probe Microanalyses of the Crystalline Components of Human and Animal Dental Calculi. *Scanning Microscopy,* 2, 1, 345-356.

Legros, R.; Balmain, N. & Bonel, G. (1987). Age-related changes in mineral of rat and bovine cortical bone. *Calcif Tissue Int,* 41, 3, 137-44.

Li, L.; Pan, H.; Tao, J.; Xu, X.; Mao, C.; Gu, X. & Tang, R. (2008). Repair of enamel by using hydroxyapatite nanoparticles as the building blocks. *Journal of Materials Chemistry,* 18, 34, 4079-4084.

Li, X. F.; Fan, T. X.; Liu, Z. T.; Ding, J.; Guo, Q. X. & Zhang, D. (2006). Synthesis and hierarchical pore structure of biomorphic manganese oxide derived from woods. *Journal of the European Ceramic Society,* 26, 16, 3657-3664.

Liou, S. C.; Chen, S. Y.; Lee, H. Y. & Bow, J. S. (2004). Structural characterization of nano-sized calcium deficient apatite powders. *Biomaterials,* 25, 2, 189-196.

Liu, D. M. (1997). Fabrication of hydroxyapatite ceramic with controlled porosity. *Journal of Materials Science-Materials in Medicine,* 8, 4, 227-232.

Liu, J. B.; Li, K. W.; Wang, H.; Zhu, M. K.; Xu, H. Y. & Yan, H. (2005). Self-assembly of hydroxyapatite nanostructures by microwave irradiation. *Nanotechnology,* 16, 1, 82-87.

Liu, Y. L.; Enggist, L.; Kuffer, A. F.; Buser, D. & Hunziker, E. B. (2007). The influence of BMP-2 and its mode of delivery on the osteoconductivity of implant surfaces during the early phase of osseointegration (vol 28, pg 2677, 2007). *Biomaterials,* 28, 35, 5399-5399.

Lopez-Macipe, A.; Gomez-Morales, J. & Rodriguez-Clemente, R. (1998). Nanosized hydroxyapatite precipitation from homogeneous calcium/citrate/phosphate solutions using microwave and conventional heating. *Advanced Materials,* 10, 1, 49-+.

Loveridge, N. (1999). Bone: More than a stick. *Journal of Animal Science,* 77, 190-196.

Lu, J. X.; Flautre, B.; Anselme, K.; Hardouin, P.; Gallur, A.; Descamps, M. & Thierry, B. (1999). Role of interconnections in porous bioceramics on bone recolonization in vitro and in vivo. *Journal of Materials Science-Materials in Medicine,* 10, 2, 111-120.

Mann, S.; Archibald, D. D.; Didymus, J. M.; Douglas, T.; Heywood, B. R.; Meldrum, F. C. & Reeves, N. J. (1993). Crystallization at Inorganic-organic Interfaces: Biominerals and Biomimetic Synthesis. *Science,* 261, 5126, 1286-92.

Manolagas, S. C. (2000). Birth and death of bone cells: Basic regulatory mechanisms and implications for the pathogenesis and treatment of osteoporosis. *Journal of Aging and Physical Activity,* 8, 3, 248-248.

Mao, Y.; Park, T. J.; Zhang, F.; Zhou, H. & Wong, S. S. (2007). Environmentally friendly methodologies of nanostructure synthesis. *Small,* 3, 7, 1122-1139.

Marra, S. P.; Daghlian, C. P.; Fillinger, M. F. & Kennedy, F. E. (2006). Elemental composition, morphology and mechanical properties of calcified deposits obtained from abdominal aortic aneurysms. *Acta Biomaterialia,* 2, 5, 515-520.

Mastrogiacomo, M.; Scaglione, S.; Martinetti, R.; Dolcini, L.; Beltrame, F.; Cancedda, R. & Quarto, R. (2006). Role of scaffold internal structure on in vivo bone formation in macroporous calcium phosphate bioceramics. *Biomaterials*, 27, 17, 3230-3237.

McLeod, K.; Kumar, S.; Smart, R. S. C.; Dutta, N.; Voelcker, N. H.; Anderson, G. I. & Sekel, R. (2006). XPS and bioactivity study of the bisphosphonate pamidronate adsorbed onto plasma sprayed hydroxyapatite coatings. *Applied Surface Science*, 253, 5, 2644-2651.

Midy, V.; Hollande, E.; Rey, C.; Dard, M. & Plouet, J. (2001). Adsorption of vascular endothelial growth factor to two different apatitic materials and its release. *J Mater Sci Mater Med*, 12, 4, 293-8.

Nakashima, S.; Yoshie, M.; Sano, H. & Bahar, A. (2009). Effect of a test dentifrice containing nano-sized calcium carbonate on remineralization of enamel lesions in vitro. *Journal of oral science*, 51, 1, 69-77.

Olszta, M. J.; Cheng, X. G.; Jee, S. S.; Kumar, R.; Kim, Y. Y.; Kaufman, M. J.; Douglas, E. P. & Gower, L. B. (2007). Bone structure and formation: A new perspective. *Materials Science & Engineering R-Reports*, 58, 3-5, 77-116.

Orsini, G.; Procaccini, M.; Manzoli, L.; Giuliodori, F.; Lorenzini, A. & Putignano, A. (2010). A double-blind randomized-controlled trial comparing the desensitizing efficacy of a new dentifrice containing carbonate/hydroxyapatite nanocrystals and a sodium fluoride/potassium nitrate dentifrice. *Journal of Clinical Periodontology*, 37, 6, 510-517.

Paine, M. L.; White, S. N.; Luo, W.; Fong, H.; Sarikaya, M. & Snead, M. L. (2001). Regulated gene expression dictates enamel structure and tooth function. *Matrix Biology*, 20, 5-6, 273-292.

Palazzo, B.; Iafisco, M.; Laforgia, M.; Margiotta, N.; Natile, G.; Bianchi, C. L.; Walsh, D.; Mann, S. & Roveri, N. (2007). Biomimetic hydroxyapatite-drug nanocrystals as potential bone substitutes with antitumor drug delivery properties. *Advanced Functional Materials*, 17, 13, 2180-2188.

Palazzo, B.; Sidoti, M. C.; Roveri, N.; Tampieri, A.; Sandri, M.; Bertolazzi, L.; Galbusera, F.; Dubini, G.; Vena, P. & Contro, R. (2005). Controlled drug delivery from porous hydroxyapatite grafts: An experimental and theoretical approach. *Materials Science & Engineering C-Biomimetic and Supramolecular Systems*, 25, 2, 207-213.

Palazzo, B.; Walsh, D.; Iafisco, M.; Foresti, E.; Bertinetti, L.; Martra, G.; Bianchi, C. L.; Cappelletti, G. & Roveri, N. (2009). Amino acid synergetic effect on structure, morphology and surface properties of biomimetic apatite nanocrystals. *Acta Biomater*, 5, 4, 1241-52.

Palmer, L. C.; Newcomb, C. J.; Kaltz, S. R.; Spoerke, E. D. & Stupp, S. I. (2008). Biomimetic systems for hydroxyapatite mineralization inspired by bone and enamel. *Chemical Reviews*, 108, 11, 4754-83.

Paschalis, E. P.; DiCarlo, E.; Betts, F.; Sherman, P.; Mendelsohn, R. & Boskey, A. L. (1996). FTIR microspectroscopic analysis of human osteonal bone. *Calcified Tissue International*, 59, 6, 480-487.

Peter, B.; Pioletti, D. P.; Laib, S.; Bujoli, B.; Pilet, P.; Janvier, P.; Guicheux, J.; Zambelli, P. Y.; Bouler, J. M. & Gauthier, O. (2005). Calcium phosphate drug delivery system: influence of local zoledronate release on bone implant osteointegration. *Bone*, 36, 1, 52-60.

Phillips, M. J.; Darr, J. A.; Luklinska, Z. B. & Rehman, I. (2003). Synthesis and characterization of nano-biomaterials with potential osteological applications. *Journal of Materials Science-Materials in Medicine*, 14, 10, 875-882.

Puleo, D. A. (2004). Bone–Implant Interface. *Encyclopedia of Biomaterials and Biomedical Engineering*, 190 - 198.

Rameshbabu, N.; Rao, K. P. & Kumar, T. S. S. (2005). Acclerated microwave processing of nanocrystalline hydroxyapatite. *Journal of Materials Science*, 40, 23, 6319-6323.

Reddi, A. H. (1994). Symbiosis of Biotechnology and Biomaterials - Applications in Tissue Engineering of Bone and Cartilage. *Journal of Cellular Biochemistry*, 56, 2, 192-195.

Rey, C.; Collins, B.; Goehl, T.; Dickson, I. R. & Glimcher, M. J. (1989). The Carbonate Environment in Bone-Mineral - a Resolution-Enhanced Fourier-Transform Infrared-Spectroscopy Study. *Calcified Tissue International*, 45, 3, 157-164.

Rey, C.; Shimizu, M.; Collins, B. & Glimcher, M. J. (1990). Resolution-enhanced Fourier transform infrared spectroscopy study of the environment of phosphate ions in the early deposits of a solid phase of calcium-phosphate in bone and enamel, and their evolution with age. I: Investigations in the upsilon 4 PO4 domain. *Calcif Tissue Int*, 46, 6, 384-94.

Rodriguez-Lorenzo, L. M.; Vallet-Regi, M. & Ferreira, J. M. (2001). Fabrication of hydroxyapatite bodies by uniaxial pressing from a precipitated powder. *Biomaterials*, 22, 6, 583-8.

Roveri, N.; Battistella, E.; Bianchi, C. L.; Foltran, I.; Foresti, E.; Iafisco, M.; Lelli, M.; Naldoni, A.; Palazzo, B. & Rimondini, L. (2009). Surface Enamel Remineralization: Biomimetic Apatite Nanocrystals and Fluoride Ions Different Effects. *Journal of Nanomaterials*, -.

Roveri, N.; Battistella, E.; Foltran, I.; Foresti, E.; Iafisco, M.; Lelli, M.; Palazzo, B. & Rimondini, L. (2008a). Synthetic Biomimetic Carbonate-Hydroxyapatite Nanocrystals for Enamel Remineralization. *Advanced Materials Research*, 47-50, 821-824.

Roveri, N.; Palazzo, B. & Iafisco, M. (2008b). The role of biomimetism in developing nanostructured inorganic matrices for drug delivery. *Expert Opinion on Drug Delivery*, 5, 8, 861-877.

Sader, M.; LeGeros, R. & Soares, G. (2009). Human osteoblasts adhesion and proliferation on magnesium-substituted tricalcium phosphate dense tablets. *Journal of Materials Science: Materials in Medicine*, 20, 2, 521-527.

Sakhno, Y.; Bertinetti, L.; Iafisco, M.; Tampieri, A.; Roveri, N. & Martra, G. (2010). Surface Hydration and Cationic Sites of Nanohydroxyapatites with Amorphous or Crystalline Surfaces: A Comparative Study. *The Journal of Physical Chemistry C*, 114, 39, 16640-16648.

Sanchez, C.; Arribart, H. & Guille, M. M. G. (2005). Biomimetism and bioinspiration as tools for the design of innovative materials and systems. *Nature Materials*, 4, 4, 277-288.

Sarikaya, M.; Tamerler, C.; Jen, A. K.; Schulten, K. & Baneyx, F. (2003). Molecular biomimetics: nanotechnology through biology. *Nature Materials*, 2, 9, 577-85.

Schmidt, H. K. (2000). Nanoparticles for ceramic and nanocomposite processing. *Molecular Crystals and Liquid Crystals*, 353, 165-179.

Shibata, Y.; He, L. H.; Kataoka, Y.; Miyazaki, T. & Swain, M. V. (2008). Micromechanical property recovery of human carious dentin achieved with colloidal nano-beta-tricalcium phosphate. *J Dent Res*, 87, 3, 233-7.

Singh, M.; Martinez-Fernandez, J. & de Arellano-Lopez, A. R. (2003). Environmentally conscious ceramics (ecoceramics) from natural wood precursors. *Current Opinion in Solid State & Materials Science*, 7, 3, 247-254.

Siva Rama Krishna, D.; Siddharthan, A.; Seshadri, S. K. & Sampath Kumar, T. S. (2007). A novel route for synthesis of nanocrystalline hydroxyapatite from eggshell waste. *J Mater Sci Mater Med*, 18, 9, 1735-43.

Sopyan, I.; Mel, M.; Ramesh, S. & Khalid, K. A. (2007). Porous hydroxyapatite for artificial bone applications. *Science and Technology of Advanced Materials*, 8, 1-2, 116-123.

Stigter, M.; Bezemer, J.; de Groot, K. & Layrolle, P. (2004). Incorporation of different antibiotics into carbonated hydroxyapatite coatings on titanium implants, release and antibiotic efficacy. *J Control Release*, 99, 1, 127-37.

Sun, W. B.; Chu, C. L.; Wang, J. & Zhao, H. T. (2007). Comparison of periodontal ligament cells responses to dense and nanophase hydroxyapatite. *Journal of Materials Science-Materials in Medicine*, 18, 5, 677-683.

Tamerler, C. & Sarikaya, M. (2007). Molecular biomimetics: utilizing nature's molecular ways in practical engineering. *Acta Biomater*, 3, 3, 289-99.

Tamerler, C. & Sarikaya, M. (2008). Molecular biomimetics: Genetic synthesis, assembly, and formation of materials using peptides. *Mrs Bulletin*, 33, 5, 504-510.

Tampieri, A.; Sprio, S.; Ruffini, A.; Celotti, G.; Lesci, I. G. & Roveri, N. (2009). From wood to bone: multi-step process to convert wood hierarchical structures into biomimetic hydroxyapatite scaffolds for bone tissue engineering. *Journal of Materials Chemistry*, 19, 28, 4973-4980.

Tancret, F.; Bouler, J. M.; Chamousset, J. & Minois, L. M. (2006). Modelling the mechanical properties of microporous and macroporous biphasic calcium phosphate bioceramics. *Journal of the European Ceramic Society*, 26, 16, 3647-3656.

Tas, A. C. (2000). Synthesis of biomimetic Ca-hydroxyapatite powders at 37 degrees C in synthetic body fluids. *Biomaterials*, 21, 14, 1429-1438.

Termine, J. D.; Kleinman, H. K.; Whitson, S. W.; Conn, K. M.; McGarvey, M. L. & Martin, G. R. (1981). Osteonectin, a bone-specific protein linking mineral to collagen. *Cell*, 26, 1 Pt 1, 99-105.

Traub, W.; Arad, T. & Weiner, S. (1989). Three-dimensional ordered distribution of crystals in turkey tendon collagen fibers. *Proc Natl Acad Sci U S A*, 86, 24, 9822-6.

Tzaphlidou, M. (2008). Bone Architecture: Collagen Structure and Calcium/Phosphorus Maps. *Journal of Biological Physics*, 34, 1-2, 39-49.

Urist, M. R. (2002). Bone: Formation by autoinduction (Reprinted from Science, vol 150, pg 893-899, 1965). *Clinical Orthopaedics and Related Research*, 395, 5-10.

Vollenweider, M.; Brunner, T. J.; Knecht, S.; Grass, R. N.; Zehnder, M.; Imfeld, T. & Stark, W. J. (2007). Remineralization of human dentin using ultrafine bioactive glass particles. *Acta Biomater*, 3, 6, 936-43.

Vriezema, D. M.; Aragonès, M. C.; Elemans, J. A. A. W.; Cornelissen, J. J. L. M.; Rowan, A. E. & Nolte, R. J. M. (2005). Self-assembled nanoreactors. *Chemical Reviews*, 105, 4, 1445-1489.

Wahl, D. A. & Czernuszka, J. T. (2006). Collagen-hydroxyapatite composites for hard tissue repair. *European Cells & Materials*, 11, 43-56.

Walsh, D.; Boanini, E.; Tanaka, J. & Mann, S. (2005). Synthesis of tri-calcium phosphate sponges by interfacial deposition and thermal transformation of self-supporting calcium phosphate films. *Journal of Materials Chemistry*, 15, 10, 1043-1048.

Walsh, D. & Tanaka, J. (2001). Preparation of a bone-like apatite foam cement. *Journal of Materials Science-Materials in Medicine*, 12, 4, 339-343.

Wang, J. W. & Shaw, L. L. (2007). Morphology-enhanced low-temperature sintering of nanocrystalline hydroxyapatite. *Advanced Materials*, 19, 17, 2364-+.

Wang, R. Z. & Weiner, S. (1998). Strain-structure relations in human teeth using Moire fringes. *Journal of Biomechanics*, 31, 2, 135-141.

Wang, X.; Zhuang, J.; Peng, Q. & Li, Y. D. (2005). A general strategy for nanocrystal synthesis. *Nature*, 437, 7055, 121-124.

Weiner, S. & Addadi, L. (1997). Design strategies in mineralized biological materials. *Journal of Materials Chemistry*, 7, 5, 689-702.

Weiner, S. & Wagner, H. D. (1998). The material bone: Structure mechanical function relations. *Annual Review of Materials Science*, 28, 271-298.

Weissen-Plenz, G.; Nitschke, Y. & Rutsch, F. (2008). Mechanisms of Arterial Calcification: Spotlight on the Inhibitors. *Advances in Clinical Chemistry, Vol 46*, 46, 263-293.

Wen, H. B.; Moradian-Oldak, J. & Fincham, A. G. (2000). Dose-dependent modulation of octacalcium phosphate crystal habit by amelogenins. *Journal of Dental Research*, 79, 11, 1902-1906.

Wesson, J. A. & Ward, M. D. (2007). Pathological biomineralization of kidney stones. *Elements*, 3, 6, 415-421.

White, S. N.; Luo, W.; Paine, M. L.; Fong, H.; Sarikaya, M. & Snead, M. L. (2001). Biological organization of hydroxyapatite crystallites into a fibrous continuum toughens and controls anisotropy in human enamel. *Journal of Dental Research*, 80, 1, 321-326.

Whittaker, D. K. (1982). Structural variations in the surface zone of human tooth enamel observed by scanning electron microscopy. *Archives of Oral Biology*, 27, 5, 383-92.

Wozney, J. M. (1992). The Bone Morphogenetic Protein Family and Osteogenesis. *Molecular Reproduction and Development*, 32, 2, 160-167.

Ye, F.; Guo, H. F. & Zhang, H. J. (2008). Biomimetic synthesis of oriented hydroxyapatite mediated by nonionic surfactants. *Nanotechnology*, 19, 24, -.

Yeon, K. C.; Wang, J. & Ng, S. C. (2001). Mechanochemical synthesis of nanocrystalline hydroxyapatite from CaO and CaHPO4. *Biomaterials*, 22, 20, 2705-12.

Yoshinari, M.; Oda, Y.; Ueki, H. & Yokose, S. (2001). Immobilization of bisphosphonates on surface modified titanium. *Biomaterials*, 22, 7, 709-715.

Zhang, Y. J. & Lu, J. J. (2007). A simple method to tailor spherical nanocrystal hydroxyapatite at low temperature. *Journal of Nanoparticle Research*, 9, 4, 589-594.

Zimmerman, A. F.; Palumbo, G.; Aust, K. T. & Erb, U. (2002). Mechanical properties of nickel silicon carbide nanocomposites. *Materials Science and Engineering a-Structural Materials Properties Microstructure and Processing*, 328, 1-2, 137-146.

5

Recent Advances in Biomimetic Synthesis Involving Cyclodextrins

Y. V. D. Nageswar, S. Narayana Murthy, B. Madhav and J. Shankar
Organic Chemistry Division-I, Indian Institute of Chemical Technology, Hyderabad-500607, India

1. Introduction

Modern bioorganic chemistry is interested in the mimicking of enzymes in their capability to bind substrates selectively and catalyze chemical reactions since biochemical selectivity will be superior to chemical selectivity in various aspects. Laboratory organic chemistry differs from that used in living systems to perform biochemical reactions. In general, organic chemists allow small reactive reagents to attack a free substrate randomly in a solution. The selectivity that is achieved is a result of selective reactivity of a particular region of the substrate or steric crowding or blocking certain approach directions. In contrast, biochemical reactions involving enzymes bind and then orient the reactants. Biochemical selectivity usually reflects such orientation, rather than the intrinsic reactivity of the substrate molecule. For instance, it is common to observe the selective oxidation of an unreactive region of a substrate molecule in an enzymatic reaction while much more reactive segments are left untouched. Enzymatic processes frequently achieve higher levels of selectivity which are not attainable by simple chemical means. Most enzyme catalyzed reactions are stereoselective, or in the choice of substrates, selective either in the type of chemical reactions performed and selective in the region of the molecule to be attacked. However, regioselectivity and stereoselectivity, in particular the formation of pure product enantiomers from achiral precursors, are aspects of enzymatic chemistry which are to be admired and imitated by synthetic chemists.

Biochemical selectivity is the result of the geometry of enzyme-substrate complexes, in which only certain substrates can fit in the enzyme and only certain points in the substrates are then in a position to be attacked. Geometric control was attained by using the reagent-substrate complexes in which a relatively rigid reagent would direct the attack into a particular region of the substrate and this is called "biomimetic control". The term "biomimetic" has since come into wider use, generally referring to any aspect in which a chemical process imitates a biochemical reaction.

Certain supramolecular hosts, with their cavities have the potential to perform novel chemical transformations, mimicking the biochemical selectivity exhibited by enzymes. Binding of substrates to these supramolecular hosts involving intermolecular interactions of non covalent nature such as hydrogen bonding, *van* der Waals forces, etc. results in host guest complexation akin to biological receptors and substrates. The formation of such inclusion complexes involves molecular recognition capability of the supramolecular hosts. In fact molecular recognition involves both binding and selection of the substrate by the host. In addition if the host bears reactive functionalities, it results in the activation of the guest molecule to under go chemical transformation of the bound substrate, wherein the role played by the intermolecular forces is significant.

These supramolecular hosts have excited interest as enzyme models catalyzing chemical reactions involving the reversible formation of host-guest complexes. Cyclodextrins acquired prominence as supramolecular hosts as they modify the properties of the included molecules. Hence they are used in a variety of industrial applications, analytical techniques and as reaction mediator (Szejtli & Osa, 1996).

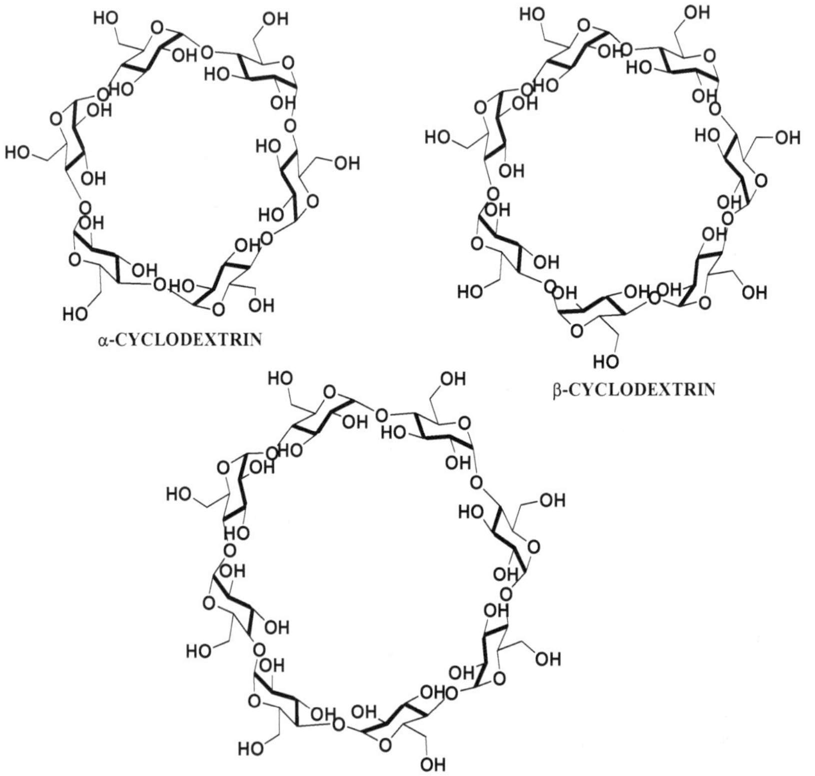

α-CYCLODEXTRIN

β-CYCLODEXTRIN

γ-CYCLODEXTRIN

Structures of α, β, and γ-CD

Cyclodextrins are produced from starch by the action of the enzyme cyclodextrin glucosyl trasferase (CGT). Cyclodextrins (CDs) are torus shaped cyclic oligosaccharides consisting mainly of 6 (α CD), 7 (β CD) and 8 (γ CD) D-glucose units. Each of the chiral glucose units is in the rigid $^4C_1$-chair conformation, giving the macrocycle the shape of a hollow truncated cone. The cone is formed by the carbon skeletons of the glucose units with glycosidic oxygen atoms in between. The primary hydroxyls of the glucose units are located at the narrow face of the cone and the secondary hydroxyls at the wider face. The primary hydroxyls on the narrow side of the cone can rotate to partially block the cavity. In contrast the secondary hydroxyls are attached by relatively rigid chains and as a consequence they can not rotate. The primary and secondary hydroxyls on the outside of the cyclodextrins make cyclodextrins water-soluble. Cyclodextrins are insoluble in most organic solvents.

Because of the relatively apolar cavity in comparison to the polar exterior, cyclodextrins can form inclusion compounds with hydrophobic guest molecules in aqueous solutions predominantly due to intermolecular interactions. In aqueous solution, the cyclodextrin cavity is occupied by water molecules in an energetically unfavorable polar-apolar association and the driving force for complex formation is the displacement of high energy water molecules by the hydrophobic guest molecule. The most important factor in complexation appears to be the "steric fit" ie., geometric compatibility between the host and the guest. However the stability of the resulting complexes varies with the size of both the guest and the host. The *Stoichiometry* of the guest to host in inclusion complexation is usually 1:1 in aqueous solution. Complexes can also be formed in DMF and DMSO, but they are less stable. However, in some cases complexation can also be formed in solid state.

Cyclodextrins with their hydrophobic cavities mimic enzymes in their capability in binding substrate selectively and catalyze the chemical reactions involving supramolecular catalysis. Cyclodextins became prominent as micro vessels for performing a variety of biomimetic synthetic reactions. Growing interest in different aspects of cyclodextrins resulted in steady increase in original research articles as well as reviews. Various methods that determine the host-guest complex formation include X-ray, fluorimetric measurements, NMR, circular dichroism, ESR, polarography, colorimetry, diffusion across semipermeable membranes and surface strain measurements. Among these methods X-ray and NMR have been established as important and reliable methods to determine molecular encapsulations. Some of the applications of CDs to attain higher selectivities in a variety of organic reactions including multi component synthesis of heterocycles are discussed.

In view of the significance attached to green chemistry and its relevance to the present day problem of global warming, the development of novel, simple, cleaner synthetic protocols is attracting attention in both academic and industrial research, resulting in an ever increasing number of publications or reports on this topic. Designing environ friendly synthetic strategies in water, minimizing the use of harmful, toxic, and flammable organic solvents and hazardous reagents/catalysts, is attaining the priority over other issues. Water has the status of universally acceptable solvent since it is economically affordable, readily available and nontoxic.

However the fundamental problem of performing organic reactions in water is that many organic substrates are hydrophobic and insoluble. These problems can be addressed if the reactions can be planned and executed by following biomimetic approaches through supra-molecular catalysis, involving host-guest complexation, in aqueous medium.

In the present context and of particular interest are water soluble hosts with hydrophobic cavities, which can mimic the enzyme-receptor relationship (enzymatic biochemical reactions). Among various possibilities, cyclodextrins offer wider scope for designing and conducting organic reactions in hydrophobic environment following microencapsulation of the substrate molecules.

To overcome the drawbacks associated with the existing synthetic methodologies, many organic transformations were attempted successfully, by using cyclodextrin as a recyclable activator in aqueous medium. Presently, it is attempted to bring some of the very recent research reports, including certain unpublished results, into this article, focusing mainly on construction of heterocyclic moieties, utilizing cyclodextrin mediated biomimetic approach, in view of the significance attached to heterocyclic chemistry.

2. Furanones

Furan-2(5H)-ones are prominent structural motifs, widely present as a subunit in many natural products isolated from a variety of sources like algae, sponges, plants, insects and animals,. Literature survey indicates that butenolide substructure is present in more than 13,000 natural products and is the core structural unit responsible to induce a wide range of biological properties such as antimicrobial, antifungal, anti-viral HIV-1, anti-inflamatory, and anticancer (De Souza, 2005). It is found in many biologically active natural products such as sarcophine and rubrolide etc., which are isolated from Ritterela rubra, (Miao & Andersen, 1991; Kotora & Negishi, 1997) a colonial tunicate. It is also present in synthetic drug molecules like benfurodil hemisuccinate (Eucilat).

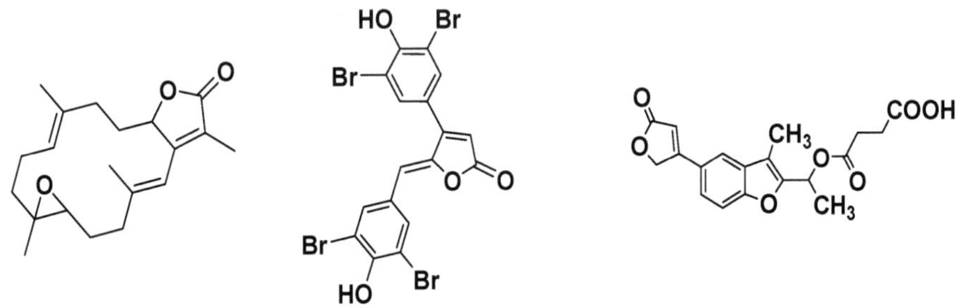

sarcophine

rubrolide

benfurodil hemisuccinate (Eucilat®)

The significant biological activity associated with butenolide synthon, attracted the attention of many researchers to develop numerous synthetic approaches for furan-2(5H)-one derivatives. The preparation of 2(5H)-furanone was also reported by refluxing furfural with hydrogen peroxide followed by oxidation resulting in a mixture of 2(3H) and 2(5H)-furanones (Cao et al., 1996). Chunling Fu et al. described a new method for the synthesis of 4-iodofuran-2(5H)-ones, involving iodolactonisation of allenoates with molecular iodine (Fu & Ma, 2005).

Sweeney et al. developed the first preparation of 3,4-bistributylstannyl 2(5H)-furanones by the reaction of TBS as well as THP protected butynoate with hexabutylditin in the presence of $PdCl_2(PPh_3)_2$ resulting in substituted acrylate intermediate, which upon treatment under a variety of conditions yielded desired furanone system (Hollingworth et al., 1996; Mabon et al., 1999 & 2002) Mauro et al. reported the synthesis of furanone synthon via ring-closing metathesis catalyzed by the first generation Grubbs' catalyst (Bassetti et al., 2005). However these methodologies suffer from certain drawbacks like use of highly volatile flammable organic solvents, costly metal catalysts and multistep protocols. In view of these limitations, development of a novel eco-friendly approach to synthesize furanones is desirable.

Nageswar et al., during their efforts towards developing biomimetic organic synthetic protocols through supra molecular catalysis, utilizing recyclable activator like β-CD, reported a simple, one pot three component, methodology for the synthesis of 3,4,5-

substituted furan-2(5H)-one derivatives from various substituted anilines, benzaldehydes and DEAD in water, in presence of β-CD. This is the first report on the biomimetic synthesis of 3, 4, 5- substituted furan-2(5H)-ones, by the supra molecular catalysis of β-CD, in water (Murthy et al., 2009).

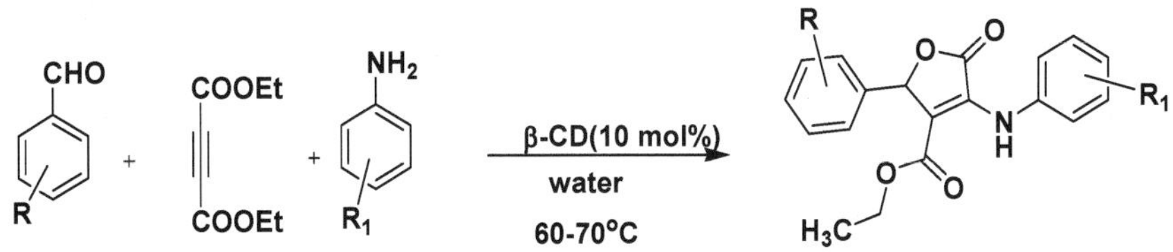

R = 4-CH_3;4-CH_2CH_3;4-OCH_2Ph;4-OCH_3;4-OCH_2CH_3;4-Cl;

R_1 = 4-CH_3;4-Cl;4-F;4-I;4-nC_4H_9;3-Cl;

Synthesis of 3, 4, 5- substituted furan-2(5H)-ones, in presence of β-CD as a supra molecular catalyst in water.

Initially, a model reaction was carried by the insitu formation of β-cyclodextrin complex of aniline in water at 50°C, followed by the addition of diethylacetylenedicarboxylate and benzaldehyde while stirring at 60–70°C to obtain ethyl 2,5-dihydro-5-oxo-2-phenyl-4-(phenylamino) furan-3-carboxylate in almost quantitative yield (85%). No product formation was observed, when the reaction was conducted in neat or in presence of water even after prolonged reaction times. The scope of this novel and interesting transformation to synthesize 3, 4, 5-substituted furan-2(5H)-one derivatives with various substituted anilines and substituted aldehydes was studied by keeping diethylacetylenedicaboxylate as a common substrate. All the reactions were clean, and the products were obtained in high yields (78-88%), with good amount of catalyst recovery. The results indicated that the substitution on the aromatic ring has a substantial role in governing the reactivity of the substrate as well as product yield. The reaction with electron donating groups like methyl, butyl on aniline gave good yield, where as in case of electron withdrawing groups, such as para-chloro and para-fluoro yields decreased. The reaction was observed to be sluggish with aliphatic amines, such as benzyl amines and n-alkyl amines. Structural identification of these products was established by spectral data. No lactone formation was observed in the absence of β-cyclodextrin, even after longer reaction times, establishing the role of β-CD. The formation of 3, 4, 5-substituted furan-2(5H)-ones, catalysed by β-CD was supported by ^1H NMR studies of the inclusion complex between aniline and β-CD. The hydrophobic environment in the cavity of β-CD facilitates the completion of the reaction via aniline/diethylethylenedicarboxylate carbanion, which is stabilized by the primary and secondary -OH groups of β-CD. This stabilized carbanion further reacts with aldehyde resulting in the formation of 3, 4, 5-substituted furan-2(5H)-one.

These reactions were conducted with a catalytic amount (10 mol %) of β-CD in water. Inclusion complex was prepared by taking β-CD and aniline in 1:1 ratio for the purpose of NMR studies. NMR spectrum of β-CD/aniline inclusion complex indicated upfield shift of aromatic protons as well as amine protons of aniline, due to the inclusion of aniline inside β-CD cavity. Apart from the upfield shift of aniline protons due to the incorporation of an aromatic ring inside the β-CD cavity, the protons located in the hydrophobic cavity of β-CD

cavity (C3-H and C5-H) were also shifted upfield due to magnetic anisotropy, caused by the aniline molecule (Grigoras & Conduruta, 2006). β-CD was recovered and reused for further runs of these reactions.
This biomimetic methodology for the synthesis of furanone derivatives involving CD as a supramolecular catalyst in aqueous medium may have wider applications in green chemistry protocols.

3. Pyrroles

The pyrrole structural motif widely occurs in nature and represents itself in many biologically important molecules such as porphyrins, alkaloids and coenzymes (Sundberg, 1996). Due to its application in many important areas, pyrrole skeleton has attracted the attention of many researchers globally. Paal-Knorr synthesis, Knorr pyrrole synthesis and Hantzsch synthesis were some of the classical approaches for the preparation of pyrrroles. Though over the years numerous synthetic strategies were reported for the preparation of pyrrole derivatives (Shindo et al., 2007; Cyr et al., 2007; Binder & Kirsch, 2006), most of them involve multistep synthetic processes, which reduce the overall yields. Even though recently a few one-step syntheses (Shiraishi et al., 1999) are reported for the preparation of pyrrroles, these suffer from several drawbacks such as use of toxic flammable organic solvents, costly transition metal catalysts and longer reaction times. To overcome these shortcomings associated with the existing methodologies, developing mild and environmentally benign synthetic protocols involving water as solvent for the synthesis of pyrrroles is desirable. Use of a recyclable catalyst as a part of green chemistry approach will be an additional advantage. Nageswar et al. during their efforts towards developing novel β-cyclodextrin-promoted synthetic strategies attempted for the first time simple versatile biomimetic approach for the synthesis of substituted pyrrroles from readily available building blocks in aqueous medium under supramolecular catalysis (Murthy et al., 2009).

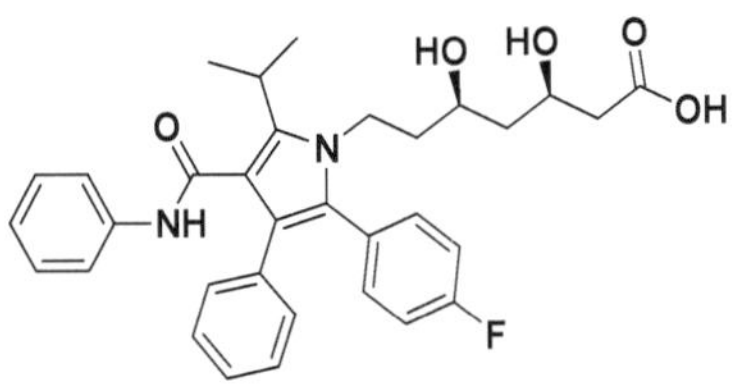

Atorvastatin

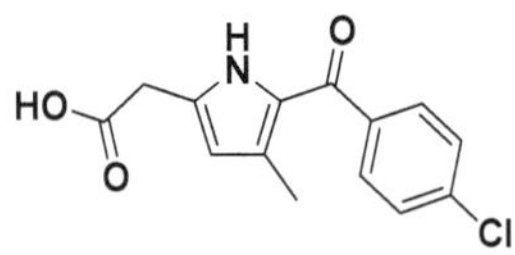

Zomepirac

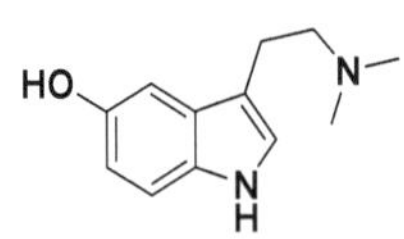

Bufotenin

Initially, phenacyl bromide is solubilised in aqueous solution containing β-CD at 50^0 C. To this β-CD-phenacyl bromide complex was added pentane-2, 4-dione followed by aniline. The entire reaction mixture was stirred at 60^0 C-70^0 C till the reaction goes for completion, giving the 1, 2, 3, 5-substituted pyrrole in excellent yield (86%). To study the scope of this interesting one pot three component biomimetic approach for the preparation of pyrrole derivatives, several reactions were carried out under similar reaction conditions, changing the amine component. 4-Methyl; 4-methoxy; 3, 4-dimethoxy; 4-chloro; 4-fluoro; 4-n butyl anilines, benzyl amine, 3-methoxy benzyl amine and 3-bromo benzyl amine were also utilized as reactants.

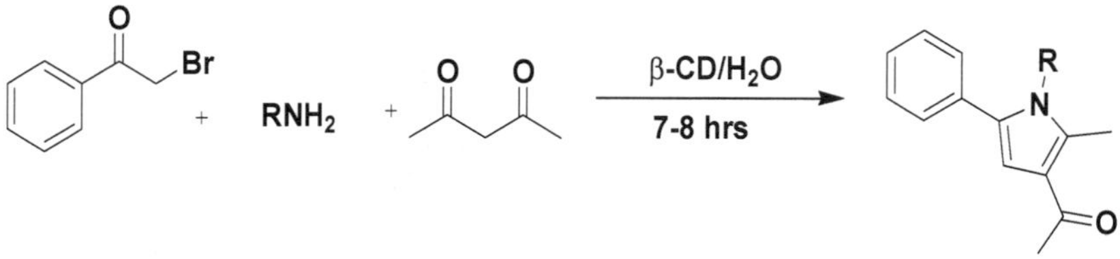

R = Ph; 4-Chloro phenyl;4-Methyl phenyl; 4-Fluoro phenyl; 4-Methoxy phenyl; 3,4-Dimethoxyphenyl; 4-n-Butylphenyl;Benzyl;3-Bromo benzyl; 3-Methoxy benzyl; 2,6-Diethyl phenyl

Synthesis of substituted pyrrole derivatives by one-pot three component approach using β-cyclodextrin as a recyclable catalyst:

It was observed that aromatic amines with electron-donating groups in *p*-position gave excellent yields, where as electron- withdrawing groups in *p*-position gave relatively reduced yields. The reactions with aliphatic amines resulted in still lower yields.

The role of β-cyclodextrin in these reactions was to solubilise and activate phenacyl bromides through hydrogen-bonding interactions, thereby promoting the reaction with pentane-2, 4-dione to complete the reaction sequence with an amine. Reaction was not observed in the absence of β-CD. β-CD was recovered and used to run subsequent cycles of the reaction. A reaction mechanism via the formation of β-CD/phenacyl bromide complex was suggested, which was further supported by the preparation and characterization studies on β-CD/phenacyl bromide inclusion complex, which was obtained by taking β-cyclodextrin and phenacyl bromide in equimolar quantities.^{1}H-NMR studies of the inclusion complex between β-CD and phenacyl bromide indicated the upfield shift of H-C(3) and H-C(5) of β-CD.

This novel, simple, and environmentally benign methodology following the biomimetic approach, reported for the first time involving β-cyclodextrin as a recyclable activator by Nageswar et al., may be a useful application to pyrrole chemistry.

4. Oxindoles

Oxindole chemistry has been extensively investigated, as it is an intermediary system between indole and isatin, two prominent structural frame works in organic chemistry. Isatin was converted to oxindole via dioxindole, first by Baeyer, establishing the relationship between the compounds. Reduction of isatin can be effected with a wide range of reducing agents such as sodium amalgam, zinc in acetic acid or zinc in hydrochloric acid or nickel catalyst. Oxidation of indoles and its derivatives by various oxidizing agents such as $KMnO_4$, HNO_3, H_2SO_4, etc. result in oxindole skeleton.

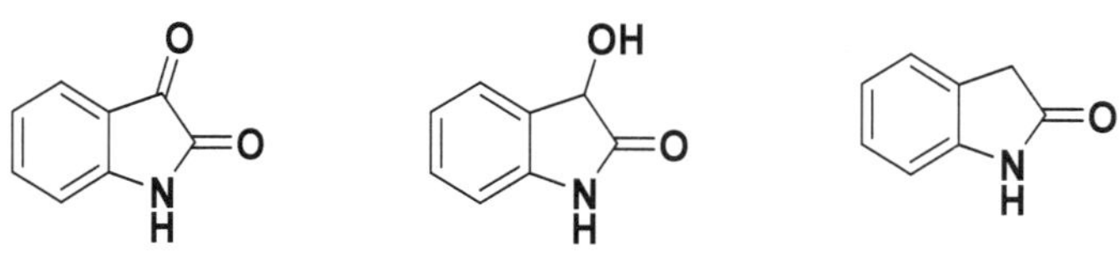

isatin **dioxindole** **oxindole**

The Baeyer's first total synthesis of oxindole from phenyl acetic acid via 2-nitrophenyl acetic acid was further modified and improved by different researchers such as Hahn, Hinsberg as well as Brunnes.

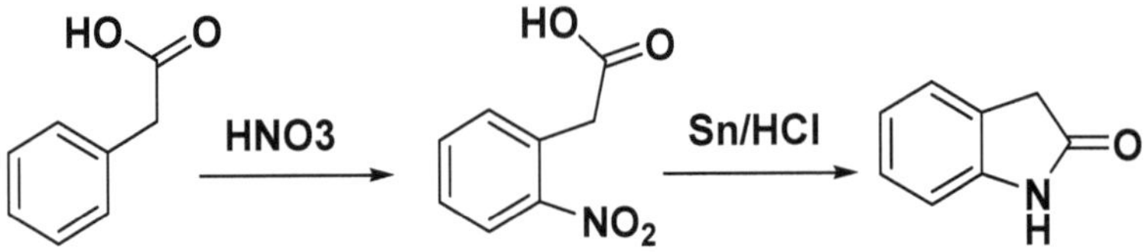

Hinsberg obtained oxindole by the reaction of aromatic amine with sodium bisulfite addition compound of glyoxal, where as Brunner prepared oxindoles by reacting an acylphenyl hydrazine in presence of alkaline reagents resulting in elimination of NH_3. In Stolle's synthesis of oxindole, α-halo acetanilide is heated with anhydrous $AlCl_3$ resulting in the cyclisation with elimination of HCl.

Recently a series of substituted oxindole derivatives were synthesized and evaluated for growth harmone releasing activity (Tokunaga et al., 2001). Gallagher et al., synthesized and reported 4-[2-(Di-n-propyl amino) ethyl]-2(3H)-indolone (SK&F 101468) as a potent and selective prejunctional dopamine receptor agonist. (Gallagher et al., 1985). A series of N-(3-piperidinyl)-2-indolines were synthesized and evaluated as a new structural class of nociceptin receptor (NOP) ligands (Zaveri et al., 2004). Spirotrypro statins A&B, isolated from the fermentation broth of Aspergillus fumigatus exhibited cell cycle inhibition and some of their biologically promising analogues were also reported (Edmondson et al., 1999).

The spirooxindole is a prominent structural component present in a number of natural products, such as coerules-cine, elacomine, horsfiline, welwitindolinone A, spirotryprostatin A, alstonisine, and surugatoxin. These compounds exhibit potent cytotoxic activity and are also known as estrogen-receptor modulators, h5-HT6 serotonin receptors, oxytocin antagonists, and antiproliferative agents. Due to their significant biological activity several synthetic methodologies have been developed for the construction of spirooxindole system. In view of the growing focus on environ friendly processes, Rao et al. revisited the synthesis of spirooxindoles by utilizing the supra molecular catalytic biomimetic approach (Sridhar et al., 2009).

Literature reports on the synthesis of spirooxindole described so far by the three component condensation reaction of isatin, malononitrile or methyl cyanoacetate, and 1, 3-dicarbonyl compounds have certain limitations as they involve the use of hazardous organic solvents, acidic or basic conditions, transition metal catalysts, surfactants, and microwave irradiation. Consequently the development of environ-friendly approaches for these spirooxindoles derivatives under neutral conditions using a recyclable activator in water is desirable.

A. Rao et al. explored the aqueous-phase synthesis of spirooxindole derivatives by the three component reaction of isatin, malononitrile, and dimedone under neutral conditions catalysed by β-cyclodextrin.

In general, these reactions were conducted via the formation of β-CD complex of isatin in water. This was followed by the successive addition of malononitrile and dimedone, and stirring at 60^0 C. The corresponding spirooxindole derivatives were obtained in excellent yields (84%-91%) after 4-6 h. This simple methodology reported by Rao et al. was compatible with several substituted isatins having different functionalities such as bromo, methyl, nitro, phenyl, and benzyl groups. It was observed that reaction of methyl cyanoacetate with isatin and dimedone under similar conditions resulted in the expected product in very good yields. All these reactions proceeded efficiently without any byproduct formation. β-cyclodextrin can be easily recovered and reused.

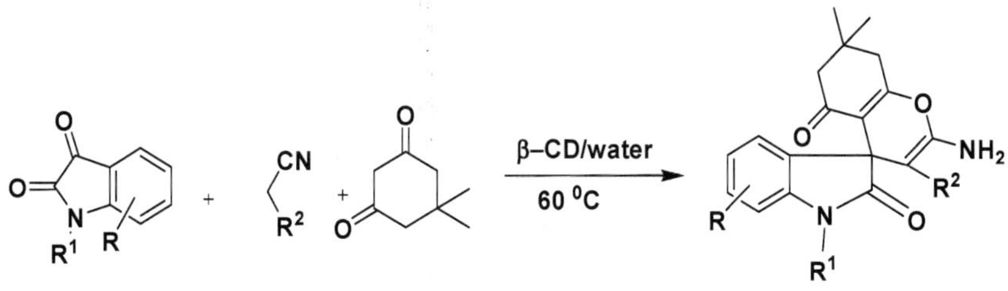

R = H, 4-Br, 6-Br, 5-CH_3,5-NO_2
R^1 = CH_3,CH_2Ph,Ph
R^2 = CN, COOMe

β-CD-catalyzed one-pot multi-component synthesis of spirooxindoles:

The scope of this methodology has been extended to the reaction of 4-hydroxy coumarin and barbituric acid under similar reaction conditions to obtain spirooxindole derivatives in impressive yields. Isolation of β-CD-isatin complex confirmed the complexation process. It was observed from ^{1}H NMR studies (D_2O) of β-CD, β-CD-isatin complex, and freeze-dried reaction mixture of isatin-malononitrile-dimedone, that there was an up-field shift of H3 and H5 protons of cyclodextrin in the β-CD–isatin complex as compared to β- CD.This proves the formation of an inclusion complex of isatin with β-CD from the secondary side of cyclodextrin. Authors observed that the spectra of the reaction mixture of the β-CD–isatin complex after the addition of malononitrile and dimedone after 2 h, showed an upfield shift of the CD H6 proton. This confirms that the reaction proceeded by the complexation of malononitrile and dimedone from the primary side of cyclodextrin and that isatin is ideally placed for the condensation with malononitrile and dimedone in the cyclodextrin cavity.

In the absence of cyclodextrin, the reaction was observed to proceed in lower yields even after longer reaction times. During complexation with β-CD the reactivity of the keto group of isatin increased due to intermolecular hydrogen bonding with the CD-hydroxyl groups. This facilitated the Knoevenagel condensation with malononitrile to form an isatylidene malononitrile, which undergoes the established sequence of reactions successively such as Michael addition of dimedone, and the cycloaddition of hydroxyl group to the cyano moiety to form the desired spirooxindole derivatives.

This neutral aqueous phase one-pot three-component biomimetic synthesis of various spirooxindole derivatives by the reaction of isatin and 1, 3-dicarbonyl compounds, is an impressive addition to green chemistry.

B. α-Hydroxyphosphonates are prominent class of biologically active compounds as well as useful reactive intermediates (Maryanoff & Reitz, 1989). In view of significant biological importance associated with α-hydroxy phophonates, this synthon has attracted enhanced research interest. These are extensively used in pharmaceutical applications such as enzyme inhibitors of renin, HIV protease and EPSP synthase (Patel et al., 1995). They also exhibited potential biological activities, such as antibacterial, antiviral, anti-inflammatory, laxative, growth hormonal, and anticancer activities (Stowasser et al., 1992). They are also used in the synthesis of 1, 2-diketones from acid chlorides, α-ketophosphonates and α-aminophosponates (Kaboudin, 2003; Firouzabadi et al., 2004; Iorga et al., 1999).

Generally the synthesis of α-hydroxy phosphonates involve the reaction of aldehydes or ketones with dialkyl or trialkyl phosphites in the presence of acidic or basic catalysts. α-Hydroxy phosphonates can also be synthesised from Tris(trimethylsilyl) phosphite but it requires elevated temperature under anhydrous reaction conditions. However, these methodologies suffer from several drawbacks such as the use of hazardous solvents, acidic conditions and metal catalysts. Consequently, the development of environfriendly biomimetic approach under neutral conditions for the synthesis of α-hydroxy phosphonates is desirable. Aqueous phase organic synthesis has recently become the focus in the development of green synthetic protocols, and it can be made more sophisticated if they can be performed under supramolecular catalysis.

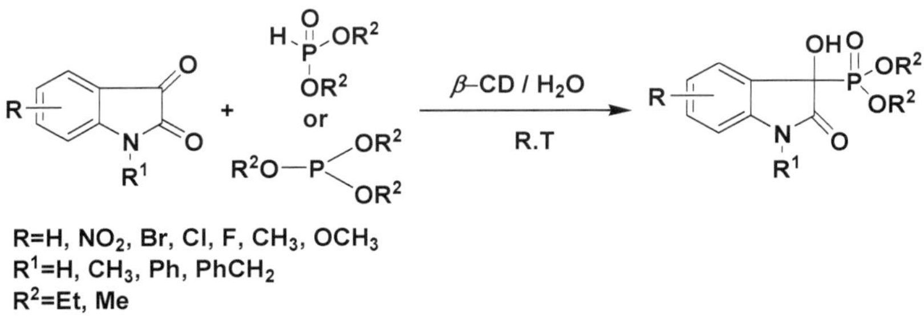

β-CD catalyzed one-pot multi-component synthesis of α¹-oxindole-α-hydroxy phosphonates

Due to the various biological activities associated with various oxindole derivatives, and α-hydroxy phosphonates, Nageswar et al. have attempted for the first time a simple aqueous phase biomimetic synthesis of α¹-oxindole-α-hydroxy phosphonates by the reaction of isatin derivatives with dialkyl or trialkyl phosphites under neutral conditions in presence of β-cyclodextrin, as a supramolecular catalyst (Shankar et al., 2010).

Initially a reaction was conducted by the *insitu* formation of the β-CD complex of the isatin in water followed by the addition of dialkyl or trialkyl phosphite. The reaction mixture was stirred at room temperature to give the corresponding α¹-oxindole-α-hydroxy phosphonates in impressive yields (86-94%). Scope of this reaction was extended to involve various substituted isatin. Reactions performed under similar conditions proceeded efficiently without the need of any metal or acid catalyst. Even though the reactions occurred in presence of α-CD and γ-CD,with lesser yields, inexpensive and easily accessible β-CD was selected as the mediator.Different substituted oxindoles synthesised by this simple and practicable methodology were characterized by their spectral data.

The catalytic efficiency of cyclodextrins for these reactions was established as no reaction was observed in the absence of cyclodextrin. Evidence for complexation between the isatin and cyclodextrin was deduced from NMR studies. A comparison of the ^{1}H NMR spectra (D_2O) of β-CD, β-CD: isatin complex revealed, the upfield shift of H3 and H5 protons of cyclodextrin in the β-CD: isatin complex as compared to β-CD. This confirmed the formation of an inclusion complex of isatin with β-CD. During complex phenomenon the keto group of isatin will be activated due to the inter molecular hydrogen bonding between CD-hydroxyl groups and isatin carbonyl, which facilitates the addition of phosphite. No by product formation was observed and the β-CD was recovered for further runs of these reactions. Thus authors developed for the first time a simple neutral aqueous phase biomimetic synthetic protocol for the preparation of various α^1-oxindole-α-hydroxy phosphonates by the reaction of the corresponding isatins with dialkyl or trialkyl phosphites in the presence of β-cyclodextrin. This novel methodology will be an useful addition to indole chemistry.

5. Thiazoles

Thiazoles are a prominent class of N-containing heterocyclic compounds of immense interest to medicinal and industrial chemists as these play a significant role in nature and have wider applications in agricultural and medicinal chemistry. For example the thiazole in vitamin B serves as an electron sink, and its coenzyme form is important for the decarboxylation of α-keto acids and is present in various natural products and herbicides. This important and useful structural motif has found application in drug development, as these exhibit diverse biological activities such as anti-glutamate, anti-Parkinson (Benazzouz et al., 1995), anti-microbial (Palmer et al., 1971), anthelmintic, anti-inflammatory (Haviv et al., 1988), anti-hyperlipidemic, anti-hypertension (Patt et al., 1992), and anti-oxidant properties as well as inhibition of enzymes such as acetylcholine esterase (Nagel et al., 1995), aldose reductase (Mylari et al., 1991), lipoxygenase (Hadjipavlou-Litina & Geronikaki,1998), ATPase (Sohn et al., 1999), and HCV helicase (phoon et al., 2001). Aminothiazoles are reported as a new class of adenosine receptor antagonists and ligands of estrogen receptors.

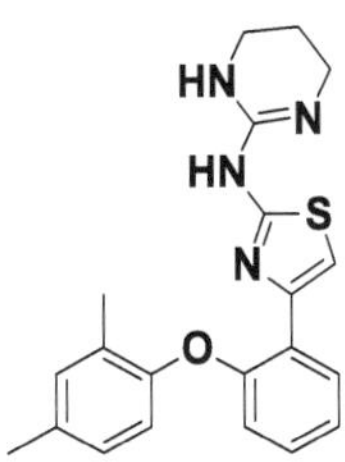

Abafungin
Broadspectrum
Anti-fungal agent

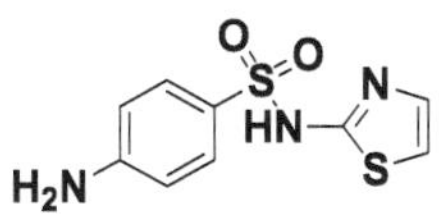

Sulfathiazole
Anti-microbial Drug

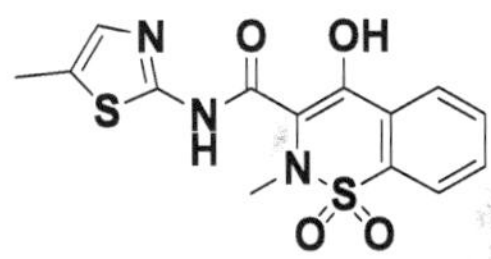

Meloxicam
Non-steroidal
Anti-inflammatory Drug

Several research groups worked extensively on thiazoles to develop various synthetic methodologies. Among these Hantzsch synthesis is the most widely used and applied, which involves the reaction of α-halo ketone or aldehyde with thioamide

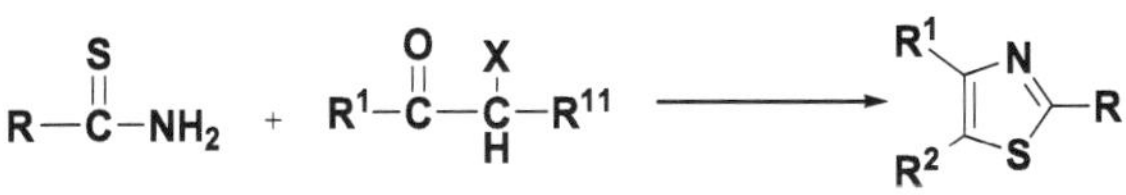

$R=NH_2$, SH, $S\text{-}NH_4$ X=Cl,Br, I

The scope for a wider selection of readily available/accessible reactants resulted in broader applicability of Hantzsch thiazole synthesis, which had fewer limitations. With a proper choice of reactants, thiazoles with alkyl, aryl or heterocyclic moieties attached to any of the three carbons of the thiazole nucleus can be prepared in this methodology. Thio amide can also be replaced by thiourea or ammonium dithiocarbamate, or dithiocarbamate, or dithiocarbamic acid or mono thio-carbamic acid or it's o-esters. Based on Hantzsch concept, some newer methods, such as cycloaddition of tosylmethyl isocyanide to thione derivatives (Bergstrom et al., 1994), oxidation of thiazoline and thiazolidine ring systems (Martin & Hu, 1999), the Ugi reaction (Kazmaier & Ackermann, 2005) and others (Mustafa et al., 2004), have been developed.

Other methodologies developed include Pd-mediated coupling process (Sapountzis et al., 2005; Lipshutz et al., 2004; Nicolaou et al., 1999), nucleophilic reactions of Lithiothiazoles (Dondoni, 1998), solid supported synthesis to generate small organic molecule libraries (Kazzouli et al., 2002) and solution phase preparation of 2-aminothiazole combinatorial libraries (Bailey et al., 1996).

Many of these synthetic methods involve the use of hazardous organic solvents, high temperatures, longer reaction times or lower yields. To overcome some of these limitations and while developing biomimetic approaches through supramolecular catalysis using cyclodextrin as a recyclable catalyst in aqueous phase, Rao et al. reported three different protocols for the synthesis of thiazole derivatives.

A. Different β-ketoesters were reacted with thiourea in presence of β-CD and NBS in water at 50 ^{0}C to obtain 4-substituted -2-amino-thiazole-5-carboxylates in excellent yields. In general these reactions were carried out by the insitu formation of β-CD complex of β-ketoesters in water at 50 ^{0}C, followed by the addition of N-bromo succinimide and thiourea. The reaction mixture was stirred for 1-2 hrs, and worked out to isolate expected products. In these reactions, the treatment of β-ketoesters with NBS may form α-bromo-β-keto esters as intermediates, which undergo cyclization with thiourea resulting in the thiazole derivatives. These reactions are simple, straight forward and high yielding protocols. The role of β-CD is to dissolve and activate the β-ketoester molecule through hydrogen-bonding, to promote the reaction. Solubility problems, longer reaction hours, low yields or mixture of products were the drawbacks when β-CD was not used. This efficient biomimetic process is a valuable addition for green chemistry, and may find wide spread applications (Narender et al., 2007).

B. Various phenyl tosylates were reacted with thiourea in presence of β-CD in water at room temperature to get 2, 4-disubstituted thiazoles in very good yields. In general, the reaction was carried out by the insitu formation of the β-CD complex of β-keto tosylate in water followed by the addition of thioamide/thiourea and stirring for 1–3 h at room temperature to give the corresponding thiazole or aminothiazole derivatives. Several examples were prepared, illustrating this simple and practical methodology. These reactions proceeded smoothly without the formation of any by products. β-CD can be easily recovered and reused. Solubility problems, longer reaction hours, lower yields, or mixture of products were the drawbacks when β-CD was not used. This simple, practicable biomimetic approach is an useful addition for green chemistry. The formation of the inclusion complex between β-ketotosylate molecule and β-CD results in chemical shift changes of cyclodextrin. The inclusion of an aromatic guest into the cyclodextrin cavity results in upfield shifts of the H-3 and H-5 of cyclodextrin, due to the ring-current effect of the aromatic ring (Demarco & Thakkar, 1970). Study of ^{1}H NMR (DMSO) of the β-CD, β-CD-phenacyl tosylate complex, and freeze-dried reaction mixtures of β-CD–phenacyl tosylate–thiourea indicated up field shift of H-3 and H-5 protons in the complex as well as in the reaction mass after 30 min. Hydrogen bonding of the tosyl group with cyclodextrin hydroxyl functionality facilitated the attack by the substrate nucleophile initiating the reaction to take place. Significance of this procedure are operational simplicity, excellent yields, and recyclability of the catalyst (Kumar et al., 2007).

C. Rao et al. reported the biomimetic synthesis of thiazole derivatives by reacting thioamide/thiourea and various substituted phenacyl bromides in presence of β-cyclodextrin in aqueous medium at 50 ºC with no other additive. In general the reactions were carried out by the insitu formation the β-cyclodextrin complex of phenacyl bromide derivatives in water followed by the addition of thiourea or thioamide to give the corresponding thiazoles and aminothiazoles. The reactions were performed smoothly without the formation of any byproducts and the expected new products were obtained in impressive yields. These thiazole derivatives were identified with the help of various analytical techniques. The role of CD in these reactions appears to be to solubilise phenacyl bromide derivatives by complexing them and activating the molecules to promote the reaction with thioamide/thiourea. In the absence of cyclodextrin the reaction has lot of drawbacks such as solubility problems, longer reaction times and very low yields. This novel methodology overcomes all these limitations, apart from formation of unwanted byproducts and will be an interesting addition to biomimetic chemistry.

6. Selenazoles

Selenazoles have been widely studied as reactive synthons as well as for their potential biological activity. Among them 1, 3- selenazoles are of pharmacological importance due to their cancerostatic and antibiotic activity (Goldstein et al., 1990; Srivastava & Robins, 1983). The C-glycosyl selenazofurin is an important example for antibacterial activity. 2-Amino-1,3-selenazoles are good superoxide anion-scavengers. Various synthetic methodologies have been developed for the selenium-containing heterocyclic compounds due to their interesting applications (Back, 1999; Wirth, 2000). These selenazoles have been synthesised mainly by the application of Hantzsch procedure.The existing protocols have a number of limitations (Koketsu et al., 2006, 2005 & 2004) such as the use of inert atmosphere, anhydrous organic solvents, basic conditions, longer reaction times, and lower yields. Selenourea, an important reactant in these methods, is an air and light sensitive compound. In view of these drawbacks there is a need to develop a mild and ecofriendly biomimetic methodology for these important compounds, using a recyclable supramolecular host.

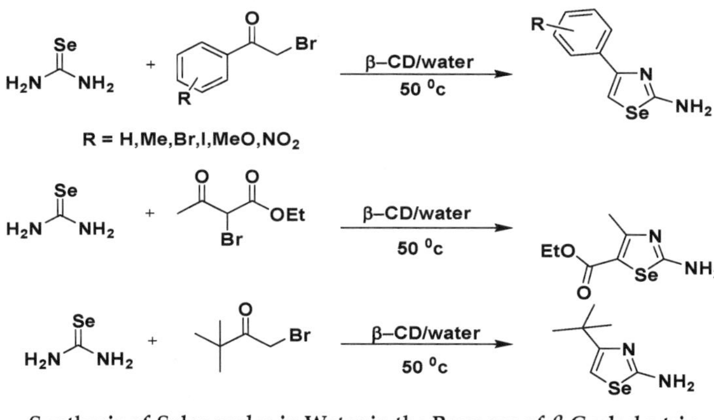

Synthesis of Selenazoles in Water in the Presence of *β*-Cyclodextrin

To overcome some of the limitations in the existing methodologies, Rama rao et al., developed simple biomimetic approach through supramolecular catalysis, for the synthesis of 2-amino-1, 3-selenazoles from α-bromoketones, and selenourea in the presence of β-cyclodextrin (Narender et al., 2007). In this investigation the reactions were conducted by the in situ formation of β-cyclodextrin complex of α-bromoketone in water at 50 °C, followed by the addition of selenourea. The reaction mixture was stirred to give the corresponding selenazoles in quantitative yields (86-95%). During the study, it was observed that the aromatic α-bromoketones (substituted phenacyl bromides) gave comparatively higher yields than those with aliphatic α-bromoketones. For example, Ethyl 2-amino-4-methyl-1, 3-selenazole-5-carboxylate was obtained in 87% yield whereas 4(4-methoxyphenyl)-2-amino-1, 3-selenazole-5-carboxylate was produced in 95% yield. The reactions proceeded without the formation of any unwanted side products. The products were characterized by spectroscopic data. β-Cyclodextrin was recovered and used for further runs. Even though these reactions take place in presence of α-cyclodextrin (α-CD), *β*-CD was used as the activator as it is inexpensive and easily available. Solubility problems, longer reaction times, lower yields were some of the drawbacks observed, when β-cyclodextrin was not used. When only catalytic amount of *β*-CD (0.1 mmol per mole of the substrate) was used it had no impact on the reaction, since the yields of the product obtained were the same as observed in the absence of *β*-CD. The study indicated the substantial role of cyclodextrin as a supra molecular catalyst in these reactions. It was also established through ^{1}H NMR studies with phenacyl bromide as a representative example. Upfield shift of H3 and H5 protons of *β*-CD in the case of *β*-CD-PB complex as compared to *β*-CD was explained as due to the screening effect of the phenyl ring of phenacyl bromide included in the hydrophobic cavity of β-CD. The upfield shifts prove the formation of an inclusion complex of phenacyl bromide with *β*-CD (D'Souza &Lipkowitz, 1998). With the addition of selenourea (after 20 and 40 min), there was a further upfield shift of the H3 and H5 protons. This increase in the upfield character of H3 and H5 protons of *β*-CD in *β*-CD-phenacylbromide complex was explained as the enhanced aromatic nature in the phenyl selenazole derivative. Thus, in this investigation, *β*-cyclodextrin appears to solubilise and activate phenacyl bromides and promote the reaction.

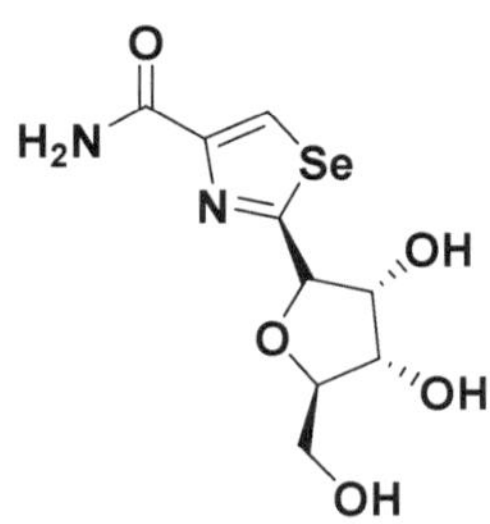

Selenazofurin

Thus the authors have investigated for the first time that selenazole formation can be promoted by *β*-cyclodextrin in water, making this methodology as a useful addition to the cyclodextrin mediated biomimetic organic synthesis.

7. Quinoline derivatives

Quinolines are N-containing heterocycles found in many natural products such as quinine, camptothecin etc, and several other drug molecules. They exhibit remarkable biological activities like anti-malarial, anti-inflammatory, anti-asthmatic, anti-bacterial, anti-hypertensive, anti-tubercular, anti-alzheimer, anti-HIV, and anti-cancer (Michael, 2007; Suresh et al., 2009). In addition, quinolines are valuable synthons, used for the preparation of nano and mesostructures with enhanced electronic and photonic properties (Zhang et al., 1999; Jenekhe et al., 2001). Therefore, quinoline ring system developed as an important target for extensive research in synthetic organic chemistry.

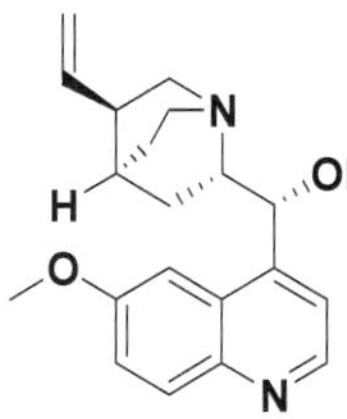

Quinine

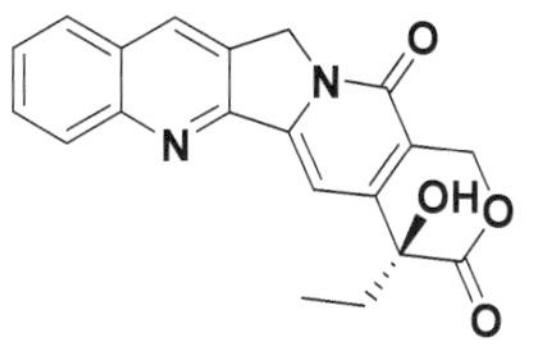

Camptothecin

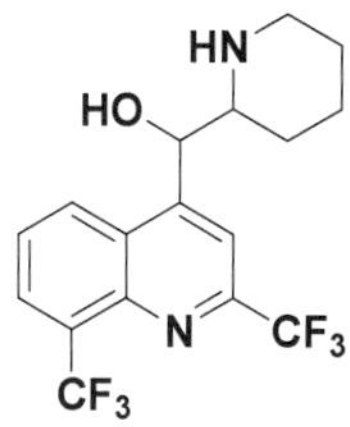

Mefloquine

Skraup, Combes, Friedlander, Doebner-VonMiller syntheses, are some of the well known methodologies for the synthesis of quinoline structural frames. Many new synthetic protocols are being reported frequently using various starting materials. Recently Gabriele (Gabriele et al., 2007) synthesized substituted quinolines from 2-aminoaryl ketones by initial reaction with Grignard reagent and further cyclization in presence of Cu/Pd catalysts. Francis (Francis et al., 2008) reported quinoline synthesis from 2-aminobenzyl alcohol and a variety of ketones catalysed by ruthenium catalysts. Xin-Yuan (Xin-Yuan et al., 2007) introduced gold catalysed quinoline synthesis under microwave-assisted conditions. Lewis acids(Hu et al., 2003; McNaughton & Miller, 2003; Zhang & Wu, 2007), Bronsted acids(Muscia et al., 2006), molecular iodine(Wu et al., 2006), proline (Jiang et al., 2008), ionic liquids (Dabiri et al., 2008) and transition metals (Martinez et al., 2007;Gabriele et al., 2007; Vieira &Alper, 2007; Cho & Ren, 2007) were some of the catalysts involved in different synthetic protocols for quinoline structural motif. However many of the aforementioned reactions require strong acids or bases, toxic flammable organic solvents, or hazardous/ expensive catalysts and elevated temperatures. These reaction conditions are also tedious and yields are low, even after prolonged reaction times.

In view of these drawbacks, it is desirable to attempt the synthesis of these bioactive molecular frame works, by environ friendly biomimetic synthetic protocols of simple nature. There are few reports (Taylor & Heindel, 1967; Hendrickson et al., 1964; James & Fanta, 1962; Bryce et al., 1983) in literature especially for the preparation of 4-substituted quinolone-2, 3-dicarboxylates. Taylor synthesized quinoline-2, 3-dicarboxylates from 2-aminobenzophenone and dimethyl acetylenedicarboxylate in benzene under reflux conditions. As 2-amino acetophenone did not react with DMAD in one pot, basic conditions (NaOMe in anhydrous MeOH) were used for the enamine adduct to cyclise in 26 hrs.

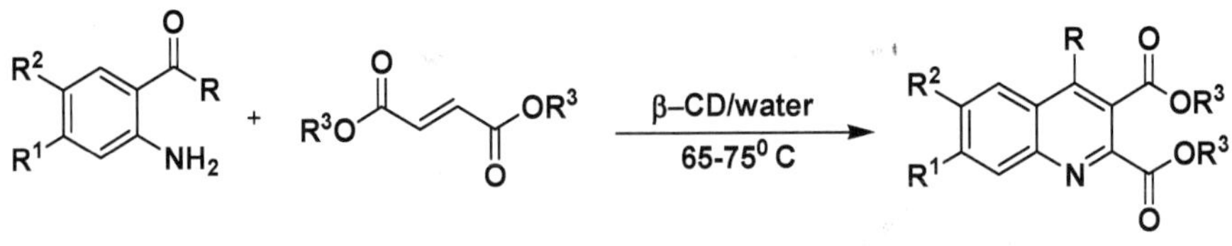

R= H,Me,Ph,2-Cl-C_6H_4; R^1=H, Br, OMe; R^2=H, Cl, OMe; R^3=Me, Et.

Synthesis of 4-substituted quinoline-2, 3-dicarboxylates by using β-cyclodextrin under neutral conditions in aqueous medium:

While exploring biomimetic approaches through supramolecular catalysis in investigating various organic transformations , Nageswar et al. attempted to prepare several substituted quinolone-2,3-dicarboxylates using β-cyclodextrin (β-CD) as a supra molecular catalyst in aqueous medium (Madhav et al., 2010).

Initially the reaction between 2-aminobenzophenone and dimethyl acetylenedicarboxylate was carried out in water catalyzed by β-CD to obtain dimethyl 4-phenylquinoline-2, 3-dicarboxylate in one pot at 75 ⁰C in 85% yield. The desired quinoline derivatives were obtained in an almost quantitative yields, in shorter reaction times. The reaction did not proceed in the absence of β-CD. Scope of the reaction was extended to include various 2-amino carbonyl compounds as substrates, and all these reactions proceeded to give the expected quinoline compounds in very good yields. Only trace of the product was isolated after longer reaction times, when 5-nitro-2-aminobenzophenone was used as a reactant. These reactions were also extended to cover diethyl acetylenedicarboxylate. Di (tert-butyl) acetylenedicarboxylate did not react under similar experimental conditions.

In general, the reactions carried out were simple, clean, and efficient. It was observed that the substitution played a significant role in governing the reactivity of the substrate. Experiments indicated that the reactions with 2-aminoacetophenone resulted in higher yields of the quinoline derivatives when compared to the reactions with 2-amino benzophenones. Among the 2-aminoacetophenones, unsubstituted 2-aminoacetophenone afforded good yield, and 4, 5-methylenedioxy-2-aminoacetophenone resulted in lower yield. Reactions with substituted 2-aminobenzophenones resulted in lower yields compared to unsubstituted 2-aminobenzophenone. Reactions with dimethyl acetylenedicarboxylate (DMAD) resulted in higher yields when compared to those with diethyl acetylenedicarboxylate (DEAD).

^{1}H-NMR studies supported the formation of complexation between 2-aminobenzophenone and β-cyclodextrin. The reactions were carried out with 0.5 equiv. of β-CD, and detailed investigation of complexation studies were undertaken with β-CD/2-aminobenzophenone in 1:1 ratio as a representative example. Comparative study of the ^{1}H-NMR of β-CD, β-CD-2-aminobenzophenone, indicated downfield shift of H-C(3) and H-C(5) of cyclodextrin in the β-CD -2-amino benzophenone and β-CD–2-amino benzophenone-DMAD complex, compared to β-CD, confirming the formation of an inclusion complex of 2-aminobenzophenone with β-CD. During complexation of 2-aminobenzophenone, β-CD solubilises the reactant, activates the carbonyl group and helps in the completion of the reaction with DMAD/DEAD. As usual β-CD can be recovered and reused. This ecofriendly biomimetic protocol for the synthesis of quinoline-2,3-dicarboxylates, is a useful addition to green chemistry.

8. Chromenes

Even though several potential applications in organic synthesis as well as bio-organic chemistry are associated with phosphonate functionality, which is a 'bioisostere' of ester moiety, derivatization through formation of phosphorus–carbon bond to obtain chromenyl phosphonates is not much explored (Moonen et al., 2004).

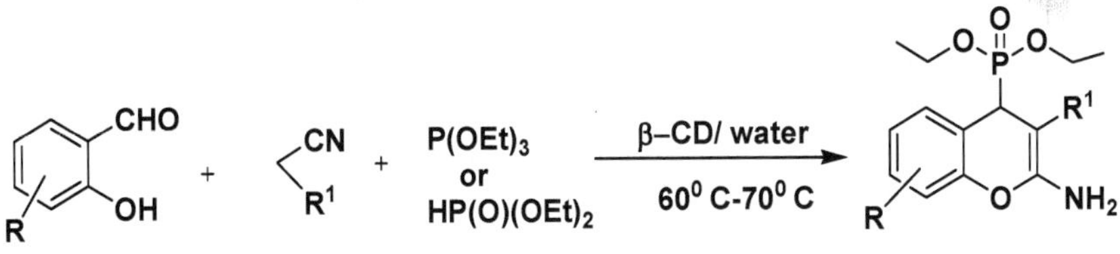

R= Cl,Br,I,OH,OMe; R^1= CN, COOEt

Synthesis of 2-amino-3-cyano-4H-chromen-4-yl phosphonate derivatives

Chromenes are a prominent class of compounds widely present in many natural products and are used in agrochemicals, cosmetics, and pigments (Ellis, 1977). Some of these 2-amino-4H-chromene derivatives are reported as Bcl-2 antagonists which are discovered through fluorescent polarization (FP) and exhibit synergy with several anticancer therapies under diverse mechanism of action (Das et al., 2009; Doshi et al., 2006). Limited number of synthetic methodologies have been reported till now for the synthesis of 2-amino-4H-chromenes by using various catalysts and additives. Indium (III) chloride was used as a lewis acid catalyst by Perumal etal in the synthesis of (2-amino- 3-cyano-4H-chromene-4-yl) phosphonic acid diethyl ester (Jayashree et al., 2009). Nageswar et al. in continuation of their efforts towards developing biomimetic organic synthetic approaches through supramolecular catalysis involving recyclable promoter such as β-CD, described a simple one pot three component preparation of 2-amino 4H-chromen-4-yl phosphonates from several substituted salicylaldehydes, malononitrile/ethyl cyano acetate and triethyl phosphate or diethyl phosphonate. This is the first report on the synthesis of these chromen phosphonate derivatives by biomimetic synthetic strategy using β-cyclodextrin in water, under neutral conditions (Murthy et al., 2010).

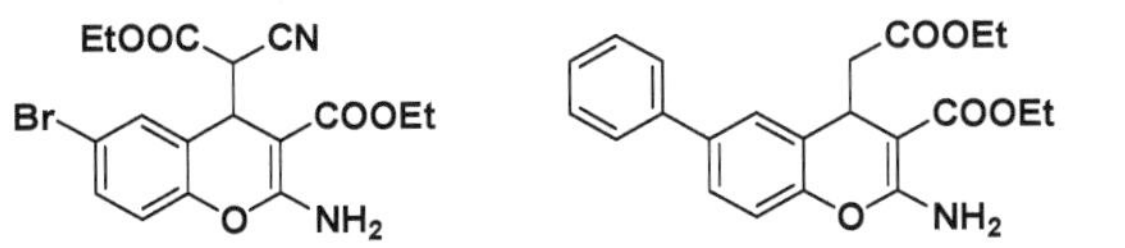

Structures of Bcl-2 protein antagonists

Initially when authors attempted the synthesis of 2-amino-4H-chromen-4-yl phosphonate derivatives in water under catalyst-free conditions, they were not successful in getting the desired product. It was observed that when salicylaldehyde was solubilised in aqueous solution of β-CD at 50⁰ C, β-CD-salicylaldehyde complex was formed and to this on addition of malononitrile followed by triethyl phosphate the corresponding 2-amino-4H-chromen-4-yl- phosphonate formed in excellent yield (88%), on stirring at 60⁰c-70⁰c for 3-4 hrs. The same reaction, when carried out by replacing malononitrile with ethyl cyano acetate under similar reaction conditions obtained ethyl-2-amino-4-(diethoxy phosphonyl)-4H-chromen-3-carboxylate in 82% yield.

The scope of this interesting reaction was extended and studied with various substituted salicylaldehydes keeping triethyl phosphate as a common substrate. It was reported that, substituents on the salicylaldehyde did not show significant effect on the product yields. However, when malononitrile was replaced with ethylcyanoacetate slight decrease in the product yields was observed. When triethyl phosphate was replaced with diethyl phosphonate as a third component in the reaction, the products were formed in lower yields in longer reaction times. All the products were characterized by spectral data. Investigations on NMR data of salicylaldehyde, β-CD, and β-CD-salicylaldehyde inclusion complex, revealed an upfield shift of 3-H and 5-H protons of the cyclodextrin in the β-CD-salicylaldehyde complex, when compared to β-CD, confirming the formation of an inclusion complex of salicylaldehyde from the secondary side of the β-cyclodextrin. The results clearly established that the reaction was proceeding through an inclusion phenomenon.

Thus an efficient, environ friendly, biomimetic synthetic approach for the preparation of 2-amino-4H-chromen - 4-yl phosphonates under neutral conditions by using β-CD as a supramolecular catalyst through host–guest complexation phenomenon was observed, which will be an useful addition to green chemistry.

9. Quinoxalines

Quinoxalines are a prominent class of nitrogen containing heterocycles, exhibiting various biological activities such as anti-viral, anti-bacterial, anti-biotic, anti- inflammatory and kinase inhibition. They are very important building blocks in the preparation of dyes, electroluminescent material, organic semiconductors, cavitands, and dehydroannulenes. Quinoxalines act as potential rigid subunits in macrocyclic receptors (Mizuno et al., 2002; Elwahy, 2000) for molecular recognition and chemically controllable switches (Crossley & Jhonston, 2002).

In general many synthetic protocals have been developed for the preparation of quinoxaline derivatives. These include condensation of 1,2-diamines and 1,2-dicarbonyl compounds(Brown, 2004),1,4-addition of 1,2-diamines to diazenylbutenes(Aparicio et al.,2006), oxidative coupling of epoxides with ene-1,2-diamines(Antoniotti & Dunach, 2002), oxidative cyclization of α-hydroxy ketones with 1,2-diamines(Raw et al., 2004; Kim et al., 2005; Robinson & Taylor, 2005; Cho et al., 2007), cyclization-oxidation of phenacyl bromides with 1,2-diamines by $HClO_4.SiO_2$ (Das et al., 2007) and by using solid phase synthesis (Wu & Ede,2001; Singh et al., 2003). Existing synthetic methodologies for quinoxaline system are rather limited in number and model when compared to their broad spectrum utility.

However these also suffered from many limitations such as use of expensive reagents, drastic reaction conditions, and complicated work-up procedures. In this context, Nageswar et al. during their work on cyclodextrin promoted biomimetic organic synthesis, developed a generally applicable and environmentally benign methodology for the synthesis of quinoxaline derivatives involving use of cyclodextrin as an efficient biomimetic catalyst (Madhav et al., 2009).

Initially, a representative reaction was conducted by the insitu formation of β-CD complex of phenacyl bromide in water at 50° C, followed by the addition of benzene-1, 2-diamine. The reaction mixture was stirred at 70° C for 2hrs resulting in 2-phenyl quinoxaline derivative. The scope of this methodology was extended to cover several substituted phenacyl bromides by reacting them with benzene 1, 2-diamine at 70° C in water in presence of CD resulting in the corresponding quinoxalines in quantitative yields (87-92%). This reaction is compatible with phenacyl bromides bearing electron-withdrawing and electron-donating substituents in the aromatic ring. All these reactions have proceeded efficiently to give impressive yields without the formation of any byproducts. This is because of the activation of phenacyl bromide by the complexation with β-cyclodextrin. The quinoxaline derivatives were isolated and identified by spectral data and by comparison with the known compounds. In all these reactions β-CD can also be recovered and used for further runs. Solubility problems, longer reaction times, lower yields were the drawbacks when β-CD was not used. The catalytic amount of β-CD (0.1 equiv) had no impact on the reaction progress, but when equimolar quantity was used yields improved.

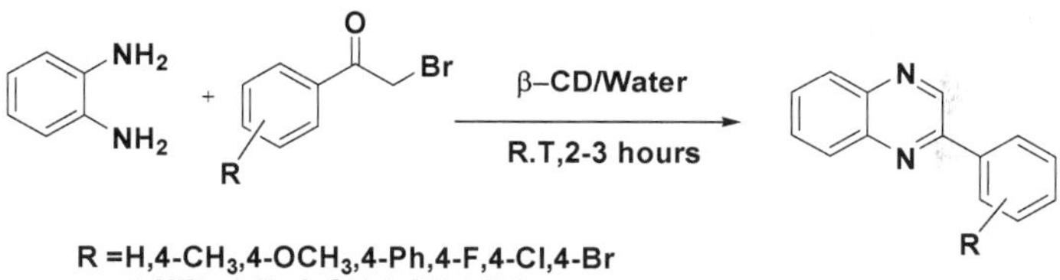

R =H,4-CH3,4-OCH3,4-Ph,4-F,4-Cl,4-Br
4-NEt2;3-Br,2-OH,4-CN,4-NO2.

Biomimetic synthesis of quinoxalines in water

β-CD solubilises phenacyl bromide by forming host-guest complex and activate carbonyl functionality to promote the reaction. Isolation of β-CD–phenacyl bromide complex and the study of ^{1}H NMR of β-CD, β-CD complex of phenacylbromide (1) and freeze-dried reaction mixture confirms the formation of CD - phenacyl bromide inclusion complex. The formation of inclusion complex from the secondary side of β-CD results in the up field shift of H3, H5 protons of β-CD phenacylbromide complex when compared to β-CD.

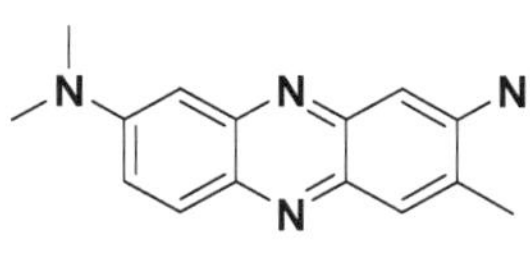

Toluylene Red

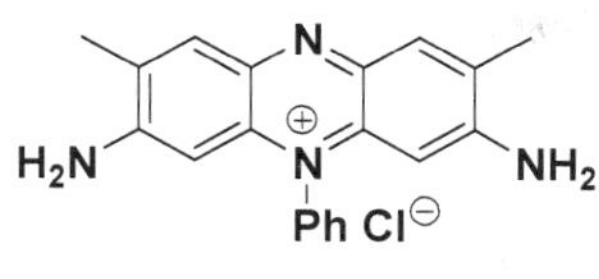

Safranin
Biological Stain

β-Cyclodextrin was proved to play a significant role by activating the phenacylbromide molecule to undergo cyclocondensation with benzene-1, 2-diamine. This straightforward simple aqueous phase approach to quinoxalines will be an useful addition to biomimetic chemistry.

10. 1, 2-disubstituted benzimidazole

Benzimidazole is a potential heterocyclic pharmacophore responsible for a number of important pharmacological properties, such as anti-pyretic, antihistaminic, anti-allergic (Nakano et al., 2000), and anti-ulcerative (Scott et al., 2002). They are also effective against various viruses like influenza, human cyto- megalovirus, and HIV. Its derivatives exhibit anti-microbial, anti-tumour activities as well as act as topoisomerase inhibitors, Factor Xa inhibitors, and selective neuropeptide YY1 receptor antagonists. Broad range of diverse activities, expressed by benzimidazole containing structures has attracted the attention of researchers across the globe.

While working on various biomimetic approaches for a broad range of heterocyclic derivatives the synthesis of 1, 2-disubstitued benzimidazoles was attempted in our laboratory (un published work Shankar et al., 2010) by reacting 2 moles of benzaldehyde with one mole of benzene 1, 2-diamine in water in presence of β-cyclodextrin at room temperature. In general, the reaction was carried out by the insitu formation of the β-CD complex of o-phenylenediamine in water followed by the addition of an aromatic aldehyde. The reaction mixture was stirred at room temperature to give the corresponding 1, 2-bis (aryl)-benzimidazoles in high yield (82%). These reactions proceeded efficiently without the need of any metal or acid catalyst. The reaction goes to completion in a short time (3.5–4.5 h). These reactions also take place with α-CD and γ-CD, with lesser yields. However, β-CD has been chosen as the mediator, since it is inexpensive and easily accessible. Scope of the reaction has been extended to cover several substituted benzaldehydes as well as benzene 1, 2-diamines. All the compounds were characterized by ^{1}H NMR, IR, and mass spectrometry. The catalytic activity of cyclodextrins for these reactions is established by the fact that no reaction was observed in the absence of cyclodextrin. Evidence for complexation between the amine and cyclodextrin is supported by 1H NMR spectroscopy. ^{1}H NMR spectra (D_2O) of β-CD, β-CD- o-phenylenediamine complex were compared. There was an upfield shift of H3 and H5 protons of cyclodextrin in the β-CD-o-phenylene diamine complex.

After the reaction, the reaction mass was cooled to room temperature and β-CD was filtered, washed with ice-cold water and dried. The recovered β-CD was further used with the same substrates as a catalyst and checked for the yields and catalytic activity of β-CD. It was observed that the yields of 1-benzyl-2-phenyl-1H-benzo[d]imidazole after two to three recycles were nearly the same. In summary, a neutral aqueous phase synthesis of various 1, 2-bis (aryl)-benzimidazoles was developed by the reaction of the corresponding o-phenylenediamine with aldehydes, under biomimetic conditions in the presence of β-cyclodextrin. These cyclodextrin-mediated aqueous phase reactions are very useful both from economical and environmental view. β-Cyclodextrin, apart from being nontoxic, is also considered as metabolically safe. This simple straightforward and environmentally benign methodology may find widespread application in organic and medicinal chemistry.

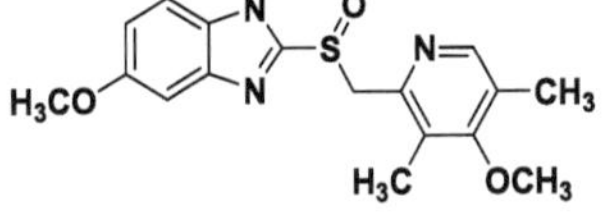

Omeprazole
Antiulcer Drug

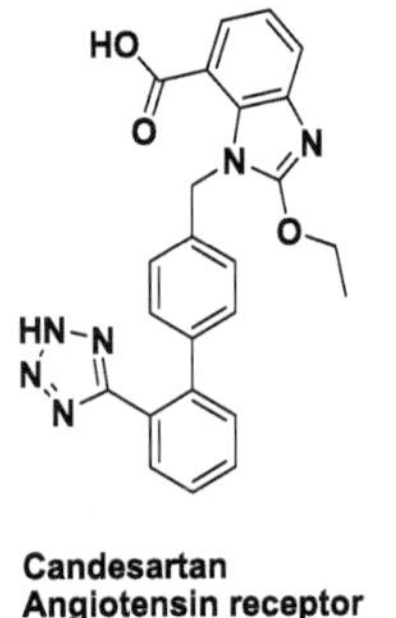

Candesartan
Angiotensin receptor antagonist TCV-116

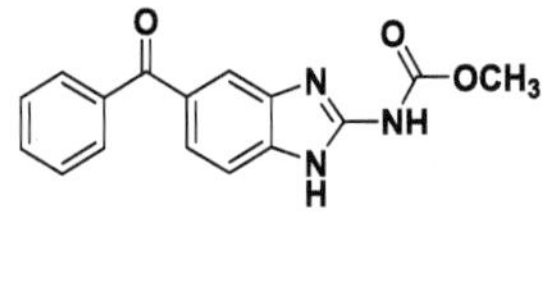

Mebendazole
Antihelmintic drug

In conclusion, we have presented here an improved methodology for the selective synthesis of 1, 2-disubstituted benzimidazoles by the condensation of o-phenylenediamine and aldehydes using β-CD as a supramolecular catalyst.

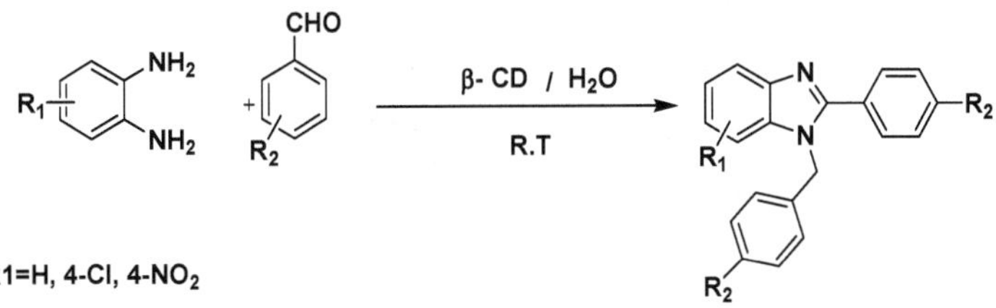

R1=H, 4-Cl, 4-NO$_2$

R2=H, 4-NO$_2$, 4-Cl, 4-CH$_3$, 4-OH, 4-OCH$_3$, 4-OEt

Synthesis of 1, 2-disubstituted benzimidazoles

11. Conclusion

The growth of literature on cyclodextrins from their discovery till now showcases the significance of cyclodextrin chemistry and their potential molecular receptor ability involving host-guest complexation and its subsequent applications in a wider arena. Cyclodextrins with their unique hydrophobic cavity, activates the guest molecules with the assistance of hydroxyl groups, to promote various organic transformations, in aqueous medium under neutral conditions. Cyclodextrins in combination with water as reaction medium will further contribute to attain new vistas in the development of novel green chemistry protocols in the future.

12. Acknowledgements

We thank CSIR, New Delhi for fellowships to S. N. M.; B.M.; J. S.

13. References

Antoniotti, S.; Dunach, E. (2002). *Tetrahedron Lett.*, 43, 2002, 3971-3973.

Aparicio, D.; Attanasi, O. A.; Filippone, P.; Ignacio, R.; Lillini, S.; Mantellini, F.; Palacios, F.; Delos Santos, J. M. (2006). *J. Org. Chem.* 71, 2006, 5897-5905.

Back, T. G. (1999). *Organoselenium Chemistry: A Practical Approach;* Oxford University Press: Oxford.

Bailey, N.; Dean, A. W.; Judd, D. B.; Middlemiss, D.; Storer, R.; Stephen, P. W.(1996). *Bioorg. Med. Chem. Lett.*, 6, 1996, 1409–1414.

Bassetti, M.; D'Annibale, A.; Fanfoni, A.; Minissi, F. (2005). *Org. Lett.* 7, 2005, 1805-1808.

Benazzouz, A.; Boraud, T.; Dubedat, P.; Boireau, A.; Stutzmann, J.-M.; Gross, C.(1995).*Eur. J. Pharmacol*, 284, 1995, 299-307.

Bergstrom, D.E,; Zhang,P; Zhou. J. (1994). *J.Chem.Soc., Perkin Trans.*1, 1994, 3029-3034.

Binder, J. T.; Kirsch, S. F.(2006). *Org. Lett.*, 8, 2006, 2151-2153.

Brown, D. J. In *Chemistry of Heterocyclic Compounds, Quinoxalines Supplements II;* Taylor, E. C., Wipf, P., Eds.; John Wiley and Sons: New Jersey, 2004.

Bryce, M. R.; Acheson, M. R.; Rees, A. J. (1983). *Heterocycles*, *20*, 1983, 489-495.

Cao, R.; Liu, C.; Liu, L. (1996). *Org. Prep. Proced. Int.*, 28, 1996, 215-216.

Cho, C. S.; Ren, W. X. (2007). *J. Organomet. Chem., 692*, 2007, 4182-4186.
Cho, C. S.; Renb, W. X.; Shim, S. C. (2007). *Tetrahedron Lett.*, 48, 2007, 4665-4667.
Crossley, J. C.; Johnston, L. A. (2002). *Chem. Commun.*, 2002, 1122-1123.
Cyr, D. J. S.; Martin, N.; Arndtsen, B. A. (2007). *Org. Lett.*, 9, 2007, 449-452.
Dabiri, M.; Salehi, P.; Mostafa, B.; Nikcheg, M. S.(2008). *Tetrahedron Lett., 49*, 2008, 5366-5368.
Das, B.; Venkateswarlu, K.; Suneel, K.; Majhi, A. (2007). *Tetrahedron Lett.* 48, 2007, 5371-5374.
Das, S. G.; Doshi, J. M.; Tian, D.; Addo, S. N.; Srinivasan, B.; Hermanson, D. L.; Xing, C. (2009). *J. Med. Chem.*, 52, 2009, 5937-5949.
Demarco, P. V.; Thakkar, A. L. (1970). *J. Chem. Soc. Chem. Commun.* 1970, 2-4.
De Souza, M. V. N. (2005). *Mini- Rev. Org. Chem.*, 2, 2005, 139-145.
Dondoni, A.(1998). *Synthesis,* 1998, 1681-1706.
Doshi, J. M.; Tian, D.; Xing, C. (2006). *J. Med. Chem.*, 49, 2006, 7731-7739.
D'Souza, Lipkowitz, K. B. (1998). *Chem. Rev., 98*, 1998, 1741-2076.
Edmondson, S.; Danishefsky, S. J.; Sepp-Lorenzino, L.; Rosen, N. (1999). *J. Am. Chem. Soc.,* 121, 1999, 2147-2155.
Ellis, G. P. (1977). *In The Chemistry of Heterocyclic Compounds.* Chromenes, Harmones, and Chromones; Weissberger, A., Taylor, E. C., Eds.; John Wiley: New York, 1977; pp 11–139. Chapter II.
Elwahy, A. H. M. (2000). *Tetrahedron*, 56, 2000, 897-907.
Firouzabadi, H.; Iranpoor, N.; Sobhani, S. (2004). *Synth. Commun.*, 34, 2004, 1463-1471.
Firouzabadi, H.; Iranpoor, N.; Sobhani, S.; Amoozgar, Z. (2004). *Synthesis*, 2004, 1771-1774.
Fu, C.; Ma, S. (2005). *Eur. J. Org. Chem.*, 2005, 3942-3945.
Gabriele, B.; Mancuso, R.; Salerno, G.; Ruffolo, G.; Plastina, P. (2007). *J. Org. Chem., 72*, 2007, 6873-6877.
Gallagher, G.; Lavanchy, P. G.; Wilson, J. W.; Hieble, J. P.; DeMarinis, R. M. (1985). *J. Med. Chem.*, 28, 1985, 1533-1536.
Goldstein, B. M.; Kennedy, S. D.; Hennen, W. J. (1990). *J. Am. Chem. Soc., 112*, 1990, 8265-8268.
Grigoras, M.; Conduruta, D. G. J. (2006). *Inclusion Phenom. Macrocycl. Chem.* 54, 2006, 101-107.
Hadjipavlou-Litina, D. J.; Geronikaki, A. A. (1998). *Drug Des. Discovery,* 15, 1998, 199-206.
Haviv, F.; Ratajczyk, J. D.; DeNet, R. W.; Kerdesky, F. A.; Walters, R. L.; Schmidt, S. P.; Holms, J. H.; Young, P. R.; Carter, G. W.(1988). *J. Med. Chem.*, 31, 1988, 1719-1728.
Hendrickson, J. B.; Rees, R.; Templeton, J. F. (1964). *J. Am. Chem. Soc., 86*, 1964, 107-111.
Hollingworth, G. J.; Perkins, G.; Sweeney, J. B. (1996). *J. Chem. Soc., Perkin Trans.1*1996, 1913-1919.
Hu, Y. Z.; Zhang, G.; Thummel, R. P. (2003). *Org. Lett.*, 5, 2003, 2251-2253.
Iorga, B.; Eymery, F.; Savignac, P. (1999). *Tetrahedron,* 55, 1999, 2671-2686.
James, D. S.; Fanta, P. E. (1962). *J. Org. Chem., 27*, 1962, 3346-3348.
Jayashree, P.; Shanthi, G.; Perumal, P. T. (2009). *Synlett,* 2009, 917-920.
Jenekhe, S. A.; Lu, l.; Alam, M. M.(2001). *Macromolecules, 34,* 2001, 7315-7324.
Jiang, B.; Dong, J. J. ; Jin, Y.; Long Du, X.; Xu, M. (2008). *Eur. J. Org. Chem.,* 2008, 2693-2696.
Kaboudin, B.(2003). *Tetrahedron Lett.,* 44, 2003, 1051-1053.
Kazmaier, U.; Ackermann, S. (2005). *Org. Biomol. Chem.*, 3, 2005, 3184-3187.
Kazzouli, S. El.; Raboin, S. B.; Mouadbib, A.; Guillaumet, G. (2002). *Tetrahedron Lett.*, 43, 2002, 3193–3196.
Kim, S. Y.; Park, K. H.; Chung, Y. K. (2005). *Chem. Commun.*, 2005, 1321-1323.
Kotora, M.; Negishi, E. (1997). *Synthesis*, 1997, 121-128.

Koketsu, M.; Mio, T.; Ishihara, H.(2004). *Synthesis,* 2004, 233-236.

Koketsu, M.; Tanaka, H.; Ishihara, H. (2005). *Chem. Lett., 34,* 2005, 1260-1261.

Koketsu, M.; Kogami, M.; Ando, H.; Ishihara, H. (2006). *Synthesis,* 2006, 0031-0036.

Kumar, V. P.; Narender, N.; Sridhar, R.; Nageswar, Y. V. D.; Rao, K. R.(2007). *Synthetic Commun.,* 37, 2007, 4331-4336.

Lipshutz, B. H.; Frieman, B.; Birkedal, H.(2004) *Org. Lett.,* 6, 2004, 2305-2308.

Mabon, R.; Richecoeur, A. M. E.; Sweeney, J. B. (1996). *J. Org. Chem.,* 64,1999,328-329.

Mabon, R.; Richecoeur, A. M. E.; Sweeney, J. B. (2002). *Tetrahedron* 58, 2002, 9117-9129.

Madhav, B.; Murthy, S. N.; Reddy, V. P.; Nageswar, Y. V. D. (2009). *Tetrahedron Lett.,* 50, 2009, 6025-6028.

Madhav, B.; Murthy, S. N.; Rao, K. R.; Nageswar, Y. V. D. (2010). *Helv. Chim. Acta.,* 93, 2010, 257-260.

Martin, L.M.; Hu, B.-H.(1999). *Tetrahedron Lett.,* 40, 1999, 7951-7953.

Martinez, R.; Ramon, D. J.; Yus, M. (2007). Eur. *J. Org. Chem.,* 2007, 1599-1605.

Maryanoff, B. E.; Reitz, A. B. (1989). *Chem. Rev.,* 89, 1989, 863-927.

McNaughton, B. R.; Miller, B. L. (2003). *Org. Lett.,* 5, 2003, 4257-4259.

Miao, S.; Andersen, R. (1991). *J. Org. Chem.,* 56, 1991, 6275-6280.

Michael, J. P.(2007). *Nat. Prod. Rep., 24,* 2007, 223-246.

Mierde, H. V.; Voort, P. V.; Vos, D. D.; Verpoort, F. (2008). *Eur. J. Org. Chem.* 2008, 1625-1631.

Mizuno, T.; Wei, W. H.; Eller, L. R.; Sessler, J. L. *J. Am. Chem. Soc.* 2002, 124, 1134-1135.

Moonen, K.; Laureyn, I.; Stevens, C. V. (2004). *Chem. Rev.,* 104, 2004, 6177-6216.

Muscia, G. C.; Bollini, M.; Carnevale, J. P.; Bruno, A. M.; Asis, S. E. (2006). *Tetrahedron Lett., 47,* 2006, 8811-8815.

Murthy, S. N.; Madhav, B.; Kumar, A. V.; Rao, K. R.; Nageswar, Y. V. D. (2009). *Tetrahedron,* 65, 2009, 5251-5256.

Murthy, S. N.; Madhav, B.; Kumar, A. V.; Rao, K. R.; Nageswar, Y. V. D. (2009). *Helv. Chim. Acta.,* 92, 2009, 2118-2124..

Murthy, S. N.; Madhav, B.; Reddy, V. P.; Nageswar, Y. V. D. (2010). *Tetrahedron Lett.,* 51, 2010, 3649-3653.

Mustafa, S.M.; Nair, V.A.; Chittoor, J. P.; Krishnapillai, S. (2004). *Mini-Rev. Org. Chem.,* 1, 2004, 375-385.

Mylari, B. L.; Larson, R.; Beyer, T. A.; Zembrowski, W. J.; Aldinger, C. E.; Dee, M. F.; Siegel, T. W.; Singleton, D. H.(1991). *J. Med. Chem.,* 34, 1991, 108-122.

Nagel, A. A.; Liston, D. R.; Jung, S.; Mahar, M.; Vincent, L. A.; Chapin, D.; Chen, Y. L.; Hubbard, S.; Ives, J. L.; Jones, S. B.(1995). *J. Med. Chem.,* 38, 1995, 1084-1089.

Narender, M.; Reddy, M. S.; Kumar, V. P.; Reddy, V. P.; Nageswar, Y. V. D.; Rao, K. R. (2007). *J. Org. Chem.,* 72, 2007, 1849-1851.

Narender, M.; Reddy, M. S.; Kumar, V. P.; Srinivas, B.; Sridhar, R.; Nageswar, Y. V. D.; Rao, K. R. (2007). *Synthesis,* 2007, 3469-3472.

Nakano, H.; Inoue, T.; Kawasaki, N.; Miyataka, H.; Matsumoto, H.; Taguchi, T.; Inagaki, N.; Nagai, H.; Satoh, T.(2000). *Bioorg. Med. Chem.,* 8, 2000, 373-380.

Nicolaou, K.C.; King, N. P.; Finlay, M. R. V .; Roschangar, F.; Vourloumis, D .; Vallberg, h.; Sarabia, F .; Ninkovic, S .; Hepworth, D. (1999). *Bioorg. Med. Chem.,* 7, 1999, 665-697.

Palmer, P. J.; Trigg, R. B.; Warrington, J. V. (1971). *J. Med. Chem.,* 14, 1971, 248-251.

Patel, D. V.; Rielly-Gauvin, K.; Ryono, D. E.; Free, C. A.; Rogers, W. L.; Smith, S. A.; DeForrest, J. M.; Oehl, R. S.; Petrillo, E. W. (1995). *J. Med. Chem.,* 38, 1995, 4557.

Patt, W. C.; Hamilton, H. W.; Taylor, M. D.; Ryan, M. J.; Taylor, D. G. Jr.; Connolly, C. J. C.; Doharty, A. M.; Klutchko, S. R.; Sircar, I.; Steinbaugh, B. A.; Bately, B. L.; Painchand, C. A.; Rapundalo, S. T.; Michniewicz, B. M.; Olzon, S. C. J.(1992). *J. Med. Chem.*, 35, 1992, 2562-2572.

Phoon, C. W.; Ng, P. Y.; Ting, A. E.; Yeo, S. L.; Sim, M. M.(2001). *Bioorg. Med. Chem. Lett.*, 11, 2001, 1647-1650.

Raw, S. A.; Wilfred, C. D.; Taylor, R. J. K. (2004). *Org. Biomol. Chem.*, 2, 2004, 788-796.

Robinson, R. S.; Taylor, R. J. K. (2005). *Synlett.*, 2005, 1003-1005.

Sapountzis, I.; Dude, H.; Lewis, R.; Gommermann, N.; Knochel, P.(2005). *J. Org .chem.*, 70, 2005, 2445-2454.

Scott, L. J.; Dunn, C. J.; Mallarkey, G.; Sharpe, M. (2002). *Drugs* , 62, 2002, 1503.

Shankar, J.; Karnakar,K.; Srinivas, B.; Nageswar, Y. V. D. (2010). *Tetrahedron Lett.*, 51, 2010, 3938-3939.

Shankar, J.; Karnakar, K.; Nageswar, Y. V. D. (2010). (Unpublished results-part of the thesis of Shankar. J.)

Shindo, M.; Yoshimura, Y.; Hayashi, M.; Soejima, H.; Yoshikawa, T.; Matsumoto, K.; Shishido, K. (2007). *Org. Lett.*, 9, 2007, 1963-1966.

Shiraishi, H.; Nishitani, T.; Nishihara, T.; Sakaguchi, S.; Ishii, Y.(1999), *Tetrahedron*, 55, 1999, 13957-13964.

Singh, S. K.; Gupta, P.; Duggineni, S.; Kundu, B. (2003). *Synlett.*, 2003, 2147-2150.

Sohn, S. K.; Chang, M. S.; Choi, W. S.; Kim, K. W.; Woo, T. W.; Lee, S. B.; Chung, Y. K.(1999). *Can. J. Physiol. Pharmacol.*, 77, 1999, 330-338.

Sridhar, R.; Srinivas, B.; Madhav, B.; Reddy, V. P.; Nageswar, Y. V. D.; Rao, K. R. (2009). *Can. J. Chem.*, 87, 2009, 1704-1707.

Srivastava, P. C.; Robins, R. K.(1983). *J. Med. Chem,. 26*, 1983, 445-448.

Stowasser, B.; Budt, K.-H.; Jian-Qi, L.; Peyman, A.; Ruppert, D. (1992). *Tetrahedron Lett.*, 33, 1992, 6625.

Sundberg, R. J.(1996). *Comprehensive Heterocyclic Chemistry,* Katritzky, A. R.; Rees, C. W. (Ed.,), 149--, Pergamon Press, Oxford.

Suresh, K. K.; Sandhya, B.; Himanshu, G.(2009). *Mini-Rev. Med. Chem., 7, 2009,* 1648-1654.

Szejtli, J.; Osa, T. (1996). In *Comprehensive Supramolecular Chemistry,* Pergamon Press. New York, 1996, Vol. 3.

Taylor, E. C.; Heindel, N. D. (1967) *J. Org. Chem., 32*, 1967, 1666-1667.

Tokunaga, T.; Hume, W. E.; Umezome, T.; Okazaki, K.; Ueki, Y.; Kumagai, K.; Hourai, S.; Nagamine, J.; Seki, H.; Taiji, M.; Noguchi, H.; Nagata, R. (2001). *J. Med. Chem.*, 44, 2001, 4641-4649.

Vieira, T. O.; Alper, H. (2007). *Chem. Commun.*, 2007, 2710-2711.

Wirth, T. (2000). *Organoselenium Chemistry. Modern Developments in Organic Synthesis;* Springer: Berlin.

Wu, J.; Xia, H. G.; Gao, K. (2006). *Org. Biomol. Chem., 4*, 2006, 126-129.

Wu, Z.; Ede, N. J. (2001). *Tetrahedron Lett.*, 42, 2001, 8115-8118.

Xin-Yuan, L.; Ding, P.; Jie-Sheng, H.; Chi-Ming, C. (2007). *Org. Lett.*, 9, 2007, 2645-2648.

Zaveri, N. T.; Jiang, F.; Olsen, C. M.;Deschamps, J. R.; Parrish, D.; Polgar, W.; Toll, L. (2004). *J. Med. Chem.*, 47, 2004, 2973-2976.

Zhang, L.; Wu, J. (2007). *Adv. Synth. Catal., 349*, 2007, 1047-1051.

Zhang, X.; Shetty, S.; Jenekhe, S. A. (1999). *Macromolecules, 32*, 1999, 7422-7429.

6

Bioinspired Assembly of Inorganic Nanoplatelets for Reinforced Polymer Nanocomposites

Tzung-Hua Lin, Wei-Han Huang, In-kook Jun and Peng Jiang
University of Florida
United States

1. Introduction

Steel and metal alloys have long been used for structural applications because they are both strong and flaw-tolerant. By contrast, ceramics, which are strong but not tolerant to surface flaws and cracks, and polymers, which are flaw-tolerant and can deform under applied stresses, are less favourable as structural materials. However, nature has resolved this dilemma by millions of years of biological evolution. For example, the nacreous layer of mollusk shells(Jackson, Vincent et al. 1988; Aksay, Trau et al. 1996; Smith, Schaffer et al. 1999), which is made up of relatively weak components (consisting of 95 volume % of brittle aragonite platelets and 5 volume % of soft biological macromolecules), shows unexpected toughness (resistance to cracking) and stiffness (resistant to deformation)(Barthelat 2007). The oriented assembly of aragonite platelets and the intricate brick-and-mortar nanostructure found in the nacreous layer have been attributed to the major reasons for the exceptional toughness and stiffness of nacres. This unusual combination of different mechanical properties inspires scientists to create strong and flaw-tolerant artificial materials that mimic the mechanical design principles found in nacres by combining platelet-like ceramic building blocks with polymeric matrices(Tang, Kotov et al. 2003; Podsiadlo, Kaushik et al. 2007; Bonderer, Studart et al. 2008).

Various bottom-up self-assembly techniques have been developed for creating biomimetic reinforced nanocomposites. Layer-by-layer (LBL) assembly of inorganic nanoplatelets and polyelectrolytes has recently been demonstrated as an efficient methodology in making reinforced polymer nanocomposites(Podsiadlo, Kaushik et al. 2007; Bonderer, Studart et al. 2008; Podsiadlo, Michel et al. 2008). The sequential adsorption of anionic montmorillonite clay platelets and poly(diallydimethylammonium) chloride polycation results in an organic-inorganic hybrid material that has ultimate tensile strength (~100 MPa) approaching to that of nacre (~130 MPa)(Tang, Kotov et al. 2003). By treating with glutaraldehyde to improve the bonding and load transfer between clay platelets and polymer matrices, nanocomposites made by LBL assembly of montmorillonite clay platelets and poly(vinyl alcohol) show even higher tensile strength (~400 MPa)(Podsiadlo, Kaushik et al. 2007). Ice-templated crystallization, gravitational sedimentation, centrifugation, as well as spin-coating have also been explored to assemble inorganic nanoplatelets into ordered structures(Almqvist, Thomson et al. 1999; Chen, Wang et al. 2008; Liu, Chen et al. 2008; Munch, Launey et al.

2008). Unfortunately, these techniques are either time-consuming or require multiple steps to infiltrate inorganic assemblies with polymer. For example, LBL assembly is a relative slow process. Hundreds of bilayers need to be deposited to form composites with micrometer-scale thickness. In addition, the inevitable agglomeration of commonly used clay restrains nanoplatelets from forming highly aligned structures and therefore weakens the mechanical properties of the resulting nanocomposites.(Liu, Chen et al. 2008)

In this chapter, we will show that ordered assemblies of nanoplatelets can be achieved by utilizing electrophoretic deposition, which is the migration of charged particles under the influence of an applied electric field and has been widely used in assembling spherical colloids into highly ordered colloidal crystals(Braun and Wiltzius 1999; Holgado, Garcia-Santamaria et al. 1999; Velev and Bhatt 2006). Organic–inorganic hybrid materials can be directly formed by electrophoretic co-deposition of inorganic platelets and organic matrix, or by sequential polymer infiltration in the interstitials of inorganic assemblies(Lin, Huang et al. 2009). Indeed, electrophoretic deposition has been extensively utilized for the deposition of ceramic particles because of its simplicity and controllability, such as bath composition and deposition parameters, and is an effective technique for rapid and scalable fabrication of nanocomposites over large areas(Zhitomirsky 2002). We will show that cathodic co-deposition of either non-ionic-type polymers or polyelectrolytes between nanoplatelets enable the deposition of organic-inorganic nanocomposites in a simple single-step approach(Grandfield and Zhitomirsky 2008; Pang and Zhitomirsky 2008; Lin, Huang et al. 2009; Lin, Huang et al. 2009). This simple electrodeposition technique will significantly reduce the cost and increase the throughput of reinforced polymer nanocomposites.

2. Experimental section

2.1 Materials and substrates

All solvents and chemicals are of reagent grade and are used without further purification. Ultrapure water (18.2 MΩ cm^{-1}) is used directly from a Barnstead water system. Ethanol (200 proof) is purchased from Pharmaco Products. Hydrochloric acid (37%), aluminum *sec*-butoxide (≥95%), and aluminum isopropoxide (≥98%) are obtained from Aldrich. Ethoxylated trimethylolpropane triacrylate monomer (ETPTA, SR 454) is obtained from Sartomer. The photoinitiator, Darocur 1173 (2-hydroxy-2-methyl-1-phenyl-1-propanone), is provided by Ciba Specialty Chemicals. Two-part polydimethylsiloxane (PDMS, Sylgard 184) is provided by Dow Corning. Polyvinyl alcohol (PVA, Mw 89,000~98,000) and polyethylenimine (PEI, Mw ~750,000) are purchased form Aldrich. Indium tin oxide (ITO) coated glass substrates with sheet resistance of 8 Ω are purchased from Delta Technologies. Gold electrodes are prepared by sputtering deposition of 20 nm of titanium and 200 nm of gold on glass slides.

2.2 Instrumentation

A kurt J. Lesker CMS-18 Multitarget Sputter is used for the sputtering deposition of titanium and gold. An EG&G Model 273A potentiostat/galvanostat (Princeton Applied Research) is used for electrophoretic deposition. Transmission electron microscopy (TEM) is performed on a JEOL 2010F TEM. Scanning electron microscopy (SEM) is carried out on a JEOL 6335F FEG-SEM. A thin layer of gold is sputtered onto the samples prior to imaging. X-ray diffraction spectra are obtained with a Philips APD-3720 equipment. A Cu $K\alpha_1$ (λ = 1.540491 Å) radiation is scanned from 10° to 70° with a scan rate of 2.4°/min. Atomic force microscopy (AFM) is carried out on a Digital Instruments Dimension 3100 unit. The zeta potential of gibbsite nanoplatelets is measured by a Brookhaven ZetaPlus Analyzer (Brookhaven Instrument Corporation). A standard spin coater (WS-400B-6NPP-Lite Spin Processor, Laurell) is used to spin-coat ETPTA monomer. The polymerization of monomer is carried out on a Pulsed UV Curing System (RC 742, Xenon). A HR4000 UV-Vis spectrometer (Ocean Optics) is used for optical transmission measurement. Tensile strength measurement are tested using an Instron model 1122 load frame upgraded with an MTS ReNew system and equipped with a 500 g load cell at a crosshead speed of 0.5 mm/min.

2.3 Synthesis of inorganic gibbsite nanoplatelets

The gibbsite nanoplatelets are synthesized by the following preparation method(Wierenga, Lenstra et al. 1998). To 1 L of ultrapure water, hydrochloric acid (0.09 M), aluminum *sec*-butoxide (0.08 M), and aluminum isopropoxide (0.08 M) are added. The mixture is stirred for 10 days and then heated in a polyethylene bottle in a water bath at 85°C for 72 h. After cooling to room temperature, dispersions of gibbsite nanoplatelets are centrifuged at 3500 g for 6 h and the sediments are redispersed in deionized water. This process is repeated for five times to remove any unreacted reactants and also concentrate the as-synthesized nanoplatelets.

2.4 Electrophoretic deposition

Electrophoretic deposition of nanoplatelets is performed in a water-ethanol mixture in a sandwich cell placed horizontally. The bottom and the top of the cell are either an ITO or a gold electrode. PDMS is used as a spacer to get an active area of 1.5×1.5 cm^2 and a cell gap of 2.2 mm.

2.4.1 Electrophoretic deposition of gibbsite nanoplatelets

The bath solution is gibbsite nanoplatelets dispersed in a water-ethanol mixture. 2 weight % of aqueous suspensions of gibbsite nanoplatelets is used. 200-proof ethanol is added into the suspensions to make the volumetric ratio of ethanol to the aqueous suspension to be 2. A constant voltage of –2.5 V (ITO vs. Au) is applied for 20 min to deposit the positively charged gibbsite nanoplatelets onto the bottom ITO working cathode. A gold electrode is used as the top counter anode.

2.4.2 Electrophoretic deposition of PVA-gibbsite nanocomposites

Electrophoretic bath solution is prepared by mixing 1 mL of 5 wt.% PVA aqueous solution, 9 mL of 2.0 wt.% gibbsite nanoplatelet aqueous solution, and 20 mL of 200-proof ethanol. Constant voltage of -2.5 V (ITO vs. Au electrode) is applied to deposit gibbsite nanoplatelets and PVA on the bottom ITO working cathode. A gold electrode is used as the top counter anode.

2.4.3 Electrophoretic deposition of PEI-gibbsite nanocomposites

Electrophoretic bath solution is prepared by mixing 2 mL of 0.3 wt.% PEI aqueous solution, 3 mL of 2.0 wt.% gibbsite nanoplatelet aqueous solution, and 10 mL of 200-proof ethanol. Constant current of 0.3 mA is applied for 15 min to deposit gibbsite nanoplatelets and PEI on the bottom gold working cathode. An ITO electrode is used as the top counter anode.

3. Gibbsite nanoplatelets

Gibbsite, aluminum hydroxide ($Al(OH)_3$), is an inorganic crystalline with stacking Al-OH layers. Each Al^{3+} is surrounded by six hydroxyl groups and can be synthesized from aqueous aluminium alkoxide solutions by hydrothermal treatment. The as-synthesized gibbsite nanoplatelets have well-defined hexagon-shape with aspect ratio of around 10, which is close to that of natural aragonite platelets found in nacre(Jackson, Vincent et al. 1988). The reaction of surface hydroxyl groups with water makes the gibbsite nanoplatelets highly charged in water and alcoholic suspensions, providing strong electrostatic repulsion responsible for the observed colloidal stability. The structure of the gibbsite crystals suggests that the acidity of the A1-OH groups at the edges is different from that on the faces. The isoelectric points for edges and faces of platelets are pH ~ 7 and pH ~ 10, respectively, resulting in an inhomogeneous charge density and causing different types of flocculation: face-to-face, edge-to-face and edge-to-edge flocculation, depending on solution pH. Gibbsite nanoplatelets have been widely used as a model system to exploit the liquid crystal phase transition in suspensions of plate-like particles(van der Kooij and Lekkerkerker 1998; van der Kooij, Kassapidou et al. 2000; van der Beek and Lekkerkerker 2004; Mourad, Wijnhoven et al. 2006). Opal-like columnar gibbsite colloidal crystals have been demonstrated by sedimentation(Brown, Clarke et al. 1998; van der Beek, Radstake et al. 2007).

A typical TEM image of purified gibbsite nanoplatelets is shown in Fig. 1. The diameter of the gibbsite nanoplatelets is estimated from TEM micrographs to be around 200 nm. TEM images also reveal the nanoplatelets tend to align parallel to the surface of TEM grids. It is very rare to find nanoplatelets oriented perpendicularly to the TEM grid surface as shown by the red arrow pointing to such a particle in Fig. 1. Thickness of nanoplatelets ranges from 10 to 15 nm, confirmed by AFM. As mentioned before, the purified gibbsite nanoplatelets are electrostatically stabilized and the zeta-potential (ζ) of the colloids in deionized water is measured to be + 40.5 ± 2.3 mV by fitting experimental data using Smoluchowski's model. This high surface charge makes the dispersions of gibbsite nanoplatelets stable and aggregated particles are rarely seen in TEM images. The selected area electron diffraction (SAED) patterns from a single platelet as shown in the inset of Fig. 1 indicate the as-made gibbsite nanoplatelets are single-crystal.

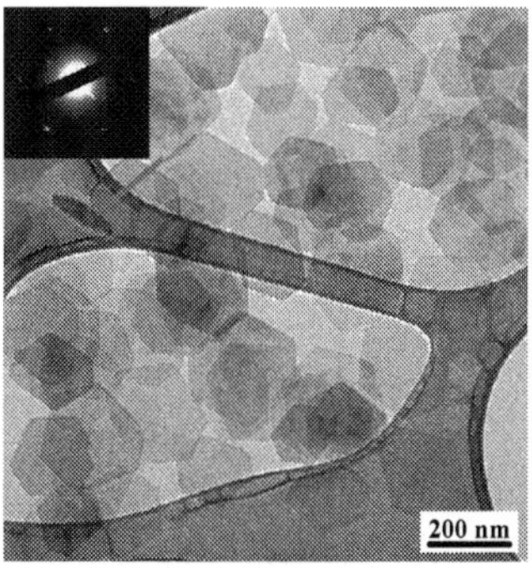

Fig. 1. TEM image of gibbsite nanoplatelets. The inset shows the electron diffraction patterns obtained from a single nanoplatelet. The red arrow points to a gibbsite nanoplatelet oriented perpendicularly to the TEM grid. Adapted from Lin, Huang et al. 2009.

4. ETPTA-gibbsite nanocomposites

4.1 Electrophoretic deposition of gibbsite nanoplatelets

Electrophoretic deposition of positively charged gibbsite nanoplatelets is performed in a water-ethanol mixture and carried out using a horizontal parallel-plate sandwich cell, which consists of an ITO working electrode on the bottom, a gold counter electrode on the top, and a PDMS spacer (~2.2 mm thick). Ethanol is used to reduce the dielectric constant of the solvent and therefore reduce the electric double-layer thickness of the nanoplatelets to promote colloidal coagulation on the gold electrode. Deionized water is added to the dispersions for bringing up the following cathodic reaction:

$$2H_2O + 2e^- \rightarrow H_2 + 2OH^- \quad E^0 = -0.828V \tag{1}$$

Since the surface of oxide particles could be positively or negatively charged, depending on solution pH, the cathodic reaction above could result in a local pH increase at the electrode surface and thus lower the surface charge of positively charged gibbsite nanoplatelets to further assist colloidal coagulation. Contrary to the cathodic reaction for the electrodeposition of gibbsite nanoplatelets, the electrodeposition of negatively charged particles may require the following anodic reaction that results in a local pH decrease at the electrode:

$$O_2 + 4H^+ + 4e^- \rightarrow 2H_2O \quad E^0 = -1.229V \tag{2}$$

Therefore, we disperse gibbsite nanoplatelets in a water-ethanol mixture with volumetric ratio of 1:2 to make the electrophoretic bath solution. The volume fraction of gibbsite particles is adjusted to $\sim 1\%$. Without ethanol, no particle deposits are observed to adhere on the working electrode after disassembling the electrophoretic cell. The addition of ethanol also facilitates to reduce cracking and porosity in the electrodeposited films. The applied electric field strength is ~ 1100 V/m. Besides parallel-plate geometry, electrodes can also be vertically inserted into the colloidal baths to conduct the electrophoretic deposition. As the gravitational sedimentation of gibbsite nanoplatelets is negligible during electrophoresis, uniform deposits are also resulted.

The deposits can be easily peeled off from the ITO surface by using a sharp razor blade, resulting in the formation of self-standing films as shown in Fig. 2A. The film is opaque and brittle. The side facing the ITO cathode is smoother than the side facing the suspension. The size of the resulting films is solely determined by the dimensions of the ITO electrode. Fig. 2A depicts a sample with 1.6×0.6 in.^{2} area deposited on a 2×1 inch^2 ITO electrode. Fig. 2B shows a top-view SEM image of the suspension-side of the sample in Figure 2A. The hexagonal gibbsite nanoplatelets are densely packed and aligned parallel to the electrode surface. The alignment of gibbsite nanoplatelets is further confirmed by the layered structure as shown in the cross-sectional SEM image of Fig. 2C. Another convincing evidence of the orientated deposition comes from the X-ray diffraction (XRD) patterns shown in Fig. 2D. Only (002) and (004) peaks are observed in the XRD spectrum. As the crystallographic *c*-axis of single-crystal gibbsite is normal to the platelet surfaces, the (002) and (004) reflection are from gibbsite platelets oriented parallel to the electrode surface(Cullity 1978). Analysis of the half-height width of the (002) peak with the Scherrer equation yields an average platelet thickness of 15.1 nm, agreeing with AFM measurement.

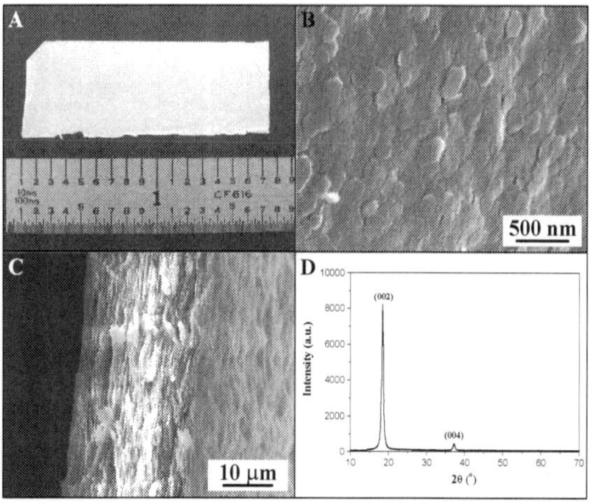

Fig. 2. Electrophoretic assembly of gibbsite nanoplatelets. (A) Photograph of a free-standing gibbsite film. (B) Top-view SEM image of the sample in (A). (C) Cross-sectional view of the same sample. (D) XRD patterns of the gibbsite film in (A). Adapted from Lin, Huang et al. 2009.

The oriented deposition of gibbsite nanoplatelets in a direct-current (dc) electric field can be understood by considering the charge distribution on the gibbsite surfaces due to different isoelectric points at faces (pH ~ 10) and edges (pH ~ 7). The pH of the bath in the electrophoretic experiments is close to 7, resulting in positively charged surfaces and almost neutral edges. Therefore, the applied electric field exerts a force only on the surfaces of the gibbsite platelets and Brownian motion could provide sufficient torque to re-orient perpendicular particles to face the ITO electrode. Once being close to the electrode, the gibbsite nanoplatelets will be forced to align parallel to the electrode surface as this orientation is more energetically favorable than the perpendicular one. If the duration of the electrophoretic process is long enough, almost all gibbsite platelets can be deposited on the ITO electrode.

4.2 Filling nanoplatelet assemblies with ETPTA

After oriented deposition, polymer-gibbsite nanocomposites can then be made by filling the interstitials between the aligned nanoplatelets with photo-curable monomers, followed by photopolymerization. We choose a non-volatile monomer, ethoxylated trimethylolpropane triacrylate (ETPTA, M.W. 428, viscosity 60 cps), to form the nanocomposites. The monomer with 1% photoinitiator (Darocur 1173, Ciba-Geigy) is spin-coated at 4000 rpm for 1 min to infiltrate the electroplated gibbsite film and then polymerized by exposure to ultraviolet radiation. The resulting nanocomposite film becomes highly transparent (Fig. 3A) due to the matching of refractive index between the gibbsite platelets and the polymer matrix. The normal-incidence transmission measurement as shown in Fig. 3B shows the free-standing nanocomposite film exhibits high transmittance (> 80%) for most of the visible wavelengths. As the reflection (*R*) from an interface between two materials with refractive index of n_1 and n_2 is governed by Fresnel's equation(Macleod 2001):

$$R = [(n_1 - n_2) / (n_1 + n_2)] \quad (3)$$

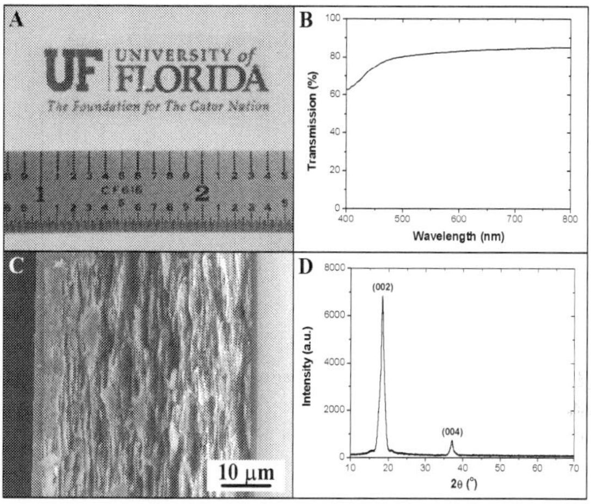

Fig. 3. Free-standing gibbsite-ETPTA nanocomposite. (A) Photograph of a transparent nanocomposite film. (B) Normal-incidence transmission spectrum of the sample in (A). (C) Cross-sectional SEM image of the same film. (D) XRD patterns of the same sample. Adapted from Lin, Huang et al. 2009.

we can estimate the normal-incidence reflection from each air-nanocomposite interface to be about 4%. Thus, the optical scattering and absorption caused by the nanocomposite itself is ca. 10%. This suggests the polymer matrix has infiltrated most interstitial spaces between the aligned gibbsite nanoplatelets. The cross-sectional SEM image in Fig. 3C shows the nanocomposite retains the layered structure of the original electroplated gibbsite film. Thin wetting layers of ETPTA (~ 1 μm thick) are observed on the surfaces of the film. The oriented arrangement of the nanoplatelets is also maintained throughout the polymer infiltration process as confirmed by the distinctive (002) and (004) peaks of the XRD spectrum shown in Fig. 3D.

4.3 Composition analysis

The ceramic weight fraction of the ETPTA-gibbsite nanocomposite film is determined by thermogravimetric analysis (TGA) as shown in Fig. 4. From the TGA curve and the corresponding weight loss rate, it is apparent that two thermal degradation processes occur. One happens at ~ 250°C and corresponds to the degradation of the polymer matrix; while another occurs at ~ 350°C and is due to the decomposition reaction of gibbsite:

$$2Al(OH)_3 \rightarrow Al_2O_3 + 3H_2O \quad (4)$$

Based on the residue mass percentage (45.65%) and assuming the ash is solely Al_2O_3, we can estimate the weight fraction of gibbsite nanoplatelets in the original nanocomposite film to be ~ 0.70. Considering the density of gibbsite (~ 2.4 g/cm^3) and ETPTA (~ 1.0 g/cm^3), the volume fraction of gibbsite nanoplatelets in the nanocomposite is ca. 0.50. The complete infiltration of ETPTA between the electroplated gibbsite platelets is further confirmed by the selective dissolution of gibbsite in a 2% hydrochloric acid aqueous solution. This results in the formation of a self-standing porous membrane with stacked hexagon-shaped pores, which are negative replica of the assembled gibbsite platelets.

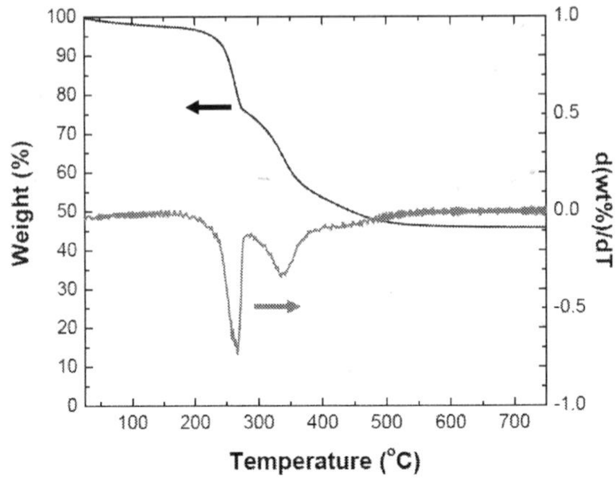

Fig. 4. Thermogravimetric analysis of a gibbsite-ETPTA nanocomposite. Adapted from Lin, Huang et al. 2009.

4.4 Mechanical test

The mechanical properties of the biomimetic polymer nanocomposites are evaluated by tensile tests. We compare the tensile strength for three types of thin films, including pure ETPTA, gibbsite-ETPTA, and TPM-modified gibbsite-ETPTA. The surface hydroxyl groups of gibbsite nanoplatelets can be easily modified by reacting with 3-(trimethoxysilyl)propyl methacrylate (TPM) through the well-established silane coupling reaction. This results in the formation of surface-modified particles with dangling acrylate bonds that can be crosslinked with the acrylate-based ETPTA matrix. The colloidal stability and the surface charge of the resulting nanoplatelets are not affected by this surface modification process as confirmed by TEM and zeta potential measurement. Fig. 5 shows the tensile stress versus strain curves for the above three types of films. The gibbsite-ETPTA nanocomposite displays ~ 2 times higher strength and ~ 3 times higher modulus when compared with pure ETPTA polymer. Even more remarkable improvement occurs when TPM-gibbsite platelets are crosslinked with the ETPTA matrix. We observe ~ 4 times higher strength and nearly one order of magnitude higher modulus than pure polymer. This agrees with early studies that reveal the crucial role played by the covalent linkage between the ceramic fillers and the organic matrix in determining the mechanical properties of the artificial nacreous composites.

We also conduct a simple calculation to evaluate if the measured mechanical properties of the gibbsite-ETPTA nanocomposites are reasonable. For a polymer matrix having a yield shear strength τ_y and strong bonding to gibbsite nanoplatelet surface (e.g., TPM-modified gibbsites), the tensile strength of the composite (σ_c) can be calculated using the volume fraction of nanoplatelets (V_p), the nanoplatelet aspect ratio (s), and the tensile strength of the nanoplatelets (σ_p) and of the polymer matrix (σ_m), as(Bonderer, Studart et al. 2008)

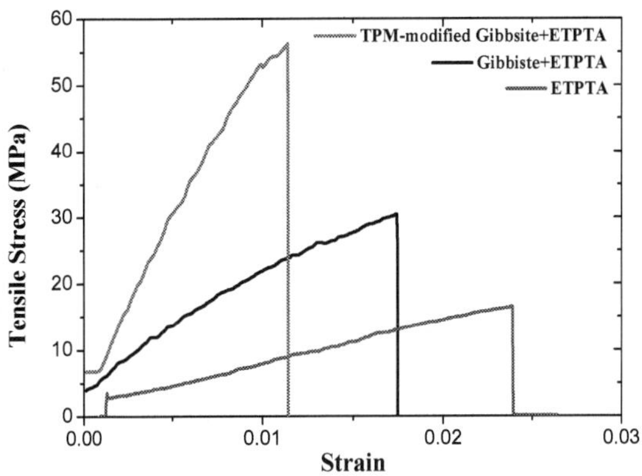

Fig. 5. Tensile stress versus strain curves for plain ETPTA film, ETPTA-gibbsite nanocomposite, and TPM-modified ETPTA-gibbsite nanocomposite. Adapted from Lin, Huang et al. 2009.

$$\sigma_c = \alpha V_P \sigma_P + (1 - V_P)\sigma_m \tag{5}$$

For the gibbsite nanoplatelet which has a relatively small aspect ratio (s ~ 12 to 18), the factor α in equation 3 can be estimated as

$$\alpha = \tau_y s / 2\sigma_P \tag{6}$$

From the above TGA analysis, the volume fraction of gibbsite nanoplatelets in the polymer nanocomposite is ~ 0.50. If we take s = 15, equation 3 can then be simplified as

$$\sigma_c = 3.75\tau_y + 0.5\sigma_m \tag{7}$$

For acrylate-based polymer (like ETPTA), the yield shear strength should be close to its tensile strength. Equation 7 can further be simplified as $\sigma_c \sim 4.25\sigma_m$. This indicates that the strength of the nanocomposite is about fourfold of the strength of the polymer matrix, agreeing with our experimental result.

5. PVA-gibbsite nanocomposites

5.1 Single-step electrophoretic deposition of PVA-gibbsite nanocomposites

The electrophoretic deposition of PVA-gibbsite nanocomposites is also carried out using the same parallel sandwich cell as described above. The high-molecular weight PVA (Mw 89,000-98,000) is neutrally charged in the electrophoretic bath and can be adsorbed on the surfaces of gibbsite nanoplatelets as water-soluble binders to cement electrodeposited gibbsite nanoplatelets together and also prevent the deposits from cracking. Fig. 6A shows a photograph of a PVA-gibbsite nanocomposite formed on an ITO cathode. The film can be easily peeled off from the electrode surface by using a sharp razor blade. The resulting self-standing film is flexible and transparent, which is different from gibbsite deposits. Optical transmission measurement at normal-incidence shows the film exhibits 60-80% transmittance for most of the visible wavelengths. Top-view SEM image in Fig. 6B illustrates the gibbsite nanoplatelets are preferentially oriented with their crystallographic *c*-axis perpendicular to the electrode surface. It is very rare to find edge-on platelets. The ordered layered structure is clearly evident from the cross-sectional SEM images as shown in Fig. 6C and 6D.

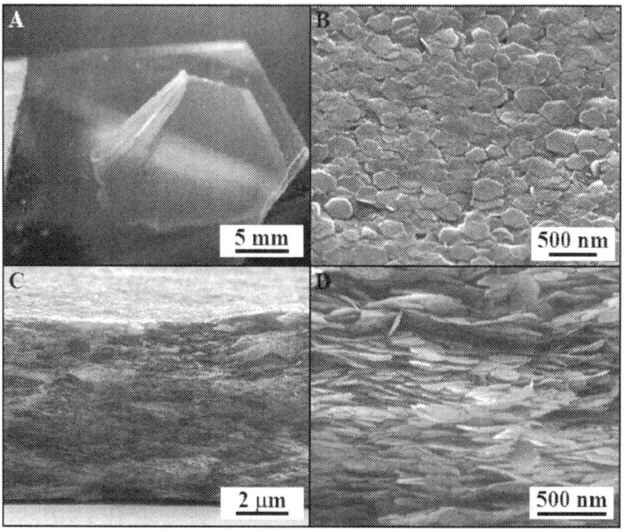

Fig. 6. Electrodeposited PVA-gibbsite nanocomposite. (A) Photograph of a composite film on an ITO electrode. (B) Top-view SEM image of the sample in (A). (C) Cross-sectional SEM image of the sample in (A). (D) Magnified cross-sectional image. Adapted from Lin, Huang et al. 2009.

5.2 XRD and TGA analysis of PVA-gibbsite nanocomposites

The oriented assembly of high-aspect-ratio gibbsite nanoplatelets is further confirmed by XRD. Fig. 7 displays a XRD spectrum of an electrodeposited PVA-gibbsite nanocomposite on an ITO electrode. The diffraction peaks from (222), (400), (441), and (662) planes of the ITO substrate are clearly appeared. Other than ITO diffraction peaks, we only observe (002) and (004) peaks from gibbsite single crystals. As the crystallographic *c*-axis of single-crystalline gibbsite is normal to the platelet surfaces, the (002) and (004) reflection are from gibbsite platelets oriented parallel to the electrode surface. This strongly supports the macroscopic alignment of gibbsite nanoplatelets in the electrophoretically deposited nanocomposites.

Thermogravimetric analysis is used to determine the weight fraction of the inorganic phase in the electrodeposited nanocomposites. Fig. 8 shows the TGA curve and the corresponding weight loss rate for the PVA-gibbsite nanocomposite film. An apparent thermal degradation process occurs at ~250°C that corresponds to the degradation of the PVA matrix and the decomposition reaction of gibbsite as shown in Equation 4. Based on the residue mass percentage (53.96%) and assuming the ash is solely Al_2O_3, we can estimate the weight fraction of gibbsite nanoplatelets in the original nanocomposite film to be 0.825.

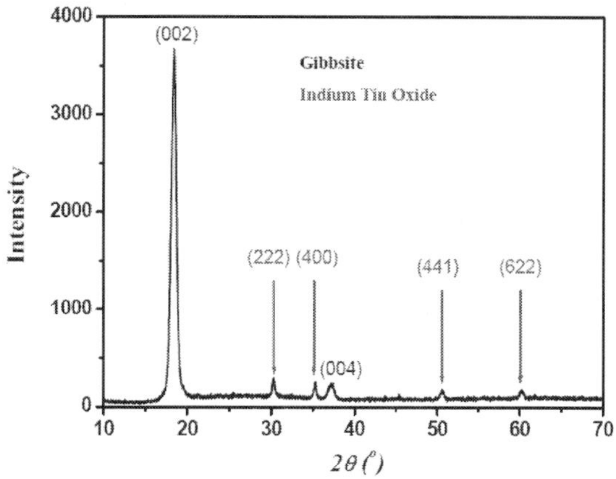

Fig. 7. XRD patterns of an electrodeposited PVA-gibbsite nanocomposite on an ITO electrode. Adapted from Lin, Huang et al. 2009.

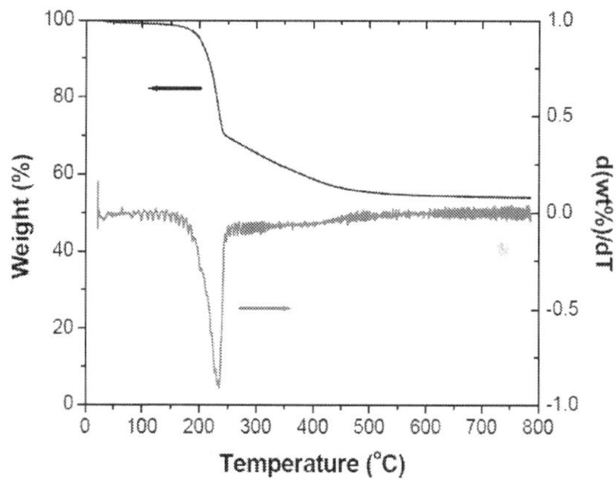

Fig. 8. Thermogravimetric analysis of PVA-gibbsite nanocomposites. Adapted from Lin, Huang et al. 2009.

6. PEI-gibbsite nanocomposites

Polyethyleneimine, which is a weak polyelectrolyte and contains amine groups, is positively charged under the electrophoretic conditions. The gibbsite nanoplatelets with a small amount of PEI are well dispersed in a water-ethanol mixture solution due to the electrostatic repulsion between particles. However, adding a larger amount of PEI leads to the agglomeration of gibbsite nanoplatelets. To allow the electrophoresis at a controlled deposition rate, as well as the formation of ordered layered structure, gibbsite nanoplatelets must be stabilized in suspensions. Therefore the influence of the PEI concentration on the stability of gibbsite is studied by measuring particle size distribution and zeta-potential.

6.1 Stability of PEI-gibbsite dispersions

To prepare the testing solution, (6 – n) mL of 2.0 wt% gibbsite solution is mixed with n mL of 0.3 wt% PEI aqueous solution, where n = 0, 1, 2, 3, 4, and 5. The weight ratio (PEI to gibbsite, R) is calculated as $(n \times 0.3)/[(6 - n) \times 2]$. Fig. 9 shows the size distribution of gibbsite nanoplatelets at different R values measured by laser diffraction. The average diameter of the as-synthesized gibbsite nanoplatelets (R = 0) is 150 nm (Fig. 9A), which is smaller than that observed from TEM images. The random mismatch of the surface of nanoplatelets to the incident laser beam reduces the effective diffraction area, resulting in a smaller average diameter. Fig. 9B shows that no significant change in the particle size distribution is observed when a small amount of PEI is added (R = 0.03). However, further increasing of PEI concentration, as shown in Fig. 9C and 9D (R = 0.075 and 0.75, respectively), leads to a larger particle diameter resulting from the flocculation of nanoplatelets. The flocculation at high polyelectrolyte concentration can be explained by the increase in ionic strength, which leads to the decrease in the electrical double-layer thickness and the instability of the colloids. Depletion flocculation also plays an important role. At a high polymer concentration, the polymer concentration gradient between the inter-particle gap and the remainder of the solution generates an osmotic pressure difference, forcing solvent flows out of the gap until particles flocculate(Dietrich and Neubrand 2001).

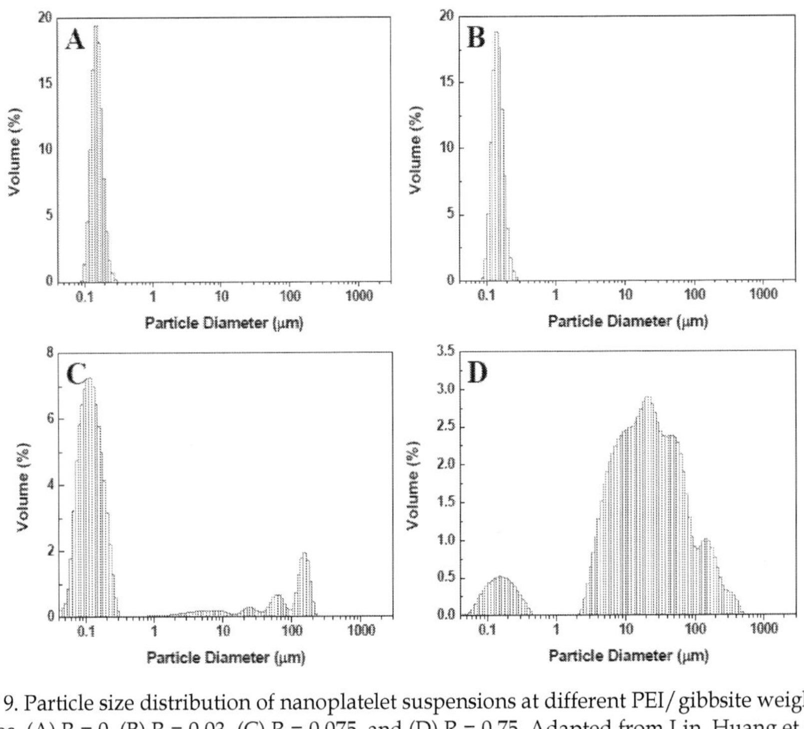

Fig. 9. Particle size distribution of nanoplatelet suspensions at different PEI/gibbsite weight ratios. (A) R = 0, (B) R = 0.03, (C) R = 0.075, and (D) R = 0.75. Adapted from Lin, Huang et al. 2009.

Electrophoretic mobility and zeta-potential of nanoplatelets in PEI-gibbsite suspensions with different R values are shown in Fig. 10. Zeta-potential is obtained by fitting experimental data using Smoluchowski's model. The increase of the electrophoretic mobility and zeta-potential when a small amount of PEI is added (R from 0 to 0.03) is due to the contribution of highly charged PEI that possesses a zeta-potential of ~+60 mV in water at neutral pH. Further increasing of PEI concentration results in the decreasing of electrophoretic mobility and zeta-potential due to the particle flocculation as shown in Fig. 9.

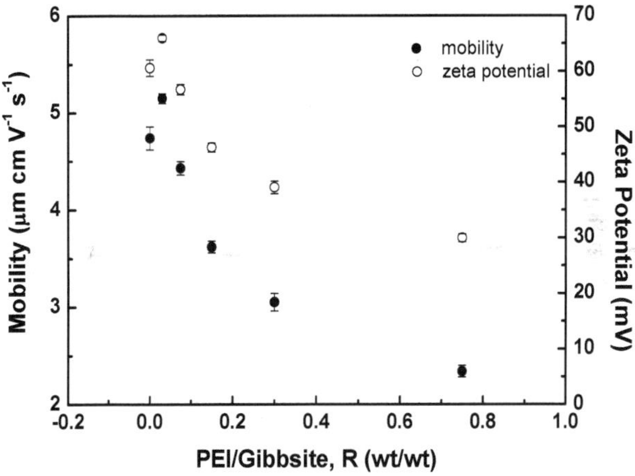

Fig. 10. Electrophoretic mobility and corresponding zeta-potential of nanoplatelets at different PEI/gibbsite weight ratio. Adapted from Lin, Huang et al. 2009.

6.2 Single-step electrophoretic deposition of PEI-gibbsite nanocomposites

The electrophoretic deposition of PEI-gibbsite nanocomposite is again performed using a parallel-plate cell. The positively charged nanoplatelets are attracted toward the bottom Au cathode by the electrical force. As gibbsite nanoplatelets have positively charged surface and almost neutral edges under the electrophoretic conditions, the electric force tends to re-orient the gibbsite nanoplatelets to face the electrode. The positively charged PEI molecules are also electrophoretically migrated toward the cathode together with gibbsite and simultaneously sandwiched between nanoplatelets, forming PEI-gibbsite nanocomposite. Ethanol is added to promote particle coagulation by squeezing the electrical double-layer thickness of the gibbsite nanoplatelets. The high pH near the cathode also helps to coagulate nanoplatelets, as well as neutralize the protonated PEI macromolecules. Top-view SEM images in Fig. 11A and 11B show that the electrodeposited nanoplatelets are preferentially oriented with their crystallographic c-axis perpendicular to the electrode surface. The hexagonal shape and the size of the platelets can be clearly seen in Fig. 11B. Cross-sectional SEM images showed in Fig. 11C and 11D provide further evidence of the ordered layered structure.

6.3 XRD and TGA analysis of PEI-gibbsite nanocomposites

XRD spectrum of the PEI-gibbsite nanocomposite on an Au electrode is shown in Fig. 12. The diffraction peak from the (002) plane of gibbsite single crystals is clearly appeared. Comparing to previous results, which show diffraction peaks from both (002) and (004) planes of gibbsite crystals, the weaker diffraction peak from (004) plane is overlapped with the strong diffraction peak of Au. The (004) diffraction peak can be clearly seen by simply replacing Au electrode with Pt (not shown here). As the (002) and (004) diffraction are originated from gibbsite platelets oriented parallel to the electrode surface, the oriented assembly of nanoplatelets is further confirmed.

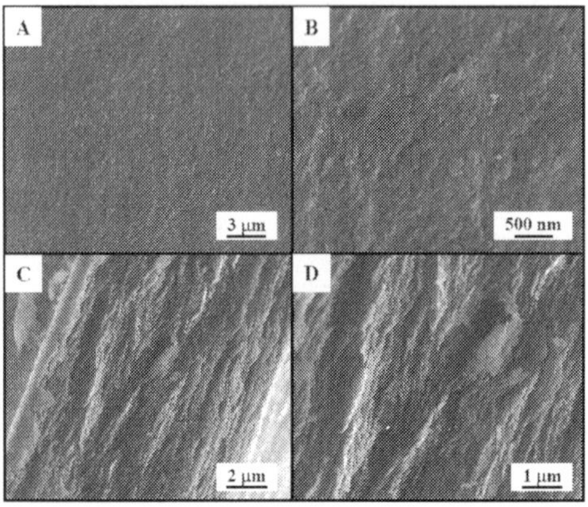

Fig. 11. SEM images of PEI-gibbsite nanocomposite. (A) Top-view image, (B) magnified top-view image, (C) cross-sectional image, and (D) magnified cross-sectional image. Adapted from Lin, Huang et al. 2009.

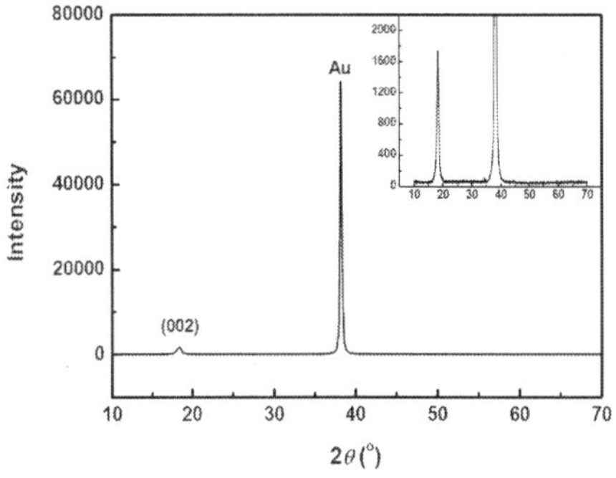

Fig. 12. XRD patterns of an electrodeposited PEI-gibbsite nanocomposite on Au electrode. Adapted from Lin, Huang et al. 2009.

TGA is carried out to determine the weight fraction of the organic phase in the nanocomposites shown in Fig. 13. An apparent thermal degradation process occurs at ~250 °C that corresponds to the degradation of the polymer matrix and the decomposition reaction of gibbsite. Based on the residual mass percentage (63.7%) and assuming the ash contains only Al_2O_3, the weight fraction of PEI in the nanocomposite film is estimated to be ~0.03, which is close to the organic content of natural nacre consisting of less than 5 wt% of soft biological macromolecules.

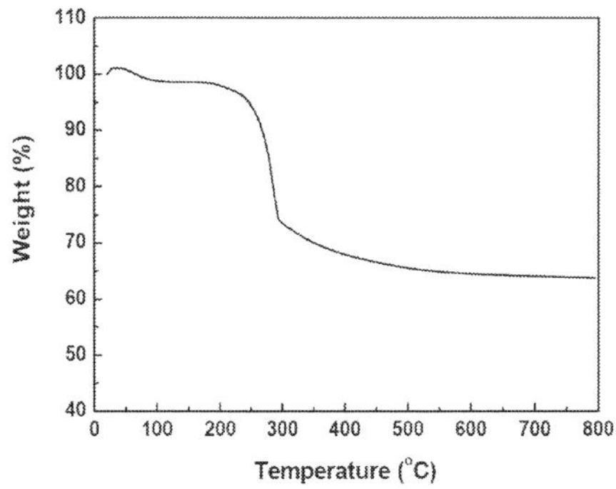

Fig. 13. Thermogravimetric analysis of an electrodeposited PEI-gibbsite nanocomposite. Adapted from Lin, Huang et al. 2009.

6.4 Mechanical test

The mechanical properties of the electrodeposited nanocomposites are evaluated using nanoindentation. This technique has been widely used in the characterization of mechanical behaviors of thin films, superhard coatings and nacres. In a nanoindentation test, a diamond Berkovich indenter is forced perpendicularly into the coating surface. The load-displacement profile is obtained during one cycle of loading and unloading, from which the hardness, H, and the reduced modulus, E_r, are calculated using the Oliver-Pharr method(Oliver and Pharr 1992). In this method, the unloading curve is fitted to the power-law relation. The contact stiffness, S, is then obtained by differentiating the power-law function at the maximum depth of penetration, h_{max}. The contact depth, h_c, can be estimated from the load-displacement profile and then the contact area, A, is obtained by using empirically determined indenter shape function, A = f(h), at h_c. Once the contact area is determined, the hardness, *H*, and reduced modulus, E_r, are obtained.

Fig. 14 shows the E_r as a function of contact depth obtained from the nanoindentation tests. The observed E_r is in the range of 2.20 to 5.17 GPa. The decrease in E_r with increasing contact

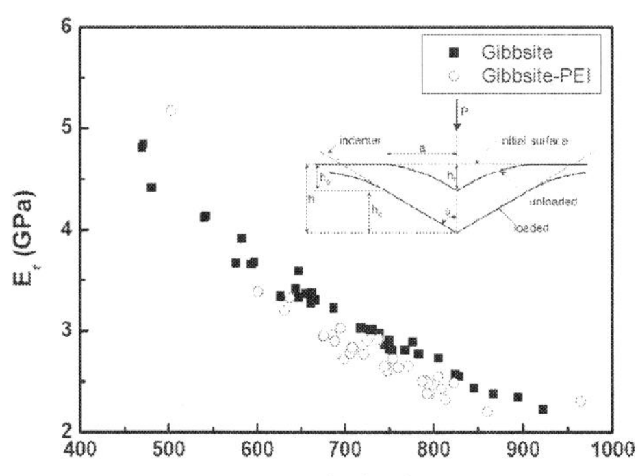

Fig. 14. Reduced modulus of pure gibbsite and PEI-gibbsite nanocomposite measured by nanoindentation. Adapted from Lin, Huang et al. 2009.

depth may be related to the indentation size effects. The size effects are explained as a result of deformation, which is mainly from crack propagation for ceramics, and factors such as surface roughness, interaction between inorganic and organic phases, and other structural details of the coatings(Page, Oliver et al. 1992; Pharr 1998). The E_r of PEI-gibbsite nanocomposite is ~0.4 GPa lower than that of pure gibbsite coating, showing the effect of the soft PEI layers in between the hard gibbsite nanoplatelets(Katti, Mohanty et al. 2006).

7. Conclusion

In conclusion, we have developed a simple and rapid electrodeposition technology for assembling gibbsite nanoplatelets into large-area, self-standing films. These nanosheets with high aspect ratio are preferentially aligned parallel to the electrode surface. The interstitials between the assembled nanoplatelets can be infiltrated with polymer to form optically transparent nanocomposites. The tensile strength and the stiffness of these biomimetic composites are significantly improved when compared to pure polymer films. The current electrodeposition technology is also promising for developing layered metal-ceramic and conducting polymer-ceramic nanocomposites that may exhibit improved mechanical and electrical properties but are not easily available by other bottom-up technologies (e.g., LBL assembly). We have also demonstrated that rapid production of nacre-like inorganic-organic nanocomposites can be achieved in a single step by electrophoretic co-deposition technology. The resulting self-standing polymer-gibbsite films are optically transparent and flexible. This technology is readily applicable to many other polyelectrolyte-nanoplatelet systems.

8. References

Aksay, I. A., M. Trau, et al. (1996). "Biomimetic pathways for assembling inorganic thin films." Science 273(5277): 892-898.

Almqvist, N., N. H. Thomson, et al. (1999). "Methods for fabricating and characterizing a new generation of biomimetic materials." Mater. Sci. Eng. C 7(1): 37-43.

Barthelat, F. (2007). "Biomimetics for next generation materials." Phil. Trans. R. Soc. A 365: 2907-2919.

Bonderer, L. J., A. R. Studart, et al. (2008). "Bioinspired design and assembly of platelet reinforced polymer films." Science 319(5866): 1069-1073.

Braun, P. V. and P. Wiltzius (1999). "Microporous materials - Electrochemically grown photonic crystals." Nature 402(6762): 603-604.

Brown, A. B. D., S. M. Clarke, et al. (1998). "Ordered phase of platelike particles in concentrated dispersions." Langmuir 14(11): 3129-3132.

Chen, R. F., C. A. Wang, et al. (2008). "An efficient biomimetic process for fabrication of artificial nacre with ordered-nano structure." Mater. Sci. Eng. C 28(2): 218-222.

Cullity, B. D. (1978). Elements of x-ray diffraction. Reading, MA, Addison-Wesley Publishing Company.

Dietrich, A. and A. Neubrand (2001). "Effects of particle size and molecular weight of polyethylenimine on properties of nanoparticulate silicon dispersions." J. Am. Ceram. Soc. 84(4): 806-812.

Grandfield, K. and I. Zhitomirsky (2008). "Electrophoretic deposition of composite hydroxyapatite-silica-chitosan coatings." Mater. Character. 59(1): 61-67.

Holgado, M., F. Garcia-Santamaria, et al. (1999). "Electrophoretic deposition to control artificial opal growth." Langmuir 15(14): 4701-4704.

Jackson, A. P., J. F. V. Vincent, et al. (1988). "THE MECHANICAL DESIGN OF NACRE." Proc. R. Soc. Lond. B 234(1277): 415-&.

Katti, K. S., B. Mohanty, et al. (2006). "Nanomechanical properties of nacre." J. Mater. Res. 21(5): 1237-1242.

Lin, T. H., W. H. Huang, et al. (2009). "Bioinspired Assembly of Colloidal Nanoplatelets by Electric Field." Chem. Mater. 21(10): 2039-2044.

Lin, T. H., W. H. Huang, et al. (2009). "Electrophoretic co-deposition of biomimetic nanoplatelet-polyelectrolyte composites." Electrochem. Commun. 11: 1635-1638.

Lin, T. H., W. H. Huang, et al. (2009). "Electrophoretic deposition of biomimetic nanocomposites." Electrochem. Commun. 11(1): 14-17.

Liu, T., B. Q. Chen, et al. (2008). "Ordered assemblies of clay nano-platelets." Bioinsp. Biomim. 3: 016005.

Macleod, H. A. (2001). Thin-Film Optical Filters. Bristol, Institute of Physics Publishing.

Mourad, M. C. D., J. Wijnhoven, et al. (2006). "Gelation versus liquid crystal phase transitions in suspensions of plate-like particles." Phil. Trans. R. Soc. A 364(1847): 2807-2816.

Munch, E., M. E. Launey, et al. (2008). "Tough, Bio-Inspired Hybrid Materials." Science 322(5907): 1516-1520.

Oliver, W. C. and G. M. Pharr (1992). "An improved technique for determining hardness and elastic-modulus using load and displacement sensing indentation experiments." J. Mater. Res. 7(6): 1564-1583.

Page, T. F., W. C. Oliver, et al. (1992). "The deformation-behavior of ceramic crystals subjected to very low load (nano)indentations." J. Mater. Res. 7(2): 450-473.

Pang, X. and I. Zhitomirsky (2008). "Electrodeposition of hydroxyapatite-silver-chitosan nanocomposite coatings." Surf. Coatings Technol. 202(16): 3815-3821.

Pharr, G. M. (1998). "Measurement of mechanical properties by ultra-low load indentation." Mater. Sci. Eng. A 253(1-2): 151-159.

Podsiadlo, P., A. K. Kaushik, et al. (2007). "Ultrastrong and stiff layered polymer nanocomposites." Science 318: 80-83.

Podsiadlo, P., M. Michel, et al. (2008). "Exponential growth of LBL films with incorporated inorganic sheets." Nano Lett. 8(6): 1762-1770.

Smith, B. L., T. E. Schaffer, et al. (1999). "Molecular mechanistic origin of the toughness of natural adhesives, fibres and composites." Nature 399(6738): 761-763.

Tang, Z. Y., N. A. Kotov, et al. (2003). "Nanostructured artificial nacre." Nat. Mater. 2(6): 413-U8.

van der Beek, D. and H. N. W. Lekkerkerker (2004). "Liquid crystal phases of charged colloidal platelets." Langmuir 20(20): 8582-8586.

van der Beek, D., P. B. Radstake, et al. (2007). "Fast formation of opal-like columnar colloidal crystals." Langmuir 23: 11343-11346.

van der Kooij, F. M., K. Kassapidou, et al. (2000). "Liquid crystal phase transitions in suspensions of polydisperse plate-like particles." Nature 406(6798): 868-871.

van der Kooij, F. M. and H. N. W. Lekkerkerker (1998). "Formation of nematic liquid crystals in suspensions of hard colloidal platelets." J. Phys. Chem. B 102(40): 7829-7832.

Velev, O. D. and K. H. Bhatt (2006). "On-chip micromanipulation and assembly of colloidal particles by electric fields." Soft Matter 2(9): 738-750.

Wierenga, A. M., T. A. J. Lenstra, et al. (1998). "Aqueous dispersions of colloidal gibbsite platelets: synthesis, characterisation and intrinsic viscosity measurements." Colloids Surf. A 134(3): 359-371.

Zhitomirsky, I. (2002). "Cathodic electrodeposition of ceramic and organoceramic materials. Fundamental aspects." Adv. Colloid Interface Sci. 97(1-3): 279-317.

7

Beyond a Nature-inspired Lotus Surface: Simple Fabrication Approach Part I. Superhydrophobic and Transparent Biomimetic Glass Part II. Superamphiphobic Web of Nanofibers

Hyuneui Lim

Department of Nature Inspired Mechanical Systems, Nano Convergence and Manufacturing Systems Research Division, Korea Institute of Machinery and Materials, 171 Jang-dong, Yuseong-gu, Daejeon, 305-343 Korea

1. Introduction

Nowadays, many people have a dream of mimicking the amazing aspects of nature, in particular their functional surfaces. In nature, there are a great many wonderful functional surfaces, such as the lotus leaf for self-cleaning, a morpho-butterfly wing for structural color, a moth eye for antireflection, the back of a stenocara beetle to capture fog, the foot of a gecko for dry adhesion, a strider's leg for water resistance, or a snake's skin as a low friction material [1]. Because biological systems change depending on the environment and circumstances, the surfaces which are always exposed to the outside are well developed for their function, especially in an optimized state. The most interesting feature is that the functional surfaces in nature have a hierarchical structure ranging from macrosize to nanosize as well as a chemical composition that facilitates low surface tension to maximize their role.

Among the numerous nature surfaces, this paper focuses on the lotus leaf, a well-known example of a superhydrophobic and self-cleaning surface [2-4]. The lotus is a plant that can grow in murky ponds. The lotus leaf is a symbol of purity in the Orient, because their leaves always remain clean and dry. This phenomenon originated from the non-wetting property of the lotus leaf. The lotus leaf has two levels of roughness structures comprised of both micrometer-scale bumps and nanometer-scale hair-like structures on the surface with a composition of wax. The trapped air on the rough surface makes water droplets bead up at a contact angle in the superhydrophobic range of 150° and then rolls off while collecting any compiled dirt due to the very low sliding angle.

In order to prove the transfer of this lotus effect to be technically feasible, there have been numerous attempts to synthesize the surface structures on the low surface tension chemical layer. Fabrication methods have been developed to create structures that mimic the superhydrophobic behavior of lotus surfaces, and these are generally categorized into one of two methods: a top-down or a bottom-up method. The top-down processes can structure patterns well according to the design for superhydrophobicity. Photolithography is one of the most important methods among the top-down processes.[5] capillary lithography [6], electron beam lithography [7], interference lithography [8], pattern transfers of natural surfaces, plasma etching without a mask [9], laser ablation [10], and electrospinning [11] are all top-down processes. The bottom-up processes include colloidal assembly [12], the sol-gel method [13], and the plasma-enhanced chemical vapor deposition of carbon nanotubes. In addition, a combination of bottom-up and top-down approaches [14,15] has been shown to be very useful when fabricating fractal microstructures and nanostructures with superhydrophobic properties.

However, the important aspect of a practical application of superhydrophobic surfaces in daily life is the durability and stability of superhydrophobic micro/nanostructures and the economic feasibility of the fabrication process. Recently, many researchers who study superhydrophobic surfaces have turned their research focus to the durability and stability of superhydrophobic micro/nanostructures and simple fabrication methods for mass production [16-17].

Another issue associated with a superhydrophobic surface is to creation of an amphiphobic surface which repels both water and organic liquids. The demand an oil-repellent surface has increased in many applications, including cell phones and touch-screen displays as well as biomedical devices. Unfortunately, an oil-repellent surface in nature has yet to be reported. Beyond the superhydrophobic lotus surface, researchers have formulated several important considerations with regard to the design of an amphiphobic surface [18,19].

In this review paper, superhydrophobic and transparent biomimetic glass and a superamphiphobic web of nanofibers are introduced. The fabrication method, advantages of biomimic surfaces, and their limitations in practical applications are discussed to help the understanding on the advance of the lotus effect. The results are mainly based on two published articles: "Simple Nanofabrication of a Superhydrophobic & Transparent Biomimetic Surface" in Chinese Science Bulletin [20], and "Superamphiphobic Web of PTFEMA Fibers via Simple Electrospinning without Functionalization" in Macromolecular Materials and Engineering [21].

2. Superhydrophobic and superhydrophilic plant leaves in nature

It is very well known that the lotus leaf, which shows a superhydrophobic property, has a dual roughness characteristic based on the microscale and nanoscale dimensions. Including the lotus leaf, there are many plants that have the ability to repel water in nature. Commonly, they have hierarchical structures on their surface. However, some plant leaves have the ability of superhydrophilicity, in which the water contact angle is less than 10°. Their surfaces can either spread water widely over a wet surface or absorb water via porous structures.

Figure 1 shows an image of superhydrophobic and superhydrophilic plant leaves. The lotus leaf and the taro leaf show a similar surface morphology with nano patterns on micro conical structures with a diameter of around 10μm, representing the superhydrophobic structure. However, the water lily shows only a microstructure having superhydrophilicity without nanoscale structures. This is very interesting because both the water lily and the lotus are aquatic plants. However, the water lily leaves are positioned on the water's surface, whereas the lotus leaves elevate several feet above it. Therefore, their surfaces are adapted to an ambient environment very intelligently.

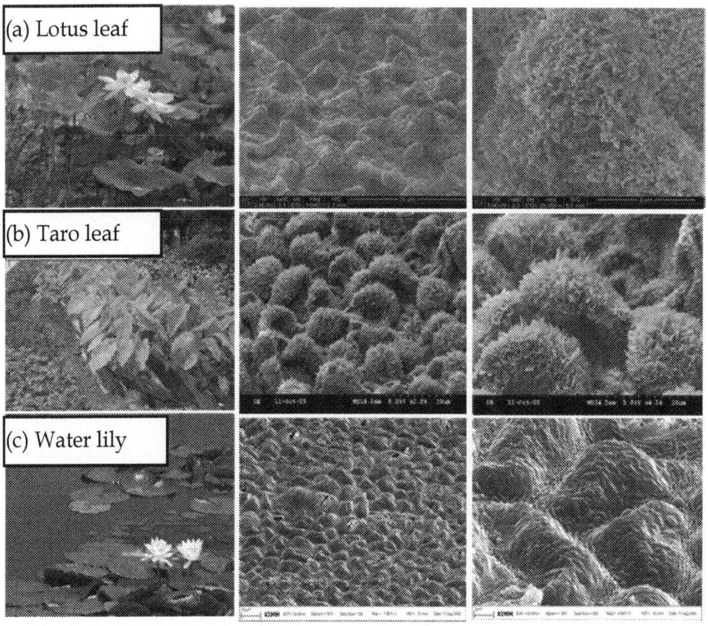

Fig. 1. Optical and SEM images of plant leaves showing the superhydrophobic and superhydrophilic characteristics: (a) lotus leaf, (b) taro leaf, and (c) water lily

Part I. Superhydrophobic and transparent biomimetic glass

A combination of colloidal lithography and plasma etching is a good candidate to create well-ordered micro/nanostructured surfaces easily. In particular, superhydrophobic and transparent glass can be created using only nanobeads smaller than 100 nm to maintain the proper level of transparency [22]. Here, a combination of colloidal lithography and plasma etching is used to fabricate superhydrophobic and transparent glass.

A schematic diagram of the fabrication process is shown in Figure 2. First, quartz glass is prepared after cleaning it by immersion in an Alconox solution (Sigma, Inc.). A water drop deposited on the cleaned dry glass surface shows a contact angle of nearly 0° without any particles of dust. Single layers of polystyrene beads were formed by spin coating as a colloidal mask. Polystyrene beads (Polysciences, Inc.) with diameters of 100 nm (S.D. = 4%) were purchased in the form of an aqueous suspension. The polystyrene bead solution was diluted to 0.6% with a mixture of methanol and triton X-100 to increase its volatility and to prevent aggregation. Spin-coating of the polystyrene nanosphere solution was performed at different spin rates for 1 minute and the quartz glass was then etched with a mixture of CF_4 and H_2 gas to enhance the etching selectivity. Finally, chemical coating of the low-surface-tension composition was done to obtain the superhydrophobic property. Additional information concerning this experimental method is available in the literature [20].

Figure 3 shows SEM images the spin-coated polystyrene beads created under several conditions, in the case 1000 rpm, 2000 rpm, 3000 rpm, 4000 rpm, and 5000 rpm, for each sample. The polystyrene beads do not spread well at a low spin rate i.e., 1000 rpm; whereas the beads are better dispersed at a relatively high spin rate i.e., 4000 and 5000 rpm. The coverage of the nanospheres derives from the balance between the spin rate and the volatility and viscosity of the colloidal suspension in the shear alignment process [23]. Among several spin rates, 3000 rpm resulted in the best spin-coated polystyrene bead layer.

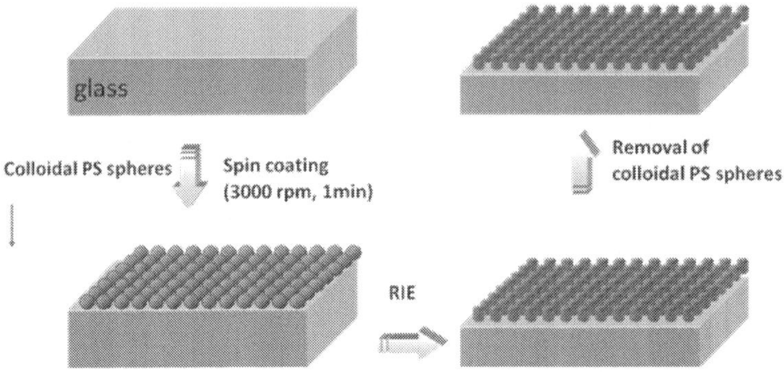

Fig. 2. Schematic diagram of the fabrication method

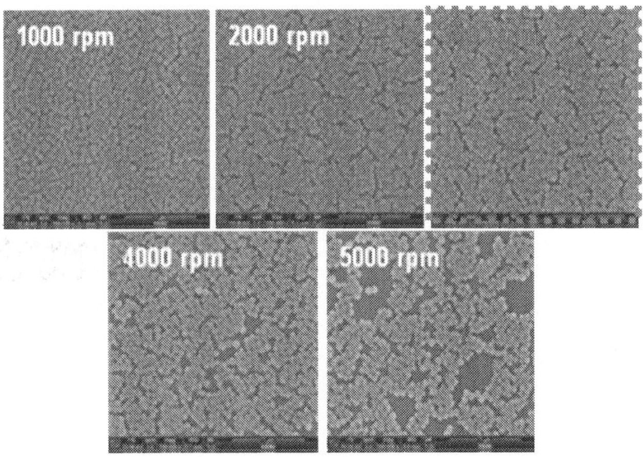

Fig. 3. SEM images of polystyrene bead layers spin-coated at different spin rates: 1000, 2000, 3000, 4000, and 5000 rpm

SEM images of polystyrene beads that were spin-coated well are shown in Figure 4. They have a single layer with close-packed and hexagonally ordered shapes. The polystyrene bead layers were also formed without defects or multiple polystyrene bead layers at an optimum spin rate, i.e., 3000 rpm.

However, for the etching process of the glass, the space between the beads of the colloidal mask requires for a reactive ion treatment on the glass surface. Therefore, spin-coated polystyrene beads were etched with CF_4 plasma for 30 seconds at a RF plasma power of 100 W to decrease the diameters of the beads. Figure 5 shows SEM images of the formed spacing between the colloidal mask beads. An interparticle distances between the beads of around 20 nm was chosen for the glass etching space.

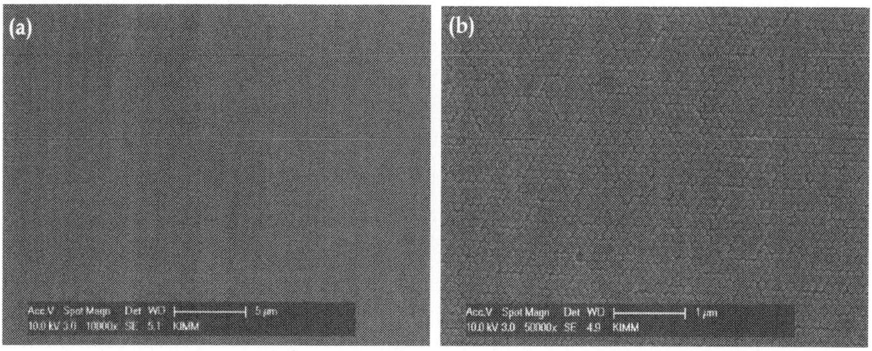

Fig. 4. SEM images of a single layer of polystyrene beads with diameters of 100 nm prepared by spin-coating at 3000 rpm: (a) an image at 10000X magnification, and (b) an image of 50000X magnification [20]

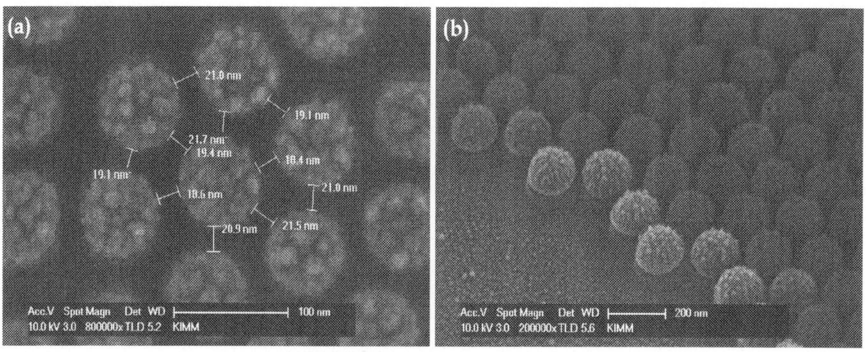

Fig. 5. SEM images of a reactive ion etching (RIE)-assisted colloidal mask of single-layered polystyrene beads treated with CF_4 plasma for 30 s; (a) top-view and (b) tilted view at 30° [20]

The nanostructures on the glass surface were formed by etching with the modified colloidal mask. Generally, glass surfaces are etched with CF_4 or SF_6 plasma. However, the use of only CF_4 plasma can lead to etching of the glass surface as well as over-etching of the 100 nm polystyrene beads, as shown in Figure 6(a). To formulate a nanostructure with a high aspect ratio, conservation of the polystyrene beads is critical during the etching process. The addition of H_2 plasma can serve as a solution and thus can protect the polystyrene beads. Figure 6(b) shows the result of the selective etching of the glass surfaces with a mixture of CF_4 plasma and H_2 plasma at a ratio of 2:1. Depending on the portion of the H_2 plasma, the selectivity between the polystyrene colloidal mask and the glass changed. When a greater amount of H_2 plasma was added, the selectivity of the etching was increased. On the other hand, the etch rate of the glass was reduced.

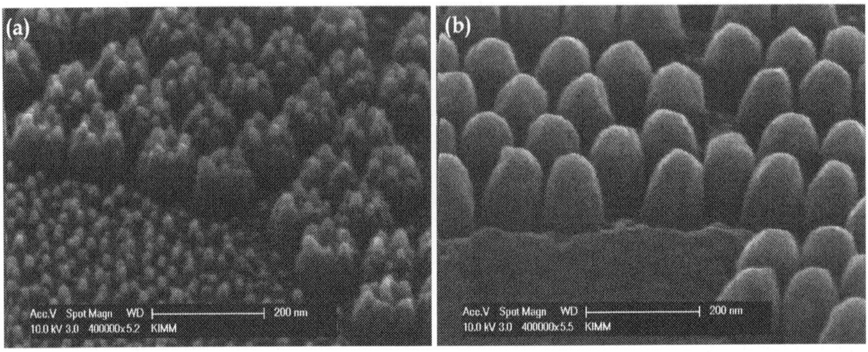

Fig. 6. SEM images of a nanostructured glass surface etched with (a) CF_4 plasma and (b) a mixture of CF_4 plasma and H_2 plasma at a ratio of 2:1 for 3 min. The SEM images were obtained at a tilted view of 30°.

Figure 7 shows the nanostructured glass surfaces according to the etching time with a mixture of CF_4 plasma and H_2 plasma at a ratio of 2:1. The heights of the nanostructures are in direct proportional to the etching time. The nanostructures on the glass surface formed a sharp end on the top and reached a height of nearly 500 nm after 11 minutes of etching. The etching rate in the given reactive ion etching condition was approximately 40 nm/min.

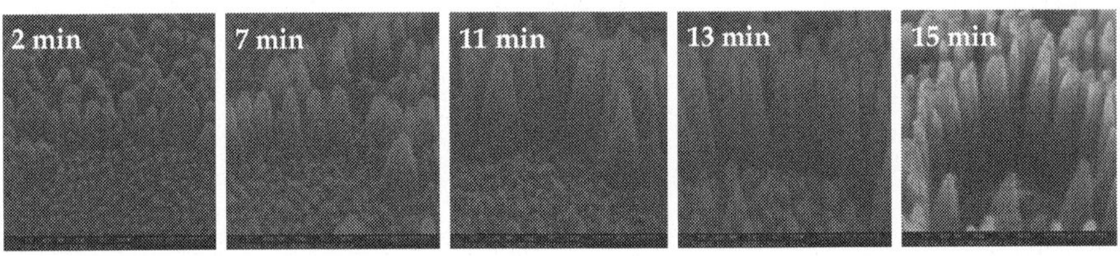

Fig. 7. SEM images of nanostructures on a glass surface etched with different etching times: 2, 7, 11, 13, and 15 min

A high-magnification image of the fabricated nanostructures is shown in Figure 8. This SEM image was obtained under environmental SEM conditions of a low pressure and a low applied voltage of 3 keV without a platinum coating. Compared to the conventional SEM images, the tower-shaped nanostructures have a sharp end on the top. This suggests that the actual shape of the nanostructures is slightly different from that shown in the SEM images when the image is obtained with a metal coating to prevent electron charging on the insulating surface of the sample. The aspect ratio the glass nanostructure was noted to be close to 4 after 10 minutes of etching.

As mention in the introduction, two main factors govern the wettability. The important factor is the chemical property of the surface. When the surface is made up of low surface energy chemicals, a geometrical surface structure enhances the hydrophobicity [24]. The geometrical surface structure of a solid is determined by the fractal structure and the roughness. Therefore, the as-prepared nanostructure glass samples must be modified chemically to obtain surface hydrophobicity.

Self-assembled monolayers (SAMs) of tridecafluoro-1,1,2,2-tetrahydrooctyltrichlorosilane (FOTS) were used as the low surface tension chemical. FOTS SAMs were deposited using a vapor-deposition method after glass etching and the removal of the remaining polystyrene beads from the top of the nanostructures. An ash process with 30 seconds of O_2 plasma following the CF_4 etching process was applied to remove the remaining polystyrene from the top of the nanostructures. The treated glass samples were then placed in a plastic container with 100 µL of FOTS droplets. Monolayer-assembled deposition was performed for 30 minutes at room temperature. The vapor deposited samples were annealed at 80°C for 1 hour to stabilize the bonding between the glass surface and the FOTS molecules as well as to increase the well-ordered packing of the FOTS molecules.

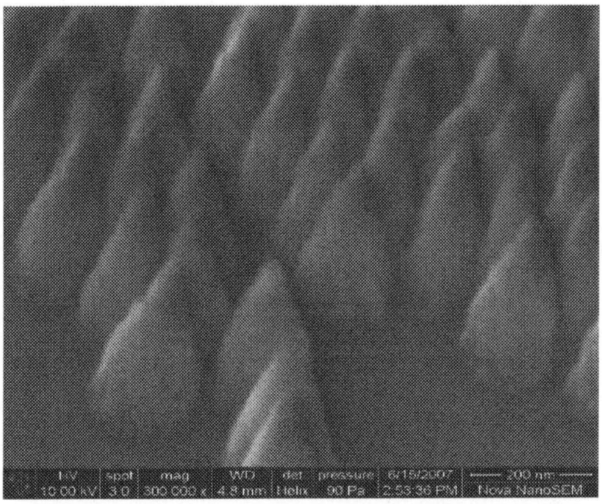

Fig. 8. SEM image of glass nanostructures after plasma etching for 10 min. The image was obtained under environmental SEM conditions without a metal coating.

Figure 9 shows the water contact angles of the nanostructured glass surfaces before and after the low-surface-tension chemical treatment. The wettability of the surfaces was measured with a contact angle analyzer (Phoenix 300, SEO Inc.) with deionized water droplets of 10 µL in volume. The water contact angle of the nanostructured glass surface was close to 4° (Figure 9(a)). The nanostructures on the surface enhanced the hydrophilicity depending on the nature of the flat glass surface. However, the nanostructured surfaces with the FOTS SAMs coating showed superhydrophobicity, with a water contact angle of nearly 150° (Figure 9(b)). Figure 9(c) clearly shows the superhydrophobicity of the fabricated glass. This superhydrophobic glass surface also shows a hexadecane contact angle of 110° given a volume of 10 µL. In the relationship between the superhydrophobic property and the height of the nanostructure, the contact angle of both the water and hexadecane increased steadily as the height of the nanostructure increased to an aspect ratio of 2.5.

In the fabrication of superhydrophobic glass, an important requirement is to retain the transparency of the glass. Therefore, only the use of a nanostructure smaller than the visible wavelength of light can enhance the wettability without leading to opacity. The transmittance of the superhydrophobic glass surface with a nanostructure diameter of 100 nm and different heights in the range of 50 nm to 1000 nm was investigated by UV-Visible spectrometry. Figure 10(a) shows the UV-Visible spectra of the nanostructured glasses with the FOTS SAMs coating and the bare quartz glass as a reference. In the range of the visible wavelength of 400 nm to 700 nm, it was determined that the antireflective phenomena known as the moth-eye antireflection effect existed. A decrease in the transmittance to less than the 500 nm wavelength was detected in several samples having a relatively high height. This may have originated from the scattering of the light given the high height of the nanostructures. However, the overall transmittance increases due to the decrease in the reflection on the nanostructured glass surface. Finally, a superhydrophobic and antireflective glass having a well-ordered nanostructure was demonstrated, as shown in Figure 10(b).

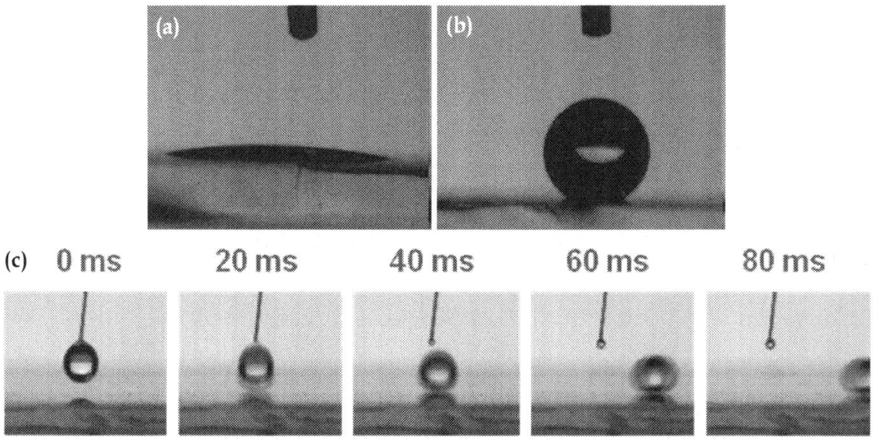

Fig. 9. Images of the water contact angles for (a) a nanostructured glass surface and (b) a nanostructured glass surface after the FOTS SAMs coating. The water contact angles are 4° and 150°, respectively [20]. (c) Sequential images of water droplets falling onto the nanostructured glass surface after the FOTS SAMs coating. The aspect ratio of the nanostructure is 4.

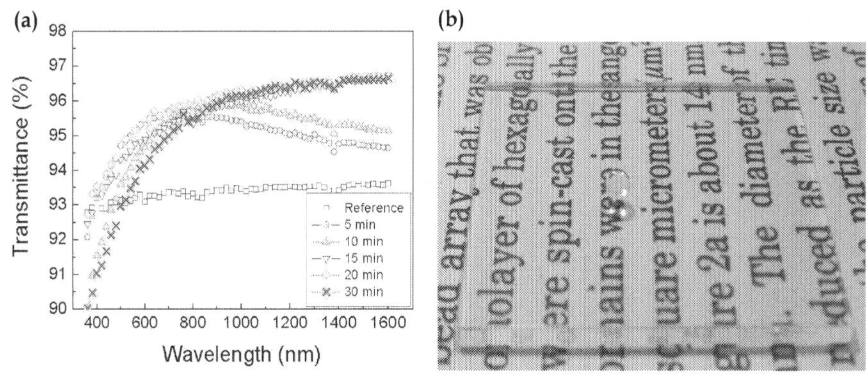

Fig 10. (a) 5 nanostructured and hydrophobic coated glasses with the different etching time and bare sample, and (b) an image of water on the superhydrophobic nanostructured glass [20]

Part II. Superamphiphobic web of Nanofibers

Currently, many researchers are interested in the demonstration of multifunctional surfaces having dual properties such as a superhydrophobicity and antireflective surface, an antifogging and antireflective surface, a switchable surface, a repellent surface capable of repelling several types of liquids, and others. Particularly, surfaces that repel water and organic liquids have recently received a great deal of attention from research and industry fields. Several important findings pertaining to amphiphobic surfaces have been reported with regard to the design of surfaces [18,19].

Two factors should be also considered in the design of a superamphiphobic surface: the chemical composition and structural morphology. For organic liquids, it is impossible to find a chemical layer that yields a contact angle greater than 90° on a flat surface [25,26]. Thus, a structural morphology must be created in which the surface curvature exhibits extreme surface resistance to wetting from all liquids. It is known that the entrapment of air beneath a re-entrant structure prevents the transition from a nonwetted state to a wetted state, even for liquids with low surface tension [27-29].

Of all the re-entrant structures, webs of microfibers and nanofibers are good candidates for a superamphiphobic surface because an electrospinning method can easily produce microfibers and nanofibers from a variety of polymeric materials [30]. In addition, the diameter of the fibers and the gap distance between the electrospun fibers can be controlled according to the processing parameters, such as the solvent, viscosity, surface tension, and electrical conductivity. Therefore, to obtain the information on robustness against wetting from low surface tension liquids, microfibers and nanofibers can form a various superamphiphobic surface. Here, an electrospun web of poly(2,2,2-trifluoroethyl methacrylate) (PTFEMA) fibers is studied to obtain an understanding of a superamphiphobic surface. The morphology of this web is modulated by changing the polymer solution concentration with other fixed processing conditions. That is, we used an applied voltage of 20 kV, a distance of 20 cm between the syringe needle tip and the collector, and a flow rate of 0.2 mL/h. A detailed description of the experimental method was introduced in earlier research, including the synthesis and electrospinning conditions of the PTFEMA as well as the characterization methods of the electrospun nanofibers web [21, 31].

A remarkable feature is that the fabrication of a web of superamphiphobic fibers was performed using a conventional electrospinning process of fluorinated polymers without any additional functionalization. A PTFEMA solution can be electrospun well with conventional processing parameters, as synthesized PTFEMA dissolves homogeneously and easily in several solvents, including Dimethyl foramide (DMF), which is an adequate solvent for electrospinning. To investigate the wetting property of the web, first the surface chemical compositions of the PTFEMA web were analyzed by XPS. An electrospun electrospun and solution casted PTFEMA sample were prepared prepared from a 26 wt% solution of DMF. The fluorine content (F/C ratio) was outstandingly high, at 0.57, and the water contact angle was 153° for the elecrospun sample, whereas the solution casting PTFEMA film showed an F/C ratio of 0.40 and a water contact angle of only 89°. The enrichment of the fluorocarbon composition and the water contact angle of the electrospun PTFEMA were caused by the surface segregation, the high ratio of the surface area to the volume, and by the rough surface morphology [32].

Figure 11 shows the superamphiphobicity of the electrospun nanofiber web. The web of PTFEMA repels both types of liquids shown in the figure, one with a surface tension of 72.8 mN/m (water colored with blue ink) and the other with a surface tension of 27.8 mN/m (hexadecane colored with red ink), while exhibiting contact angles greater than 150°.

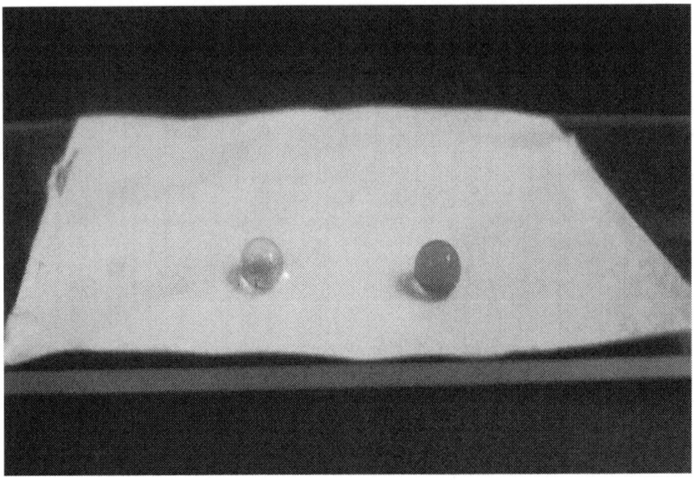

Fig. 11. Photograph of 6 μL droplets of hexadecane (colored with red ink) and 6 μL droplets of water (colored with blue ink) on an electrospun web of PTFEMA fibers with a 26 wt% polymer solution concentration concentration [21]

All of the electrospun webs of PTFEMA fiber are typical superhydrophobic surfaces, showing water contact angles that exceed 150°. However, the wetting response of the low surface tension liquid hexadecane differed depending on the morphology of the fiber webs. The sample prepared from the 26 wt% solution had the thinnest fiber diameter of approximately 500 nm and the narrowest diameter distribution, ranging from 300 nm to 700 nm; its surface repels hexadecane with a high contact angle of around 154°, as shown in Figure 12(a). However, Figure 12(b) shows that the fiber web electrospun with a 24 wt% concentration is different in terms of the fiber diameter and hexadecane contact angle. The 24 wt% sample had an average diameter of 600 nm and considerable variation in its fiber diameters, with some very thick fiber diameters of around 2000 nm or 3000 nm. In addition, the hexadecane droplet collapses with a contact angle of approximately 25° despite the fact that its surface exhibits superhydrophobicity.

The interaction between hexadecane and a web of PTFEMA fiber was investigated to confirm the wetting property of the 24 wt% samples. We obtained SEM images to determine how the morphology of the web changes after soaking the fiber web with hexadecane. As shown in Figure 13, an appreciable change was not detected after the soaking test, which proves that PTFEMA does not react with or dissolve in hexadecane.

The robustness parameter was studied to elucidate the wetting and nonwetting phenomena of hexadecane on superhydrophobic nanofiber webs with different fiber diameters. We used the robustness equation developed by Tuteja and Choi to reveal the relationships among the robustness, the fiber diameter, and the degree of porosity [19]. A detailed explanation of the robustness of fiber web samples is available in the literature [21]. The calculated robustness shows how the hexadecane droplet is sustained on the 26 wt% sample and why it collapses on the 24 wt% sample.

Figure 14 shows a summary of the hexadecane robustness and contact angle in relation to the gap distance and fiber radius depending the PTFEMA solution concentration. When the apparent contact area is identical, a thinner fiber and lower porosity increase the robustness. The 24 wt% sample shows low robustness, explaining why the hexadecane droplet collapsed although it had a high water contact angle. The 26 wt% sample had the highest level of robustness, keeping the hexadecane droplet intact for more than 8 hours. Figure 14 suggests that the 28 wt% sample and the 30 wt% sample repel the hexadecane droplet for quite a long time. The assumption that the diameter and gap distance of the fibers on the nanofiber surface are homogeneous in terms of the robustness equation implies that the 24 wt% sample has a relatively high level of robustness. However, local variation in both the fiber diameter and the distribution in our samples caused local weak spots to arise with a

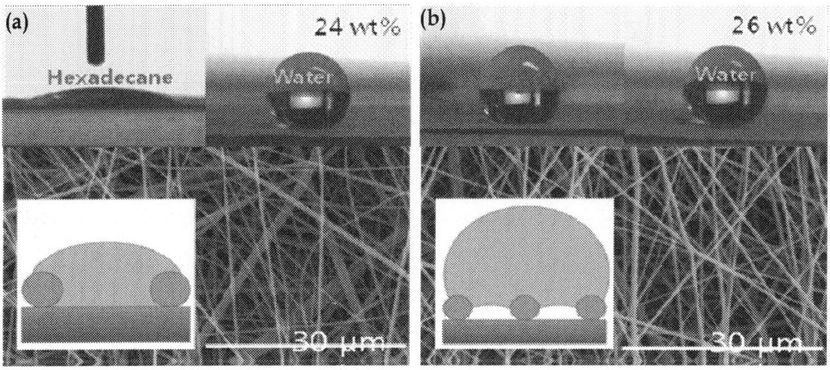

Fig. 12. Hexadecane and water contact angle images, SEM images, and schematic diagram of a nanofiber web with a hexadecane droplet. PTFEMA fibers were electrospun with different polymer solution concentrations: (a) 24 wt% and (b) 26 wt%. The volume of both the hexadecane and the water was 6 µL [21].

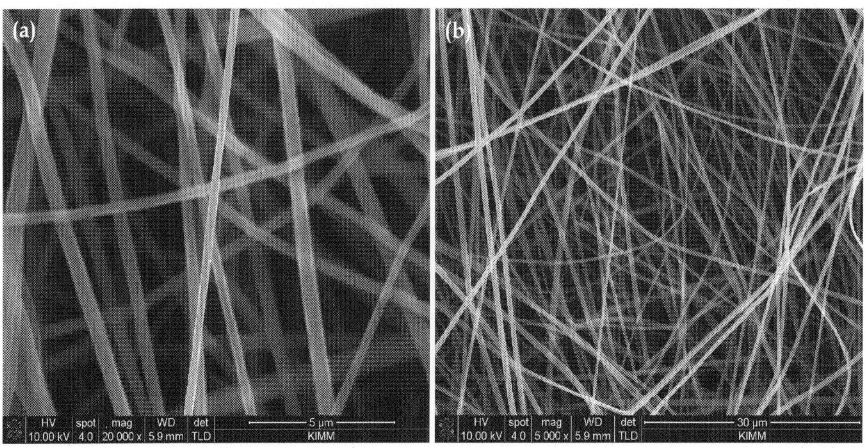

Fig. 13. SEM images of PTFEMA fibers electrospun from 24 wt% after soaking with hexadecane: (a) 5000X magnification, and (b) 20000X magnification

low level of robustness, and the droplet consequently collapsed in those areas. This lower local robustness of the 24 wt% sample can govern the collapse of the hexadecane droplet. From these results, that control of the wettability against high and low surface tension liquids can be attained by modulating the morphology of the surface, even though the chemical composition is identical. Therefore the fiber diameter and the porosity should be carefully designed to yield a high contact angle and a high level of robustness, as the porosity is related to the contact angle: that is, a high porosity value yields a low contact area and, consequently, a high contact angle.

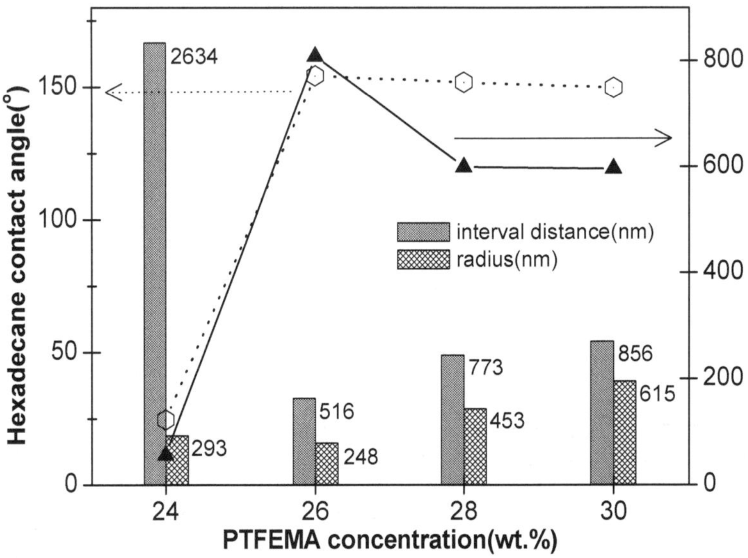

Fig. 14. The relationship between the hexadecane contact angles and the robustness with the gap distance between the fibers and the fiber radius of an electrospun web of the PTFEMA fibers with different polymer solution concentrations of 24 wt%, 26 wt%, 28 wt%, and 30 wt%. The volume of hexadecane was 6 μL in all cases [21].

3. Conclusions

Two types of nature-inspired lotus surfaces were demonstrated. A superhydrophobic and transparent biomimetic surface and a superamphiphobic electrospun nanofibers web were prepared by simple fabrication methods involving a combination of colloidal lithography and plasma etching for the former and a conventional electrospinning method with traditional processing parameters for the latter. The dual functional surfaces were introduced simply by starting with the mimicking of the lotus leaf. The simple nanostructuring process yielded a superhydrophobic structure with an antireflective property. Our study on repellence against hexadecane and water wetting reveals that a small, uniform fiber diameter and interval distance can induce a high level of robustness on a low surface tension liquid.

At present, many researchers are making a great effort to realize an artificial lotus leaf with advanced functions. Some of these results have moved beyond simply a lotus leaf. However, an artificial lotus leaf remains associated with problems related to its practical application. The most dissimilar aspect between nature and artificiality by humans is the ability to regenerate. We have a long way to go in this respect compared to nature. However, our attempts to live together with nature using nature-inspired technology bring sustainability and comfort to human life.

4. Acknowledgements

This work was supported by a grant (No. 2008-E032) from the Korea Ministry of Knowledge Economy. And the author thanks to the group members, especially Dr. Wandoo Kim, Dr. Seungmuk Ji, and Joonsik Park.

5. References

[1] Bhushan B. Biomimetics:Lessons from Nature - an Overview. Phil. Trans. R. Soc. A, 2009, 367: 1445-1486
[2] Neinhuis C, Barthlott W. Characterization and Distribution of Water Repellent, Self-cleaning Plant Surfaces. Ann Bot., 1977, 79: 667-677
[3] Genzer J, Efimenko K. Recent Developments in Superhydrophobic Surface and their Relevance to Marine Fouling: A Review. Biofouling, 2006, 22(5): 339-360
[4] Li X-M, Reinhoudt D, Crego-Calama M. What Do We Need for a Superhydrophobic Surface? A Review on the Recent Progress in the Preparation of Superhydrophobic Surfaces. Chem. Soc. Rev.,2007, 36: 1350-1368
[5] Martines E, Seunarine K, Morgan H, Gadegaard N, Wilkinson C D W, Riehle M O. Superhydrophobicity and Superhydrophilicity of Regular Nanopatterns. Nano Lett, 2005, 5: 2097-2103
[6] Suh K Y, Jon S. Control over Wettability of Polyethylene Glycol Surfaces using Capillary Lithography. Langmuir, 2005, 21: 6836-6841
[7] Kanamori Y. Roy E. Chen Y. Antireflection sub-wavelength gratings fabricated by spin-coating replication. Microelectron. Eng, 2005, 78-79: 287-293
[8] Gombert A, Glaubitt W, Rose K, Dreibholz J, Blasi B, Heizel A, Sporn D, Doll W, Wittwer V. Subwavelength-Structured Antireflective Surfaces on Glass. Thin Solid Films, 1999, 351: 73-77
[9] Minko S, Muller M, Motornov M, Nitschke M, Grundke K, Stamm M. Two-level Structured Self-adaptive Surfaces with Reversibly Tunable Properties. J. Am. Chem. Soc., 2003, 125: 3896-3900
[10] Noh J., Lee J.-H., Na S., Lim H., Jung D.-H. Fabrication of Hierarchically Micro- and Nano-structured Mold Surfaces Using Laser Ablation for Mass Production of Superhydrophobic Surfaces. Jpn. J. Appl. Phys., 2010, 49: 106502
[11] Ma M L, Hill R M, Lowery J L, Fridrikh S V, Rutledge G C. Elec-trospun Poly(Styrene-block-dimethylsiloxane) Block Copolymer Fibers Exhibiting Superhydrophobicity. Langmuir, 2005, 21: 5549-5554
[12] Gu G, Dang H, Zhang Z, Wu Z. Fabrication and Characterization of Transparent Superhydrophobic Thin Films based on Silica Nanoparticles. Appl. Phys. A, 2006, 83: 131-132

[13] Hosono E, Fujihara S, Honma I, Zhou H S. J. Superhydrophobic Perpendicular Nanopin Film by the Bottom-up Process. Am. Chem. Soc., 2005, 127: 13458-13459
[14] Sun T, Wang G J, Liu H, Feng L, Jiang L, Zhu D B. Suh K Y, Jon S. Control over the Wettability of an Aligned Carbon Nanotube Film. J. Am. Chem. Soc., 2003, 125: 14996-14997
[15] Zhu L B, Xiu Y H, Xu J W, Tamirisa P A, Hess D W, Wong C P. Superhydrophobicity on Two-tier Rough Surfaces Fabricated by Con-trolled Growth of Aligned Carbon Nanotube Arrays Coated with Fluorocarbon. Langmuir, 2005, 21: 11208-11212
[16] Zimmermann J., Reifler F. A., Fortunato G., Gerhardt L.-C., Seeger S. A Simple, One-Step Approach to Durable and Robust Superhydrophobic Textiles. Adv. Funct. Mater. 2008, 18: 3662-3669
[17] Lim H. S., Baek J. H., Park K., Shin H. S., Kim J., Cho J. H. Multifunctional Hybrid Fabrics with Thermally Stable Superhydrophobicity. Adv. Mater. 2010, 22, 2138-2141.
[18] Liu Y., Xiu Y., Hess D. W., Wong, C. P. Silicon Surface Structure-Controlled Oleophobicity. Langmuir, 2010, 26: 8908-8913
[19] Tuteja A., Choi W., Mabry J. M., McKinley G. H., Cohen R. E. Robust omniphobic surfaces. PNAS, 2008, 105: 18200-18205
[20] Lim H., Jung D.-H., Noh J.-H., Choi G.-R., Kim W.-D. Simple Nanofabrication of a Superhydrophobic & Transparent Biomimetic Surface. Chinese Sci. Bull., 2009, 54: 3613-3616
[21] Choi G.-R., Park J., Ha J.-W., Kim W.-D., Lim H. Superamphiphobic Web of PTFEMA Fibers via Simple Electrospinning without Functionalization. Macromol. Mater. Eng., 2010, 295:995-1002.
[22] Sun C-H, Gonzalez A, Linn N C, Jing P, Jiang B. Templated Biomi-metic Multifunctional Coatings. App. Phys. Lett., 2008, 92: 051107-051109
[23] Min W.-L., Jiang P., Jiang B. Large-Scale Assembly of Colloidal Nanoparticles and Fabrication of Periodic Subwavelength Structures. Nanotechnology 2008, 19: 475604.
[24] Quere D. Rough Ideas on Wetting. Physica A, 2002, 313: 32-37
[25] Li X.-M., Reinhoudt D., Crego-Calama M. What do we need for a superhydrophobic surface? A review on the recent progress in the preparation of superhydrophobic surfaces. Chem. Soc. Rev. 2007, 36: 1350-1368
[26] Onda T., Shibuichi S., Satoh N., Tsujii K. Super-Water-Repellent Fractal Surfaces. Langmuir, 1996, 12: 2125-2127
[27] Tuteja A., Choi W., Ma M., Mabry J. M., Mazzella S. A., Rutledge G. C., McKinley G. H., Cohen R. E. Designing Superoleophobic Surfaces. Science, 2007, 318, 1618-1622
[28] Ahuja A., Taylor J. A., Lifton V., Sidorenko A. A., Salamon T. R., Lobaton E. J., Kolodner P., Krupenkin T. N. Nanonails: A Simple Geometrical Approach to Electrically Tunable Superlyophobic Surfaces. Langmuir, 2008, 24: 9-14
[29] Leng B., Shao Z., With G., Ming W. Superoleophobic cotton textiles. Langmuir 2009, 25: 2456-2460
[30] Ramakrishna S., Fujihara K., Teo W.-E., Lim T.-C., Ma Z., An introduction electrpspinning and nanofibers, World scientific publishing Singapore 2005, Ch. 3.
[31] Ha J.-W., Park I. J., Lee S.-B., Antireflection Surfaces Prepared from Fluorinated Latex Particles. Macromolecule, 2008, 41: 8800-8806
[32] Hunley M. T., Harber A., Orlicki J. A., Rawlett A. M., Long T. E. Effect of Hyperbranched Surface-Migrating Additives on the Electrospinning Behavior of Poly(methyl methacrylate). Langmuir, 2008, 24: 654-657

8

Learning from Biosilica: Nanostructured Silicas and Their Coatings on Substrates by Programmable Approaches

Ren-Hua Jin[1,2] and Jian-Jun Yuan[1]
[1]*Synthetic Chemistry Lab., Kawamura Institute of Chemical Research*
[2]*JST-CREST*
Japan

1. Introduction

Silica-based materials are important for a wide range of technological applications, such as catalysts, polymeric fillers, coatings, chemical and biological separations, sensors, photonic and electronic devices, bio-encapsulation, enzyme immobilization, bioimaging, drug delivery, and so on (Davis, 2002). Recently, silica synthesis with the control of nanostructures and surface chemistry has been demonstrated to be important to improve the performance for various applications. For example, self-assembled surfactants have been used as templates for the controlled synthesis of mesoporous silicas (Kresge et al., 1992). Fibrous or tubular silicas could be synthesized by templating organogelators (van Bommel et al., 2003). However, these silica productions often involve hash and environmentally unfriendly conditions, such as high or low pH, high temperature and/or pressure, long reaction time, use of toxic and/or expensive organic solvents, as well as multiple steps and complex protocols. Moreover, precise control over the silica nanostructure and morphology still remains a major technical challenge, despite recent advances (Yang et al., 1997).
In contrast, silica biomineralization occurs in water under ambient conditions for various biological systems such as diatoms and sponges, producing exquisite hierarchical structures and multiple morphologies with precise nanoscale control (Schröder et al., 2008; Hildebrand, 2008). Marine organisms produce more than 6 gigatonnes of silicon each year to build their silica skeletons (Tréguer et al., 1995). As a typical example, diatom is eukaryotic single-celled algae with cell walls of being intricately and ornately shaped on the nanometer scale. Such cell wall structure is species-specific, indicating the molecular control of intracellular processes by which organics direct mineral formation (Kröger & Poulsen, 2008). The architecture and organic-silica composite nature of diatom wall exhibit remarkable mechanic strength and serve as protector armor against phytoplankton predators (Smetacek, 1999). The diatom is important for the biological cycling of both silicon and carbon, with about 20% of total photosynthetic CO_2 fixation. This is equivalent to the photosynthetic activity of all rainforests combined (Field et al., 1998). The recent studies on diatom wall also indicate that (*i*) the cell wall of *Thalassiosira weisflogii* acts as a proton buffer for improving the CO_2 acquisition via an extracellular carbonic anhydrase (Milligan & Morel, 2002), and (*ii*) the square lattice of hole pattern in the girdle band region of the cell wall of *Coscinodiscus*

granii acts as a photonic crystal, which may aid in light harvesting for photosynthesis (Fuhrmann et al., 2004).

In this article, we will first give a brief introduction to the biosilica formation with an emphasis on the role of self-assembled organic matrix (i.e. polyamines) for the formation of complex nanostructure and precise nanopattern of biosilicas. The second section provides a comprehensive overview of our recent work on the multiple morphogenesis of silicas by programmable self-assembly of linear polyethyleneimine (PEI). Finally, we will briefly discuss some researches currently under progress and the potential technological applications of our biomimetic PEI-directed silica nanomaterials.

2. Biosilica formation mediated with self-assembled organic matrix

Biological organisms are able to take up silicon from the environment in soluble form as silicic acid, store it in cell and catalyze its polymerization into silica with precise structure architecture down to nanoscale (Hildebrand, 2008). Among these processes, self-assembled organic matrix has been assumed to play key roles for directing the biosilicification in diatoms, sponges and higher plants (Perry & Keeling-Tucker, 2000; Schröder et al., 2008). Sponges synthesize silica in specifically differentiated cells to form a skeletal element (or spicule). Each spicule contains a central macroscopic organic core, or axial filament of protein, that is wholly included within the biosilica (Weaver & Morse, 2003). By demineralizing the surrounding silica with a buffered hydrofluoric acid solution, the axial protein filaments occluded within the spicules can be isolated. Morse and co-workers discovered that this axial filament consists predominantly of a cathepsin L-ralated enzyme, and termed silicatein (Shimizu et al., 1998; Cha et al., 1999; Weaver & Morse, 2003; Brutchey & Morse, 2008). The native silicatein isolated from axial filaments as well as recombinant protein demonstrate the activity for forming silica from soluble silicon alkoxide precursor in solution (Shimizu et al., 1998; Cha et al., 1999). Also the studies using biocatalytically active recombinant silicatein showed that silica formation in sponges is an enzymatic process (Krasko et al., 2000; Schröder et al., 2006). Furthermore, recent studies confirmed the mechanism of self-assembly of silicatein monomers to oligomers and long protein filaments (Croce et al., 2004; Murr & Morse, 2005; Croce et al., 2007). The results from SAXS examination indicated that the axial filament is formed from a very high degree of organization (hexagonal) of the protein units (Croce et al., 2004; 2007). Müller and co-workers found that silicatein is present not only in the axial filament but also on the surface of the spicules (Müller et al., 2006), supporting the view that growth of spicules occurs through apposition of lamellar silica layer with a distance of 0.2-0.5 μm from each other (Müller et al., 2005).

Diatom cell wall is constructed in a petri-dish-like fashion with a top half overlapping the slightly smaller bottom half. Silica mineralization takes place inside the diatom protoplast within a specialized membrane-bound compartment termed silica deposition vesicle (SDV) (Sumper & Kröger, 2004). Biosilicas from all diatom species investigated so far has turned out to be a composite material composed of silica, proteins and long-chain polyamines (Sumper & Kröger, 2004; Kröger & Poulsen, 2008). Three families of proteins have been identified in the cell wall of marine diatom *C. fusiformis,* termed frustulins, pleuralins and silaffins (Pohnert, 2002). Frustulins are a group of calcium-binding glycoproteins being assumed to play a role in cell adhesion to surfaces, gliding of pennate diatoms, and protection against desiccation (Kröger et al., 1994; 1996). The pleuralins (HF-extractable proteins) are highly acidic molecules, comprising a proline-rich region and several repeats of a proline-, serine-, cysteine, aspartate-rich domain (Kröger et al., 1997). Immunoelectron microscopy studies revealed that frustulins and pleuralins are not involved in silica formation because they become associated with the biosilica only after its deposition on the cell surface (van de Poll et al., 1999; Kröger & Wetherbee, 2000). Silaffins (proteins with silica affinity) are a group of low molecular polypeptides, which can be extracted from the diatom cell wall using anhydrous HF (Kröger et al., 2002). Silaffins were found to be mainly composed of serine and lysine residues. Using a milder extraction condition (a slightly acidic, aqueous ammonium fluoride solution), native silaffins (termed natSil, Figure 1A) have been isolated from C. *fusiformis.* (Kröger et al., 2002). In the native silaffins, all the serine units are found to be phosphorylated, and all the lysine units are either methylated or covalently linked with a long-chain polyamine (Kröger et al., 1999; 2001; 2002). Silaffin NatSil-1A is extremely active in promoting silica precipitation in vitro, causing silica

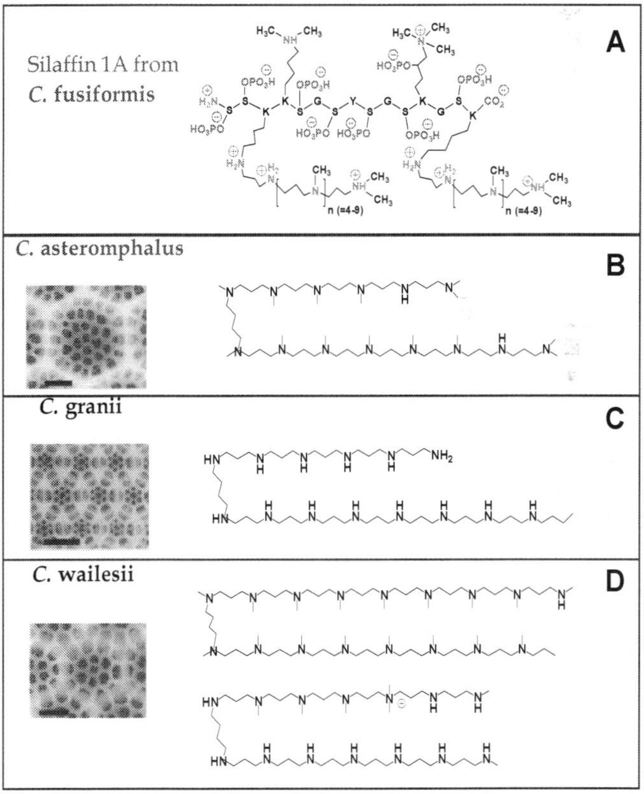

Fig. 1. Diatoms and their organic components active for silica deposition and pattern formation. (A) chemical structure of native silaffin-1 of C. fusiformis. (B), (C) and (D) SEM images and polyamines isolated from the differently pattered cell walls of diatoms C. asteromphalus, C. granii and C. wailesii, respectively. The bars: 1 μm (B-D).

precipitation within a few minutes by accelerating polycondensation of silicic acid and acting as a flocculating agent (Kröger et al., 2002; Poulsen et al., 2003). The supermolecular aggregates self-assembled from Silaffin-1 A in solution were estimated to comprise 700 peptide molecules, which appears to serve as a template for silicic acid polycondensation (Brunner et al., 2004).

Long chain polyamines (LCPA) were found to be characteristic constituent of biosilica from all genera of diatoms analyzed so far (Sumper & Kröger, 2004). The cell wall silica from most diatom species studied to date has a roughly equivalent content of silaffins and LCPA. The studies also showed that some of diatoms, *C. asteromphalus*, *C. granii*, and *C. wailesii*, appear to contain only LCPA (Sumper, 2002). In biosilicas, LCPA could exist in peptide-bound or peptide-free state. In diatom *C. fusiformis* polyamines with about 5-10 N-methylpropylamine units are attached to lysine residues of Silaffin NatSil-1A (Figure 1A). The attached polyamines are important for imparting the zwitterionic structures to NatSil due to their cationic property, which has been proposed to be an essential prerequisite for silica biomineralization. Furthermore, as the active functional groups on the silaffins appear to be the LCPA, polyamines alone can also promote silica formation in a similar way to silaffins in the presence of inorganic phosphate or other polyvalent anions (Kröger et al., 2000).

Recently, Sumper and co-workers have revealed that the polyamines from different diatom species exhibit different molecular structure, indicating that polyamines are species-specific for creating species-specific silica nanostructures (Sumper & Lehmann, 2006). Structural variations of polyamines include the overall chain length, the degree of methylation, the positions of secondary and tertiary amino functionalities and the site-specific incorporation of quaternary ammonium functionalities. A selection of typical polyamine structures covering these features and their corresponding silica nanopattern are shown in Figure 1B, C and D. Moreover, polyamines have also been proposed to play key roles for nanopattern formation of diatoms. By examining the silica formation guided by self-assembled emulsion droplets from polyamine-phosphate system, Sumper found that hexagonal network silica was produced by using polyamine-stabilized silica sol as the silicon source (Sumper, 2004). In contrast, silica nanoparticles were obtained if silicic acid was used as source. Polyamines are likely to not only stabilize silica sols but also induce a phase-separation, producing (hexagonal) pattern silica. Thus, both the supramolecular self-assembly and the presence of polyamines are important to control both the rate and mechanism of silica precipitation and formation of the elaborate patterns.

3. Multiple morphogenesis of silicas from programmable self-assembly of linear PEIs

3.1 Linear PEIs, crystallization and crystalline morphology

PEI can be divided into branched and linear PEIs according to their chain architecture. Commercial branched PEIs are obtained by cationic ring-opening polymerization of aziridine (ethylene imine) in water or water-alcohol mixture with a protonic acid as catalyst. The branched PEI is a polyamine containing primary, secondary and tertiary amine groups, which has a high cationic charge density in water and a branched structure. The branched PEIs have been widely used in many industrial fields, such as water treatment flocculants, paper production, dye fixation in textile processing, pigment dispersant, coatings, pressure sensitive adhesives, and so on. Recent studies have demonstrated the applications of branched PEI in medicinal chemistry, for example as most efficient nonviral vectors for gene delivery. In contrast, linear PEIs obtained from the hydrolysis of linear polyoxazoline in acidic and basic conditions (Saegusa et al., 1975; Jin & Motoyoshi, 1999), are highly crystalline owing to its linear structure. Different to the branched one, linear PEI is composed of only secondary amine. Linear PEI is difficult to dissolve into water and normal organic solvents (except methanol) at room temperature due to the crystalline structure (Yuan & Jin, 2005a). We have been able to design linear PEI backbone into various chain architectures (Figure 2). About two decades ago, Chatani and co-workers did the pioneering works on the understanding of crystalline structure of linear PEI (Chatani, et al., 1981; 1982; 1983). Depending on the humid atmosphere, four crystalline phases consisting of anhydrate, hemihydrate, sesquihydrate, and dihydrate per EI unit have been confirmed. Linear PEI chains adopt a double-stranded helical conformation by forming parallel array in the anhydrate, while all-trans planar-zigzag conformations are adopted by the fully extended form for the hemihydrate, sesquihydrate, and dehydrate. Recently, the crystalline structure and the phase transition of the linear PEI were further studied by Hashida et al (Hashida et al., 2002) and Hasegawa et al (Kakuda et al., 2009), mainly based on the new-developed spectroscopy methods. Compared to the wide applications of branched PEI in industrial and academical research fields, linear PEI seems to be only used in the laboratory in a very limited field. Recently, linear PEIs have been attempted to be used for gene delivery (Hsiue et al., 2006), biosensors based on ferrocene modification (Merchant et al., 2009) and electrochemically responsive thin film (Schmidt et al., 2009), mainly based on the long-chain secondary amine property. In contrast, the nature and characteristics of crystalline structure of linear PEI have not been exploited for materials application, due to that the self-assembled information programmed in the crystalline structure of linear PEI has not been discovered until our recent findings (Yuan & Jin, 2005a). Our interest in linear PEI started from our studies on the synthesis, micelle/vesicle/ emulsion self-assembly and silica-based hybrid materials of chain-architecture-controlled polyoxazolines (Jin, 2002a; 2002b; 2003a; 2003b; 2003c; 2004). For example, star architecture consisting of a small benzene core and densely-six-armed poly(methyloxazoline) has been observed to be able to self-assemble in situ into a superstructured colloidal crystalline polymer in the reaction solution (Jin, 2003b). The hydrophobic-hydrophilic amphiphilic star block copolyoxazolines have been designed to control porphyrin moieties in the different sites of self-assembled micelles (Jin, 2002a). By hydrolyzing one of block from star block polyoxazoline into polyethyleneimine, we can produce micelles with porphyrin core and cationic shell in water and reverse micelles with cationic core and porphyrin-funcationalized shell in organic media (Jin, 2003c).

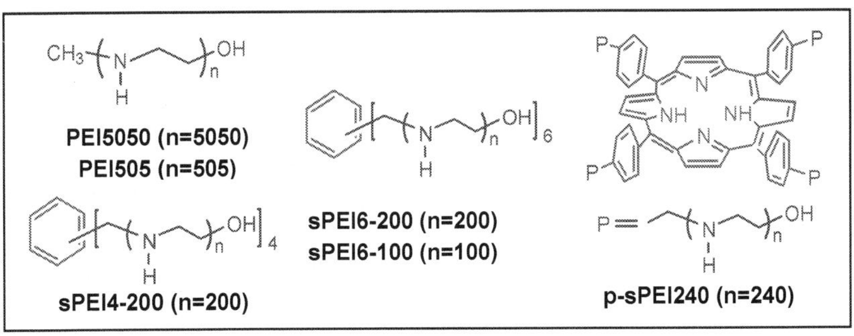

Fig. 2. Linear PEIs with various chain architectures.

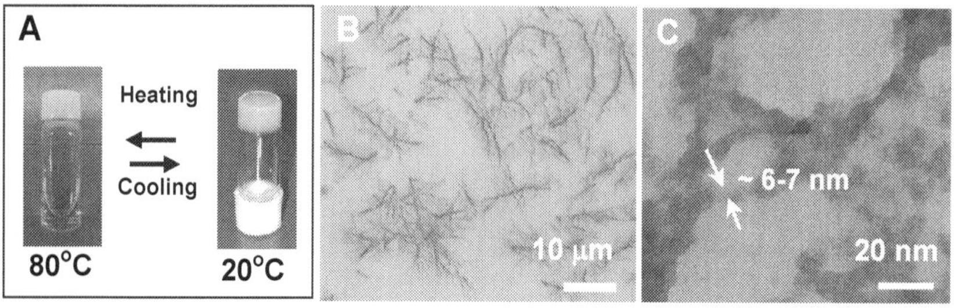

Fig. 3. Fibrils self-assembled from linear PEI in water. (A) Reversible hydrogelation of **PEI5050** with 1 wt% concentration in water by heating-cooling cycles. (B) Optical microscope image of branched fibrous bundles of crystalline **PEI5050** in water (1 wt%). (C) TEM image of fibrous aggregates of 0.25 wt% **PEI5050** in water.

The breakthrough of the linear PEI-directed inorganic materials synthesis came from the discovery of crystalline morphology of linear PEI in water media (Yuan & Jin, 2005a). We found that linear PEI do not dissolve in water at room temperature, but is highly soluble upon heating at 80°C (Figure 3A). It is interesting that the hydrogelation occurred upon naturally cooling the hot aqueous solutions of PEI to room temperature, and such hydrogelation is completely reversible by heating-cooling cycles (Figure 3A). The XRD studies on the 5 wt% **PEI5050** hydrogel indicated the diffraction patterns at 2θ of 13.5, 20.3, 27.2 and 27.9° due to the dihydrate crystalline structures of PEI. This is consistent to the earlier studies from Chantani et al (Chatani et al., 1983). This novel thermoreversible hydrogel from linear PEI shows the tunable gel-sol transition temperatures from about 43 to 79°C, depending on the PEI concentrations and solution conditions. Linear PEI could gelate neat water with a concentration as low as about 0.25 wt%, indicating that one EI unit could gelate 956 water molecules. Such high ability to gelate water is unusual for physical hydrogel from normal polymers. Thus we assumed that the self-assembled nanostructure from linear PEI should play vital role for strongly gelate water molecules. Microscopy studies supported this assumption. Direct observation by optical microscopy on a small piece of **PEI5050** hydrogel with 1.0 wt. % concentration revealed that the aggregates are composed of fibrous bundles on the micrometer scale (Figure 3B). It seems likely that many crystalline unit nanofibers organized into the branched bundles. TEM studies indicated that the unit nanofibers were about 6-7 nm in width (Figure 3C). Our further experiments confirmed that star-like PEIs with linear backbones could also gelate water in the similar way as that of linear PEI (**PEI5050**) by forming fibrous crystalline structure; in contrast, the branched PEI just forms molecularly dissolved solution under similar conditions. This result indicated that linear backbone is prerequisite conditions in the formation of PEI fibrous crystalline structures. This physical and ice-cream-like hydrogel could be chemically cross-linked by glutaraldehyde to improve the mechanical properties. This is the first finding of fiber-like crystalline morphology for linear PEI in water-based media upon naturally cooling a hot solution. There have been a number of studies on the modification of linear PEI by attached the hydrophobic or hydrophilic blocks (Akiyama et al., 2000), but the crystalline morphology studies are extremely rare. Recently, Menzel and co-workers reported the thermal gelation of amphiphilic PEI with end-capped by alkyl chains (alky-PEI), and cryo-SEM observation revealed the fibrous network structure of the alkyl-PEI crystalline hydrogels (Navarro et al., 2009). This is consistent with our earlier results.

3.2 PEI nanofiber-templated silica deposition

Marine sponges produce structured spicule by templating self-organized organic fibers, which simultaneously serve as template, scaffold and catalyst for silica mineralization. Inspired by this silica formation in nature, we explored to use our self-assembled crystalline PEI nanofiber as biomimetic template for silica deposition (Jin & Yuan, 2005a; Yuan & Jin, 2005b; Yuan et al. 2006) (Figure 4A). The silica deposition was simply achieved by mixing an aqueous dispersion of **PEI5050** nanofiber, ethanol and TMOS at 20°C for 40 min. TEM observation clearly demonstrated the formation of PEI@silica nanofibers with a width of about 20-23 nm (Figure 4B). This hybrid nanofiber has well-defined core-shell structure composed of an axial, crystalline PEI filament core of about 5-7 nm in diameter and a silicified shell of about 7 nm. Silica tube could be obtained by calcining the PEI@silica hybrid nanofiber at 500°C to remove the organic components (Figure 4C). The representative samples of PEI@silica nanofibers and silica nanotubes after calcination at 700°C showed BET surface area of about 71 and 298m²/g, respectively, indicating that removal of organic PEI (i.e., nanotube formation) contributes greatly to the increase in surface area. We also found that silica deposition templated by this unique PEI nanofiber could occur at a significantly fast rate. Elemental analysis on the PEI@silica sample from 10 min silica deposition showed 74 wt% silica content.

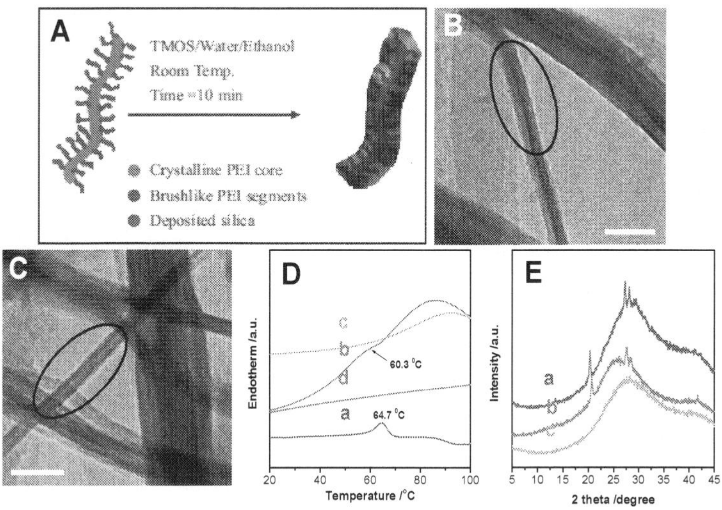

Fig. 4. Silica mineralization by templating self-assembling PEI nanofiber. (A) Schematic representation of PEI nanofiber serving as biomimetic template for controlled silica deposition. (B) TEM image of unit PEI@silica nanofiber prepared by using aggregates of 2 wt% **P5050** as template and TMOS as silica source. (C) TEM image of silica nanotube obtained by calcining (B) at 500°C. The bars are 50 nm for B and C. (D) DSC traces of **PEI5050** under different environments: (a) aqueous aggregate of 2 wt% **PEI5050**, (b) PEI@silica composite, (c) PEI@silica composite after ethanol washing, (d) the second heating run of (b). (E) XRD patterns of (a) aqueous aggregate of 2 wt% **PEI5050**, (b) PEI@silica composite and (c) PEI@silica composite after ethanol washing.

No nontemplated silica formation was observed, indicating that the silica deposition proceeds exclusively and site selectively on the surface of fibrous PEI aggregates. Self-organized PEI nanofiber with a crystalline core serves as a template for shape direction, and the amorphous shell with brushlike PEI segments acts as the catalyst/scaffold for silica deposition at ambient conditions. This mechanism has been confirmed by the combined studies of ^{1}H NMR, XRD and DSC. ^{1}H NMR study on a dilute dispersion of PEI nanofibers in D_2O confirmed the existence of brushlike PEI shell on the surface of crystalline PEI core. DSC measurements demonstrated a melting peak at 60.0°C for crystalline PEI in PEI@silica hybrid nanofiber, which is similar to that before silica deposition (Figure 4D). In addition, the same diffraction peaks (2θ) at 20°, 27°, and 28°, ascribed to a dihydrated PEI crystal (NCH_2CH_2/H_2O=1:2) with a zigzag conformation, were obtained by XRD measurement on samples before and after silica deposition (Figure 4E). Both DSC and XRD investigation confirm the template role of crystalline PEI nanofiber upon silica deposition.

To design model systems for mimicking silica biomineralization, Menzel and co-workers (Menzel et al. 2003) reported using linear PEI with a degree of polymerization of 8-9 for silica deposition. This low-molecular-weight linear PEI was dissolved into 10^{-5} M HCl solution and the silicification was performed at pH4.3. This experiment confirmed the strong accelerating effect for silicification of linear PEI as a molecular polyamine. However, no characteristic morphogenesis was addressed under the silica deposition conditions investigated, since self-assembled crystalline nanofiber morphology of linear PEI, which could be transcribed into silica, is not available at pH4.3. Recently, Patel et al (Patel et al., 2009) reported silica formation onto nanofibers of linear PEI blended with poly(vinyl pyrrolidone) obtained via electrospinning. Schiraldi and co-workers (Johnson et al., 2009) described the production of linear PEI/clay aerogel and the subsequent mineralization of this composite by condensation of tetramethyl orthosilicate (TMOS). In both cases of PEI-mediated silica mineralization depending on electrospinning fibers and aerogel, however, the characteristic nanostructures due to the PEI crystalline property have not been exploited.

Our processing for shaped silicas is remarkably different from conventional silica-fiber formation based on the fibrous aggregates from small-molecule gelators (van Bommel et al., 2003), in which a solution deposition of silica (nontemplated silica) is normally unavoidable because an acidic or basic catalyst is present in solution. Later, a surface mechanism was proposed for silica deposition by designing an organogelator possessing a gelating cholesterol moiety and a catalytic benzylamine residue (van Bommel & Shinkai, 2002), with the silica formation occurring merely on the gel-fiber surface. However, the silicification was performed in organic media, and seems to be relatively low in efficiency, because a long deposition time (1 week) and heat treatment are needed. Recently, Shimizu and co-workers demonstrated direct silica deposition without the aid of solution catalysis by using tubular fibers consisting of peptidic lipids with secondary ammonium hydrochloride residues on the surface of the tubular assemblies (Ji et al., 2004). This approach can produce hollow silica cylinders with very thin walls (4.5-8.0 nm) but still requires a longer deposition time (1 week). The organogelators and lipids used for such silica formation are costly, thus restricting their widespread adoption. Also, organogelator-derived silicas generally lack the possibility of multiple morphogenesis and hierarchical architecture of silicas because of the small molecular size of the gelators.

Compared to organic alkoxysilane, using sodium silicate as silica source is cost-effective and environmentally benign. Such an inorganic silica source does not produce organic by-products. By using self-assembled PEI nanofiber as structure directing templates, we have successfully achieved fibrous PEI@silica hybrid structures by using commercial water glass as source (Figure 5). The nanostructure and morphologies could be controlled by adjusting polymer concentrations and pH values of the aqueous solution of sodium silicate (Zhu & Jin, 2008).

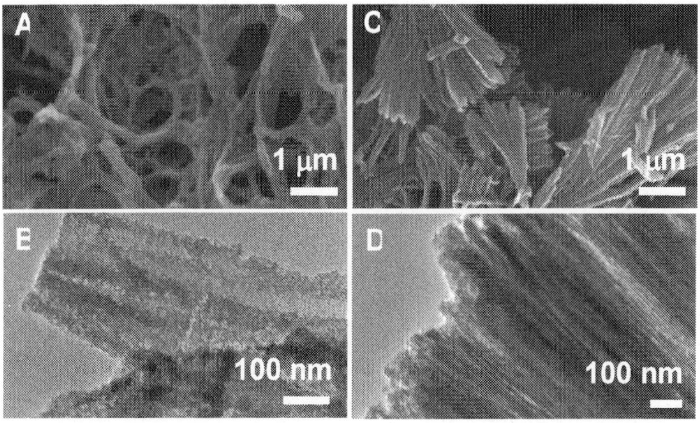

Fig. 5. Fibrous PEI@silicas synthesized by using water glass as source. (A) SEM and (B) TEM images of PEI@silica formed by the mediation of 1 wt% of **PEI5050**; (C) SEM and (D) TEM images of PEI@silica obtained by the mediation of **sPEI6-200.**

3.3 Morphological control of silicas by adjusting the self-assembly of linear PEI

Different to the conventional biomimetic silicification systems based on molecular self-assembly (Cha et al., 2000; Patwardhan et al., 2005; Pouget et al., 2007; Yuan et al., 2007), linear PEI-directed silica formation featured with multiple morphogenesis and well-controlled hierarchical architectures through programmed self-assembly of PEI macromolecules with linear backbones. The self-assembly of crystalline PEI aggregates could be controlled by a programmable adjustments of some simple parameters, including polymer chain architecture and molecular weight, concentrations, additives, media, physical field and so on. The programmed PEI aggregates are transcribed into silicas with multiple morpholognesis by performing a biomimetic silicification.

3.3.1 PEI concentration

One of extremely simple method for adjusting PEI self-assembly is to change the concentrations of PEI in water (Yuan & Jin, 2005b). The concentration effect of silica morphogenesis was addressed by performing silicification reaction on the aggregates from **PEI505** with concentrations from 5.0 to 0.1 wt% using TMOS as silica source under room temperature for 40 min (Figure 6). It was found that silicas produced from **PEI505** with concentrations from 2.0-5.0 wt% show fiber-based bundles with a size of several micrometers. Obviously, the bundles tend to expand in a two-dimensional way, and became looser when the concentrations of **PEI505** decrease. Further decreasing PEI concentration to $\leq$ 1.0 wt% leads to morphological transformation of silicas from the fiber bundles into curved leaf-like film. Silicas prepared from **PEI505** aggregates of 0.5 wt% concentration show leaf lamellae composed of interwoven nanofibers, meaning that the silica film grew by linking separate fibers to each other (Figure 6). The silica film mediated by 0.25 wt% **PEI505** was thicker and the fiber structure still could be resolved. When **PEI505** concentration decreased to 0.1 wt%, the silica film shows a smooth surface without fiber structure. It was assumed that the formation of a thick silica film, which is supported by fiber-to-fiber linking, is associated with the presence of a large amount of PEI chain that are attached to the surface of crystalline PEI aggregates. ^{1}H NMR studies indicated that the relative contents of amorphous brush on the crystalline PEI fibril dramatically increased as the PEI concentrations deceased from 0.3 to 0.05 wt%. This means that PEI aggregates obtained from lower concentrations would favor to offer much more brush sites on crystalline PEI surface, where the promoted silicification reaction led to the formation of silica film structure.

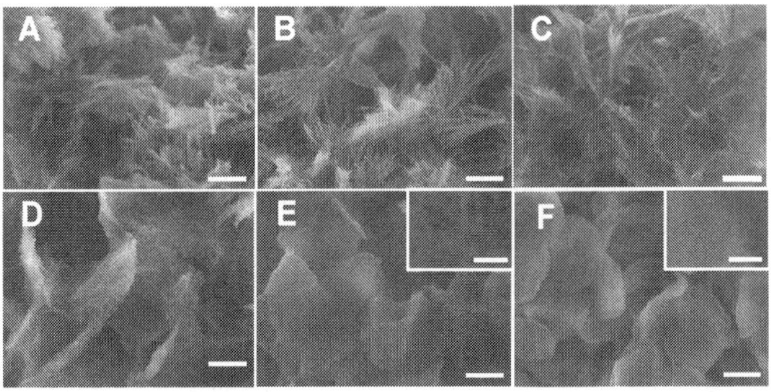

Fig. 6. Morphological dependence of PEI@silicas on the concentrations of **PEI505**. SEM images of PEI@silicas synthesized by **PEI505** aggregates with the concentrations of 5, 3, 2, 0.5, 0.25 and 0.1 wt% for (A), (B), (C), (D), (E) and (F), respectively. Bars are 5 μm for A-F and 500 nm for insets of E and F.

3.3.2 Polymer architecture

Multiple morphogenesis of silicas could be generated by designing and using the linear PEI with different chain architectures (Jin & Yuan, 2005a). As shown in Figure 7A and B, silicas templated by using **PEI5050** aggregates with concentrations of 2 and 0.25 wt% exhibited the expanded bundle and leaf morphologies, respectively. In contrast, a six-armed star PEI with a small benzene core (**sPEI6-100**) directed the formation of silicas with dramatically different morphologies. A fibrous framework was created by using 2 wt% **sPEI6-100** aggregates as templates (Figure 7C). High-magnification observation reveals that larger fibers are composed of thinner nanofibers. When the concentration of **sPEI6-100** decreased to 0.25 wt%, silicification produced silicas with looser bundle morphologies (Figure 7D). Each silica bundle was observed to be composed of well-defined nanofibers with the length of tens of micrometer and the diameters of about 30-50 nm. Compared to **PEI5050** (simple linear architecture), **sPEI6-100** (small benzene core with six-arm star architecture) demonstrated the enhanced ability to form self-assembled aggregates and subsequent silicas with well-defined unit nanofiber structure. It is very interesting that the silica asters were achieved by using a star PEI with porphyrin core (**p-sPEI4-240).** The asters could have more than five silica arms, which expands towards three-dimensional directions (Figure 7E). The arms become wider towards the outer of silica asters. Each arm shows serrate end, indicating that the arms are densely organized with unit nanofibers. The silicas obtained from the lower content of **p-sPEI4-240** (0.25 wt%) still retained the aster morphology.

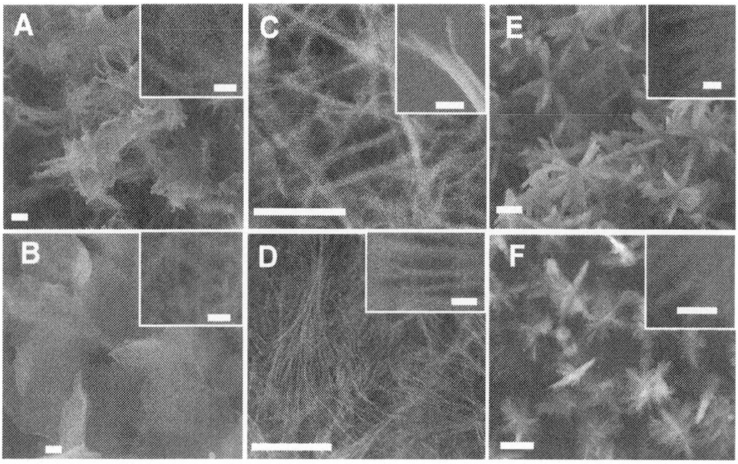

Fig. 7. Shaping silicas by designing linear PEI backbone into star architecture. SEM images of PEI@silicas prepared by using **PEI5050** with concentrations of 2.0 wt% (A) and 0.25 wt% (B); using **sPEI6-100** with concentrations of 2.0 wt% (C) and 0.25 wt% (D) and **p-sPEI4-240** with concentrations of 2.0 wt% (E) and 0.25 wt% (F). The bars are 2 μm for (A-D) and 100 nm for each inset.

3.3.3 Media for PEI crystallization

By taking advantage of methanol being a good solvent for dissolving crystalline PEI at room temperature, we developed the strategy to generate shaped silicas by using methanol as a mediator to adjust the programmed self-assembly of crystalline PEI (Jin &Yuan, 2005b). This methanol-programmed approach could both enrich the shape generation of silicas and offer potential advantages of ambient processing of PEI aggregates, which would be of particular interest in view of applications such as bioactive component immobilization and surface patterning of silicate-based materials. It was found that the silica morphologies could be controlled accurately by simply adjusting the amount of methanol addition. Compared to the obvious nanofiber structure of silica (Figure 8A) formed in neat water, aqueous medium with 50 vol% methanol addition mediated the silica particles composed of beautiful unit ribbons (Figure 8B). The unit ribbons have a typical width of 1-2 micrometers and a length of more than 10 micrometers. Such simple methanol-mediated approach has been also extended to star PEI for achieving the new silica morphologies (Jin & Yuan, 2006). For example, 0.5 wt% **sPEI4-200** aggregates mediated the formation of very large and curved silica films composed of unit nanofibers (Figure 8C). In contrast, 50 vol% methanol addition in media for assembling **sPEI4-200** aggregates led to the formation of well-defined fan-like silicas with very dense aggregation of unit fibers (Figure 8D). 0.3 wt% **sPEI4-200** in a medium with 30 vol% methanol content directed fanlike silicas with relatively loose aggregation and flowerlike silicas with loose petals (Figure 8F). In contrast, only nanofiber-based silica films formed when using neat water as media (Figure 8E) under the same conditions. We also found that such morphological changes with methanol addition did not depend on the heating history of PEI aggregates formation, indicating that methanol-water media composition merely determined the PEI self-assembly. We propose that the addition of methanol in media could retard the nucleation of PEI crystalline, and thus the growth of crystallites was limited within relatively small domains. This slow and suppressed aggregation and/or crystallization process would be favorable to construct the ribbon-like or fan-like structure. This assumption was supported by our experimental observation. The aggregate formation in neat water media was observed to take several minutes when cooling the hot solutions of **PEI5050** or **sPEI4-200**, whereas the complete aggregation in the methanol-modulation process usually needs several hours, especially for the systems with higher methanol contents.

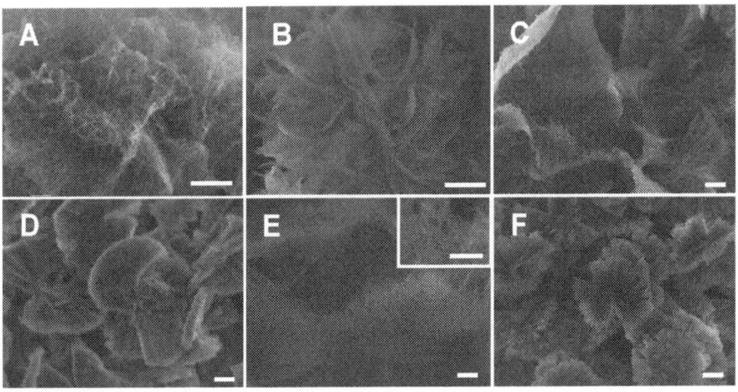

Fig. 8. Control of PEI@silica morphology by MeOH mediation. PEI@silicas were synthesized by using aggregates: (A) 1.0 wt% **PEI5050** in water; (B) 1.0 wt% **P5050** in a mixture of water-MeOH (1/1 in volume ratio); (C) 0.5 wt% **sPEI4-200** in water; (D) 0.5 wt% **sPEI4-200** in a mixture of water-MeOH (1/1 in volume ratio); (E) 0.3 wt% **sPEI4-200** in water; (F) 0.3 wt% **sPEI4-200** in a mixture of water-MeOH (30 vol% MeOH). The bars are 2 μm for A-F and 500 nm for the inset of E.

3.3.4 Acid additives

The ethyleneimine units of PEI could associate with acidic molecules by hydrogen bonding interaction to form complexes. Therefore, such complexation could also be used to control the PEI aggregation and subsequent direct silica morphologies (Jin & Yuan, 2007a). We selected the acid molecules of HCl, poly(ethylene glycol) bis(carboxymethyl) (BA) and tetra(p-sulfophenyl)porphyrin (TSPP) with functional protons 1, 2 and 4 in one molecule. Given that protonated segments of linear PEI are freely soluble in water, the partial protonation of linear PEI could allow the modification of crystalline aggregates of PEI, leading to the formation of new structure and morphology. The silicas formed without HCl addition showed silica network with dense nanofiber structure (Figure 9A). In contrast, silicification of 1 wt% **PEI5050** aggregates prepared from 10^{-5} M HCl produced silicas composed of relatively looser network structure and unit nanofibers with increased diameter (Figure 9B). This could be attributed to the formation of PEI nanofibers with increased density or thickness of PEI amorphous shell due to the suitable protonation degree of PEI backbone by HCl addition. Further increase of the concentration of HCl was found to damage the nanofiber structure of silica. The silicas mediated by the aggregates prepared in 10^{-2} M HCl solution showed olive-like shape (Figure 9C). Many silica nanofibers of about 1 μm length grew from the surface of the particles. Obviously, HCl addition in increased amount is capable of directing 3-demensional silica structures composed of silica nanofibers.

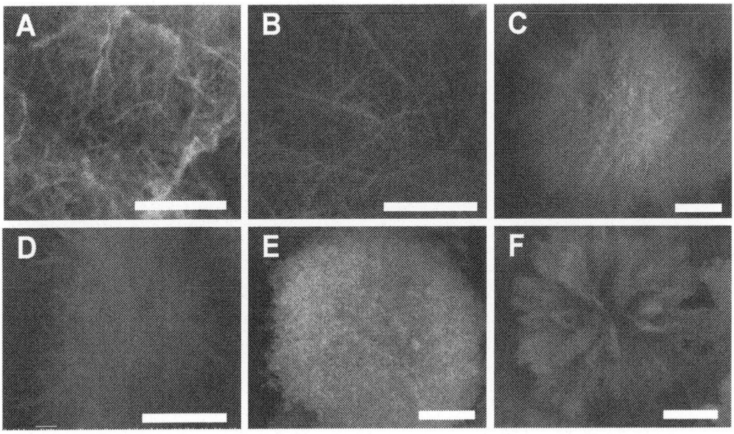

Fig. 9. Shaped PEI@silicas synthesized by templating **PEI5050** aggregates without acid additive (A) and with the mediation of 10^{-5} M HCl (B), 10^{-2} M HCl (C), 10^{-2} M BA600 (D), 10^{-2} M BA250 (E) and TSPP ([EI]/[TSPP]=1200/1, 30 vol% MeOH addition) (F). The **PEI5050** concentrations are 1.0 and 0.3 wt% for (A-E) and (F), respectively. The bars are 2 μm for each case.

Different to inorganic HCl, addition of bifunctional organic acids, poly(ethylene glycol) bis(carboxymethyl) ethers with molecular weights of ca. 250 and 600 (denoted as BA250 and BA600) could adjust the properties and morphologies of the crystalline aggregates of linear PEI, by physical cross-linking via formation of hydrogen bonding. Upon silificifying the aggregates self-assembled from PEI by addition of 10^{-2} M BA600 (Figure 9D) and BA250 (Figure 9E), it was found that micro-scaled plate-like silica particles were formed. However, the nanostructures of particles showed the difference between BA600 and BA250 addition. The silica particles from BA250 addition appear much denser in comparison with the silicas mediated by BA600 association, and almost no fibrous structure could be observed from the silica particles obtained from BA250.

A four-armed star PEI with porphyrin core (**p-sPEI4-240**) can direct silica into a beautiful aster structure (Jin & Yuan, 2005a), which is dramatically different to silica mediated from simple linear PEI. The specific aggregation of porphyrin residues was assumed to play the important role for affording the 3-D self-assembly of PEI crystalline unit. This assumption was exploited to design the silica morphology by incorporating TSPP (a porphyrin possessing four sulfonic groups) into linear PEI. By silicifying **PEI505** aggregates formed in an aqueous system containing 30 vol% methanol, 0.3 wt% **PEI505** and a trace of TSPP (in a molar ratio of EI/TSPP at 1200/1), the beautiful flower-like silica particles with micrometer size were achieved (Figure 9F). In the flower-like particles, many silica petals with the width of 500-1000 nm and the length of several micrometers grew from the center in a radiation way. Clearly, the participation of TSPP in the self-assembly of crystalline aggregates of **PEI505** efficiently promoted the formation of 3-D silica structure (flower-like). This is consistent with the formation of 3-D aster silicas from **p-sPEI4-240**.

In addition to the impressive shape control, another important merit for TSPP mediation is that this process simultaneously produced the photo-functionalized hybrid silicas materials. The UV-vis spectrum of the stock solution of PEI and TSPP in methanol showed a typical spectroscopic line due to the molecular state of porphyrin. In contrast, the spectroscopic line of the trapped TSPP in the shaped silicas changed remarkably; the soret band became very broad with a red-shift from 418 to 423 nm, and the Q-bands also shifted toward longer wavelengths, indicating that the porphyrin residues are in a stacking state in the shaped silica. For silicas mediated from TSPP addition, we suggested that two sets of interactions could be a cooperative trigger to induce subtle PEI self-assembly. One set is the association of TSPP with PEI by hydrogen bonding interaction, and the other set is the aggregation between prophyrin planes by π-π stacking. These shaped silicas with PEI/TSPP are expected to be used in photonic, electronic and catalytic fields due to the porphyrin functions.

3.3.5 Metal ions as additives

Metal cations should be efficient candidates for regulating the nucleation and growth of LPEI crystals with defined morphologies, as PEI is a strong coordinator to form complexes (Zhu et al., 2007). The PEI aggregates with the mediation of metal ions were prepared by slowly cooling hot aqueous solutions of PEI containing three groups of metal cations with different valences (monovalent cations: Li^+, Na^+, K^+; divalent cations: Cu^{2+}, Co^{2+}, Zn^{2+}, Mn^{2+}; trivalent cations: Al^{3+}, Eu^{3+}, Fe^{3+}, In^{3+}). The silicification was performed by mixing the aggregates with TMOS and methanol at room temperature for 40 min. It was found that bulky, turbine-like and urchinlike silica, were produced by mediation of Na^+, Cu^{2+} and Al^{3+} with the ratios of EI to metal ions of 20/1, respectively (Figure 10A, B and C). It seems that the Na^+ ion suppressed fiber formation completely. The cross-sectional transmission electron microscopy (TEM) image for Cu^{2+}-mediated silica revealed that the unit blade of turbine-like is about 200 nm in width, and 20 nm in thickness. The urchin-like silicas from Al^{3+} addition showed a globular shape with numerous fine, needlelike fibers approximately 20 nm in width. Recently, detailed studies on the formation of 2-D turbine-like structures were performed by selecting $M^{II}(p\text{-TolSO}_3)_2$ as additives (Matsukizono et al., 2009). All silica structures from mediation of Cu^{II}, Fe^{II}, Ni^{II}, Co^{II}, Zn^{II}, Mn^{II} are composed of leaf-like units of 200 nm width, which are bundled and grew in radial fashion to form 2-D turbine-like microstructures with a diameter of 5-6 μm. In contrast, for non-coordinative ion, tetraethylammonium p-toluenesulfonate salts ($NEt_4(p\text{-TolSO}_3)$), only fibrous aggregates were observed. It is clear that these 2-D structures were induced by the coexisting metal salts with coordinative ability. The interactions between metal ions and amine groups seem to be the main factor for promoting 2-D shaped structures. Further studies indicated that the turbine structure could be controlled by changing the ratios of $[EI]/[M^{II}]$ (Figure 10D, E and F) and self-assembly time of PEI-M^{II} in water (Figure 10G, I and J). At 1000/70 of $[EI]/[Ni^{II}]$, 2-D turbine-like structures are obtained. These well-shaped structures became more swollen as Ni^{II} ions decreased from 70 to 40 mM. Further decrease of Ni^{II} concentration down to 20 mM leads to the formation of rougher aggregates of blade-like components in a more randomly bundled fashion, which is similar to those obtained from non-metal containing linear PEI aqueous solutions. In this system, growing times of PEI crystalline precipitates influenced the silica structures. For examples, the crystalline precipitates formed after 80 min lead to structured silica with two narrow fan-like edges. After that, new sheets were generated in both sides of each edge and these edges grew in a fan-like fashion with time. Finally, the fan closed to form turbine-like structures after 140 min.

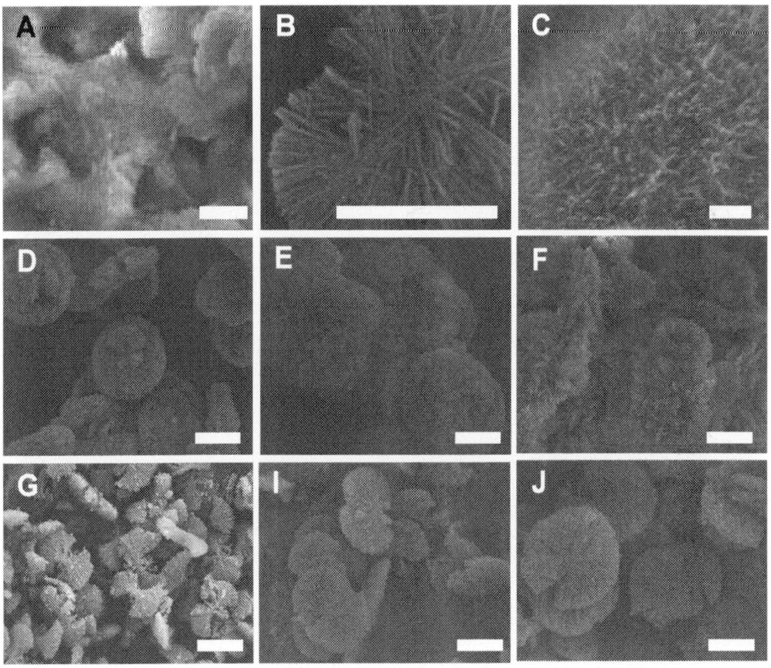

Fig. 10. SEM images of shaped silicas from self-assmebled PEI aggregates mediated from metal ions. (A), (B) and (C) are synthesized by the mediation of Na^+, Cu^{2+} and Al^{3+}, respectively, with the molar ratio of EI to metal ions of 20/1. (D), (E) and (F) are prepared by templating the aggregates from **PEI5050** solution containing $Ni^{II}(p\text{-}TolSO^3)^2$ with the concentrations of 70, 40 and 20 mM of Ni^{II} ions ([EI]=1000mM), respectively. (G), (I) and (J) are morphological evolution of silica altered by pre-structured **PEI5050** formed in Zn^{II}(p-TolSO3)2 aqueous solutions ([EI]=1000 mM, [Zn]=60 mM) at times of 80, 110 and 140 min, respectively. The bars are 2 μm for each case.

3.3.6 Physical field

The programmed self-assembly of linear PEI could be also simply adjusted by changing the physical field for the formation of crystalline PEI (Yuan & Jin, unpublished results). Using external physical field is of great interest due to that we don't need design and synthesize new polymer for shaping silica into complex morphologies and hierarchical nanostructure, which is relatively complex and time-consuming. Silica network composed of nanofibers of about 30 nm width was formed by silicifying the crystalline aggregates formed by naturally cooling the 1.0 wt% **PEI5050** hot solution (80°C) to room temperature (Figure 11A). In contrast, the width of fibrous silicas increased to about 500 nm - 1 μm when PEI aggregates were prepared by cooling the same hot solution with slow rate (Figure 11B). Obviously, the slowly cooling process enables the PEI molecules to have longer time to crystallize into objects with lager size. On the other hand, we also tried to freeze the molecular solution of PEI by immersing hot solution of PEI into mixture of ice-water and acetone-dry ice (-70°C). After the temperature of frozen PEI solution was naturally back to room temperature, the PEI aggregation occurred. It is interesting that the sample from ice freeze showed the formation of silica plate (Figure 11C), and freeze from acetone-dry ice resulted in bulk-like silica composed of folded film (Figure 11D).

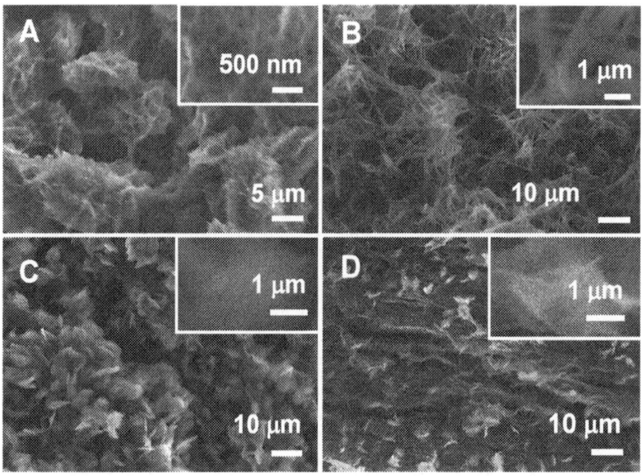

Fig. 11. Shaping silicas by physical field. (A) was prepared by using aggregates formed by naturally cooling 80°C aqueous solution of **PEI5050** to room temperature; (B) was obtained by templating the aggregates formed by keeping 80°C aqueous solution of **PEI5050** at 50°C for 1 h and then naturally down to room temperature; (C) and (D) were formed by using PEI aggregates prepared by immersing 80°C aqueous solution of **PEI5050** into a bath of ice-water and acetone/dry ice, respectively, and then allowing iced samples back to room temperature naturally. All samples have the same concentration of 1.0 wt% **PEI5050.**

3.3.7 Fluorescent silica nanoparticles with controlled diameters

Well-defined silica nanoparticles with controlled size and tunable functions are interesting especially for biomedical applications. Conventional Stöber method (Stöber et al. 1968) for the synthesis of silica nanoparticles requires harsh conditions and needs care for particle control. Recently, there have been some reports describing the biomimetic synthesis of silica spheres mediated by bio-polyamines or synthetic linear or dendrimer polyamines (Knecht & Wright, 2004; Li et al., 2009), however, the precise particles size control and facile functionalization still is a challenge. By simply adjusting the media compositions for PEIs with linear backbone, we are able to generate the uniformed silica nanoparticles functionalized with acidic dyes by one-port manner (Jin & Yuan, 2007b). By optimizing

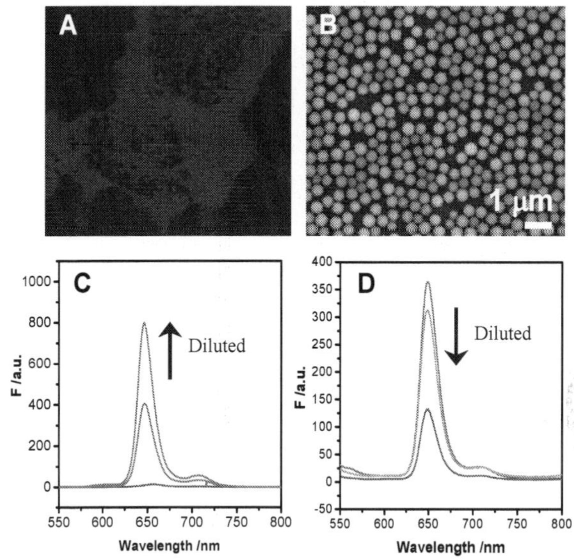

Fig. 12. Uniformed silica nanoparticles synthesized by the mediation of linear poly(ethyleneimine)s and dyes. (A) Fluorescent microscopic and (B) SEM images of silica nanoparticles prepared by using **sPEI4-50**/TSPP (1200/1 in molar ratio). (C) Fluorescence spectra of **sPEI4-50**/TSPP solution and (D) TSPP-entrapped silica spheres with diluting the concentrations.

medium composition of methanol/water to be 7/3 in volume, the linear-backbone-based PEIs with different architectures and/or addition of TSPP directed the formation of monodisperse silica nanospheres with silicification reaction time of 1 h at room temperature (Figure 12A and B). The diameters of silica nanoparticles could be controlled from 50 to 700 nm by adjusting the polymer architectures, additives or solution conditions for silica mineralization. The attractive feature in our approach is that photofunctional dyes could be simultaneously and simply encapsulated into the resulting silica spheres. The precursor PEI/TSPP (1200/1) and silica nanoparticles by silicifying precursor PEI/TSPP showed the same peak position of absorption spectra, indicating that the porphyrin residues entrapped in the silica spheres exist as molecularly distributed state (i.e., isolated without stacking). This is very different to that of aster- and flower-like silicas prepared from **p-sPEI-240** and **PEI505**/TSPP (1200/1 in molar ratio), respectively. Fiber-based 3-D silicas were synthesized by templating the crystalline PEI aggregates formed in pure water (**p-sPEI-240**) or in methanol/water (5/5 in vol., **PEI505**/TSPP). In contrast, the silica nanoparticles were formed by using a medium of methanol/water (7/3 in vol.), in which PEI do not crystallize due to the excess presence of methanol. To further understand the spectroscopic properties of these silica nanoparticles, the dependence of intensities of absorption and emission on the concentrations was examined. We found that absorption intensities of both PEI/TSPP precursor and PEI/TSPP/silica nanoparticles increased with increasing concentrations (Jin & Yuan, 2007b). However, the emissions of PEI/TSPP precursor and PEI/TSPP/silica nanoparticles in methanol showed different behavior upon concentration change. The emission intensity (at 650 nm) of the original methanol solution of PEI/TSPP precursor is very weak, compared to those from diluted solutions (Figure 12C). This is due to the dynamic-induced self-quenching of TSPP at higher concentration, suggesting that porphyrin residues are not tethered to the star polymer and thus are in movement with collision. However, the emission intensity of the PEI/TSPP/silica nanoparticles in methanol increased upon increasing concentrations (Figure 12D), indicating that TSPP residues with PEI were almost completely encapsulated in the silica nanospheres and existed as isolated state. The dye entrapped into silica nanospheres did not show bleach even dispersed in methanol for over one year. Thus these novel TSPP-functionalized silica nanoparticles would be superior to some of conventional dye-encapsulated silica nanoparticles based on Stöber routes by either using silica source with chemically-bonded-dyes or physically doping dyes into silica network, in which dye incorporation is not easily controllable (Chan et al., 2004).

3.4 Linear PEI for mineralization of other oxides, metals and salts

Titanium oxides, as one of the most useful semiconductors, have been applied in a wide area due to their many promising properties. Conventional process has made progress on tailoring TiO_2 into precisely controlled nanostructure, however titania deposition normally occurred under harsh conditions. Inspired by biosilica formation, biomimetic synthesis of titania materials have been attempted by using various biologically-derived molecules or synthetic polyamines (Brutchey & Morse, 2008). However, it remains difficult to construct TiO_2 materials with definite morphologies (i.e. fiber-like) and characteristic function by this process. Our recent work demonstrated that well-shaped fibrous networks of PEI@TiO_2 hybrids (Figure 13) could be controllably prepared in an aqueous solution at room temperature by using crystalline PEI aggregates as a regulator and water-soluble titanium bislactate as source (Zhu & Jin, 2010). Fibrous hybrids were found to be composed of anatase nano crystallites (Figure 13B and C) and linear PEI with a regularly-layered structure. The morphologies and structures of TiO_2-PEI hybrids depended on pH of reaction systems and concentrations of PEI and titania source. Recently, Zhao and co-workers also described using fibrous PEI aggregates as template to direct the low-temperature formation of nano-branched aluminum–magnesium hydroxide (Xiang et al., 2008).

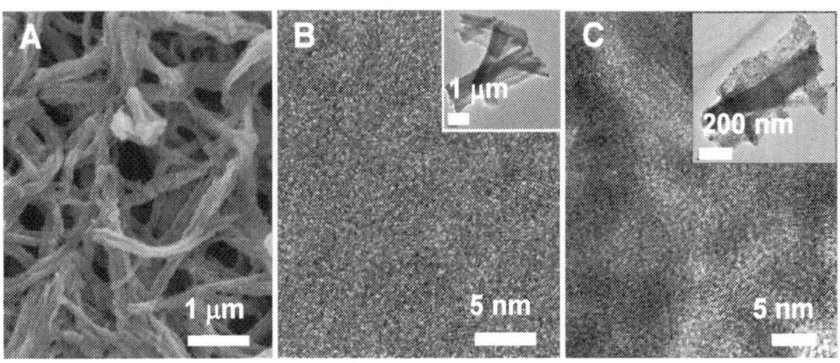

Fig. 13. (A) SEM image of fibrous PEI@titania hybrids synthesized by simple and efficient aqueous process regulated by linear polyethyleneimine aggregates, (B) TEM (inset) and HRTEM image of synthesized PEI@titania, indicating the formation of very tiny crystalline domains and (C) TEM (inset) and HRTEM images of fibrous titania formed by calcining PEI@titania at 500 °C.

On the other hand, polymers with linear PEI backbone have been also examined to mineralize metals into various structure and morphologies. For example, with the use of low-molecular-weight linear PEI or alkylated PEI (with repeated units of EI of around 8) to serve as a reducing agent and a protective agent, $HAuCl_4$ was reported to be induced to form gold nanoparticles and nanoplates through either a thermal process or room temperature (Chen et al., 2007). We are interested in using high-molecular-weight linear PEI with self-assembled crystalline property for reduction and stabilization of metal ion. By simply mixing the aqueous dispersion of crystalline PEI aggregates with $AgNO_3$ aqueous solution at room temperature, an Ag nanoparticles-PEI paste could be obtained. The macroporous silver frameworks have been achieved by calcining the Ag nanoparticles-PEI pastes (Jin & Yuan, 2005c). We found that the porous silver frameworks could be tunable into dome-like shapes with the inner chambers or monoliths with shape-preservation by simply adjusting some synthesis parameters.

Recently, Taubert and co-workers (Shkilnyy et al., 2008) reported that PEI could be an efficient template for the controlled mineralization of calcium phosphate. It was found that spherical calcium phosphate/polymer hybrid particles were formed at pH values above 8 through a mineralization-trapping pathway, where small calcium phosphate particles formed at the initial step were stabilized by protonated PEI. Comparative studies revealed that branched and linear PEIs did not show significant difference for calcium phosphate mineralization, since PEIs were only used as pH-responsive cationic polymer for modifying crystal growth of calcium phosphate. Self-assembling property of linear PEI due to aqueous crystallization was not involved in the morphological creation of calcium phosphate, as seen in the mineralization of silica, titania or metals.

3.5 PEI@oxides as nanoreactors for generating metal nanoparticles

One of important characters of our PEI@oxides materials are that the PEI occluded in hybrids is still available for subsequent chemical reactions, leading to the facile synthesis of novel composite materials. The central PEI entrapped in the silica fiber could be used as a nanoreactor to synthesize metallic nanostructures (Yuan et al. 2006). The reduction of Na_2PtCl_4 was simply performed by keeping an aqueous mixture of PEI@silica nanofiber and Na_2PtCl_4 for 30 min at room temperature and then aged at 80°C for another 30 min, without any additive reducing agents. XRD measurement indicated the formation of a face-centered cubic (fcc) lattice of the platinum crystal structure. HRTEM studies demonstrated the formation of Pt@silica nanocables with the Pt central nanowires of about 3 nm in width (Figure 14A). Surprisingly, when irradiated with a strong electron beam, the Pt nanowire in the silica nanotube broken into individual nanoparticles (Figure 14B). The in situ formation of Pt and Au nanoparticles in PEI@silica prepared using water glass as silica source has also been successfully achieved (Zhu & Jin, 2008). These metal nanoparticles functionalized silica materials were expected to have potentials for catalysis or optic application. Furthermore, PEI residues in the PEI@TiO_2 hybrids have been also exploited to reduce Na_2PtCl_4 into Pt nanoparticles by simply mixing PEI@TiO_2 with the reactants at room-temperature (Zhu & Jin, 2010). TEM studies indicated that the fibrous morphologies remained undestroyed after the formation of metallic nanoparticles (Figure 14E). The further HRTEM images showed that the Pt nanoparticles in situ formed have a typical diameter of about 3 nm, are homogeneously distributed in the hybrid fibers (Figure 14F). These nanostructured TiO_2 doped with Pt nanoparticles revealed visible light responsible photocatalytic power in decolorization of dyes.

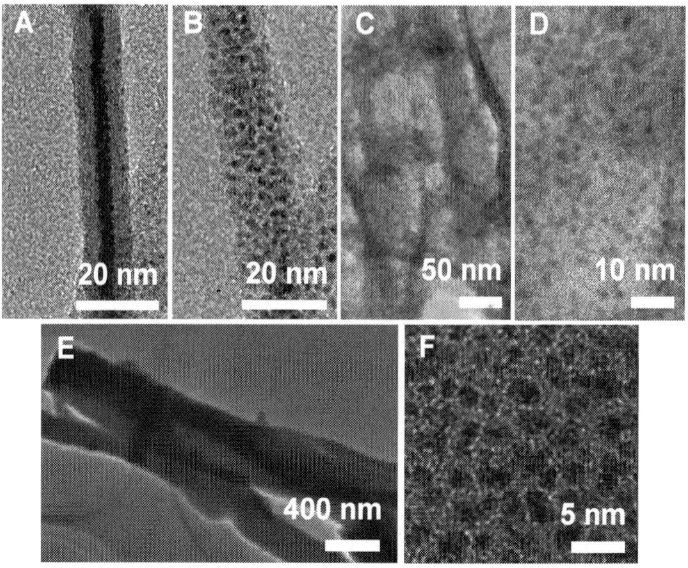

Fig. 14. PEI@silica or PEI@titania hybrids as microreactors for *in situ* formation of Pt nanoparticles. (A and B) PEI@silica hybrid from TMOS source; (C and D) PEI@silica hybrids from water glass as source; (E and F) PEI@titania hybrids.

4. Concluding remarks and future outlook

It is important for device and sensor application to biomimetically construct nanostructured ceramic surface on substrates. It has been a number of reports describing the biomimetic formation of silica (Yang et al., 2009; Rai & Perry, 2009) and titania (Kharlampieva et al., 2008) film on the solid substrates. Although some reports have been successful to control film thickness, particles packing, or patterns, constructing the silica film with high-degree controllable nanostructure on the arbitrary substrates is still a challenge. Very recently, we have successfully constructed the silica nanograss on the arbitrary substrates with any shapes by extending the programmed self-assembly of linear PEI from solution (silica powder) to interface (silica nanograss) (Figure 15) (Jin & Yuan, 2009). Such a process has been expanded for the formation of nanofiber-based titania surface, which demonstrated the photoresponsive surface wettability (Yuan & Jin, 2010a). These novel interface materials with controlled nanostructure and surface morphology are expected to have potential applications as microreactors, sensors, microfluidic devices, surface with designer wettability (Yuan & Jin, 2010a; 2010b) and so on. Moreover, the further functionalization of such silica nanograss is possible by exploiting the chemistry of PEI and conventional silica, allowing our interface materials to be applicable in a wide variety of emerging nanotechnology. On the other hand, although the biomimetic silicas have many amazing features including ambient-conditions synthesis, potentially precise control over nanostructure and good biocompatibility, the commercial application still remains a big challenge. One of major reason is that most of currently-developed systems for biomimetic silica formation are not easy to scale up, and suffer from high cost, low reproducibility and relatively poor morphogenesis. Recently, we have optimized the conditions to achieve a low-cost and reproducible synthesis of several hundred gram scale of silica nano ribbons. Silicification was performed in neat water under room temperature by using a cheap, commercially-available silica source. This achievement on biomimetic silica synthesis would make it possible to develop the related technological applications in a wide range of fields.

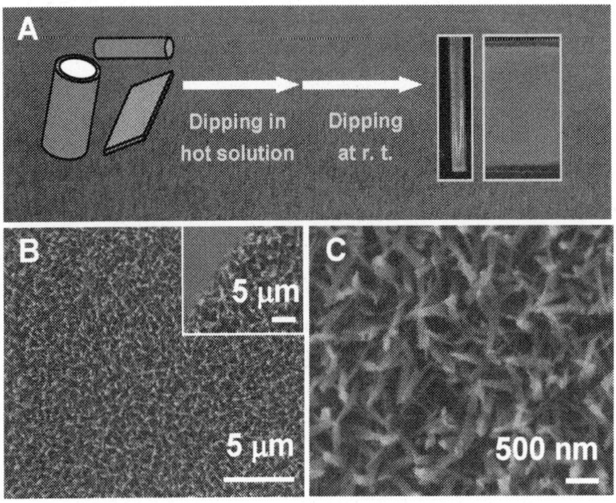

Fig. 15. PEI@silica nanograss on arbitrary substrates with. (A) two-step processing for growing the PEI@silica nanoribbons on substrates; (B) a representative SEM image of PEI@silica nanograss, the inset is a cross-section image of nanograss; (C) high-magnification SEM image of PEI@silica nanograss, indicating the blade-like morphology

5. References

Akiyama, Y.; Harada, A.; Nagasaki, Y. & Kataoka, K. (2000). Synthesis of poly(ethylene glycol)-block-poly(ethylenimine) possessing an acetal group at the PEG end, *Macromolecules*, 33, 5841-5845.

Brunner, E.; Lutz, K. & Sumper, M. (2004). Biomimetic synthesis of silica nanospheres depends on the aggregation and phase separation of polyamines in aqueous solution, *Phys. Chem. Chem. Phys.*, 6, 854-857.

Brutchey, R.L. & Morse, D.E. (2008). Silicattein and the translation of its molecular mechanism of biosilicification into low temperature nanomaterial synthesis, *Chem. Rev.*, 108, 4915-4934.

Cha, J.N.; Shimizu, K.; Zhou, Y.; Christiansen, S.C.; Chmelka, B.F.; Stucky, G.D. & Morse, D.E. (1999). Silicatein filaments and subunits from a marine sponge direct the polymerization of silica and silicones in vitro, *Proc. Nat. Acad. Sci. USA*, 96, 361-365.

Cha, J.N.; Stucky, G.D.; Morse, D.E. & Deming, T.J. (2000). Biomimetic synthesis of ordered silica structures mediated by block copolypeptides, *Nature*, 403, 289-292.

Chan, Y.; Zimmer, J.P.; Stroh, M.; Steckel, J.S.; Jain, R.K. & Bawendi, M.G. (2004). Incorporation of luminescent nanocrystals into monodisperse core-shell silica microspheres, *Adv. Mater.*, 16, 2092-2097.

Chatani, Y.; Tadokoro, H.; Saegusa, T. & Ikeda, H. (1981). Structural studies of poly(ethylenimine). 1. Structures of two hydrates of poly(ethylenimine): sesquihydrate and dehydrate, *Macromolecules*, 14, 315-321.

Chatani, Y.; Kobatake, T.; Tadokoro, H. & Tanaka, R. (1982). Structural studies of poly(ethylenimine). 2. Double-stranded helical chains in the anhydrate, *Macromolecules*, 15, 170-176.

Chatani, Y.; Kobatake, T. & Tadokoro, H. (1983). Structural studies of poly(ethylenimine). 3. Structural characterization of anhydrous and hydrous states and crystal structure of the hemihydrate, *Macromolecules*, 16, 199-204.

Chen, C.C.; Hsu, C.H. & Kuo, P.L. (2007). Effects of alkylated polyethylenimines on the formation of gold nanoplates, *Langmuir*, 23, 6801-6806.

Croce, G.; Frache, A.; Milanesio, M.; Marchese, L.; Causà, M.; Viterbo, D.; Barbaglia, A.; Bolis, V.; Bavestrello, G.; Cerrano, C.; Benatti, U.; Pozzolini, M.; Giovine, M. & Amenitsch, H. (2004). Structural characterization of siliceous spicules from marine sponges, *Biophys. J.*, 86, 526-534.

Croce, G.; Viterbo, D.; Milanesio, M. & Amenitsch, H. (2007). A mesoporous pattern created by nature in spicules from Thetya aurantium sponge, *Biophys. J.*, 92, 288-292.

Davis, M.E. (2002). Ordered porous materials for emerging applications, *Nature*, 417, 813-821.

Field, C.B.; Behrenfeld, M.J.; Randerson, J.T. & Falkowski, P. (1998). Primary production of the biosphere: integrating terrestrial and oceanic components, *Science*, 281, 237-240.

Fuhrmann, T.; Landwehr, S.; El Rharbi-Kucki, M. & Sumper, M. (2004). Diatoms as living photonic crystals, *Appl. Phys. B*, 78, 257-6028.

Hashida, T.; Tashiro, K.; Aoshima, S. & Inaki, Y. (2002). Structural investigation on water-induced phase transitions of poly(ethylene imine). 1. Time-resolved infrared spectral measurements in the hydration process, *Macromolecules*, 35, 4330- 4336.

Hildebrand, M. (2008). Diatoms, Biomineralization processes, and genomics, *Chem. Rev.*, 108, 4855-4874.

Hsiue, G.H.; Chiang, H.Z.; Wang, C.H. & Juang, T.M. (2006). Nonviral gene carriers based on diblock copolymers of poly(2-ethyl-2oxazoline) and linear polyethyleneimine, *Bioconj. Chem.*, 17, 781-786.

Ji, Q.; Iwaura, R.; Kogiso, M.; Jung, J.H.; Yoshida, K. & Shimizu, T. (2004). Direct sol-gel replication without catalyst in an aqueous gel system: from a lipid nanotube with a single bilayer wall to a uniform silica hollow cylinder with an ultrathin wall, *Chem. Mater., 16*, 250-254.

Jin, R.H. & Motoyoshi, K. (1999). Porphyrin-centered water-soluble star-shaped polymers: poly(N-acetylethylenimine) and poly(ethylenimine) arms, *J. Porphyrins Phthalocyanines*, 3, 60-64.

Jin, R.H. (2002a). Controlled location of porphyrin in aqueous micelles self-assembled from porphyrin centered amphiphilic star poly(oxazolines), *Adv. Mater.*, 14, 889-892.

Jin, R.H. (2002b). Silica-polyoxazoline hybrid with nanosized hollow enclosing porphyrin in hybrid walls, *Chem. Commun.*, 198-199.

Jin, R.H. (2003a). Self-assembly of porphyrin-centered amphiphilic star block copolymer into polymeric vesicular aggregates, *Macromol. Chem. Phys.*, 204, 403-409.

Jin, R.H. (2003b). Colloidal crystalline polymer generated in situ from growing star poly(oxazolines), *J. Mater. Chem.*, 13, 672-675.

Jin, R.H. (2003c). Functional polymeric micelles formed from a novel cationic star block copolymer, *ChemPhysChem*, 4, 1118-1121.

Jin, R.H. (2004). Water soluble star block poly(oxazoline) with porphyrin label: a unique emulsion and its shape direction, *J. Mater. Chem.*, 14, 320-327.

Jin, R.H. & Yuan, J.J. (2005a). Synthesis of poly(ethyleneimine)s-silica hybrid particles with complex shapes and hierarchical structures, *Chem. Commun.*, 1399- 1401.

Jin, R.H. & Yuan, J.J. (2005b). Simple synthesis of hierarchically structured silicas by poly-(ethyleneimine) aggregates pre-organized by media modulation, *Macromol. Chem. Phys.*, 206, 2160-2170.

Jin, R.H. & Yuan, J.J. (2005c). Fabrication of silver porous frameworks using poly(ethyleneimine) hydrogel as a soft sacrificial template, *J. Mater. Chem.*, 15, 4513-4517.

Jin, R.H. & Yuan, J.J. (2006). Shaped silicas transcribed from aggregates of four-armed star polyethyleneimine with a benzene core, *Chem. Mater.*, 18, 3390-3396.

Jin, R.H. & Yuan, J.J. (2007a). Hierarchically structured silica from mediation of linear poly(ethyleneimine) incorporated with acidic/basic additives, *Polym. J.*, 39, 464-470.

Jin, R.H. & Yuan, J.J. (2007b) One-pot and rapid synthesis of uniformed silica spheres via mediation of linear poly(ethyleneimine)s and dyes, *Polym. J.*, 39, 822- 827.

Jin, R.H., & Yuan, J.J. (2009) Biomimetically controlled formation of nanotextured silica/titania films on arbitrary substrates and their tunable surface function, *Adv. Mater.*, 21, 3750-3753.

Johnson, J.R.; Spikowski, J. & Schiraldi, D.A. (2009). Mineralization of clay/polymer aerogels: a bioinspired approach to composite reinforcement, *ACS Appl. Mater. Interfaces*, 1, 1305-1309.

Kakuda, H.; Okada, T. & Hasegawa, T. (2009). Temperature-induced molecular structural changes of linear polyethylene imine in water studied by mid-infrared and near-infrared spectroscopies, *J. Phys. Chem. B*, 113, 13910-13916.

Kharlampieva, E.; Tsukruk, T.; Slocik, J.M.; Ko, H.; Poulsen, N.; Naik, R.R.; Kröger, N. & Tsukruk, V.V. (2008). Bioenabled surface-mediated growth of titania nanoparticles, *Adv. Mater.*, 20, 3274-3279.

Knecht, M.R. & Wright, D.W. (2004). Dendrimer-mediated formation of multicomponent nanospheres, *Chem. Mater.*, 16, 4890-4895,

Krasko, A.; Lorenz, B.; Batel, R.; Schröder, H.C.; Müller, I.M. & Müller, W.E.G. (2000). Expression of silicatein and collagen genes in the marine sponge Suberites domuncula is controlled by silicate and myotrophin, *Eur. J. Biochem.*, 267, 4878-4887, 4855-4874.

Kresge, C.T.; Leonowicz, M.E.; Roth, W.J.; Vartuli, J.C. & Beck, J.S. (1992). Ordered mesoporous molecular sieves synthesized by a liquid-crystal template mechanism, *Nature*, 359, 710-712.

Kröger, N.; Bergsdorf, C. & Sumper, M. (1994). A new calcium-binding glycoprotein family constitutes a major diatom cell wall component, *EMBO J.*, 13, 4676- 4683.

Kröger, N.; Bergsdorf, C. & Sumper, M. (1996). Frustulins: domain conservation in a protein family associated with diatom cell walls, *Eur. J. Biochem.*, 239, 259-284.

Kröger, N.; Lehmann, G.; Rachel, R. & Sumper, M. (1997). Characterization of a 200-kDa diatom protein that is specifically associated with a silica-based substructure of the cell wall, *Eur. J. Biochem.*, 250, 99-105.

Kröger, N.; Deutzmann, R. & Sumper, M. (1999). Polycationic peptides from diatom biosilica that direct silica nanosphere formation, *Science*, 286, 1129-1132.

Kröger, N. & Wetherbee, R. (2000a). Pleuralins are involved in theca differentiation in the diatom Cylindrotheca fusiformis, *Protist*, 151, 263-273.

Kröger, N.; Deutzmann, R.; Bergsdorf, C. & Sumper, M. (2000b). Species-specific polyamines from diatoms control silica morphology, *Proc. Natl. Acad. Sci. U.S.A.*, 97, 14133-14138.

Kröger, N.; Deutzmann, R. & Sumper, M. (2001). Silica-precipitating peptides from diatoms: The chemical structure of silaffin-1A from Cylindrotheca fusiformis, *J. Bio. Chem.*, 276, 26066-27070.

Kröger, N.; Lorenz, S.; Brunner, E. & Sumper, M. (2002). Self-assembly of highly phosphorylated silaffins and their function in biosilica morphogenesis, *Science, 298,* 584-586.

Kröger, N. & Poulsen, N. (2008). Diatoms-from cell wall biogenesis to nanotechnology, *Ann. Rev. Gene.*, 42, 83-107.

Li, X.; Yang, T.; Gao, Q.; Yuan, J. & Cheng, S. (2009). Biomimetic synthesis of copolymer-silica nanoparticles with tunable compositions and surface property, *J. Colloid Interface Sci.*, 338, 99-104.

Matsukizono, H.; Zhu, P.X.; Fukazawa, N. & Jin, R.H. (2009). Turbine-like structured silica transcribed simply by pre-structured crystallites of linear poly(ethyleneimine) bounded with metal ions, *CrystEngComm*, 11, 2695-2700.

Menzel, H.; Horstmann, S.; Behrens, P.; Bärnreuther, P.; Krueger, I. & Jahns, M. (2003). Chemical properties of polyamines with relevance to the biomineralization of silica, *Chem. Commun.*, 2994-2995.

Merchant, S.A.; Tran, T.O.; Meredith, M.T.; Cline, T.C.; Glatzhofer, D.T. & Schmidtke, D.W. (2009). High-sensitivity smperometric biosensors based on ferrocene-modified linear poly(ethylenimine), *Langmuir,* 25, 7736-7742.

Milligan, A.J. & Morel, F.M.M. (2002). A proton buffering role for silica in diatoms. *Science,* 297, 1848-1850.

Müller, W.E.G.; Rothenberger, M.; Boreiko, A.; Tremel, W.; Reiber, A. & Schröder, H.C. (2005). Formation of siliceous spicules in the marine demosponge Suberites domuncula, *Cell and Tissue Res.*, 321, 285-297.

Müller, W.E.G.; Belikov, S.I.; Tremel, W.; Perry, C.C.; Gieskes, W.W.C.; Boreiko, A. & Schröder, H.C. (2006). Siliceous spicules in marine demosponges (example Suberites domuncula), *Micron,* 37,107-120.

Murr, M.M. & Morse, D.E. (2005). Fractal intermediates in the self-assembly of silicatein filaments, *Proc. Nat. Acad. Sci. USA*, 102, 11657-11662.

Navarro, S.; Shkilnyy, A.; Tiersch, B.; Taubert, A. & Menzel, H. (2009). Preparation, characterization, and thermal gelation of amphiphilic alkyl-poly(ethyleneimine), *Langmuir,* 25, 10558-10566.

Patel, P.A.; Eckart, J.; Advincula, M.C.; Goldberg, A.J. & Mather, P.T. (2009). Rapid synthesis of polymer-silica hybrid nanofibers by biomimetic mineralization, *Polymer,* 50, 1214-1222.

Patwardhan, S.V.; Clarson, S.J. & Perry, C.C. (2005). On the role(s) of additives in bioinspired silicification, *Chem. Commun.*, 1113-1121.

Perry, C.C. & Keeling-Tucker, T. (2000). Biosilicification: The role of the organic matrix in structure control, *J. Bio. Inorg. Chem.*, 5, 537-550.

Pohnert, G. (2002). Biomineralization in diatoms mediated through peptide- and polyamine-assisted condensation of silica, *Angew Chem. Int. Ed.*, 41, 3167- 3169.

Pouget, E.; Dujardin, E.; Cavalier, A.; Moreac, A.; Valery, C.; Marchi-Artzner, V.; Weiss, T.; Renault, A.; Paternostre, M. & Artzner, F. (2007). Hierarchical architectures by synergy between dynamical template self-assembly and biomineralization, *Nat. Mater.*, 6, 434-439.

Poulsen, N.; Sumper, M. & Kröger, N. (2003). Biosilica formation in diatoms: Characterization of native silaffin-2 and its role in silica morphogenesis, *Proc. Natl. Acad. Sci. U.S.A.*, 100, 12075-12080.

Rai, A. & Perry, C.C. (2009). Fabrication of tuneable thickness silica films on solid surfaces using amines and proteins, *Silicon*, 1, 91-101.

Saegusa, T.; Kobayashi,S. & Yamada, A. (1975). Graft copolymerization of 2-methyl-2-oxazoline onto chloromethylated polystyrene and hydrolysis of graft copolymer to a chelating resin of poly(styrene-g-ethylenimine), *Macromolecules,* 8, 390- 396.

Schmidt, D.J.; Cebeci, F.C.; Kalcioglu, Z.I.; Wyman, S.G.; Ortiz, C.; Vliet, K.J.V. & Hammond, P.T. (2009). Electrochemically controlled swelling and mechanical properties of a polymer nanocomposite, *ACS Nano,* 3, 2207-2216.

Schröder, H.C.; Boreiko, A.; Korzhev, M.; Tahir, M.N.; Tremel, W.; Eckert, C.; Ushijima, H.; Müller, I.M. & Müller, W.E.G. (2006). Co-expression and functional interaction of silicatein with galectin: Matrix-guided formation of siliceous spicules in the marine demosponge Suberites domuncula, *J. Bio. Chem.*, 281, 12001- 12009.

Schröder, H.C.; Wang, X.; Tremel, W.; Ushijima, H. & Müller, W.E.G. (2008). Biofabrication of biosilica-glass by living organisms, *Nat. Prod. Rep.*, 25, 455-474.

Shimizu, K.; Cha, J.; Stucky, G.D. & Morse, D.E. (1998). Silicatein α: Cathepsin L-like protein in sponge biosilica, *Proc. Nat. Acad. Sci. USA,* 95, 6234-6238.

Shkilnyy, A.; Friedrich, A.; Tiersch, B.; Schone, S.; Fechner, M.; Koetz, J.; Schlapfer, C.-W. & Taubert, A. (2008). Poly(ethylene imine)-controlled calcium phosphate mineralization, *Langmuir,* 24, 2102-2109.

Sumper, M. (2002). A phase separation model for the nanopatterning of diatom biosilica, *Science,* 295, 2430-2433.

Sumper, M. & Kröger, N. (2004a). Silica formation in diatoms: The function of long-chain polyamines and silaffins, *J. Mater. Chem.*, 14, 2059-2065.

Sumper, M. (2004b). Biomimetic patterning of silica by long-chain polyamines, *Angew Chem. Int. Ed.*, 43, 2251-2254.

Sumper, M. & Lehmann, G. (2006). Silica pattern formation in diatoms: Species-specific polyamine biosynthesis, *ChemBioChem,* 7, 1419-1427.

Smetacek, V. (1999). Diatoms and the ocean carbon cycle, *Protist,* 150, 25-32.

Stöber, W.; Fink, A. & Bohn, E. (1968). Controlled growth of monodisperse silica spheres in the micron size range, *J. Colloid Interface Sci.*, 26, 62-69.

Tréguer, P.; Nelson, D.M.; van Bennekom, A.J.; DeMaster, D.J.; Leynaert, A. & Quéguiner, B. (1995).The silica balance in the world ocean: a re-estimate, *Science*, 268, 375-379.

van Bommel, K.J.C. & Shinkai, S. (2002). Silica transcription in the absence of a solution catalyst: the surface mechanism, *Langmuir*, 18, 4544-4548.

van Bommel, K.J.C.; Friggeri, A. & Shinkai, S. (2003). Organic templates for the generation of inorganic materials, *Angew Chem. Int. Ed.*, 42, 980-999.

van de Poll, W.H.; Vrieling, E.G. & Gieskes, W.W.C. (1999). Location and expression of frustulins in the pennate diatoms Cylindrotheca fusiformis, Navicula pelliculosa, and Navicula salinarum (Bacillariophyceae), *J. Phycol.*, 35, 1044-1053.

Weaver, J.C. & Morse, D.E. (2003). Molecular biology of demosponge axial filaments and their roles in biosilicification, *Micro. Res. Tech.*, 62, 356-367.

Yang, H.; Coombs, N. & Ozin, G.A. (1997). Morphogenesis of shapes and surface patterns in mesoporous silica, *Nature*, 386, 692-695.

Yang, S.H.; Park, J.H.; Cho, W.K.; Lee, H.-S. & Choi, I.S. (2009). Counteranion-directed, biomimetic control of silica nanostructures on surfaces inspired by biosilicification found in diatoms, *Smal*, 5, 1947-1951.

Yuan, J.J. & Jin, R.H. (2005a). Fibrous crystalline hydrogels formed from polymers possessing a linear poly(ethyleneimine) backbone, *Langmuir*, 21, 3136-3145.

Yuan, J.J. & Jin, R.H. (2005b). Multiply shaped silica mediated by aggregates of linear poly(ethyleneimine), *Adv. Mater.*, 17, 885-888.

Yuan, J.J.; Zhu, P.X.; Fukazawa, N. & Jin, R.H. (2006). Synthesis of nanofiber-based silica networks mediated by organized poly(ethylene imine): structure, properties, and mechanism, *Adv. Funct. Mater.*, 16, 2205-2212.

Yuan, J.J.; Mykhaylyk, O.O.; Ryan, A.J. & Armes, S.P. (2007). Cross-linking of cationic block copolymer micelles by silica deposition, *J. Am. Chem. Soc.*, 129, 1717-1723.

Yuan, J.J. & Jin, R.H. (2010a). Bioinspired synthesis of continuous titania coat with tunable nanofiber-based network structure on linear polyethyleneimine-covered substrates, *Langmuir*, 26, 4212-4218.

Yuan, J.J. & Jin, R.H. (2010b). Water motion and movement without sticking, weight loss and cross-contaminant in superhydrophobic glass tube, *Nanotechnology*, 21, 065704.

Zhu, P.X. & Jin, R.H. (2007). Polyethyleneimine aggregates regulated by metal cations acting as biomimetic organic reactors for silica architectures, *Small*, 3, 394-398.

Zhu, P.X. & Jin, R.H. (2008). Environmentally benign and cost-effective silicification: From water glass to nanostructured silica by poly(ethyleneimine) mediation, *J. Mater. Chem.*, 18, 313-318.

Zhu, P.X. & Jin, R.H. (2010). Simple and efficient aqueous process for nanostructured fibrous TiO2 regulated by linear polyethyleneimine aggregates, *Eur. J. Inorg. Chem.*, 3, 476-482.

Xiang, T.; Zhao, L.; Li, Y.; Lei, Z.; Jin, S.; Li, S.; Li, Y. & Liang, Y. (2008). Template formation of aluminum-magnesium hydroxide nano-branches on linear poly(ethylene imine), *Mater. Lett.*, 62, 1627-1629.

9

Biomimetic Fiber-Reinforced Compound Materials

Tom Masselter and Thomas Speck
Plant Biomechanics Group Freiburg (PBGF),
Faculty of Biology, Botanic Garden,
University of Freiburg
Germany

1. Introduction

During the last years, many efforts have been made to transfer results of quantitative analyses of functional morphology and biomechanics in plants into technical applications. These attempts have been increasingly successful as is proven by the increasing number of biomimetic products on the market (e.g. paints based on the Lotuseffect® among many others, see Bar-Cohen (2006) and Masselter et al. (2010a)), of which the top 100 biomimetic products have generated about 1 billion Euros in 2005 to 2008 (Bushan, 2009). These successes are the result of the long period over which the form-structure-function relationships of the plants have been investigated and understood. Of the broad spectrum of biomimetic products, fiber-reinforced composites represent some of the most successful biomimetic technical applications. The potential of developing biomimetic fiber-reinforced compound materials is very high because 1) the fiber-matrix structure in plants is comparable to those in technical materials and 2) the complex fiber-matrix structures in plants are organized in at least five hierarchical levels (Masselter et al., 2009b, 2010a; Speck T. et al., 2007), from the molecular scale over the nanoscale and microscale to macroscale (Jeronimidis, 2000a). Quantitative analysis of this hierarchical structuring of plants is generally being increasingly recognized as one of the most important keys for understanding the form-structure-function relationships in plants (see Fratzl, 2007). This method allows interpreting and abstracting the interaction between the structural components in plants that possess different mechanical properties and in consequence, building a new generation of lightweight but stiff fiber-reinforced biomimetic compound materials (Masselter 2009b, 2010a,b; Speck, O. et al., 2005; Speck, T. et al., 2007; Speck, T. & Speck, O. 2008).
In a biomimetic project, dealing with the development of fiber-reinforced compound materials the most important assets are the biological concept generators, which can be linear (unbranched) or branched, thereby mirroring the structures that are present in technics. Branched structures as Y- and T-shaped branched components are very common in many fields of technical applications (Fig. 1). In plants, these branchings have to bear high static and dynamic loads that form a complex overlay of different loading modes: bending, compression-tension and torsion (Jeronimidis, 2000b). In technics, similar loads often drastically decrease the life time of a technical component causing wear and material fatigue

(Fig. 1C). This situation is further complicated by the need to join these technical structures together by welding or riveting. These joints represent potential failure regions as notch stresses are often very high in these regions (Mattheck, 2007). What's more, producing these joinings is time-consuming and costly. In plants, branchings are developed and shaped in a manner so that notch stresses present in 'joints' (i.e. stem-branch attachments) are diverted and distributed, so that similar zones of weakness do not develop (Mattheck, 1990, 2007; Mattheck & Tesari 2002; Schwager et al., 2010).

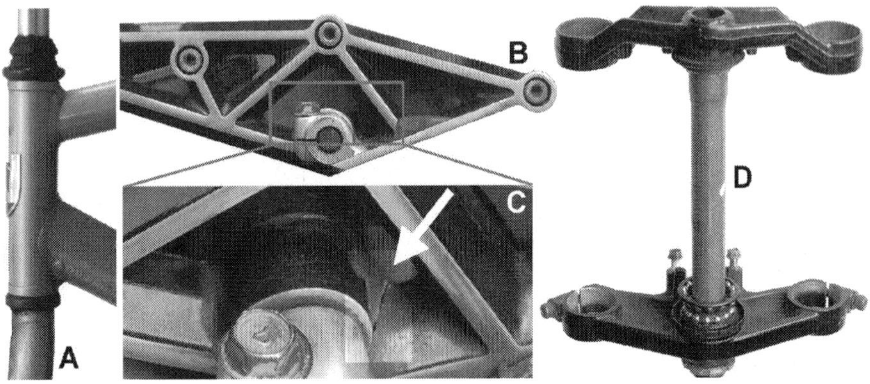

Fig. 1. Supporting structures in bicycle and motorbike engineering. (A) Headset of bicycle, (B),(C) subframe of motorbike with failure (arrow), (D) metal fork bridge of motorbike. © PBGF.

Generally speaking, plants are ‚ideal' concept generators for improving branched or unbranched technical structures since:

- Plants typically 'avoid' critical notch stresses
- Plants are lightweight structures
- Plants possess interesting mechanical properties like for example high stiffness and strength combined with a benign fracture behavior and good damping
- The laminated configuration of technical fiber-reinforced compound materials and the structure of some plant stems are highly comparable (Fig. 2, Ehrenstein, 2006; Speck T. et al., 2007)

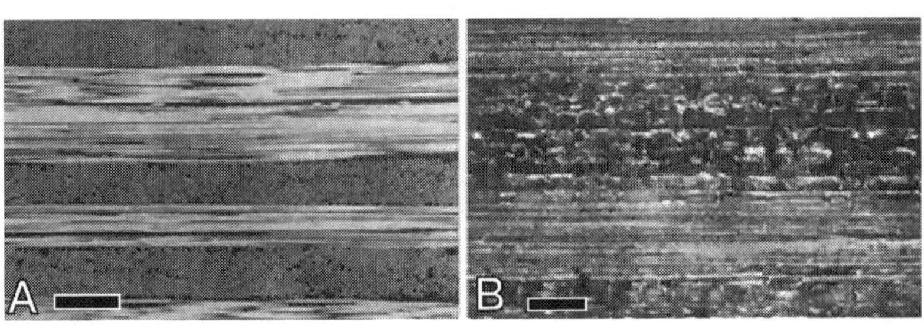

Fig. 2. Section of carbon-fiber-reinforced laminate (A) and bamboo stem wall (B) (from Ehrenstein, 2006). Scale bars = 200 μm.

2. Biomimetic fiber-reinforced compound materials and structures

2.1 Linear ‚unbranched' structures

2.1.1 Wood: Hierarchical structuring and microfibril angle

There exist numerous applications in which wood, wood pulp and natural fibers are used as components in the manufacturing of composites (e.g., Gindl & Jeronimidis 2004) for improving mechanical, thermal or other beneficial properties. Until now, the potential of using the hierarchical structure of wood as concept generator for developing innovative biomimetic fiber-reinforced compound materials has still been too little utilized (Fratzl, 2002b, 2007), even though wood is an excellent example for a complex structure that has led to several biomimetic applications (see below). The hierarchical structure of wood is well visible, including stem, tissue (Fig. 3A), cell (Fig. 3B,C) and ultrastructural level (Fig. 3D). Microfibril angles, i.e., the angles between the microfibrils and the longitudinal axis of wood tracheids, range typically between 0 and 30 degrees (Fig. 3D).

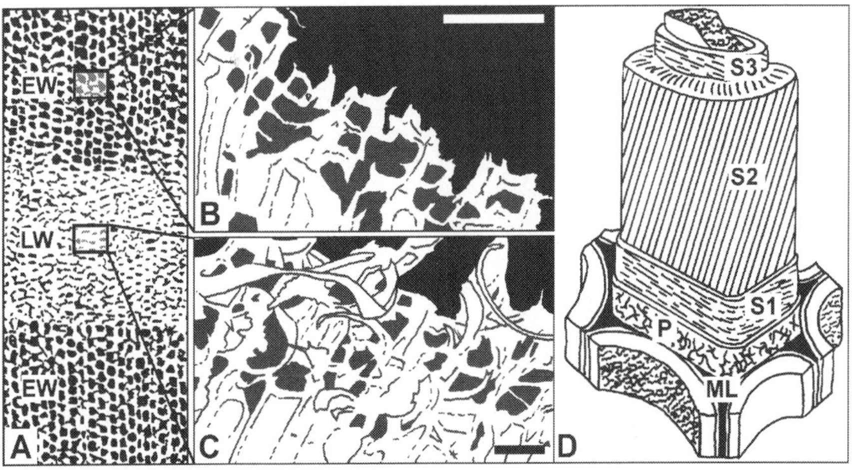

Fig. 3. Schematic drawing showing the hierarchical structure of spruce wood. (A) Tissue-level: cross-section of spruce wood; earlywood (EW) can be dinstiguished from the denser latewood (LW), (B, C) cell level: cellulose microfibril angle differs in (B) (0°) and (C) (50°) resulting in a plane fracture surface (B) or a highly structured fracture surface (C) in which tracheids and part of the tracheid wall are torn out, (D) ultrastructural level: different layers of a wood fiber tracheid can be distinguished: ML: middle lamella, P: pectin layer, S1-3: cell wall layers 1-3. The layer S2 represents approx. 80% of the overall thickness. Scale bars: (B) 100 µm; (C) 50 µm. Redrawn from Fratzl (2002a), Lichtenegger et al. (1999), Reiterer et al. (2001) and Vincent (2003). © PBGF.

When loaded under tension parallel to the longitudinal axis of the tracheids, spruce wood may show a markedly different fracture behavior (Fig. 3B, C) depending on the values of the fiber angle in the S2 wall of the fibers (Jeronimidis, 1979, 1980a,b, Fig. 3D). When the angles are well above 0°, the lignin between the helically arranged cellulose microfibers in the cell wall fractures (Fig. 3C) (Reiterer et al., 2001). This mechanism allows the tracheids to elongate, dissipates large amounts of energy and leaves the cellulose microfibers intact, so that they are still able to carry a load. Other interesting mechanical properties of wood for biomimetic applications are its low density, a high Young's modulus for resisting compressive forces, high fracture stress for resisting lateral forces and a large fracture strain to survive bending.

In a GFRP (glass-fiber reinforced plastic) with helically wound fibrous tubes, failure modes are very similar (Fig. 4A) to the failure modes of spruce wood (Gordon & Jeronimidis, 1980). There is a maximum of the work of fracture for a winding angle of 15° if subjected to three-point bending and tension. Initial failure is due to the resin between the fibers failing in shear (Fig. 4B). After that, the fibers rotate toward the longitudinal axis of the tubes, increasingly shearing the matrix and giving rise to further failures (Fig. 4B). This extends the strain before final failure and absorbs a large amount of energy. Both effects are of high interest for technical implementations. The findings of Gordon & Jeronimidis (1980) led to a patented composite material (Fig. 4C), which represents a different way of building a system of tubes with helically arranged fibers by using corrugation, with an optimal fiber angle α of about 15 degrees.

The potential fields of technical implementation are manifold, above all in the automotive industry and particularly in aerospace (Fig. 5) (Mangalgiri, 1999; Zhang et al., 2007). In new airplanes like the A380, compound materials contribute to 20-22% of the weight (Quilter, 2004). Carbon-fiber reinforced plastic, glass-fiber reinforced plastic and quartz-fiber reinforced plastic are used extensively in the wings, the fuselage sections, the tail and the doors (http://aero-defense.ihs.com).

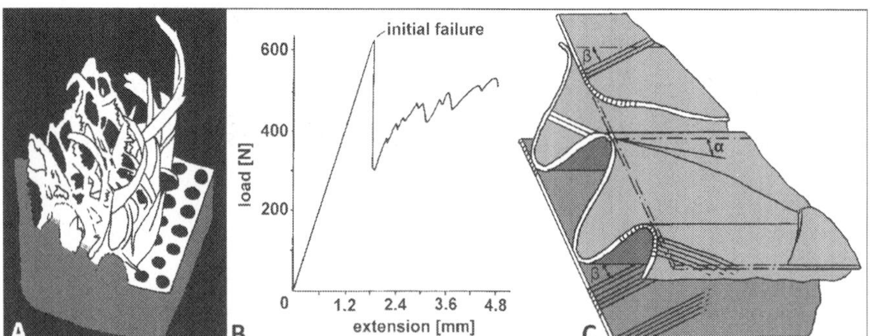

Fig. 4. Biomimetic glass-fiber reinforced plastics (GFRP). (A) Fracture morphology for GRFP with macrofibers, (B) force-displacement curve for GFRP, (C) patented composite material using optimized orientation of the reinforcing fibers to a corrugated medium. Redrawn from Caplin et al. (1983) and Gordon & Jeronimidis (1980). © PBGF.

2.1.2 Autonomous actuation and self-adaptation

Passive actuation systems in plants are of special interest for a biomimetic transfer as no active movements have to be abstracted and transferred into a technical application. Passive movements of plants or plant organs are mainly caused by changes in environmental conditions that act on dead tissues and cells (Dawson et al., 1997; Elbaum et al., 2007). Cell wall swelling or shrinking is effectuated by a combination of stiff cellulose fibrils that are embedded in different angles in a pliant and highly swellable matrix. Through this

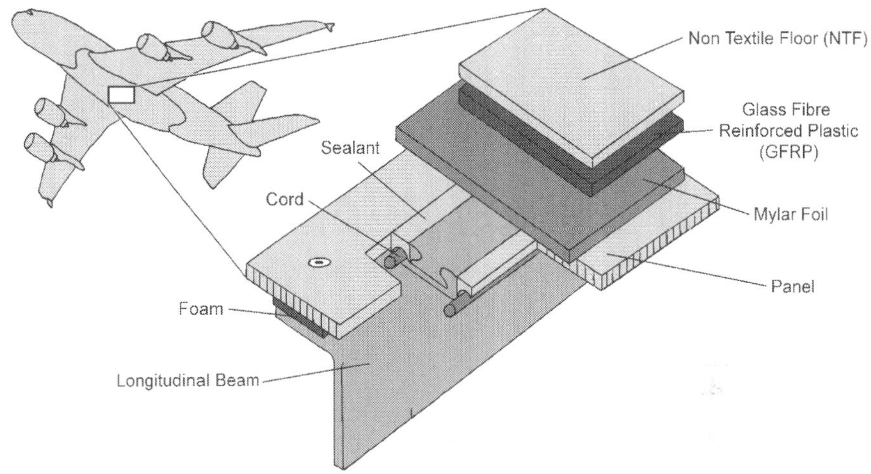

Fig. 5. Sandwich structure of the fuselage in a modern aircraft. Redrawn from http://www.airbus.com © PBGF.

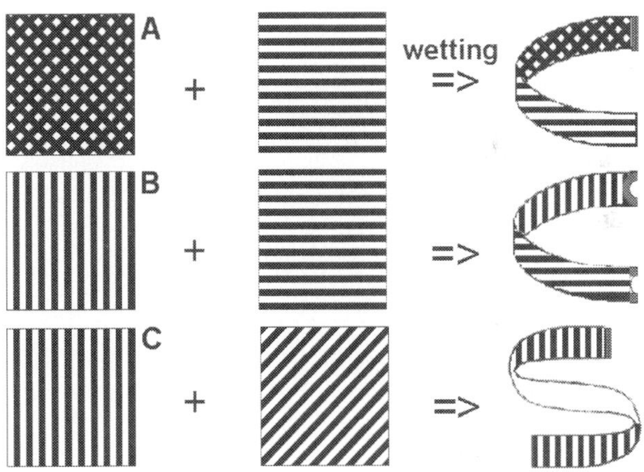

Fig. 6. Actuation principles of compound layer models. Different movements can be achieved by hydrating a swelling layer depending on its joining to a non-swelling layer. (A) Bending in a layer in which the fibers are parallel in one layer and in the other randomly organized, (B) rolling and bending in a bimorph layer with fibers and swelling direction of the two layers at an angle of 90°, (C) twisting and torsion in a similar bimorph layer with 45° angle. Redrawn from Stahlberg & Taya (2006). © PBGF.

structure, plants can generate various actuators by combining tissue layers consisting of cells with different swelling behavior and therefore elongation when wetted or dry. This actuator may cause bending, rolling and bending, twisting and torsion of plant organs (Fig. 6) and can cause large deformations. The modes of deformation depend on the relative

orientation of the cellulose microfibrils and the relative swelling direction of the two tissue layers (Fig. 6).
One of these actuation principles can be observed in wheat awns (Fig. 7A-C). These elongate structures are attached to the wheat fruit (Fig. 7A). By a passive movement, they assist in the dispersion and mobility of the fruit. In the adaxial side of the awn, the cap, the cellulose microfibrils are almost parallel to the longitudinal axis of the awn, on the abaxial side, the ridge, the microfibers are randomly organised (Fig. 7B). A change in humidity in the daily cycle causes differential swelling of the two sides and bending of the awns, by which the awned fruits dig themselves into the ground. As there are hooks on the abaxial side of the awns, preventing them from going upward (out of the soil) the fruits are pushed deeper in the ground (Fig. 7C) with every wetting-desiccation cycle (Burgert & Fratzl, 2009; Elbaum et al., 2007; Fratzl et al., 2008)

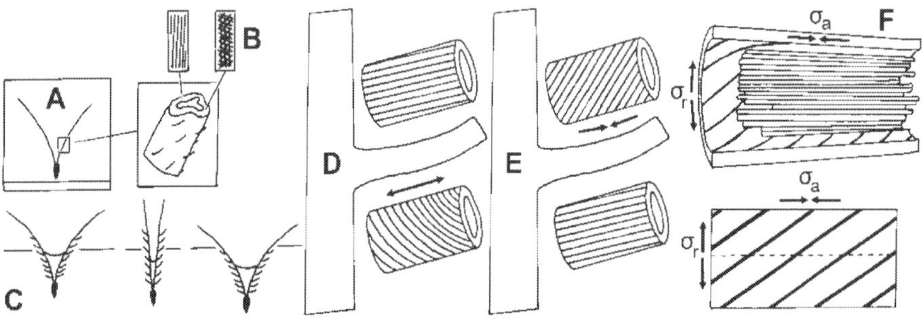

Fig. 7. Passive actuation systems in plants. (A) Dispersal unit of wheat with awns, (B) layers with axioparallel fibers (adaxial layer) and randomly organized fibers (abaxial layer) that cause bending (C) in daily cycles (open at day (dry) and closed by night (wet) due to a change in moisture. These cycles push the fruit in the ground. (D) Uprighting of a conifer branch by compression wood at the lower side of the branch. The angles in the microfibrils in normal wood (above) and compressive wood (below) are markedly different. Hygroscopic swelling increases the length of the compression wood tracheids causing an upright bending of the branch. (E) Uprighting of an angiosperm tree branch by tension wood in the upper side of the branch. (F) Model of the functioning principle of tension wood. Swelling of the gelatinous G-layer fibers (horizontal tubes at upper image) creates circumferential hoop stresses σ_r in the tracheid that are converted into axial tensile stresses σ_a shortening the length of the tracheid. The ratio between the axial tensile stresses σ_a and the radial stresses σ_r depends on the angle of the microfibrils. Redrawn from Burgert & Fratzl (2009), Elbaum et al. (2007) and Goswami et al. (2008). © PBGF.

Compression wood (Fig. 7D) as well as tension wood (Fig. 7E) can also act as actuators, by changing the curvature of the axis of a branch (Fig. 7D,E). In compression wood, swelling leads to an axial elongation of the wood (Fratzl et al., 2008). In tension wood, swelling leads to a reduction in axial length, depending in both cases on the angle of the cellulose microfibrils in the cell wall of the tracheid of wood fibers respectively. In tension wood, if the structure is exposed to humidity, the axioparallel G-layer fibers swell, leading to circumferential hoop stresses and inducing tensile stresses in and shortening of the cell wall, which causes actuation of a movement and a change of curvature of the branch (Burgert & Fratzl, 2009; Fratzl et al., 2008; Jeronimidis, 1980a).

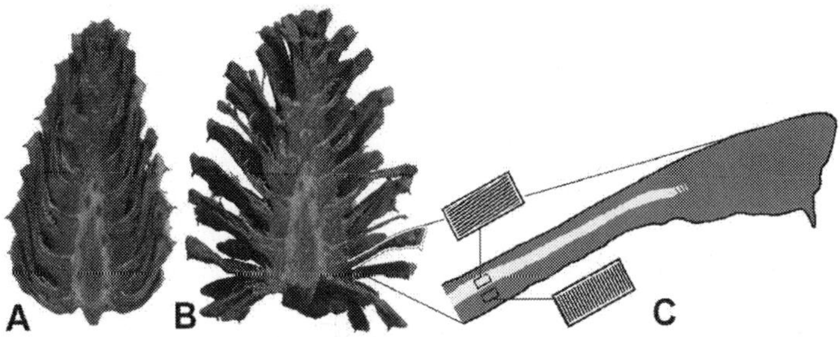

Fig. 8. Opening and closure of pine cones (*Pinus nigra*) due to changing moisture conditions. (A) Closed, wet state, (B) opened, dry state, (C) longitudinal schematic section displaying the differing directions of the fibers at the lower and the upper part of the seed scale leading to rolling and bending of the scale. © PBGF.

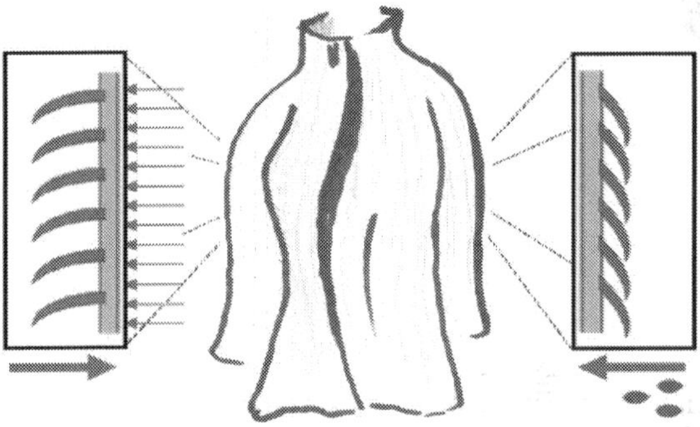

Fig. 9. Biomimetic clothing using an actuation principle similar to that of the pine cones to regulate ventilation and insulation. © PBGF.

In technical implementations, i.e. in fiber-reinforced compound materials, a wide range of potential movements and shape-shifts can be attained (Burgert & Fratzl 2009; Fratzl et al., 2008) using these actuation principles. One example of such a structure is the development of a biomimetic garment using the large displacement generated by moisture in pine cones (Fig. 8). These biological structures open up and close depending on the humidity of the environment (Fig. 8A,B). The orientation of the cellulose microfibrils in the cell walls of the upper side of the scale is almost parallel to the longitudinal axis of the scale; the microfibrils in the cell walls in the lower side of the scales are oriented almost perpendicular to the longitudinal axis of the scale (Burgert & Fratzl, 2009; Dawson et al., 1997, Fig. 8C). When the seeds are ripe, the cells in the scales die and desiccation causes a differential shrinking of the scale cells and an abaxial bending of the scales. This leads to an opening of the cone and allows the release of the anemochorous seeds.

Using the 'pine cone effect', an innovative self-adaptive clothing with small flaps that open and close depending on the moisture content of the environment (i.e., the sweatiness of the wearer) was developed by Julian Vincent from the University of Bath and Veronika Kapsali from the London College of Fashion (Fig. 9). Similar to its biological concept generator, the garment consists of two layers: one swellable layer with a dual structure, possibly wool combined with thin spikes each only 1/200th of a millimeter wide. This layer opens up when it is wetted and closes when it dries, thereby reducing its permeability and increasing the insulation. The wearer is protected against splash water and rain by an additional second layer.

Functioning has been demonstrated by developing a prototype using this relatively simple actuation principle which has the added advantage of being very failsafe and therefore highly reliable. Potential implementations are manifold because the novel biomimetic structural material is adequate for use in athletic performance, comfort wear, fabrics in the health sector, agriculture, building, packaging and upholstery.

2.1.3 External actuation and elastic architecture

Passive movements in plants are induced by external forces. This allows for movements of high complexity, including multiplanar simultaneous deformation. An excellent example is the fold-flap system present in the flower of the Bird-of-Paradise (*Strelitzia reginae*, Fig. 10, Lienhard et al., 2009, 2010; Poppinga et al., 2010a,b).

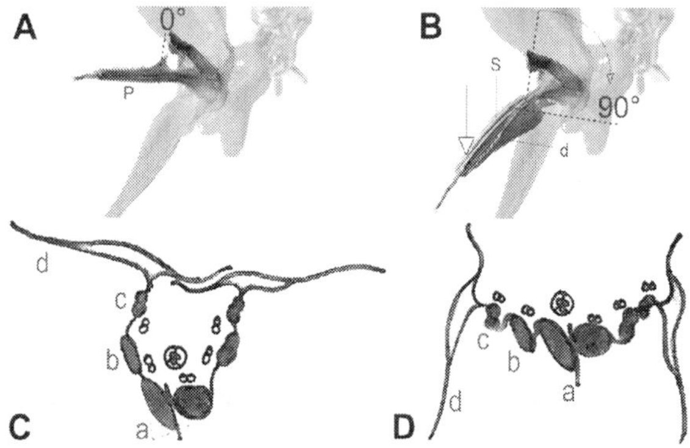

Fig. 10. Actuation principle of *Strelitzia reginae*. (A) Original (closed) position of the perch (p), (B) if the perch is bent down, the perch lamina (d) rotates and flaps sideways at an angle of approx. 90°, inducing opening of the flower and exposure of stamina and style (s), (C) schematic cross-section through the perch, with the closed lamina (d) and the top ribs (c), the middle ribs (b) and the compound lower rib at its bottom (a), (D) same cross-section as in C, in opened position. © PBGF and itke University of Stuttgart.

The flower of *S. reginae* has evolved a special landing platform -the perch- (Fig. 10A) for its pollinators, which are small birds. If a bird lands on the specially structured perch (p) to feed on nectar, the perch is bent down (Fig. 10B). The perch is composed of two petals and consists of stiff fibrous ribs (Fig. 10C, D) attached to a lamina (d) which is a thin and flexible parenchymatous tissue. When this composite structure is bent down, torsional buckling occurs, the lamina is simultaneously bent sideways, and the previously enclosed stamina (s) and style become exposed and pollen can be transferred to the bird's feet. When no force acts on the perch, i.e., the bird takes off, the deformation of the perch is reversed and the initial state is restored. This cycle can be repeated up to three thousand times with an almost identical force-displacement curve (Poppinga et al., 2010a,b). The mechanical behavior in bending is based on the interaction of the deforming fibrous ribs and the flexible lamina changing its curvature.

This can be abstracted in a first step by physical demonstrators consisting of a plastic rod with a rectangular plastic lamina glued vertically in longitudinal direction on top of the rod, forming a structure that shows similar torsional behavior when bent. In a next step computer simulations via Finite Element modeling are carried out (Fig. 11). These simulations allow for a detailed understanding of the abstracted systems, a mechanical analysis of developing stresses and strains under deformation and an evaluation of the potential technical applicability of the structures (Lienhard et al., 2009, 2010; Poppinga et al., 2010a).

The technical implementations of such systems are for example façade-shading systems (Fig. 12), which are patented under the name Flectofin™. The Flectofin™ principle uses the coupling of two main elements. A supporting rod acts as backbone element and has a rectangular cross-section. The rod can be easily bent in the direction of the smaller cross-section. The lamina or fin is a thin shell element that is attached perpendicular to the rectangular rod. The sideways bending and finally 90° flapping of the fin is a failure mode initiated by torsional buckling when bending the backbone (compare Figs. 10 and 11). As a result the curvature of the fin is changed to produce a double bent shell, which provides higher stiffness for the whole system (see Fig. 12).

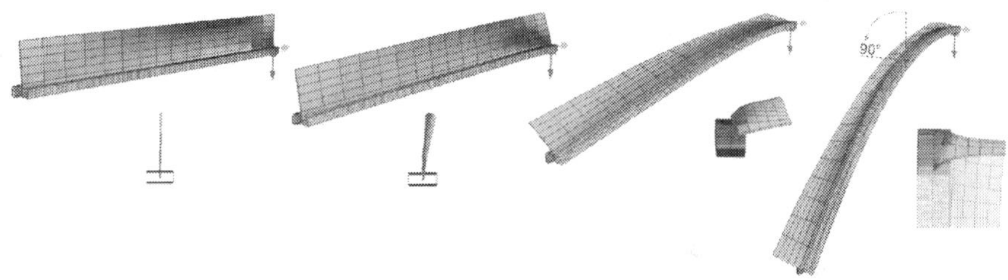

Fig. 11. Simulation of the abstracted kinetic structure in a finite element model. © itke University of Stuttgart.

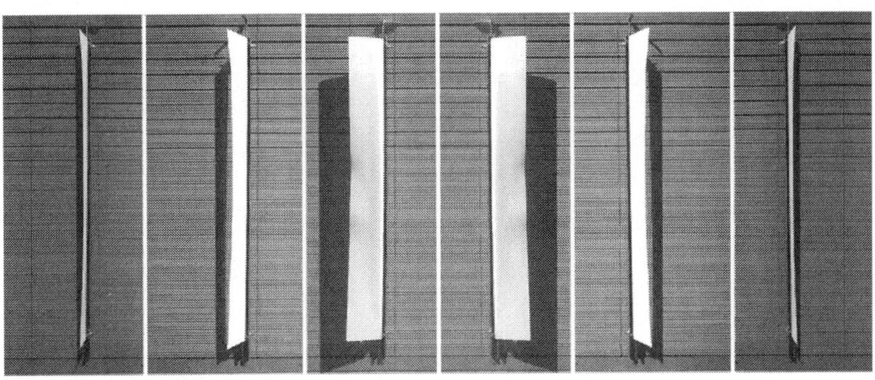

Fig. 12. Demonstrator for a façade shading system able to bend sideways up to an angle of 90° inspired by the kinetic system found in the flower of *Strelitzia reginae*. Torsional buckling and displacement of the lamina are induced by slightly bending the supporting rod. © itke University of Stuttgart.

The Flectofin™ principle can be applied to various technical purposes. Possible application fields range from technical microflaps for functional coatings to large scale adaptive façade shading systems in architecture. It also can be used for prevention of or retaining of humidity, improving microclimates and working conditions for people and machines.

2.1.4 Morphological and mechanical gradients

Biological structures can incorporate a wide range of morphological gradients, e.g., in size of particles (coarse-fine), density of fibers, fiber angle, cell wall thickness, cell sizes, etc. Often these morphological gradients are complex and render the structural basis of mechanical gradients such as stiffness, hardness, breakage, damping and wear behavior. Understanding the morphological-mechanical relation of these gradients and their hierarchical arrangement in biological structures may help in improving the mechanical performance of biomimetic compound materials composite technical structures and avoid failure such as delamination. Gradients at stem, tissue, cellular and subcellular level can be found in recent plants (e.g. *Washingtonia robusta,* Rüggeberg et al., 2008, 2009) or *Arundo donax* (Spatz et al., 1997, Rüggeberg et al., 2010) as well as in fossil species (e.g., *Medullosa* sp., see Speck, T. & Masselter, 2008).

2.1.4.1 Washingtonia robusta

Morphological-mechanical gradients are present on different hierarchical levels in the Mexican fanpalm, *Washingtonia robusta* (Fig. 13). At stem level to tissue level, the vascular bundles with their fiber caps are distributed unevenly in the cross-section of the cortex and of the central cylinder (Fig. 13). The number of vascular bundles and the size and structure of the fiber caps changes from the center to the periphery. The fiber caps are built of homogeneously thick-walled fibers and therefore are very stiff at the stem periphery, thus providing high flexural stiffness to the stem. The fiber caps located in the center of the trunk show morphological gradients that lead to a transition of stiffness from the center to the periphery of the fiber cap (Fig. 14). The fiber cap is stiffest near the phloem (ph) and the stiffness decreases toward the periphery of the fiber cap (f) as the ratio cell wall thickness to cell diameter decreases (Rüggeberg et al., 2008, 2009). These stiffness gradients could be beneficial for stem damping.

The mechanical gradients present in this plant are interesting for a technical implementation as they improve damping and may also prevent fracture due to delamination (Fig. 15) when the structure is submitted to cyclic or sudden loading.

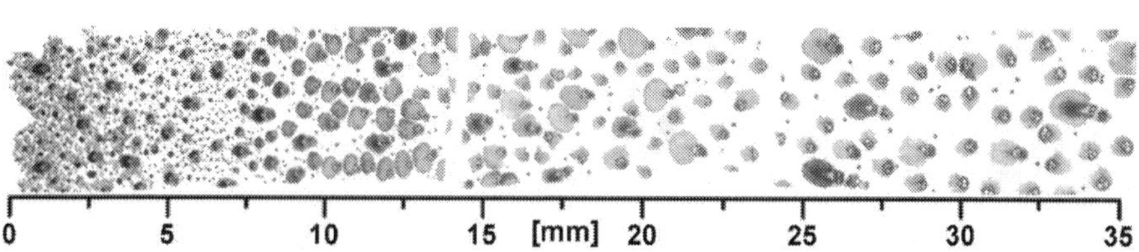

Fig. 13. Cross-section of cortex and outer central cylinder of the stem of the fanpalm *Washingtonia robusta.* Numbers indicate the distance from the outer edge of the trunk. The darker areas represent the vascular bundles with fiber caps embedded in a parenchymatous ground tissue. © Markus Rüggeberg. Source: Rüggeberg et al., 2009.

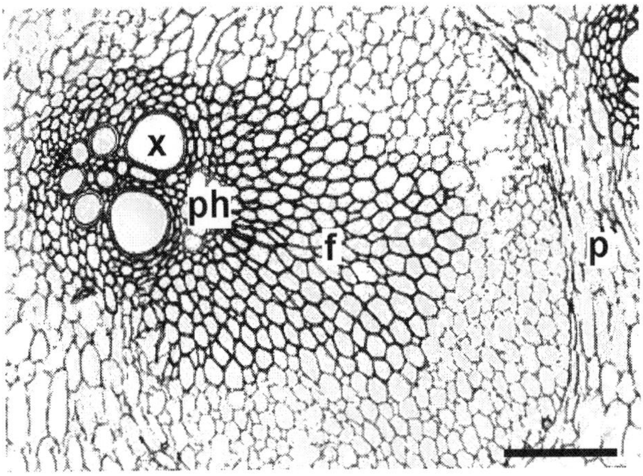

Fig. 14. Cross-section of vascular bundle with fiber cap in the stem cortex of the fan palm *Washingtonia robusta*. f: fiber cap, x: xylem, ph: phloem, p: parenchymatous cortex. Scale bar: 250 µm. © Markus Rüggeberg. Source: Rüggeberg et al., 2008.

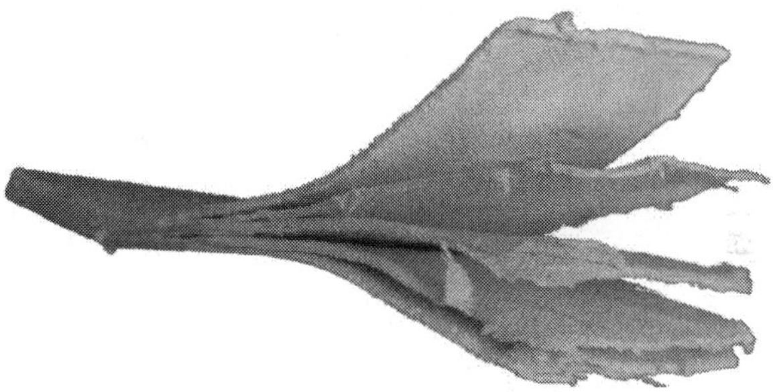

Fig. 15. Delaminated technical composite structure © PBGF.

Prevention of delamination is an important issue for many technical structures because catastrophic failures can occur, as for example during the demolition of a windmill in Denmark in 2009. One of the blades of this windmill delaminated, leading to an unbalance in the wheel and to a delamination of the other blades, ultimately causing the destruction of both the wind wheel and the tower of the windmill (http://www.bt.dk).

2.1.4.2 Medullosa sp.

Fossil plants can have stem morphologies that are no longer existent and those can be quite different from extant stems. In well preserved fossil plants like the Carboniferous seed plant *Medullosa*, gradients at different hierarchical levels can be distinguished. At stem level, the number as well as the size and type of the fiber bundles change from the stem centre to the periphery (Fig. 16). At tissue level, the outer primary cortex shows two gradients from its inner side to its outer side: (1) a decrease of the cross-sectional area of the sclerenchymatous fiber bundles that are embedded in a parenchymatous ground tissue and (2) an increase of the lignification of the cell walls of the parenchymatous cells of the ground tissue (Fig. 17A).

At cellular level, resin ducts in the ground tissue of the inner cortex have two morphological gradients (Fig. 17 B,C). The first gradient is a decrease of the cell wall thickness from the resin duct to the parenchymatous ground tissue of the inner cortex. The second gradient consists of a decrease of the cellular lumen from the inner side of the duct toward its periphery followed by a subsequent increase of the cellular lumen in the inner cortex tissue surrounding the duct. In fossil plants that cannot be tested mechanically, the stem, tissue and cell structure on different hierarchical levels can be assumed to have mechanical implications. This is supported by numerous studies, e.g., Masselter et al., 2006, 2007, 2009a; Rowe & Speck, 1998; Speck & Rowe, 1994, 1998, 1999, 2003.

Gradients are already incorporated in some materials as, e.g., a functionally graded material consisting of a nickel-alumina joint (Bruck et al., 2002). Gradients in the microstructure link the very stiff alumina (Al_2O_3) with a Young's modulus of about 300 GPa to the much more flexible nickel with a Young's modulus of about 2 GPa. This leads to different stress-strain relationships in the various parts of the graded microstructure and a customized gradient for optimal performance can be determined (Bruck et al., 2002). Natural concept generators can further improve the transition regions between stiff and flexible materials by 1) introducing continuous gradients instead of discrete transitions between different material layers and 2) by optimization at different hierarchical levels (Speck & Masselter, 2008).

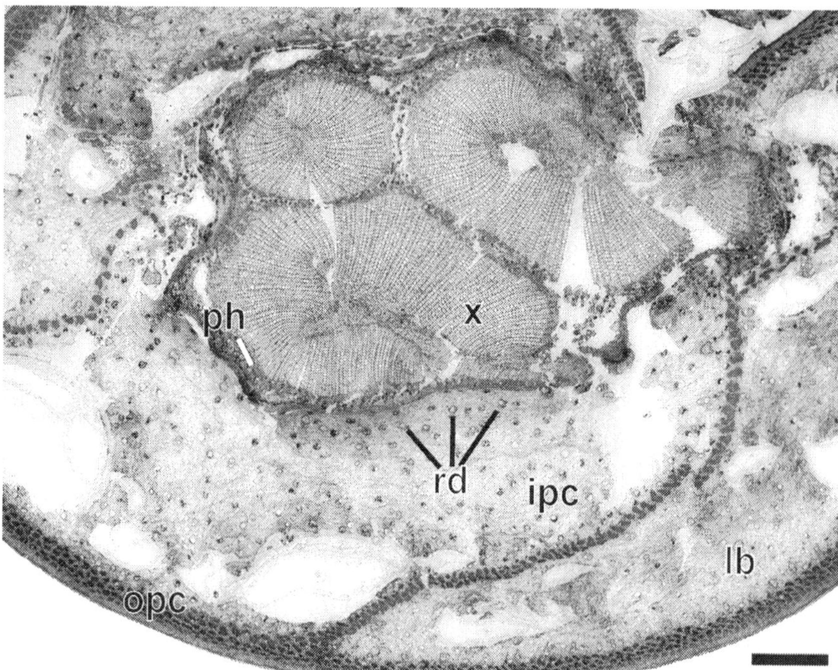

Fig. 16. Cross-section of a stem of *Medullosa* sp. with xylem (x), phloem (ph), inner primary cortex (ipc), leaf bases (lb), resin ducts (rd) and an outer primary cortex (opc). Scale bar: 5 mm. © PBGF.

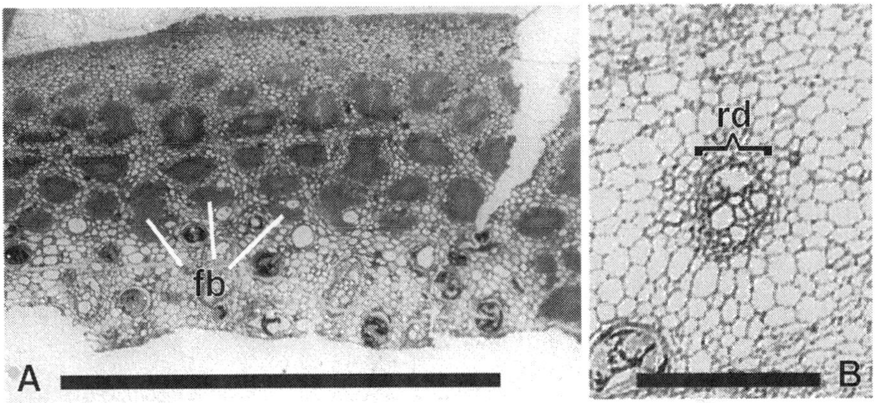

Fig. 17. Cross-section of a stem of *Medullosa* sp. (A) Detail of the outer primary cortex with densely arranged fiber bundles (fb), (B) detail of a resin duct (rd) with surrounding parenchymatous cortex tissue. Scale bars: A: 5 mm, B: 1 mm. © PBGF.

2.1.5 Heat insulation and flame retardancy

Heat insulation is an important issue when considering the high and increasing costs for energy and the ecological consequences of increasing energy consumption. Biological concept generators can be barks from trees (Fig. 18A), which can show a very good flame retardancy and heat insulation (Bauer et al., 2008, 2010). Increased flame retardancy and heat insulation is of interest for many technical applications. Recent investigations of the Plant Biomechanics Group in Freiburg suggested that in addition to the moisture content, the factors thickness, internal air cavities and surface structuring of the bark improve flame retardancy and heat insulation (Bauer et al., 2008, 2010). Potential technical implementations of these findings are the optimization of wood and bark panels (Fig. 18B), but also the development of new biomimetic insulation materials.

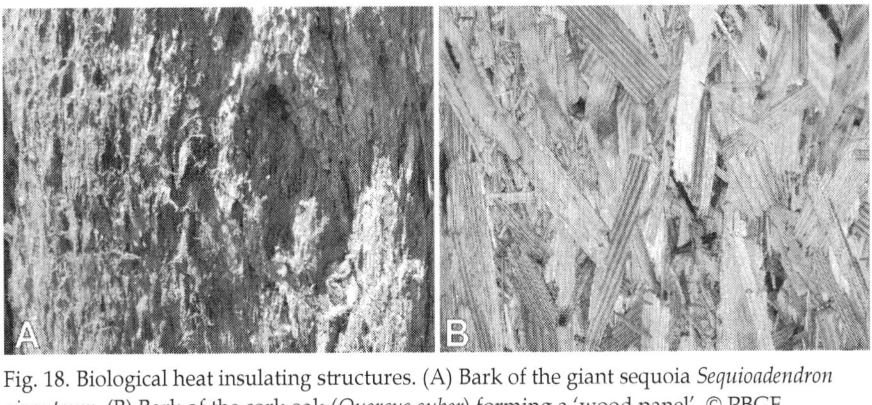

Fig. 18. Biological heat insulating structures. (A) Bark of the giant sequoia *Sequioadendron giganteum*, (B) Bark of the cork oak (*Quercus suber*) forming a 'wood panel'. © PBGF.

2.1.6 Impact damping

Many arborescent plants possess dual damping properties, e.g. vibration damping in their stems and leafs and impact damping in their fruits (Fig. 19). Impact damping is an important technical issue as many containers need protection from sudden shocks like crashes, drops or ballistic impacts. Some examples are the containments of hazardous goods, various types of protection helmets and hulls for electronic devices (e.g., mobiles) or car bodies. In order to optimize such technical structures, different biological concept generators with high energy dissipation upon impact are currently being investigated, such as petioles of the rhubarb (Huber et al., 2009) as well as fruits and nuts like the pumello, *Citrus maxima,* the coconut and the macadamia nut (Fischer et al., 2010; Seidel et al., 2009, 2010). When testing rhubarb petioles with an impact pendulum, the vascular bundles remain intact and are strained while the cortex structures and the parenchyma are destroyed, thereby dissipating a high amount of impact energy (Huber et al., 2009).

In the pumello (Fig. 19A) the deformation of the hierarchically structured thick spongy peel is mainly responsible for the energy dissipation upon impact (Fischer et al., 2010; Seidel et al., 2009, 2010). The tough outer layer of *Macadamia* nuts (Fig. 19C), the testa, is an example of a puncture material reinforced by densely packed stone cells (Seidel et al., 2009, 2010), while the *Coconut* (Fig. 19B) presents an interesting sandwich structure of a flexible middle layer of loosely interconnected fibers (mesocarp) and a stiff inner layer (endocarp) with densely arranged stone cells, thereby providing physiological and mechanical protection of the embryo by incorporating both good impact damping and puncture resistance (Speck T. et al., 2009).

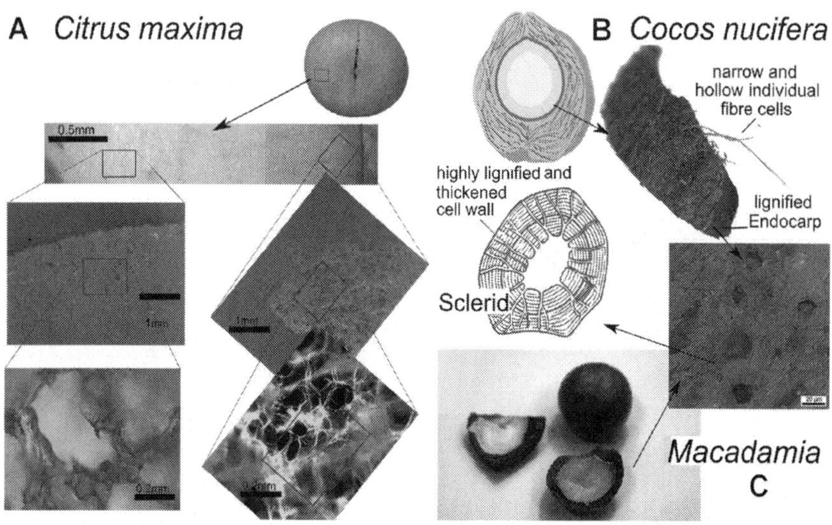

Fig. 19. Biological role models for shock-absorbing structures. (A) Highly damping spongy gradient structure in the peel of pumello (*Citrus maxima*), (B) combination of fibrous damping structure and tough shell in the fruit wall of coconut (*Cocos nucifera*), (C) entirely tough shell of fruits of *Macadamia* sp. © PBGF.

The hierarchical aspects of the organisation of these biological role models let them serve as concept generators for technical materials with a combination of solid layers with spongy fiber-reinforced structures, thereby ensuring good energy dissipation, shock-protection and puncture resistance (Fig. 20).

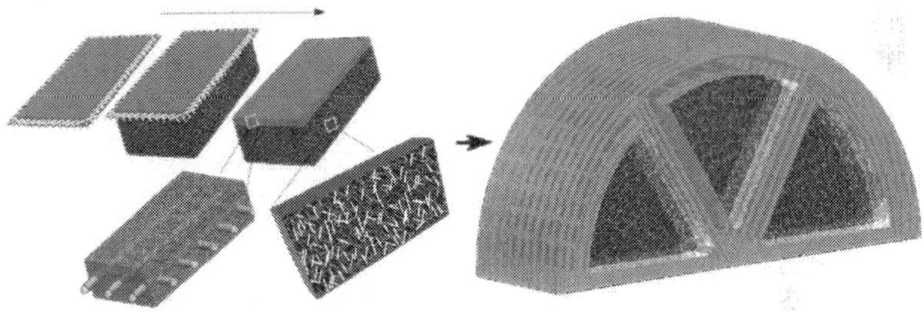

Fig. 20. Idea for biomimetic shock-absorbing structures developed on the basis of the biological concept generators (see Fig. 19). © Foundry Institute RWTH Aachen.

2.1.7 Vibration damping

Another important issue in many technical applications is vibration damping. This is the case for shock-absorbing pallets, which have to provide damping for the payloads, which often consist of delicate goods, like switch cabinets holding high-end computers. In a joint R&D project of the Plant Biomechanics Group Freiburg with the ITV Denkendorf and the company Rittal GmbH & Co. KG Herborn, a prototype of a shock-absorbing pallet with optimized mechanical characteristics was developed. At the beginning of the biomimetic project there was a technical problem: a shock-absorbing pallet with improvable damping properties and a material mix that makes it complicated or (nearly) impossible to recycle (Fig. 21). In order to solve these shortcomings, a screening for biological concept generators with excellent vibration damping was performed. The culms of bamboo, the spines of the

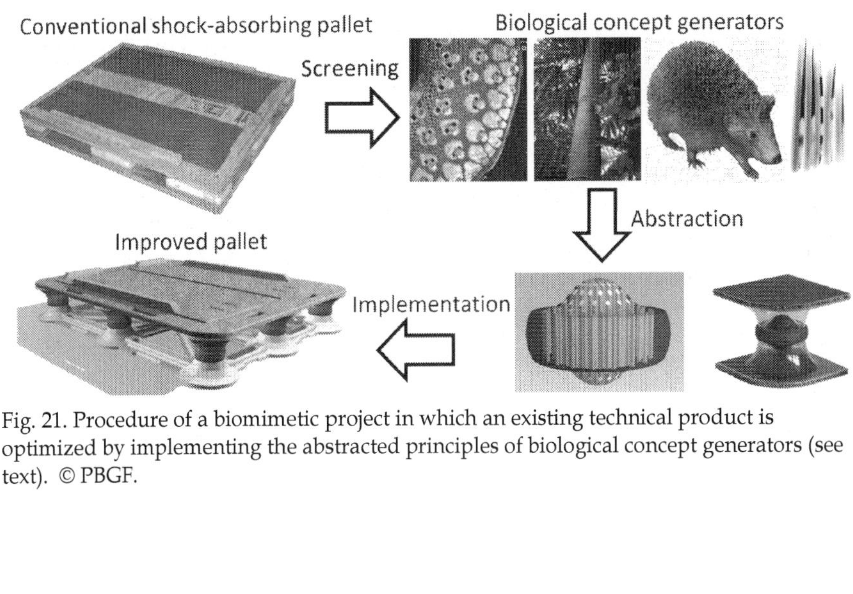

Fig. 21. Procedure of a biomimetic project in which an existing technical product is optimized by implementing the abstracted principles of biological concept generators (see text). © PBGF.

hedgehog and the quills of the porcupine were identified as potential concept generators. In a next step, the concept generators were tested as to their mechanical properties, the form-structure-function relationship was analyzed, and the principles were abstracted and implemented in a technical structure. Thereby, a shock-absorbing pallet with optimized damping properties and good recyclability was developed (Fig. 21, see Masselter et al. (2008) for a detailed description).

2.1.8 Flexible hulls

An additional approach for a transfer of concepts based on biological role models into technical applications consists of using structural changes in tissues that are induced by ontogenetic growth processes. In the Carboniferous seed plant *Lyginopteris oldhamia*, secondary growth leads to stresses and strains in the outer cortex, which becomes highly strained and is ultimately sloughed off (Fig. 22, Masselter et al., 2006, 2007). Of major

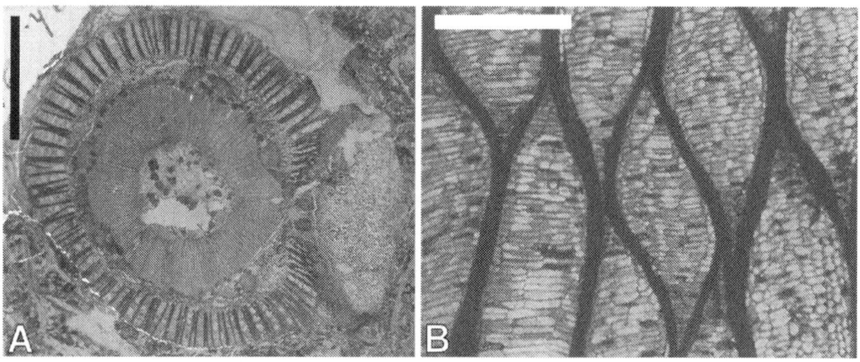

Fig. 22. *Lyginopteris oldhamia*. (A) Cross-section of the stem, (B) detail of strained outer primary cortex of the stem. Scale bars: (A) 5mm, (B) 1mm © PBGF.

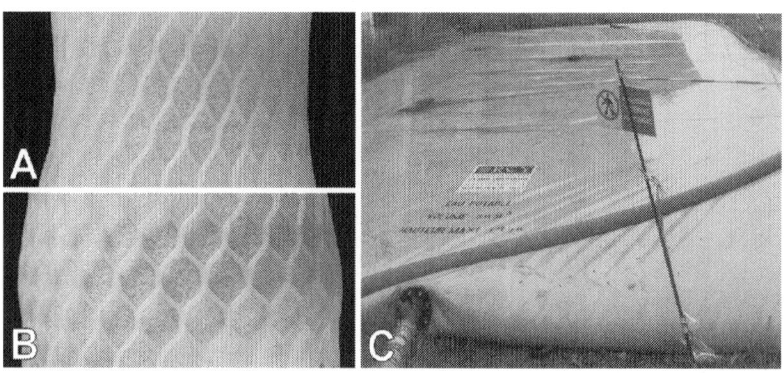

Fig. 23. Potential technical implementation for flexible hull structures. (A, B) Demonstrators combining a cellular matrix consisting of closed-cell foams and inextensible fibers, (A) undeformed state, (B) deformed state, (C) conventional flexible tank as an example for a potential technical application. © PBGF.

interest are 1) the morphological-mechanical gradients, (2) the special organization of the parenchymatous/sclerenchymatous cortex and the fact that (3) the expansion of this cortical tissue is a gradual process while the sloughing is a more ‚abrupt' failure event. By integrating similarly arranged fiber-reinforced materials (Fig. 23A,B) into the hulls of conventional flexible tanks (Fig. 23C), an increase in extensibility could be achieved while the outer ‚overall' shape is retained. Other potential applications include structures with improved safety if exploding, as the tearing of the biomimetic hull structured according to the biological role model consumes a lot of energy and could therefore dampen the explosion impact.

2.1.9 The Technical Plant Stem

The ‚Technical Plant Stem' can be considered as a kind of 'summary' for the linear fiber-reinforced composites as this biomimetic product incorporates various mechanical optimizations discussed above, e.g., vibration damping, light weight, a benign fracture behavior, impact damping and high flexural stiffness.. Three of the five biological concept generators for the 'Technical Plant Stem' that are suitable for a transfer into biomimetic products are shown in figure 24. The cross-sections show the extreme lightweight construction of *Equisetum hyemale* as well as the morphological/mechanical gradients in *Arundo donax* and the interlocking of tissues in *Equisetum giganteum.* These morphological structures significantly influence the mechanical properties of these plants (Spatz & Emanns, 2004; Spatz et al., 1997, 1998). Biomechanical analyses by the Plant Biomechanics Group in Freiburg proved that the biological concept generators possess interesting mechanical characteristics (Spatz et al., 1997; Speck O. & Spatz, 2004; Speck O. et al., 2005).
After quantitatively analyzing, understanding and abstracting these principles, prototyping of a biomimetic structure took place and the ‚Technical Plant Stem' was developed (Milwich et al., 2006, 2007). Optimizations that were introduced into the 'Technical Plant Stem' are the following: gradients within the culm, optimized fiber orientation, gradual bonding of fibers and matrix, interlocking of tissues, lightweight construction and helical wall reinforcements (Fig. 25).

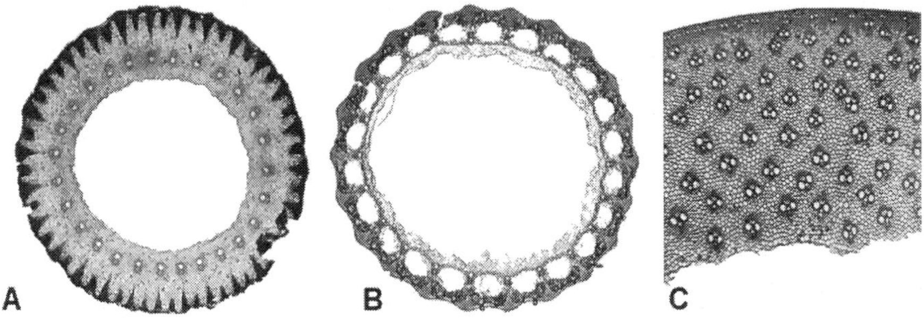

Fig. 24. Three of the five biological concept generators for the 'Technical Plant Stem'. (A) Cross-section of the stem (diam. 12 mm) of the Brazilian Giant Horsetail (*Equisetum giganteum*), (B) cross-section of the stem (diam. 6 mm) of the Dutch rush (*Equisetum hyemale*), (C) cross-section of the stem wall (width 4.3 mm) of the Giant Reed (*Arundo donax*). © PBGF.

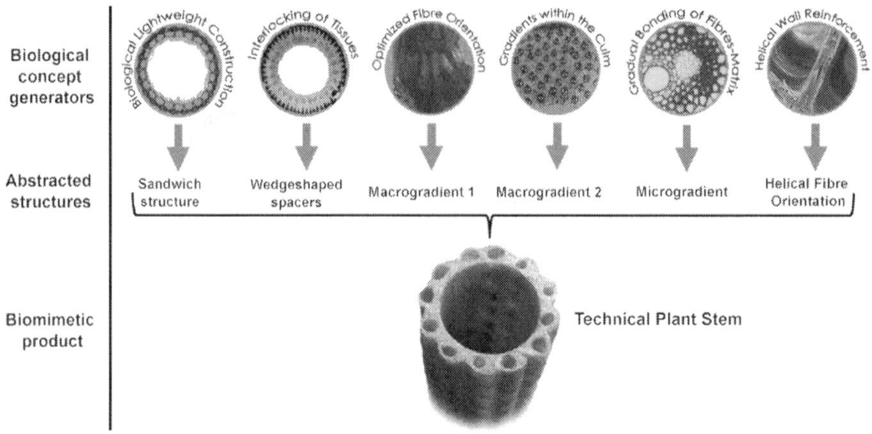

Fig. 25. Procedure of a biomimetic project in which a novel biomimetic product is developed by implementing the abstracted principles of several biological concept generators. © PBGF.

The potential fields of technical implementations range from the automotive industry (Fig. 1) to aerospace (Fig. 5) and also include architecture as well as sports equipment and special technical structures such as windmills or prostheses.

2.2 Branched fiber-reinforced structures

2.2.1 Biological concept generators

Y-shaped and T-shaped branchings that are present in technical structures are also found in branched arborescent plants. These branchings are optimized for fracture toughness (Jungnikl et al., 2009). Due to their special morphological organization, arborescent monocotyledons (Fig. 26A,B) and columnar cacti (Fig. 26C) hold a high potential for transfer into technical implementation. The stem-branch attachments of these plants are very different from those of gymnosperms and of most dicotyledon trees. A new biomimetic project for analysing the regions of stem-branch attachments of arborescent monocotyledons and columnar cacti and for transferring the results in technical applications has started in 2009 at the PBGF in cooperation with the Institute for Textile Technology and Process Engineering (ITV) Denkendorf, the Botanic Garden of the TU Dresden and the Institute for Lightweight Structures and Polymer Technology (ILK) of the TU Dresden.

The morphology of the stem-branch attachments found in arborescent monocotyledons and columnar cacti differs in its arrangement on several hierarchical levels. At stem level, the region of the stem-branch attachment is thickened by anomalous secondary growth in *Dracaena* (Fig. 26A) while the attachment is unthickened in *Freycinetia insignis* (Fig. 26B). In contrast, in the genus *Cereus*, the base of the branch is very small and the branch becomes thicker distally (Fig. 26C). At tissue level, the structure, the arrangement and the course of (groups of) fiber bundles (Fig. 26D,E) are of major influence on the biomechanical properties of the plant stems. These arrangements can be analyzed by using computer tomography, by maceration or by serial sectioning. At tissue and cellular level, the structure and course of individual fibers can be analyzed by using light microscopy and confocal laser microscopy. These methods allow to study the structure and gradients in the contact region between the fiber bundles and the cellular matrix of the parenchymatous ground tissue.

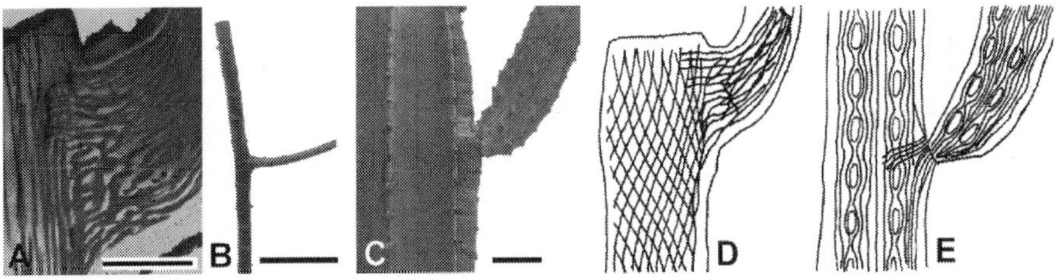

Fig. 26. Biological concept generators for branched technical structures. Longitudinal section of the stem-branch attachment region of *Dracaena marginata* (A) as well as an external view of the stem-branch attachment of *Freycinetia insignis* (B) and in *Cereus* sp. (C). Schematic drawing of the arrangement of fibrous bundles or wood strands, respectively, in the stem-branch attachment region of *Dracaena* sp. (D) and *Cereus* sp. (E). Scale bars: (A): 5mm; (B),(C):50 mm. © PBGF.

Biomechanical tests include breaking experiments in which a force is applied to a lateral twig until this twig breaks (Fig. 27A), using similar methods as described in detail in Beismann et al. (2000). This setup allows determining the force necessary to break the twig and the fracture toughness as well as the stress and strain at fracture. In many of the tested specimens, the resulting force displacement curve (Fig. 27B) shows a benign fracture behavior with a long plastic range, which is interesting for developing innovative branched technical structures. The structural analysis and the mechanical tests are complemented by FE-analyses (Fig. 28A) (Masselter et al., 2009, 2010a,b; Schwager et al., 2010).

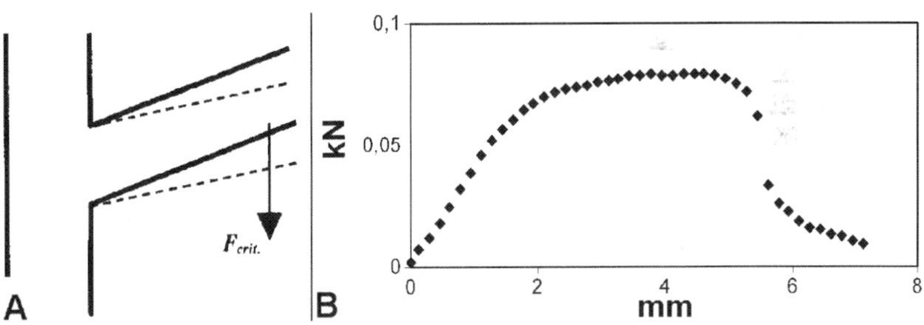

Fig. 27. Breaking experiment, schematic drawing of the geometry of a stem-branch attachment (A). The solid line represents a lateral twig before bending, the dashed line represents a lateral twig shortly before fracture, F_{crit} is the critical force necessary to break the twig. Exemplary force-displacement curve (B) measured for *Dracaena reflexa* using the setup shown in (A). © PBGF.

2.2.2 Technical implementation

Due to the fibrous composite structure of the biological concept generators, the braiding technique is predestined to transfer the branched biological role models into biomimetic products and to manufacture circular preforms (Fig. 28B). State-of-the-art braiding techniques such as the overbraiding technique or the 3D-rotary braiding technique are being further developed by the ITV Denkendorf and the ILK Dresden as they can be used for producing braided branchings (Cherif et al., 2007; Drechsler, 2001, Fig. 28C).

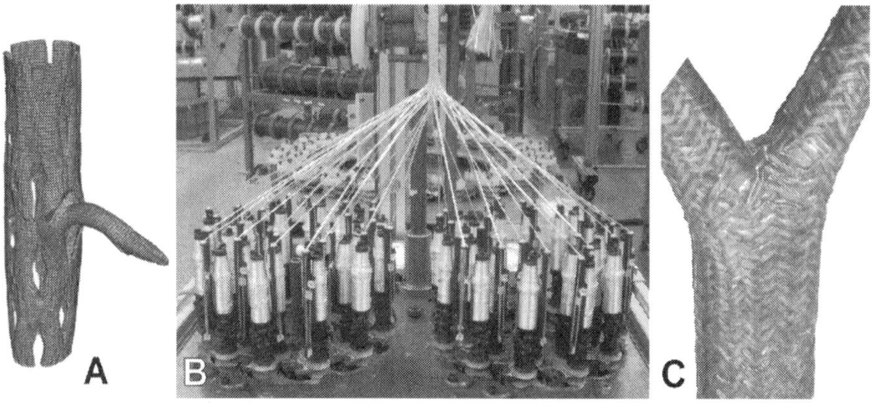

Fig. 28. (A) Simulated notch stresses in a stem-branch attachment region of a columnar cactus, (B) double braiding unit for producing branched braidings and (C) prototype of a braided Y-shaped preform. © (A) ILK Dresden, (B, C) ITV Denkendorf.

2.2.3 Technical applications for branched structures

A potential technical transfer is given for example in automotive engineering by developing optimized branched lightweight fiber-reinforced compound structures with minimized notch stresses following the studies of Claus Mattheck (Mattheck 1990, 2007, 2010, Mattheck & Tesari 2002, see Fig. 29)

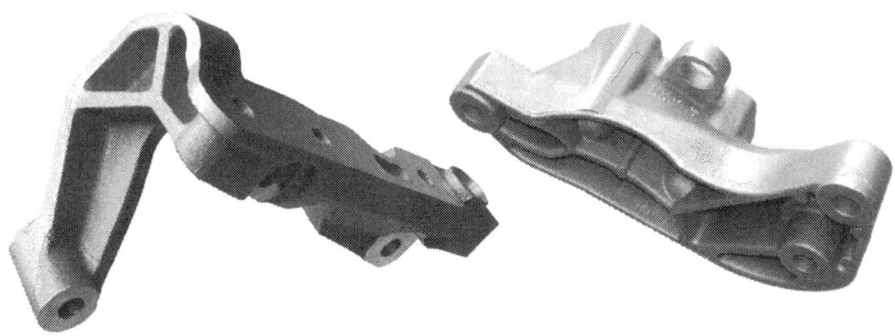

Fig. 29. Supporting structures in cars (Opel). © Claus Mattheck, KIT, Karlsruhe.

3. Acknowledgements

We gratefully acknowledge the German Research Foundation (DFG) for funding the projects on branched biomimetic structures and impact damping structures within the Priority Programme SPP 1420. We are grateful to the German Ministry for Education and Research for funding the project on elastic architecture within the framework BIONA 'Bionic innovations for sustainable products and technologies'. We would also like to thank the publisher Hanser Fachbuchverlag for the kind permission to reproduce Figure 2.

Furthermore, we are grateful for being allowed to use figure 29 by permission of Claus Mattheck. We acknowledge Jean Galtier from the CNRS in Montpellier for providing the peels of *Medullosa* sp. (Fig.16). We would like to thank Markus Rüggeberg, his co-authors, as well as the journal 'Proceedings of the Royal Society B' for the kind permission to reproduce figure 13 and 14.

4. References

Bar-Cohen, Y. (2006). *Biomimetics: biologically inspired technologies*. Taylor and Francis, ISBN 978-0849331633, Boca Raton, Florida.

Bauer, G.; Speck, T.; Liehr, A.W. & Speck, O. (2008). Wärmeisolierung von Baumrinde: Neue Ansätze für bionische Dämmmaterialien. In: *Bionik: Patente aus der Natur*, Kesel, A.B. & Zehren, D. (Eds.), 48-56, GTBB, ISBN 9783000271939, Bremen.

Bauer, G.; Speck, T.; Blömer, J.; Bertling, J. & Speck, O. (2010). Insulation capability of the bark of trees with different fire adaptation. *J. Mater. Sci.*, 45, 21, (Nov. 2010) 5950-5959, ISSN 0022-2461.

Beismann, H.; Wilhelmi, H.; Baillères, H.; Spatz, H.-C.; Bogenrieder, A. & Speck, T. (2000). Brittleness of twig bases in the genus *Salix*: fracture mechanics and ecological relevance. *J. Exp. Bot.*, 51, 344, (March 2000) 617-633, ISSN 0022-0957.

Bruck, H.A.; Evans, J.J. & Peterson, M.L. (2002). The role of mechanics in biological and biologically inspired materials. *Exp. Mech.*, 42, 4, (April 2006) 361-371, ISSN 1741-2765.

Burgert, I. & Fratzl, P. (2009): Actuation systems in plants as prototypes for bioinspired devices. *Phil. Trans. R. Soc. A*, 367, (April 2009) 1541-1557, ISSN 1471-2962.

Bushan, B. (2009). Biomimetics. *Phil. Trans. R. Soc. A*, 367, (April 2009) 1433-1444, ISSN 1471-2962.

Caplin, J.; Gordon, J.E. & Jeronimidis, G. (1983): Composite material, U.S. Patent No. 4409274.

Cherif, C.; Diestel, O. & Gries, T. (2007). *Textile Halbzeuge und Halbzeugfertigung," Textile Verbundbauweisen und Fertigungstechnologien für Leichtbaustrukturen des Fahrzeug- und Maschinenbaus*, Progress-media Verlag, Dresden.

Dawson, C.; Vincent, J.F.V. & Rocca, A.M. (1997). How pine cones open. *Nature*, 390, (Dec. 1997) 668, ISSN 1476-4687.

Drechsler, K. (2001). Composites im Flugzeug- und Automobilbau. *Conference proceedings of Denkendorfer Kolloquien, Technische Textilien*, Denkendorf, 2001.

Ehrenstein, G.W. (2006). *Faserverbund-Kunststoffe: Werkstoffe, Verarbeitung, Eigenschaften*. Hanser Fachbuchverlag, ISBN 978-3446227163, Muenchen.

Elbaum, R.; Zaltzman, L.; Burgert, I. & Fratzl, P. (2007). The role of wheat awns in the seed dispersal unit. *Science*, 316, (May 2007) 884-886, ISSN 1095-9203.

Fischer, S. F.; Thielen, M.; Loprang, R.R.; Seidel, R.; Speck, T.; Fleck, C. & Bührig-Polaczek, A. (2010). Pummelos as Concept Generators for Biomimetically-Inspired Low Weight Structures with Excellent Damping Properties. *Adv. Biomater.* (in press).

Fratzl, P. (2002a). Characterising natural fibre composites with hierarchical structure. *Fibre Diffr. Rev.*, 10, (April 2002) 31-39, ISSN 1463-8401.

Fratzl, P. (2002b). Von Knochen, Holz und Zähnen. *Physik Journal,* 1, 5, (May 2002) 49-55, ISSN 1617-9439.

Fratzl, P. (2007). Biomimetic materials research: what can we really learn from nature's structural materials? *J. R. Soc. Interface,* 4, 15, (Aug. 2007) 637-642, ISSN 1742-5662.

Fratzl, P.; Elbaum, R. & Burgert, I. (2008). Cellulose fibrils direct plant organ movements. *Faraday Discuss.,* 139, 275-282, ISSN 1359-6640.

Gindl, W. & Jeronimidis, G. (2004). Wood pulp fiber reinforced melamime-formaldehyde composites. *J. Mater. Sci.,* 39, 9, (Mai 2004) 3245-3247, ISSN 0022-2461.

Gordon, J.E. & Jeronimidis, G. (1980). Composites with high work of fracture. *Phil. Trans. R. Soc. A,* 282, 1411, (Jan. 1980) 545-550, ISSN 1471-2962.

Goswami, L.; Dunlop, J.W.C.; Jungnikl, K.; Eder, M.; Gierlinger, C.; Coutland, G.; Jeronimidis, G.; Fratzl, P. & Burgert, I. (2008). Stress generation in the tension wood of poplar is based on the lateral swelling power of the G-layer. *Plant J.,* 56, 4, (Jul. 2008) 531-538, ISSN 1365-313X.

Huber, T.; Graupner, N. & Müssig, J. (2009). As tough as it is delicious? A mechanical and structural analysis of red rhubarb (*Rheum Rhabarbarum*). *J. Mater. Sci.,* 44, 15, (Aug. 2009) 4195-4199, ISSN 1573-4803.

Jeronimidis, G. (1979). Morphological aspects of wood fracture. In: *Proc. ICM-3 Cambridge, Mechanical Behaviour of Materials, Vol. 3;* Miller, K.J. & Smith, R.F. (Eds.), 329-340, Cambridge.

Jeronimidis, G. (1980a). Wood, one of nature's challenging composites. In: *Mechanical Properties of Biological Materials, 34th Symposium of the Society for Experimental Biology* Vincent J.F.V. & Currey, J.D. (Eds.), 377-395, Cambridge University Press, Cambridge.

Jeronimidis, G. (1980b). The fracture behaviour of wood and the relations between toughness and morphology. *Proc. R. Soc. B,* 208, 1173, (Jul. 1980) 447-460, ISSN 1471-2954.

Jeronimidis, G. (2000a). Structure-property relationships in biological materials. In: *Structural biological materials,* Elices, M. (Ed.), 3-16, Elsevier Science, ISBN 0080434169, Oxford.

Jeronimidis, G. (2000b). Design and function of structural biological materials. In: *Structural biological materials,* Elices, M. (Ed.), 19-29, Elsevier Science, ISBN 0080434169, Oxford.

Jungnikl, K.; Goebbels, J.; Burgert, I. & Fratzl, P. (2009). The role of material properties for the mechanical adaptation at branch junctions. *Trees,* 23, 3, (Jun 2009) 605-610, ISSN 1432-2285.

Lichtenegger, H.C.; Reiterer, A.; Stanzl-Tschegg, S. & Fratzl, P. (1999). Variation of cellulose microfibril angles in softwoods and hardwoods - a possible strategy of mechanical optimization. *J. Struct. Biol.,* 128, 3, (Dec. 1999) 257-269, ISSN 1047-8477.

Lienhard, J.; Poppinga, S.; Schleicher, S.; Masselter, T.; Knippers, J. & Speck, T. (2009). Abstraction of plant movements for deployable structures in architecture. In: *Proceedings of the 6th Plant Biomechanics Conference,* Thibaut, B. (Ed.), 389-397, Ecofog, Cayenne, French Guyana.

Lienhard, J.; Poppinga, S.; Schleicher, S.; Speck, T. & Knippers, J. (2010). Elastic architecture: nature inspired pliable strcutures. In: *Design and Nature V*, Brebbia, C.A. (Ed.), 469 - 477, WIT Press, ISBN 9781845644543, Southampton, Boston.

Mangalgiri, P.D. (1999). Composite materials for aerospace applications. *Bull. Mater. Sci.*, 22, 3, (May 1999) 657-664, ISSN 0250-4707

Masselter, T.; Barthlott, W.; Bauer, G.; Bertling, J.; Cichy, F.; Ditsche-Kuru, P.; Gallenmüller, F.; Gude, M.; Haushahn, T.; Hermann, M.; Immink, H.; Knippers, J.; Lienhard, J.; Luchsinger, R.; Lunz, K.; Mattheck, C.; Milwich, M.; Mölders, N.; Neinhuis, C.; Nellesen, A.; Poppinga, S.; Rechberger, M.; Schleicher, S.; Schmitt, C.; Schwager, H.; Seidel, R.; Speck, O.; Stegmaier, T.; Tesari, I.; Thielen, M. & Speck, T. (2010a). Biologically inspired products. In: Bar-Cohen, Y. (ed.), *Nature based Innovation*, CRC Press, Pasadena (in press), peer-reviewed.

Masselter, T.; Haushahn, H.; Schwager, M.; Milwich, M.; Nathanson, R.; Gude, M.; Cichy, F.; Hufenbach, W.; Neinhuis, C. & Speck, T. (2010b). Biomimetic fibre-reinforced composites inspired by branched plant stems. In: *Design and Nature V*, Brebbia, C.A. (Ed.), 411 - 420, WIT Press, ISBN 9781845644543, Southampton, Boston.

Masselter T.; Milwich, M.; Monnerat, H.; Scharf, U.; Hartel, M. & Speck, T. (2008). Bio-inspired solutions for technical problems: biomimetic cable entries and shock-absorbing pallets. In: *Design and Nature IV*, Brebbia, C.A. (Ed.), 51-58, WIT Press, ISBN 1746-448X, Southampton, Boston.

Masselter, T.; Rowe, N.P.; Galtier J. & Speck, T. (2009a). Secondary growth and deformation of stem tissues in the Lower Carboniferous seed fern *Calamopitys*. *Int. J. Plant Sci.*, 170, 9 (Nov. 2009) 1228-1239, ISSN 1058-5893.

Masselter, T.; Rowe, N.P. & Speck, T. (2007). Biomechanical reconstruction of the Carboniferous seed fern *Lyginopteris oldhamia:* implications for growth form reconstruction and habit. *Int. J. Plant Sci.*, 168, 8 (Oct. 2007) 1177-1189, ISSN 1058-5893.

Masselter, T. & Speck, T. (2009b). From stems to sticks - what can we learn for biomimetics from natural fibre-reinforced structures? In: *Proceedings of the 6th Plant Biomechanics Conference*, Thibaut, B. (Ed.), 375-366, Ecofog, Cayenne. French Guyana.

Masselter, T; Speck, T. & Rowe, N.P. (2006). Ontogenetic reconstruction of the Carboniferous seed plant *Lyginopteris oldhamia*. *Int. J. Plant Sci.*, 167, 1 (Jan. 2006) 147-166, ISSN 1058-5893.

Mattheck, C. (1990). Engineering components grow like trees. *Materwiss. Werksttech.*, 21, 4 (Apr. 1990) 143-168, ISSN 0933-5137.

Mattheck, C. (2007). *Secret design rules of nature - Optimum shapes without computers*, Verlag Forschungszentrum Karlsruhe GmbH, ISBN 9783923704620, Karlsruhe.

Mattheck, C. (2010). *Denkwerkzeuge nach der Natur*, Verlag Karlsruher Institut für Technologie, ISBN 9783923704736, Karlsruhe.

Mattheck, C. & Tesari, I. (2002). Konstruieren wie die Natur. Bauteile wachsen wie Bäume und Knochen, *Konstruieren und Giessen*, 27, 2, 4-9.

Milwich, M.; Planck, H.; Speck, T. & Speck, O. (2007). Der technische Pflanzenhalm: ein bionisches Schmaltextil. *Melliand Textilberichte - Band- und Flechtindustrie*, 44, 34–38, ISSN 0005-4925.

Milwich, M.; Speck, T.; Speck, O.; Stegmaier, T. & Planck, H. (2006). Biomimetics and technical textiles: solving engineering problems with the help of nature's wisdom. *Am. J. Bot.*, 93, 10, (Oct. 2006) 1455-1465, ISSN 1537-2197.

Poppinga, S.; Lienhard, J.; Masselter, T.; Schleicher, S.; Knippers, J. & Speck, T. (2010a). Biomimetic Deployable Systems in Architecture. In: *WCB 2010, IFMBE Proceedings 31,* Lim, C.T. & Goh, J.C.H. (Eds.), 40-43, Springer, ISBN 9783642145155, Heidelberg, Germany.

Poppinga, S.; Masselter, T.; Lienhard, J.; Schleicher, S.; Knippers, J. & Speck, T. (2010b). Plant movements as concept generators for deployable systems in architecture. In: *Design and Nature V,* Brebbia, C.A. (Ed.), 403 - 409, WIT Press, ISBN 9781845644543, Southampton, Boston.

Quilter, A. (2004). Composites in Aerospace applications. *Aircraft Maint. Technol.*, 16, 1, (Oct. 2004) 14-16, ISSN 1072-3145.

Reiterer, A.; Lichtenegger, H.C.; Fratzl, P. & Stanzl-Tschegg, S. (2001). Deformation and energy absorption of wood cell walls with different nanostructure under tensile loading. *J. Mater. Sci.*, 36, 19, (Oct. 2001) 4681-4686, ISSN 0022-2461.

Rowe, N.P. & Speck, T. (1998). Biomechanics of plant growth forms: the trouble with fossil plants. *Rev. Palaeobot. Palynol.*, 102, 1-2, (Jul. 1998) 43-62, ISSN 0034-6667.

Rüggeberg, M.; Burgert, I. & Speck, T. (2010). Structural and mechanical design of tissue interfaces in the giant reed *Arundo donax*. *J. R. Soc. Interface,* 7, 44, (Mar. 2010) 499-506, ISSN 1742-5662.

Rüggeberg, M.; Speck, T. & Burgert, I. (2009). Structure-function relationships of different vascular bundle types in the stem of the Mexican fanpalm (*Washingtonia robusta*). *New Phytol.*, 182, 2, (Jul. 2009) 443-450, ISSN 1469-8137.

Rüggeberg, M.; Speck, T.; Paris, O.; Lapierre, C.; Pollet, B.; Koch, G. & Burgert, I. (2008). Stiffness gradients in vascular bundles of the palm *Washingtonia robusta*. *Proc. R. Soc. B,* 275, 1648, (Oct. 2008) 2221-2229, ISSN 1471-2954.

Schwager, H.; Haushahn, T.; Neinhuis, C.; Speck, T. & Masselter, T. (2010). Principles of branching morphology and anatomy in arborescent monocotyledons and columnar cacti as concept generators for branched fibre-reinforced composites. *Adv. Biomater.* (in press)

Seidel, R.; Bührig-Polaczek, A.; Fleck, C. & Speck, T. (2009). Impact resistance of hierarchically structured fruit walls and nut shells in view of biomimetic applications. In: *Proceedings of the 6th Plant Biomechanics Conference,* Thibaut, B. (Ed.), 406-411, Ecofog, Cayenne, French Guyana..

Seidel, R.; Thielen, M.; Schmitt, C.; Bührig-Polaczek, A.; Fleck, C. & Speck, T. (2010). Fruit walls and nut shells as an inspiration for the design of bio-inspired impact resistant hierarchically structured materials. In: *Design and Nature V,* 421-430, Brebbia, C.A. (Ed.), WIT Press, ISBN 9781845644543, Southampton, Boston.

Spatz, H.-Ch.; Beismann, H.; Brüchert, F.; Emanns, A. & Speck, T. (1997). Biomechanics of the giant reed *Arundo donax*. *Phil. Trans. R. Soc. B,* 352, 1349, (Jan. 1997) 1–10, ISSN 1471-2954.

Spatz, H.-Ch. & Emanns, E. (2004). The mechanical role of the endodermis in *Equisetum* plant stems. *Am. J. Bot.*, 91, 11, (Nov. 2004) 1936-1938, ISSN 1537-2197.

Spatz, H.-Ch.; Köhler, L. & Speck, T. (1998). Biomechanics and functional anatomy of hollow-stemmed sphenopsids. I. *Equisetum giganteum* (Equisetaceae). *Am. J. Bot.*, 85, 3, (Mar. 1998) 305-314, ISSN 1537-2197.

Speck, O.; Milwich, M.; Harder, D. & Speck, T. (2005). Vom biologischen Vorbild zum technischen Produkt: der "Technische Pflanzenhalm". *Museo,* 22, 96-103.

Speck, O. & Spatz, H.-Ch. (2004). Damped oscillations of the giant reed *Arundo donax* (Poaceae). *Am. J. Bot.*, 91, 6, (Jun. 2004) 789-796, ISSN 1537-2197.

Speck, T.; Harder, D. & Speck O. (2007). Gradient materials and self-repair: learning technology from biology. *VDI-Report,* B4284, 1-13.

Speck, T. & Masselter, T. (2008). Learning from the past for the future: fossil plants as concept generators for biomimetic materials and structures. In: *Bionik: Patente aus der Natur,* Kesel, A.B. & Zehren, D. (Eds.), 14-23, GTBB, ISBN 9783000271939, Bremen.

Speck, T. & Rowe, N.P. (1994). Biomechanical analysis of *Pitus dayi*: early seed plant vegetative morphology and its implications on growth habit. *J. Plant Res.*, 107, 1088, (Dec 1994) 443-460, ISSN 0918-9440.

Speck, T. & Rowe, N.P. (1998). Modelling form and function in fossil plants. *Rev. Palaeobot. Palynol.,* 102 (special issue), 1-114, ISSN 0034-6667.

Speck, T. & Rowe, N.P. (1999). A quantitative approach for analitically defining size, growth for and habit in living and fossil plants. In: *The evolution of plant architecture,* Kurmann M.H. & Hemsley, A.R. (Eds.), 447-449, Kew: Royal Botanic Gardens, ISBN 9781900347723, Kew.

Speck, T. & Rowe, N.P. (2003). Modelling primary and secondary growth processes in plants: a summary of the methodology and new data from an early lignophyte. *Phil. Trans. R. Soc. B,* 358, 1437, (Sept. 2003) 1473-1485, ISSN 1471-2970.

Speck, T. & Speck, O. (2008). Process sequences in biomimetic research, In: *Design and Nature IV,* Brebbia, C.A. (Ed.), 3-11, WIT Press, ISBN 1746-448X, Southampton, Boston.

Speck, T.; Speck, O.; Masselter, T. & Seidel, R. (2009). Verpacken, Auspacken und Schützen nach dem Vorbild der Natur: Biologische Verpackungen und Behälter als Ideengeber für bionische Entwicklungen, In: *Blasformen 2009, VDI- Berichte Kunststofftechnik,* 4299, 1-19, VDI Verlag GmbH, ISBN 9783182342991, Düsseldorf, Germany.

Stahlberg, R. & Taya, M. (2006). What can we learn from nastic plant structures? The phytomimetic potentiality of nastic structures. *Proc. SPIE,* Vol. 6168, (Mar. 2006), 616802, ISSN 0277-786X.

Vincent, J.F.V. (2003). Biomimetic modelling. *Phil. Trans. R. Soc. B,* 358, No. 1437 (Sept. 2003), 1597-1603, ISSN 1471-2970.

Zhang, Y.; Vassilopoulos, A.P. & Keller, T. (2007). Fatigue Behaviour of Adhesively Bonded Pultruded Gfrp. In: *Experimental Analysis of Nano and Engineering Materials and Structures,* Gdoutos, E.E. (Ed.), 203-204, Springer, ISBN 9781402062384, Dordrecht.

http://aero-defense.ihs.com/NR/rdonlyres/AEF9A38E-56C3-4264-980C-D8D6980A4C84/0/444.pdf 20.07.2010, 15:37

http://www.airbus.com/store/mm_repository/pdf/att00014197/media_object_file_fast_44_p2_p7.pdf 22.06.2010, 10:36

http://www.airbus.com/fileadmin/documents/Airbus_Technical_Data/AC/AC_A380_01NOV2008.pdf 22.11.2009, 10:43

http://www.bt.dk/nyheder/vindmoelle-eksploderet, 20.01.2010, 9:43

10

Creating Scalable and Addressable Biomimetic Membrane Arrays in Biomedicine

Jesper Søndergaard Hansen and Claus Hélix Nielsen
Technical University of Denmark and Aquaporin A/S
Denmark

1. Introduction

Biomimetic membrane arrays that mimic biological cell membranes, with the ability to support membrane protein or peptide reconstitutions, are increasingly being recognised as an important platform for biomedical applications. High-throughput screening (HTS) systems based on membrane arrays may become an important alternative to cell-based screening of potential drug candidates on membrane protein targets (Fang *et al.*, 2006). The advantages of such membrane arrays are the ability to address specific drug-on-target interactions and to identify potential unintended effects on cell membrane properties or interactions with secondary unwanted proteins. The transport properties of channel proteins or peptides may also be utilized in novel sensor based platforms such as stochastic sensors for detection of organic molecules in solutions for use in medicine or environmental monitoring (Ashkenasy *et al.*, 2005; Capone *et al.*, 2007; Gu *et al.*, 1999; Nikolelis & Siontorou, 1996).

Provided that the effective membrane area can be scaled sufficiently, protein channel-based membrane arrays may be applied in larger scale biomedical applications. An example is aquaporins, which are water selective proteins that function to filter water, for example in the mammalian kidney. Aquaporin-based large scale biomembranes may be envisaged as the new generation hemodialysis systems for kidney patients, or be applied in general water purification systems.

Biomimetic membrane peptide or protein based arrays are however not currently applied in commercial biomedical or biotechnological applications. While creation of a single lipid bilayer membrane across a Teflon aperture is a well-established technique, the creation of biomembrane arrays comprises a relatively new concept in the scientific field of biomimetics. The reasons are amongst others associated with the inherent difficulties of reproducible creating planar suspended membranes and a generally low stability of established biomembranes. Moreover, amongst the general challenges in biomimetic membrane design is scale up of membrane effective areas to create stable and addressable membrane arrays with long lifetimes (> days).

This chapter will give an overview of recent advances in the development of planar biomimetic membrane arrays, and will discuss strategies and general challenges for creating stable and scalable biomembranes for use in biomedical applications.

2. Biomimetic membrane design

Current planar membrane designs include vertically and horizontally positioned arrays in a chamber or device, which typically relies on membrane arrays being established either by manual, robotics or microfluidic techniques. The choice of design may depend on the nature of the membrane molecule to be incorporated (peptide or protein) and the biomedical application in question.

2.1 Membrane array scaffolds

The fabrication method as well as membrane array geometries are important parameters to consider when designing chambers and devices for sensor and separation applications based on biomimetic membrane arrays.
Membrane proteins function among others to facilitate passive-mediated or active transport of small molecules and substances across the membrane, or function as receptors mediating intracellular signal transduction pathways upon extracellular ligand binding to the receptor. To utilize membrane protein function in model membrane designs, suspended membranes may be created that allow for transport processes to take place across the artificially made membranes. A membrane scaffold supporting planar suspended membrane array formations is illustrated in Fig. 1A.
To create medical screening platforms or microarray assays, the multi aperture scaffold may further be embedded in a polymer-matrix to create individually well-defined wells as is known from microtiter plates or immobilized soluble protein dot-blot microarrays. The design illustrated in Fig. 1B shows a composite half-sandwich scaffold design with well-defined wells. The matrix may be designed to be porous to maintain ion and solute diffusion across the established membranes. This is necessary if electrophysiological measurements of receptor or protein channel properties are included in the design as a read-out parameter.

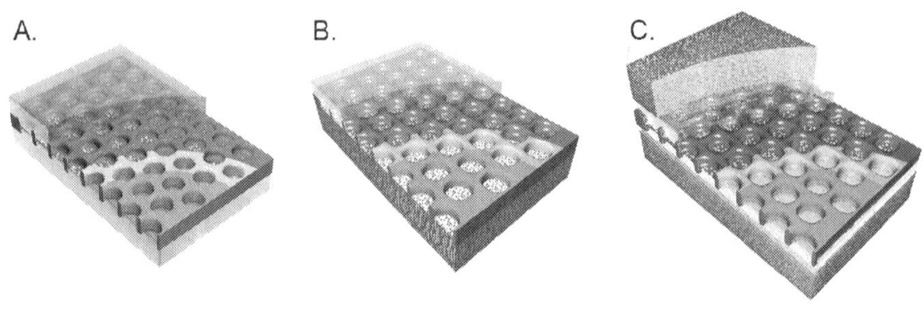

Fig. 1. Biomimetic membrane array designs using micro-structured ethylene tetrafluoroethylene (ETFE) as scaffold. A) ETFE membrane scaffold for freely suspended planar membrane arrays. B) Composite half-sandwich membrane scaffold consisting of an ETFE partition partly embedded in a porous support structure to create individually well-defined wells (grey). C) Complete composite scaffold sandwich structure. Shown in the illustrations are the ETFE membrane scaffold (green), surface modifications of the ETFE scaffold (yellow), biomimetic membranes (red), proteins (white), aqueous layers or hydrogel polymers (transparent) and porous supportive structures (grey).

To support applying a hydrostatic or an osmotic pressure across the membrane, separation applications based on protein channel properties require that the established biomimetic membrane arrays are stabilized by a complete sandwich composite structure (Fig. 1C). As illustrated in Fig. 1, the membrane array scaffold can be created as a modular design based on the actual aperture scaffold and from this design multi composite/encapsulated scaffolds may be created depending on the design criteria.

Single aperture partitions can be created by various mechanical methods such as micro drilling, needle puncturing (Ginsburg & Noble, 1974), heated wire (Benz *et al.*, 1975; Montal & Mueller, 1972; Wonderlin, Finkel & French, 1990) or electrical sparks (Minami *et al.*, 1991). However, common for these methods are that they are generally not suitable for fabricating scaffolds comprising an array of apertures. The reasons are that these methods cannot produce consistent aperture sizes and position the produced apertures closely and precisely, and moreover these techniques have tendencies to create groin and burr edges that do not support stable membrane formations.

Methods described suitable for the fabrication of membrane scaffold arrays include hot embossing of silicon wafers (Heyderman *et al.*, 2003), lithography techniques (Le Pioufle *et al.*, 2008; Mayer *et al.*, 2003; Suzuki, Le Pioufle & Takeuchi, 2009), UV excimer laser ablation (O'Shaughnessy *et al.*, 2007; Sandison & Morgan, 2005) and CO_2-laser ablation (Vogel *et al.*, 2009). The ability to produce consistently sized and closely positioned apertures are important parameters to enable successful formation of stable membranes in array. Of the three mentioned techniques for creating highly defined aperture arrays, the CO_2 laser ablation technique is likely the most versatile and cost efficient technique. It has the ability to ablate Teflon films with different thicknesses (micrometers to >1 mm), enable fast scaffold production times (milliseconds-seconds) and support easy scale up. Fig. 2 shows rectangular and hexagonal aperture scaffolds, respectively, micro-structured with the CO_2 laser ablation technique.

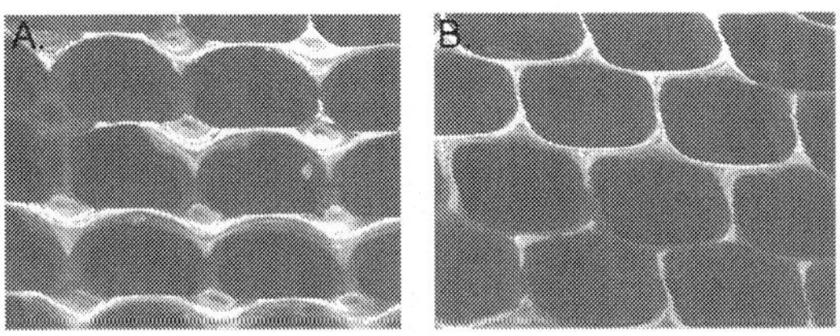

Fig. 2. Scanning electron microscopy images of CO_2 laser fabricated ETFE multi-aperture scaffolds. Images show middle sections of A) Rectangular 8×8 aperture array and B) Hexagonal 8×8 aperture array. EFTE micro structuring was performed as described by Vogel *et al.* (Vogel *et al.*, 2009).

2.2 Chamber designs for membrane array formation

There exist numerous chamber designs to encompass a membrane array scaffold, albeit there are common features relating to the strategy of membrane formation. Fig. 3 schematically illustrates some of the chamber design strategies recently developed in our laboratory, and we will discuss current trends and common features in chamber designs from these examples.

The vertical chamber design strategy (Fig. 3A, D) is a classical chamber design approach originally described for painting or folding a lipid bilayer across a Teflon partition aperture (Montal & Mueller, 1972; Mueller & Rudin, 1969). This design provides easy access to the chambers via wells from the top of the chamber and to each side of the established membranes. This allows for addition of solutes (e.g. creation of osmotic gradients), substances (e.g. ligands), transmembrane peptides, membrane proteins, liposomes or proteoliposomes close to established membranes. At the same time it allows for sample collecting via the accessible top chamber wells. In this manner, the horizontal chamber design has, among others, been applied to characterize vesicle fusion events with planar artificially made membranes (Kendall & MacDonald, 1982; Perin & MacDonald, 1989; Woodbury & Hall, 1988a; Woodbury & Hall, 1988b; Zimmerberg, Cohen & Finkelstein, 1980b). The hydrophilic dye calcein was used as a traceable marker that was encapsulated into lipid synaptic vesicles and added to one side of the membrane (Zimmerberg, Cohen & Finkelstein, 1980a). Membrane fusion events with the established planar membrane resulted in calcein release to the other side of the membrane, which could subsequently be sampled and the fluorescent calcein content quantified (Zimmerberg *et al.*, 1980a).

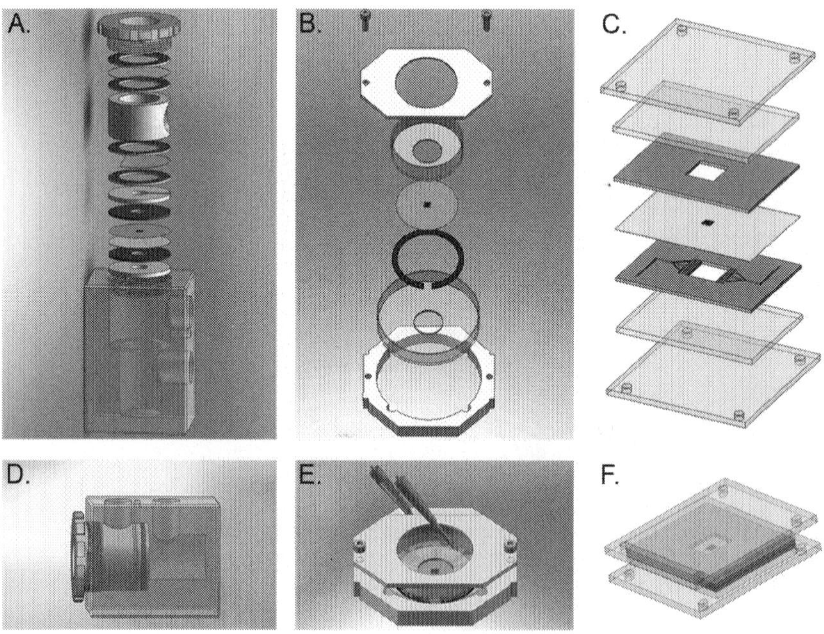

Fig. 3. Chamber designs for creating biomimetic membrane arrays A), D) Automation technique chamber design strategy for establishing vertically oriented membrane arrays (Hansen *et al.*, 2009b). B), E) Horizontal chamber design that supports combined optical-electrical measurements of established biomimetic membranes (Hansen *et al.*, 2009a). C), F) Automated microfluidic chamber design for microfluidic filling and establishment of biomembrane arrays (Kamila Pszon-Bartosz *et al.*, manuscript in submission).

We recently developed a vertical chamber based on the classical design (Fig 3A, D), where the membrane formation strategy was modified to comprise a novel membrane array formation technique; the so called automation technique for the establishment of vertically positioned membrane arrays (Hansen *et al.*, 2009b). Electrophysiological recordings across the membrane demonstrated that functionally membrane arrays were created in this design. Moreover, this technique supported membrane formations of 5×5, 8×8 and 30×21 arrays having average aperture diameters of 300 µm (Hansen *et al.*, 2009b).

In general, the vertical chamber design allows for electrophysiological recordings across the membrane, but the simultaneous visualization of established membranes by surface sensitive techniques such as fluorescence microscopy is not straightforward in this design. Therefore, the current trends in chamber design are directed towards the development of horizontal chambers that fit, or can be adapted, into modern array scanners (Le Pioufle *et al.*, 2008; Suzuki *et al.*, 2009) or fluorescent microscope stages (Hemmler *et al.*, 2005; Wilburn, Wright & Cliffel, 2006). Such designs are typically created to support more than one read-out parameter such as having voltage-clamp read-outs combined with optical imaging.

Membrane array formation in horizontal chambers is typically carried out manually by painting the membrane array across the scaffold or by applying microfluidic techniques to establish fully automated membrane formations. The rationale behind manually painting membranes onto scaffold arrays is that it may be adapted to robotic-based membrane deposition techniques, such as robotic array spotters or printers, or be re-designed to include microfluidic membrane formation techniques.

The chamber fabrication time and the material costs are important parameters to ensure that biomimetic membrane based arrays are made economically feasible for the pharmaceutical industry or creating commercially available medical point-of-care microdevices. Therefore, preferred biomimetic membrane designs comprise single-use chambers or microarray devices that are based on low-cost materials, easy to produce and which are easy and efficient to handle. Our suggestions of how to meet these design criteria are illustrated in Fig 3B-F. Fig 3B, 3E illustrate a single-use chamber design based on clamping membrane scaffold arrays between 35-mm and 50-mm culture dishes, whereas Fig. 3C, 3F show a fully automated and closed microfluidic device based on poly(methyl methacrylate) (PMMA), in which all materials are cut and micro structured by CO_2 laser ablation.

2.3 Considerations of membrane design criteria

Membrane design criteria should preferably be defined on the basis of the biotechnological application in question. A commonly accepted membrane quality criterion is that established membranes should exhibit >1 Giga-Ohm sealing resistance in order to achive low ion leakage. (Reimhult & Kumar, 2008). This is however a somewhat misleading membrane quality criterion. Ohmic sealing that may be obtained for a given membrane is inversely related to the effective membrane area, meaning that >1 Giga-Ohm seals cannot practically be achieved with large membrane arrays. Instead, for large biomimetic membrane arrays it therefore makes more sense to define membrane quality as membranes having a large effective area as evidenced by a large value for the electrical capacitance and low ionic permeability as evidenced by a low value for the electrical conductance compared to the effective membrane area.

Another important design criterion for biotechnological/pharmacological applications may be peptide or protein reconstitution yield, because this likely depend on the application.

Less peptides or proteins are likely needed to create a sensitive screening platform in drug discovery compared to creating a membrane based separation technology. Thus when setting up design criteria, strategies and goals for the peptide or protein reconstitution yield need to be taken into consideration.

Additional design criteria for HTS systems or mass transfer flow applications may include a high perforation level of the membrane scaffold material so that the artificial membrane platform is scalable to meet various requirements for individual technical applications (Hansen *et al.*, 2009b). For example functional membrane units can be arranged in arrays to facilitate rapid screening (e.g. by microplate readers).

Membrane stability is a key parameter to be considered for biomimetic membrane based devices. There is a general consensus that biomimetic membranes should have lifetimes for > 1 day (Reimhult & Kumar, 2008). This will also depend on the application in question and on whether a membrane-based assay relies on the end user to create the membrane arrays as a step in the assay protocol, or if the membranes will be fully assembled in ready-to-use devices before reaching the end user. In addition, the membranes or precursor membrane solutions should exhibit transportation robustness and be storable for defined time periods.

The methodology for membrane formation should be considered during the design of novel biomimetic sensor and separation platforms. This may also relate to cost efficiency and feasibility to enter a competitive market. Membrane formations by robotic spotting techniques is likely more expensive than microfluidic-based membrane formations, but robotic deposition techniques may be designed for an application where the total cost would still allow for a competitive product. Thus biomimetic membrane device fabrication processes and materials costs should be considered as a whole during product development.

3. Formation of functionally stable and scalable membrane arrays

Although, it is straightforward to set up specific design criteria for a given biomimetic based platform technology, there are several inherent challenges of biomimetic membrane formations that tend to make it difficult or challenging to meet defined design criteria in practice. Challenges with poor membrane stability, limited scalability and low membrane formation reproducibility must be solved in order to create a general commercially available biomimetic membrane based platform technology.

3.1 Biomimetic membrane stability

Poor membrane stability is a recognized challenge with artificially made membranes. This is an even more pronounced general challenge when working with arrays of biomimetic membranes. To understand why poor membrane stability is a general challenge, it is necessary to realize the properties and dimensions that apply for artificial biomimetic membranes.

The lipid bilayer is only a few nanometers thick and varies with the acyl chain length from 4-10 nm for natural occurring phospholipid species (Lewis & Engelman, 1983; White & Thompson, 1973). The partition scaffold is typically in the range of 20 to 50 micrometers in thickness, meaning that the aperture scaffold is thousand times thicker than the lipid bilayer. Lipid bilayers established across partition apertures are therefore surrounded by an annulus of thick parent lipid solution to compensate for the dimension differences between scaffold and bilayer thickness (White, 1972) (Fig. 4). Solvents such as alkanes (e.g. *n*-decane) are typically used to precondition the scaffold to membrane formations; so called partition prepainting. It is believed that the solvent of the preconditioning step and/or the solvent present in the lipid bilayer slowly diffuses from the annulus, resulting in membrane destabilization and eventually membrane collapse (Malmstadt, Jeon & Schmidt, 2008).

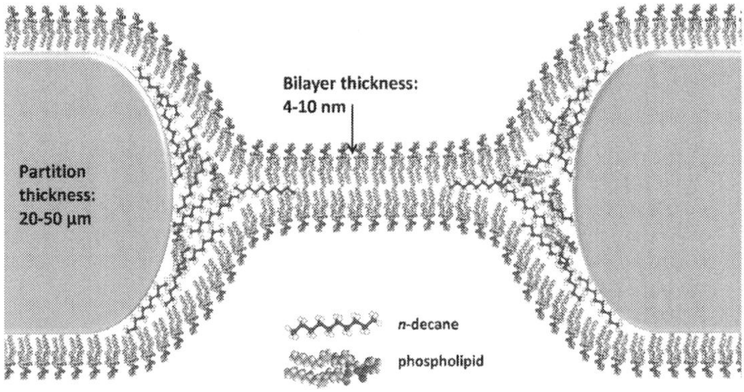

Fig. 4. Schematic illustration of typical dimensions of a lipid bilayer and partition aperture. Typical lipid bilayer thicknesses are 4-10 nanometers (nm), whereas partition thicknesses generally range from 20 to 50 micrometers (μm). The figure is not drawn to scale.

Malmstadt *et al.* showed that membrane stability may be significantly increased (> days) by stabilizing the membrane surroundings by hydrogel encapsulation, which was explained to result from a slowing down of the solvent diffusion out of the annulus, thereby prolonging the membrane lifespan (Malmstadt *et al.*, 2008). This approach is promising and may also be crucial for creating stable and portable devices.

We noticed that the typical partition preconditioning step resulted in inhomogeneous coverage of the preconditioning solution on the partition. Since the membrane stability is dependent on sufficient hydrophobic interactions between the bilayer forming solution and the partition scaffold we speculated that a more homogenous surface pretreatment coverage could result in increased membrane stability (Hansen *et al.*, 2009b). To investigate this, we developed an airbrush technique to homogenously cover the partition with preconditioning solution. This resulted in a markedly increased reproducibility in membrane formation, but did not increase the membrane lifetimes correspondingly (Hansen *et al.*, 2009b).

Ries *et al.* showed that the membrane electrical characteristics, dynamics of membrane formation and the membrane stability are strongly dependent on the partition substrate (Ries *et al.*, 2004). Inspired by this, we studied the effect of covalently modifying the partition substrate using surface plasma polymerization (Perry *et al.*, submitted). By this technique we were able to increase the membrane stability significantly. Using double-sided *n*-hexene partition surface modifications we were able to increase membrane lifetimes from an average of 100 min (Hansen *et al.*, 2009b) to average membrane lifetimes of approx. 70 hours, while 20% of established membranes lasted 140 hours (Perry *et al.*, submitted). These results underline that long term stability of established biomimetic membranes is critically dependent on a sufficient interaction with the hydrophobic surface of the partition and the bilayer forming solution.

Another approach to increase membrane stability has been based on biomimetic membranes consisting of semi-synthetic or synthetic biomimetic polymers. It was recently demonstrated that 8×8 arrays of triblock copolymers could successfully be established by the automation technique for creating biomimetic membrane arrays (Gonzalez-Perez *et al.*, 2009). Membrane stability could be achieved with lifetimes up to 23 hours. Also cross-linkable lipids have been suggested to being able to increase membrane stability (Benz, Praß & Ringsdorf, 1982; Daly *et al.*, 2006; Shenoy *et al.*, 2005), but more work is needed to show if this strategy may sufficiently increase membrane lifetimes.

Besides the membrane annulus and the biomimetic membrane composition, the aperture diameter is also a crucial determining factor for membrane stability. The membrane stability generally increases with decreasing aperture diameters. This has motivated designs based on nano-sized biomimetic membrane arrays (Han *et al.*, 2007; Hemmler *et al.*, 2005; Studer & Tiefenauer, 2007). The nano-sized aperture diameters should in principle favour long lived membranes, but they may also increase the risk of creating non-functional membranes, because the nanoscale aperture diameter may preclude sufficient membrane thinning.

An impressive silicone nitride chip array comprising 960,000 nano-membranes has been developed (Han *et al.*, 2007). The membrane lifetimes achieved using this technique were up to 144 hours. These lifetimes are comparable to our best membrane array lifetimes using plasma polymerization as pretreatment. In comparison the total membrane effective area of 0.045 cm^2 for the previously described 8×8 arrays is about 150 times larger than the total membrane area in the silicon nano-membrane chip array. Practical use of small nano-sized chip arrays could be in microelectronic devices or novel nanotechnology applications.

While membrane stabilities of > 1 day can be achieved with recent advances in biomimetic membrane research, it is still difficult to create storable and transportable biomimetic membrane devices. However, recent developments in membrane encapsulation strategies suggest that robust portable biomimetic membranes may be created (Jeon, Malmstadt & Schmidt, 2006; Kang *et al.*, 2007; Malmstadt *et al.*, 2008; Oliver *et al.*, 2008; Uto *et al.*, 1994). Efforts are none the less still required to create a general stable and transportable biomimetic membrane design.

3.2 Membrane array scalability

A general biomimetic membrane platform supporting different biotechnological applications would preferably be scalable to meet various application requirements. Fig. 5 illustrates scalability in biomimetic design. Biomimetic membrane scalability is not straightforward, and also represents a new concept in formation of biomimetic membrane arrays. The tendency in biomimetic membrane work has actually been to scale down the designs. The reason is likely related to the inherent membrane instability, but recent advances in membrane stability (as discussed in section 3.1) have led to the acceptance that scaling up the arrays may indeed be practically feasible. In this relation, we recently demonstrated that scaling up from rectangular 8×8 arrays (64 membranes) to rectangular 24×24 (576 membranes) or hexagonal 24×27 (648 membranes) arrays may actually provide an overall higher membrane stability evidenced by significant longer lifetimes (Hansen *et al.*, 2009a).

An emerging concept, relying on a high degree of membrane scalability, is novel separation technologies based on reconstitution of functional membrane protein channels. A study of the solute transport characteristics and permeability of aquaporin water selective channels incorporated into polymer vesicles indicated that the water permeability and salt rejection of aquaporin based biomimetic membranes would potentially represent a novel separation

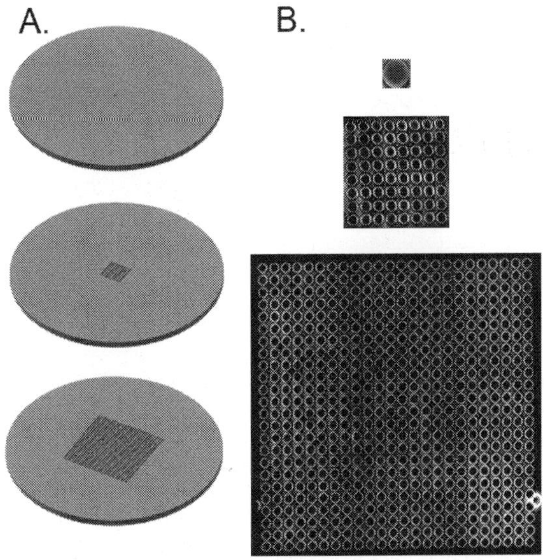

Fig. 5. Illustration of scalability of biomimetic membranes A) Schematic presentation of scalable aperture scaffolds with 300 μm diameter apertures supporting establishment of suspended biomembranes. B) Fluorescent images of established membranes in ETFE microstructured scaffolds corresponding to panel A). Established lipid membranes of 1,2-diphytanoyl-*sn*-glycero-3-phosphocholine were doped with the fluorescent lipid analogue 1-oleoyl-2- [6-[(7-nitro-2-1, 3-benzoxadiazol-4-yl) amino]hexanoyl]-*sn*-glycero-3-phosphocholine (NBD-PC) for visualization. Membranes shown in panel B) were established in the chamber design depicted in Fig. 3B and 3E. The membranes of panel B) are not shown to scale.

technology that would be able to exceed current reverse osmosis and forward osmosis membranes in performance (flux and salt-rejection) (Kumar *et al.*, 2007). Novel membrane protein based separation technologies may be explored, provided that the biomimetic membrane effective area can be scaled sufficiently. Extended research activities in biomimetic membrane scalability is therefore required to produce first generation biomimetic membrane based separation technologies.

3.3 Membrane addressability in membrane arrays

Biomimetic membrane arrays offer a platform for generating large membrane protein arrays, where a lot of information can be achieved with extremely low sample volumes (Suzuki & Takeuchi, 2008). A unique feature of biomimetic membrane arrays is that it offers the opportunity of multiplexed measurements on several levels within the same technology platform.

The trend in biomimetic membrane design is to create chambers that support electrical recordings of membrane, protein or peptide electrical properties combined with fluorescence microscopy. The most straightforward designs include voltage-clamp measurements of an entire array to ensure that functional membranes are established

(Hansen *et al.*, 2009a; Hemmler *et al.*, 2005; Wilburn *et al.*, 2006). In principle the electrical voltage clamp recordings could be adapted to individually address the membrane electrical properties of a membrane array. The concept of multiplexed electrical recordings was explored in a proof-of-concept study by Suzuki *et al.*, demonstrating that each well of a 96-wells microplate format could be electrically addressed (Suzuki *et al.*, 2009). Each well of the 96-wells plate however comprised a membrane array of 3×3 membranes, and individually membrane addressability was not addressed in this study, but would in principle be achievable in the presented design.

A solution to enable individual addressability of membranes of a biomimetic membrane array could be achived by creating a microelectrode array that would be positioned beneath the membrane scaffold. A microelectrode array has been successfully created for electrochemical detection of soluble enzyme activities (Lin *et al.*, 2008). Although the microelectrode array was demonstrated using immobilized soluble proteins, there is no principal hindrance in adapting this concept to biomimetic membrane array designs. Fig. 6 schematically illustrates how such microelectrode arrays may be envisaged to be adapted in biomimetic membrane designs in order to create individually addressable membranes.

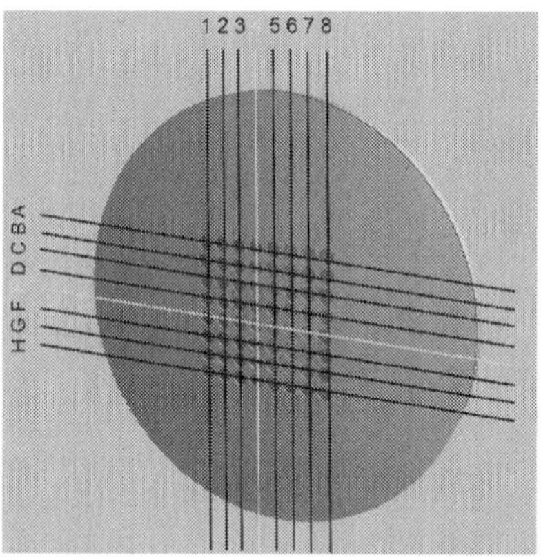

Fig. 6. Schematic illustration of how electrical multiplexing of biomimetic membrane arrays may be designed. Shown are the aperture partition (green), biomimetic membranes (red), electronic grid (black and yellow lines). The yellow lines show the individually addressed membrane of the array (where line E crosses line 4).

Electrical membrane array multiplexing using microelectrode arrays combined with in situ fluorescence assays would offer results read-out on two levels. The latter has been demonstrated on solid supported protein immobilized G-protein coupled receptor (GPCR) microarrays, where receptor-ligand interactions could be detected using fluorescently-labelled ligands (Fang, Frutos & Lahiri, 2002; Fang, Lahiri & Picard, 2003).

A third level of biomimetic membrane readouts could be created by detection of small solutes, ions or other substances transported across the membrane facilitated by proteins or peptides reconstituted into the biomimetic membrane arrays. Hemmler *et al.* demonstrated this principle in practice by visualizing transport of the aqueous calcein fluorescent dye across individual membranes reconstituted with α-hemolysin membrane protein pores (Hemmler *et al.*, 2005). Next generation of individually addressable membrane arrays could be envisaged to comprise ligand-receptor assays, where extracellular binding of ligand to receptors would lead to a secondary signaling pathway on the other side that subsequently would lead to a fluorescent or colorimetric signal, which could be quantified. For microfluidic devices the chamber outlets could be connected in line with fluorescence or absorbance detection, or alternatively connected to HPLC instruments for quantifying solutes or molecules. Functional demonstration of such novel conceptual ideas are however still to be proven in practice.

To sum up, a lot of information may be achieved with extremely low sample volumes from a single biomimetic membrane array by designing platforms that enable multiple results read-out. Such design strategies may aim at combining microelectrode multiplexing, in situ fluorescence assays and quantification of transport processes across the membranes by sample collecting followed by solute determination or concentration measurements.

3.4 Incorporation of membrane peptides and proteins into membrane arrays

Functional incorporation of membrane molecules into biomimetic membranes is essential to create peptide or membrane protein based sensor or separation applications using biomimetic membrane arrays.

Small fusiogenic membrane spanning depsipeptides or peptides generally insert spontaneously into established membranes, and may in many instances be dissolved in aqueous buffers, or other solvents (e.g. alcohols), that can be added directly to established membranes (Zagnoni *et al.*, 2007). The ease of incorporation is one of the main reasons why they are often used to demonstrate that functional biomimetic membranes have been successfully established. In this sense incorporation of small fusiogenic peptides constitute a quality control parameter for functional biomimetic membrane formation. Moreover, some fusiogenic peptides may be relevant in biotechnological and biomedical applications such as for creation of ion-sensing electrodes or biosensors for detection of small solutes and analyte molecules (Borisenko, Zhang & Woolley, 2002; Capone *et al.*, 2007; Frant & Ross, 1970; Nikolelis & Siontorou, 1996; Schar-Zammaretti *et al.*, 2002).

In contrast, medium to large membrane proteins (35-500 kDa), especially α-helical membrane proteins, do generally not readily self-insert into pre-established membranes (Zagnoni *et al.*, 2007). Although, the light-driven α-helical proton-pump bacteriorhodopsin (BR) as well as several *E. coli* outer membrane (β-barrel) porins (e.g. OmpA, OmpF and FomA) may be reconstituted into planar membranes directly from a detergent solubilized state (Arora *et al.*, 2000; Pocanschi *et al.*, 2006; Schmitt, Vrouenraets & Steinem, 2006), this is general not applicable for most membrane proteins. Therefore, a general reconstitution methodology is required for incorporation of membrane proteins into biomimetic membranes preserving correct protein function (e.g. ensuring correct orientation in the membrane).

Another, largely unresolved challenge is how to reconstitute different proteins into individual membranes to create large membrane protein microarrays, as is known from commercially available DNA microarrays or immobilized protein dot-blot arrays.

4. Biomedical application of biomimetic membranes

The function of a biomimetic membrane array depends not only of successful reconstitution of membrane proteins in stable host lipid/polymer membranes. Also the sensitivity or signal-to-noise ratio in the output-signal of the device must be high in order to allow for detection of analyte concentrations down to the single-molecule level. Thus sufficient amplification of the signal is vital for biomedical application of biomimetic membrane devices. This amplification generally arises as an intrinsic amplification in the biomimetic membrane material per se combined with external amplification.

Due to the relative ease by which pA currents can be resolved many biomimetic membrane based sensor platforms have built on incorporation of ion channels (Nielsen, 2009). The linear gramicidins present a versatile system that can be easily engineered. The preferred conformation of gramicidin in lipid bilayers is a $\beta^{6.3}$ helical fold of the pentadecapeptide. Upon dimerization of two gramicidin monomers from each opposing lipid monolayers an ion conducting dimer permeable to monovalent cations is formed. This system has revealed many basal features of ion channel function, for reviews see (Andersen & Koeppe, 2007; Koeppe & Andersen, 1996). In a freestanding bilayer gramicidin monomers diffuse randomly in each monolayer leaflet and dimerization is a random process. When a transmembrane potential is applied over a membrane separating two aqueous electrolyte compartments dimerization is evident as discrete amplitude changes in the recorded current-trace corresponding to appearance and disappearance of ion conducting dimers.

Sensors based on matrices with engineered gramicidin channels have been presented (Cornell *et al.*, 1997; Wiess-Wichert *et al.*, 1997). These sensors operate by changing the conformational equilibrium between gramicidin monomers and dimers. Concretely the sensors are built with a lower lipid monolayer tethered to an electrode and a mobile upper lipid monolayer where each monolayer leaflet contains engineered gramicidins. The gramicidins in the lower monolayer are covalently tethered to the electrode substrate whereas the upper monolayer gramicidins are covalently linked to specific antibodies moieties which can recognize specific analyte molecules. Another set of antibodies are covalently linked to the upper headgroup of bilayer spanning bolalipids with the lower bolalipid headgroup linked to the electrode substrate. This arrangement effectively anchors the bolalipid-linked antibodies relative to the gramicidin monomer-linked antibodies in the upper monolayer.

If no analyte molecules are present, the conformational equilibrium between monomers and dimers results in a randomly fluctuating current with a mean value effectively dependent on the total gramicidin concentration. When an analyte is present it may cross-link antibodies attached to the mobile outer layer channels with those attached to membrane spanning bolalipid-based tethers. The result is a decreased mean value of the fluctuating current as the outer monomers now are 'captured' by the analyte mediated crosslinking and therefore not available for dimerization with their immobilized lower monolayer channel partners. The increase in the effective transmembrane resistance (equivalent to a decrease of membrane admittance) with time provides a means to estimate the concentration of the analyte.

Gramicidin channels are low molecular weight peptides and unique in the sense that channel function (i.e. transfer of ions across the membrane) depends on dimerization of two (identical) monomers. In general membrane spanning ion channels are high molecular weight oligomeric structures with large hydrophilic moieties where the oligomeric interactions may depend only on weak interactions. However, recently the voltage-gated HERG potassium channel has been successfully reconstituted in biomimetic membranes tethered on mercury showing that large 'bulky' channel forming oligomeric proteins can be functional in a confined cushion geometry (Becucci *et al.*, 2008).

Ion channel gating (i.e. opening and closing of the ion conducting pathway) is a result of complex conformational changes in the protein. Although our structural understanding of ion channel gating is still limited, sensing devices based on detecting ion channel gating has been proposed. For example the ligand-gated nicotinic acetylcholine receptor (nAchR) ion channel (with acetylcholine as the 'natural' ligand) has been reconstituted in free-standing lipid bilayers (Boheim *et al.*, 1981; Eray *et al.*, 1995) as well as in lipopetide supported biomimetic membranes (Schmidt *et al.*, 1998). Using nAchR modified with two bispecific antibodies the channel remains open until both antibodies bind to the same antigen (Eray *et al.*, 1995).

Also the rectifying voltage gated Kv1.5 potassium channel has been reconstituted in free standing and solid supported membranes (Dhoke *et al.*, 2005; Matsuno *et al.*, 2004). The current/voltage relations display symmetric sigmoidal shapes. This highlights one of the major challenges in biomimetic membrane design based on reconstituted ion channels. The sigmoidal I/V relationship indicates that approximately half of the channels are inserted so they are rectifying the ionic current in one direction and the other half is rectifying currents in the opposite direction. For some application orientational randomness is problematic as membrane proteins generally have distinct intracellular and extracellular binding sites - thus for a sensor based on ligand detection directional control over protein insertion is imperative. However by careful optimization reconstitution procedures a more or less pronounced unidirectionality may be achieved.

The application of gated ion channels in biosensors exemplifies how signal amplification occurs both intrinsically (e.g. the binding of a single ligand gives rise to currents with 10^6 ions/second per channel) and externally though e.g. the I/V conversion and amplification of the current signal in voltage-clamp amplifiers. As we gain more insight into channel gating through more high-resolution structures of ion channel proteins in various conformational states the use of complex ion channel proteins in biomimetic membrane sensors may evolve from an 'all-or-nothing' type of response to more complex read-outs based on detecting ion channel sub-conductance states.

Ion channels represent one important class of biomedical 'targets'. Another important class is comprised of GPCRs. GPCRs generally detect molecules outside the cell and initiate downstream signalling in the form of a cascade of biochemical reactions leading to changes in cellular function. Since GPCRs are targets for more than 50% of all medicinal drugs there is a huge interest in understanding GPCR mediated signalling. Although the signalling process is generally well-described it is also very complex because it can involve several GPCRs simultaneously and the signalling may also occur by other pathways not requiring G-proteins. Also different ligands can result in different signals from the same GPCR depending on the cell type and *vice versa:* the same ligand can result in different signals in different cells. This complexity presents a major obstacle in our understanding of GPCRs but recently an elegant biosensing method has pointed to a way of overcoming some of the complexities. The sensor is based on coupling ion channels with GPCRs. Thus when the GPCR binds an agonist, its conformation changes, and this changes the structure of the coupled ion channel. (Moreau *et al.*, 2008). The conformational change in the GPCR is thus transduced into a change in ion channel current. In order to make this (and other ion channel based methods) technologically feasible electrical measurements must be integrated with membrane array designs allowing for parallel current recordings.

Another strategy is to take advantage of the electrical properties of bilayers and use them as insulating surfaces. Any defect in this surface is easily detectable as a change in impedance and as the defect locations create strong non-specific binding sites the sensitivity of such a device is high (Steltze, 1993). Impedance analysis on supported lipid bilayers can also be used to dissect the action of channel forming peptides e.g. the bee venom melittin (Becucci *et al.*, 2006a), the potassium specific valinomycin (Becucci *et al.*, 2005), and channel forming proteins e.g. the bacterial outer membrane porin Omp F (Becucci, Moncelli & Guidelli, 2006b) on the bilayer. This approach has also been used in black polymer membranes (BPMs) where protein driven energy transduction was realized by incorporation of cytochrome c oxidase (COX) (Ho *et al.*, 2004).

Light driven transport across membranes constitutes a particular interesting biosensing mechanism behind the design of membranes for energy conversion and advanced photoresponsive/optical devices (LaVan & Cha, 2006). BR and halorhodopsin (HR) are examples of light-driven ion pumps for protons (Oesterhelt & Stoeckenius, 1973) and chloride (and other halide) ions respectively (Essen, 2002; Schobert & Lanyi, 1982). BR occurs natually in highly ordered two-dimensional arrays (purple membranes) in *Halobacterium salinarium* (Oesterhelt & Stoeckenius, 1973). BR may be reconstituted in proteoliposomes (Kayushin & Skulachev, 1974; Oesterhelt & Schuhmann, 1974) but direct adsorption of purple membrane fractions onto suitable substrates takes direct advantage of the natural two-dimensional layout of BR in the native membrane (Ganea *et al.*, 1998). This approach has been refined by forming lipid membranes on a porous alumina substrate and then adsorbing purple membrane patches onto the membrane (Horn & Steinem, 2005). Also HR (Essen, 2002; Varo, 2000) has been reconstituted in proteoliposomes (Duschl, McCloskey & Lanyi, 1988) and lipid bilayer membranes (Bamberg, Hegemann & Oesterhelt, 1984).

Biomimetic sensing with reconstituted rhodopsins rely on an optical input, but changes in optical properties of supported biomimetic membranes may also be used as output signal. For example the application of supported membranes in the design of biosensors mounted on electro-optical devices is attracting considerable interest. Using surface plasmon resonance (SPR) allows for real-time measurements of ligand binding to immobilized proteins (Löfås & Johnsson, 1990) and thus opens for the possibility to detect ligand binding to membrane spanning proteins. Immunosensing can be seen as a special case of ligand binding sensing and detection of *Staphylococcus* enterotoxin B (SEB) in milk has been demonstrated in a microfluidic system with supported bilayer membranes with biotinylated anti-SEB IgG (Dong, Scott Phillips & Chen, 2006).

Although most work on biomimetic membrane sensors is based on incorporating membranes proteins, some sensor designs may also be realized in protein free systems. A recent example is a membrane supported by nanoporous aluminium oxide providing a high surface area and a protective environment against dewetting (Largueze, Kirat & Morandat, 2010). The membrane contains polyethylene-glycol (PEG) conjugated lipids as hydrating, protective and tethering agents and ubiquinone which is a naturally occurring redox lipophilic mediator embedded within the acyl chains of the lipid bilayer. The sensing system is based on cyclic voltammetry and can detect alterations of lipid membranes that are induced by the addition of surfactants (exemplified by the commonly used non-ionic detergent: Triton X-100). Biomedical application of this system could for example be screening of pulmonary surfactant candidates, monitoring enzymatic degradation by lipases, and studying peptide bilayer insertion.

Another method relies in the use of infrared absorption spectroscopy (IRAS) measurements. A recent study combining IRAS and voltage-clamp has demonstrated changes in specific regions in spectra obtained with solvent containing biomimetic membranes formed with

D_2O in the electrolyte solutions providing insight into membrane formation (Hirano-Iwata *et al.*, 2009). An OD stretching peak (arising from D_2O) appeared immediately after lipid application (painting). The band intensity increased with time with a concomitant decrease in bandwidth which could reflect gradual changes in the ordering of interfacial water molecules. Also specific bands could be assigned to CH_x stretching modes of acyl chains. The intensity of these bands was about ten times higher than that of the C=O modes of PC. Thus these CH_x bands likely arose from *n*-decane rather than from phospholipid acyl chains. The band intensities decreased with time, suggesting that *n*-decane was slowly expelled. These results demonstrate that IRAS can detect self-thinning of the lipid solution to form biomimetic membranes, the resulting expulsion of the *n*-decane solvent, and reordering of interfacial D_2O. By extending this methodology combined IRAS-voltage-clamp may be used to detect spectroscopic signals due to specific conformational changes in lipid acyl chains induced by pharmaceutical compounds as well as a biomedical screening assay for investigating the properties of naturally occurring (antioxidant) membrane residing solvents e.g. ubiquinone.

5. Future research

By virtue of mimicking cellular membranes, model systems based on one or few lipid species and reconstituted proteins have attracted considerable interest in biomedical research since the first appearance of black lipid membranes in the 1960ties. With the recent advances in nanotechnology over the last two decades this interest has now manifested itself in laboratory model devices with multiparameter detection of membrane dynamics and protein function. Recent developments in membrane design have led to the concept of biomimetic membrane arrays that may provide powerful HTS assays in drug discovery and in creation of novel separation technologies based on membrane peptide and protein function.

A reason that biomimetic membrane array devices are not already commercially available is related to the difficulty of creating stable and transportable devices. Although, major efforts have resulted in increased biomimetic membrane stability and lifetimes (several days to weeks), further improvements are still required. Especially transportation robustness needs further attention. With further developments in multi composite materials, sandwich structuring and encapsulation strategies storable and transportable biomimetic membrane based biomedical devices appear feasible.

While general protocols for reconstitution small fusiogenic membrane-spanning depsipeptides and peptides are relatively well-established, general reconstitution strategies are urgently required for controlled and reliable incorporating medium to large membrane proteins (35-500 kDa) that do not reliable self-insert into established biomimetic membrane arrays. Moreover, designs that support reconstitution of different membrane proteins into individual membranes would enable fabrication of membrane peptide or protein microarrays similar to current DNA microarrays and protein dot-blot arrays.

With the recent advances in biomimetic membrane array design and with further developments of biomimetic designs to comprise laboratory-on-a-chip (LOC) and micro-total-analysis systems (μTAS) the ultimate goal of industrially fabricated devices for drug-discovery, toxicologial testing, and other biomedical/pharmaceutical applications based on biomembrane function seem within reach.

6. References

Andersen, O.S. & Koeppe, R.E., 2nd (2007): Bilayer thickness and membrane protein function: an energetic perspective *Annu Rev Biophys Biomol Struct* 36: 107-30.

Arora, A., Rinehart, D., Szabo, G. & Tamm, L.K. (2000): Refolded outer membrane protein A of Escherichia coli forms ion channels with two conductance states in planar lipid bilayers *J Biol Chem* 275(3): 1594-600.

Ashkenasy, N., Sanchez-Quesada, J., Bayley, H. & Ghadiri, M.R. (2005): Recognizing a single base in an individual DNA strand: a step toward DNA sequencing in nanopores *Angew Chem Int Ed Engl* 44(9): 1401-4.

Bamberg, E., Hegemann, P. & Oesterhelt, D. (1984): Reconstitution of halorhodopsin in black lipid membranes *Prog Clin Biol Res* 164: 73-9.

Becucci, L., Carbone, M.V., Biagiotti, T., D'Amico, M., Olivotto, M. & Guidelli, R. (2008): Incorporation of the HERG potassium channel in a mercury supported lipid bilayer *J Phys Chem B* 112(4): 1315-9.

Becucci, L., Leon, R.R., Moncelli, M.R., Rovero, P. & Guidelli, R. (2006a): Electrochemical investigation of melittin reconstituted into a mercury-supported lipid bilayer *Langmuir* 22(15): 6644-50.

Becucci, L., Moncelli, M.R. & Guidelli, R. (2006b): Impedance spectroscopy of OmpF porin reconstituted into a mercury-supported lipid bilayer *Langmuir* 22(3): 1341-6.

Becucci, L., Moncelli, M.R., Naumann, R. & Guidelli, R. (2005): Potassium ion transport by valinomycin across a Hg-supported lipid bilayer *J Am Chem Soc* 127(38): 13316-23.

Benz, R., Frohlich, O., Lauger, P. & Montal, M. (1975): Electrical capacity of black lipid films and of lipid bilayers made from monolayers *Biochim Biophys Acta* 394(3): 323-34.

Benz, R., Praß, W. & Ringsdorf, H. (1982): Black Lipid Membranes from Polymerizable Lipids *Angewandte Chemie International Edition in English* 21(S5): 869-880.

Boheim, G., Hanke, W., Barrantes, F.J., Eibl, H., Sakmann, B., Fels, G. & Maelicke, A. (1981): Agonist-activated ionic channels in acetylcholine receptor reconstituted into planar lipid bilayers *Proc Natl Acad Sci U S A* 78(6): 3586-90.

Borisenko, V., Zhang, Z. & Woolley, G.A. (2002): Gramicidin derivatives as membrane-based pH sensors *Biochim Biophys Acta* 1558(1): 26-33.

Capone, R., Blake, S., Restrepo, M.R., Yang, J. & Mayer, M. (2007): Designing nanosensors based on charged derivatives of gramicidin A *J Am Chem Soc* 129(31): 9737-45.

Cornell, B.A., Braach-Maksvytis, V.L., King, L.G., Osman, P.D., Raguse, B., Wieczorek, L. & Pace, R.J. (1997): A biosensor that uses ion-channel switches *Nature* 387(6633): 580-3.

Daly, S.M., Heffernan, L.A., Barger, W.R. & Shenoy, D.K. (2006): Photopolymerization of mixed monolayers and black lipid membranes containing gramicidin A and diacetylenic phospholipids *Langmuir* 22(3): 1215-22.

Dhoke, M.A., Ladha, P.J., Boerio, F.J., Lessard, L.B., Malinowska, D.H., Cuppoletti, J. & Wieczorek, D.S. (2005): Porous membranes for reconstitution of ion channels *Biochim Biophys Acta* 1716(2): 117-25.

Dong, Y., Scott Phillips, K. & Chen, Q. (2006): Immunosensing of Staphylococcus enterotoxin B (SEB) in milk with PDMS microfluidic systems using reinforced supported bilayer membranes *Lab on a Chip* 6: 675-681.

Duschl, A., McCloskey, M.A. & Lanyi, J.K. (1988): Functional reconstitution of halorhodopsin. Properties of halorhodopsin-containing proteoliposomes *J Biol Chem* 263(32): 17016-22.

Eray, M., Dogan, N.S., Reiken, S.R., Sutisna, H., Van Wie, B.J., Koch, A.R., Moffett, D.F., Silber, M. & Davis, W.C. (1995): A highly stable and selective biosensor using modified nicotinic acetylcholine receptor (nAChR) *Biosystems* 35(2-3): 183-8.

Essen, L.O. (2002): Halorhodopsin: light-driven ion pumping made simple? *Curr Opin Struct Biol* 12(4): 516-22.

Fang, Y., Frutos, A.G. & Lahiri, J. (2002): Membrane protein microarrays *J Am Chem Soc* 124(11): 2394-5.

Fang, Y., Hong, Y., Webb, B. & Lahiri, J. (2006): Applications of biomembranes in drug discovery *MRS bulletin* 31(7): 5.

Fang, Y., Lahiri, J. & Picard, L. (2003): G protein-coupled receptor microarrays for drug discovery *Drug Discov Today* 8(16): 755-61.

Frant, M.S. & Ross, J.W., Jr. (1970): Potassium ion specific electrode with high selectivity for potassium over sodium *Science* 167(920): 987-8.

Ganea, C., Tittor, J., Bamberg, E. & Oesterhelt, D. (1998): Chloride- and pH-dependent proton transport by BR mutant D85N *Biochim Biophys Acta* 1368(1): 84-96.

Ginsburg, S. & Noble, D. (1974): The activation enthalpies for ion conductance systems in lipid bilayer membranes *Journal of Membrane Biology* 18(1): 163-176.

Gonzalez-Perez, A., Stibius, K.B., Vissing, T., Nielsen, C.H. & Mouritsen, O.G. (2009): Biomimetic Triblock Copolymer Membrane Arrays: A Stable Template for Functional Membrane Proteins *Langmuir* 25(18): 10447-10450.

Gu, L.Q., Braha, O., Conlan, S., Cheley, S. & Bayley, H. (1999): Stochastic sensing of organic analytes by a pore-forming protein containing a molecular adapter *Nature* 398(6729): 686-90.

Han, X., Studer, A., Sehr, H., Geissbühler, I., Di Berardino, M., Winkler, F.K. & Tiefenauer, L.X. (2007): Nanopore Arrays for Stable and Functional Free-Standing Lipid Bilayers *Advanced Materials* 19(24): 4466-4470.

Hansen, J.S., Perry, M., Vogel, J., Groth, J.S., Vissing, T., Larsen, M.S., Geschke, O., Emneus, J., Bohr, H. & Nielsen, C.H. (2009a): Large scale biomimetic membrane arrays *Anal Bioanal Chem* 395(3): 719-27.

Hansen, J.S., Perry, M., Vogel, J., Vissing, T., Hansen, C.R., Geschke, O., Emneus, J. & Nielsen, C.H. (2009b): Development of an automation technique for the establishment of functional lipid bilayer arrays *Journal of Micromechanics and Microengineering* 19(2): 025014.

Hemmler, R., Bose, G., Wagner, R. & Peters, R. (2005): Nanopore unitary permeability measured by electrochemical and optical single transporter recording *Biophys J* 88(6): 4000-7.

Heyderman, L.J., Ketterer, B., Bächle, D., Glaus, F., Haas, B., Schift, H., Vogelsang, K., Gobrecht, J., Tiefenauer, L., Dubochet, O., Surbled, P. & Hessler, T. (2003): High volume fabrication of customised nanopore membrane chips *Microelectronic Engineering* 67-68: 208-213.

Hirano-Iwata, A., Oshima, A., Onodera, K., Aoto, K., Taira, T., Yamaguchi, R., Kimura, Y. & Niwano, M. (2009): Self-formation of bilayer lipid membranes on agarose-coated silicon surfaces studied by simultaneous electrophysiological and surface infrared spectroscopic measurements *Applied Physics Letters* 94.

Ho, D., Chu, B., Lee, H. & Montemagno, C. (2004): Protein-driven energy tranduction across polymeric biomembranes *Nanotechnology* 15: 1084-1094.

Horn, C. & Steinem, C. (2005): Photocurrents generated by bacteriorhodopsin adsorbed on nano-black lipid membranes *Biophys J* 89(2): 1046-54.

Jeon, T.J., Malmstadt, N. & Schmidt, J.J. (2006): Hydrogel-encapsulated lipid membranes *J Am Chem Soc* 128(1): 42-3.

Kang, X.F., Cheley, S., Rice-Ficht, A.C. & Bayley, H. (2007): A storable encapsulated bilayer chip containing a single protein nanopore *J Am Chem Soc* 129(15): 4701-5.

Kayushin, L.P. & Skulachev, V.P. (1974): Bacteriorhodopsin as an electrogenic proton pump: reconstitution of bacteriorhodopsin proteoliposomes generating delta psi and delta pH *FEBS Lett* 39(1): 39-42.

Kendall, D.A. & MacDonald, R.C. (1982): A fluorescence assay to monitor vesicle fusion and lysis *J Biol Chem* 257(23): 13892-5.

Koeppe, R.E., II & Andersen, O.S. (1996): Engineering the gramicidin channel *Annu. Rev. Biophys. Biomol. Struct.* 25: 231-258.

Kumar, M., Grzelakowski, M., Zilles, J., Clark, M. & Meier, W. (2007): Highly permeable polymeric membranes based on the incorporation of the functional water channel protein Aquaporin Z *Proc Natl Acad Sci U S A* 104(52): 20719-24.

Largueze, J.-B., Kirat, K.E. & Morandat, S. (2010): Preparation of an electrochemical biosensor based on lipid membranes in nanoporous alumina *Colloids and Surfaces B: Biointerfaces* 79: 33-40.

LaVan, D.A. & Cha, J.N. (2006): Approaches for biological and biomimetic energy conversion *Proc Natl Acad Sci U S A* 103(14): 5251-5.

Le Pioufle, B., Suzuki, H., Tabata, K.V., Noji, H. & Takeuchi, S. (2008): Lipid bilayer microarray for parallel recording of transmembrane ion currents *Anal Chem* 80(1): 328-32.

Lewis, B.A. & Engelman, D.M. (1983): Lipid bilayer thickness varies linearly with acyl chain length in fluid phosphatidylcholine vesicles *Journal of Molecular Biology* 166(2): 211-217.

Lin, Z., Takahashi, Y., Kitagawa, Y., Umemura, T., Shiku, H. & Matsue, T. (2008): An addressable microelectrode array for electrochemical detection *Anal Chem* 80(17): 6830-3.

Löfås, S. & Johnsson, B.J. (1990): A novel hydrogel matrix on gold surfaces in surface plasmon resonance sensors for fast and efficient covalent immobilization of ligands *Chem. Soc. Chem. Commun.*: 1526-1528.

Malmstadt, N., Jeon, J. & Schmidt, J. (2008): Long-Lived Planar Lipid Bilayer Membranes Anchored to an In Situ Polymerized Hydrogel *Advanced Materials* 20(1): 84-89.

Matsuno, N., Murawsky, M., Ridgeway, J. & Cuppoletti, J. (2004): Solid support membranes for ion channel arrays and sensors: application to rapid screening of pharmacological compounds *Biochim Biophys Acta* 1665(1-2): 184-90.

Mayer, M., Kriebel, J.K., Tosteson, M.T. & Whitesides, G.M. (2003): Microfabricated teflon membranes for low-noise recordings of ion channels in planar lipid bilayers *Biophys J* 85(4): 2684-95.

Minami, H., Sugawara, M., Odashima, K., Umezawa, Y., Uto, M., Michaelis, E.K. & Kuwana, T. (1991): Ion channel sensors for glutamic acid *Anal Chem* 63(23): 2787-95.

Montal, M. & Mueller, P. (1972): Formation of bimolecular membranes from lipid monolayers and a study of their electrical properties *Proc Natl Acad Sci U S A* 69(12): 3561-6.

Moreau, C.J., Dupuis, J.P., Revilloud, J., Arumugam, K. & Vivaudou, M. (2008): Coupling ion channels to receptors for biomolecule sensing *Nat Nanotechnol* 3(10): 620-5.

Mueller, P. & Rudin, D.O. (1969): Translocators in bimolecular lipid membranes: their role in dissipative and conservative bioenergetic transduction *Curr Topics Bioenergetics* 3: 157–249.

Nielsen, C.H. (2009): Biomimetic membranes for sensor and separation applications *Anal Bioanal Chem* 395: 697-718.

Nikolelis, D.P. & Siontorou, C.G. (1996): Ammonium ion minisensors form self-assembled bilayer lipid membranes using gramicidin as an ionophore. Modulation of ammonium selectivity by platelet-activating factor *Anal Chem* 68(10): 1735-41.

O'Shaughnessy, T.J., Hu, J.E., Kulp, J.L., 3rd, Daly, S.M. & Ligler, F.S. (2007): Laser ablation of micropores for formation of artificial planar lipid bilayers *Biomed Microdevices* 9(6): 863-8.

Oesterhelt, D. & Schuhmann, L. (1974): Reconstitution of bacteriorhodopsin *FEBS Lett* 44(3): 262-5.

Oesterhelt, D. & Stoeckenius, W. (1973): Functions of a new photoreceptor membrane *Proc Natl Acad Sci U S A* 70(10): 2853-7.

Oliver, A.E., Kendall, E.L., Howland, M.C., Sanii, B., Shreve, A.P. & Parikh, A.N. (2008): Protecting, patterning, and scaffolding supported lipid membranes using carbohydrate glasses *Lab Chip* 8(6): 892-7.

Perin, M.S. & MacDonald, R.C. (1989): Fusion of synaptic vesicle membranes with planar bilayer membranes *Biophys J* 55(5): 973-86.

Pocanschi, C.L., Apell, H.J., Puntervoll, P., Hogh, B., Jensen, H.B., Welte, W. & Kleinschmidt, J.H. (2006): The major outer membrane protein of Fusobacterium nucleatum (FomA) folds and inserts into lipid bilayers via parallel folding pathways *J Mol Biol* 355(3): 548-61.

Reimhult, E. & Kumar, K. (2008): Membrane biosensor platforms using nano- and microporous supports *Trends Biotechnol* 26(2): 82-9.

Ries, R.S., Choi, H., Blunck, R., Bezanilla, F. & Heath, J.R. (2004): Black Lipid Membranes: Visualizing the Structure, Dynamics, and Substrate Dependence of Membranes *Journal of Physical Chemistry B* 108(41): 16040-16049.

Sandison, M.E. & Morgan, H. (2005): Rapid fabrication of polymer microfluidic systems for the production of artificial lipid bilayers *Journal of Micromechanics and Microengineering* 15(S139-S144).

Schar-Zammaretti, P., Ziegler, U., Forster, I., Groscurth, P. & Spichiger-Keller, U.E. (2002): Potassium-selective atomic force microscopy on ion-releasing substrates and living cells *Anal Chem* 74(16): 4269-74.

Schmidt, E.K., Liebermann, T., Kreiter, M., Jonczyk, A., Naumann, R., Offenhausser, A., Neumann, E., Kukol, A., Maelicke, A. & Knoll, W. (1998): Incorporation of the acetylcholine receptor dimer from Torpedo californica in a peptide supported lipid membrane investigated by surface plasmon and fluorescence spectroscopy *Biosens Bioelectron* 13(6): 585-91.

Schmitt, E.K., Vrouenraets, M. & Steinem, C. (2006): Channel activity of OmpF monitored in nano-BLMs *Biophys J* 91(6): 2163-71.

Schobert, B. & Lanyi, J.K. (1982): Halorhodopsin is a light-driven chloride pump *J Biol Chem* 257(17): 10306-13.

Shenoy, D.K., Barger, W.R., Singh, A., Panchal, R.G., Misakian, M., Stanford, V.M. & Kasianowicz, J.J. (2005): Functional reconstitution of protein ion channels into planar polymerizable phospholipid membranes *Nano Lett* 5(6): 1181-5.

Steltze, M. (1993): On the application of supported bilayers as receptive layers for biosensors with electrical detection *J. Phys. Chem.* 97: 2974-2981.

Studer, A. & Tiefenauer, L. (2007): Stable planar lipid bilayers in nanopores *European Cells and Materials* 14(Suppl. 3): 33.

Suzuki, H., Le Pioufle, B. & Takeuchi, S. (2009): Ninety-six-well planar lipid bilayer chip for ion channel recording fabricated by hybrid stereolithography *Biomed Microdevices* 11(1): 17-22.

Suzuki, H. & Takeuchi, S. (2008): Microtechnologies for membrane protein studies *Anal Bioanal Chem* 391(8): 2695-702.

Uto, M., Araki, M., Taniguchi, T., Hoshi, S. & Inoue, S. (1994): Stability of an Agar-Supported Bilayer Lipid Membrane and Its Application to a Chemical Sensor *Analytical Sciences* 10(6): 943-946.

Varo, G. (2000): Analogies between halorhodopsin and bacteriorhodopsin *Biochim Biophys Acta* 1460(1): 220-9.

Vogel, J., Perry, M., Hansen, J.S., Bolinger, P.Y., Nielsen, C.H. & Geschke, O. (2009): A support structure for biomimetic applications *Journal of Micromechanics and Microengineering* 19(2): 025026.

White, S.H. (1972): Analysis of the torus surrounding planar lipid bilayer membranes *Biophys J* 12(4): 432-45.

White, S.H. & Thompson, T.E. (1973): Capacitance, area, and thickness variations in thin lipid films *Biochim Biophys Acta* 323(1): 7-22.

Wiess-Wichert, C., Smetazko, M., Valina-Saba, M. & Schalkhammer, T. (1997): A new analytical device based on gated ion channels: A peptide-channel biosensor *J. Biol. Screening* 2: 11-18.

Wilburn, J.P., Wright, D.W. & Cliffel, D.E. (2006): Imaging of voltage-gated alamethicin pores in a reconstituted bilayer lipid membrane via scanning electrochemical microscopy *Analyst* 131(2): 311-6.

Wonderlin, W.F., Finkel, A. & French, R.J. (1990): Optimizing planar lipid bilayer single-channel recordings for high resolution with rapid voltage steps *Biophys J* 58(2): 289-97.

Woodbury, D.J. & Hall, J.E. (1988a): Role of channels in the fusion of vesicles with a planar bilayer *Biophys J* 54(6): 1053-63.

Woodbury, D.J. & Hall, J.E. (1988b): Vesicle-membrane fusion. Observation of simultaneous membrane incorporation and content release *Biophys J* 54(2): 345-9.

Zagnoni, M., Sandison, M.E., Marius, P., Lee, A.G. & Morgan, H. (2007): Controlled delivery of proteins into bilayer lipid membranes on chip *Lab Chip* 7(9): 1176-83.

Zimmerberg, J., Cohen, F.S. & Finkelstein, A. (1980a): Fusion of phospholipid vesicles with planar phospholipid bilayer membranes. I. Discharge of vesicular contents across the planar membrane *J Gen Physiol* 75(3): 241-50.

Zimmerberg, J., Cohen, F.S. & Finkelstein, A. (1980b): Micromolar Ca^{2+} Stimulates Fusion of Lipid Vesicles with Planar Bilayers Containing a Calcium-Binding Protein *Science* 210(4472): 906-908.

11

Cerasomes: A New Family of Artificial Cell Membranes with Ceramic Surface

Jun-ichi Kikuchi and Kazuma Yasuhara
Nara Institute of Science and Technology (NAIST)
Japan

1. Introduction

Organic–inorganic hybrid materials have attracted much attention in the field of materials science because of their great potential for use in a wide variety of applications through fusion of individual organic and inorganic properties (Schmidt, 1994; Mackenzie, 1994; Sanchez et al., 2001; Schottner, 2001). Up to the present time, various kinds of material combinations and synthetic strategies have been developed. The sol–gel method is one of the most powerful techniques to prepare hybrid materials and has provided moderate preparative conditions for the construction of inorganic oxide frameworks that are derived from hybrid materials (Sakka, 2005). In particular, the preparation of novel materials with organized nanostructures is a fascinating research subject in the field of hybrid materials (Ulman, 1996; Ozin, 2000; Dabbs & Aksay, 2000; Scott et al., 2001; van Bommel et al., 2003; Cölfen & Mann, 2003). These approaches are generally based on sol–gel techniques that utilize the presence of molecular assemblies as templates, such as rod-like micelles (Yanagisawa et al., 1990; Kresge et al., 1992; Inagaki et al., 1999), block-copolymers (Krämer et al., 1998; Melosh et al., 1999; Ryoo et al., 2000), microemulsions (Sims et al., 1998; Feng et al., 2000), organogels (Ono et al., 1998), cast films of bilayer membranes (Sakata & Kunitake, 1990) and bilayer vesicles (Hubert et al., 2000). Thus, the properties of nanohybrids depend on their nanostructures, especially the structure at the interface between the inorganic and organic components. Pre-organization by employing non-covalent interactions between an organic template and an inorganic precursor is known to be very important. However, the interface between the organic and inorganic components in these hybrids seems to be structurally ambiguous and more difficult to control at the molecular level than the individual component structures. Additionally, most of these materials are composed of inorganic components alone, and the organic portions are simply employed as templates.

In contrast, a novel class of layered organic–inorganic nanocomposites composed of amphiphilic molecules with a covalent bond between the silicate and the surfactant has been developed in recent years (Huo et al., 1996; Shimojima et al., 1997; Moreau et al., 2001; Ruiz-Hitzky et al., 2002; Zhang et al., 2004). These materials offer great potential because the hybrid precursors can form three-dimensional networks during the self-assembling process, whereby inorganic layers and organic moieties are covalently linked with stable Si–C bonds.

We recently developed cerasomes, a novel type of organic–inorganic nanohybrid, through a combination of sol–gel reactions and self-assembling of lipidic organotrialkoxysilanes in aqueous media to form vesicles covered with silicate surfaces (Katagiri et al., 1999). A cerasome is composed of a spherical lipid-bilayer membrane having an internal aqueous compartment, like so-called liposomes formed with phospholipids or synthetic lipids (Torchilin & Weissig, 2003; Kunitake, 1992), but is additionally covered with a silicate, surface framework (Fig. 1). While liposomes are widely used as biomembrane models and functional nanocapsules, their morphological instability is always a serious challenge for practical applications. It is hoped that cerasomes will overcome this limitation through the existence of a surface, silicate layer. Moreover, we can say that a cerasome is a novel organic–inorganic nanohybrid having a precisely designed nanostructure. That is, the thicknesses of both the organic and inorganic layers of a cerasome are attributed to the molecular structure of the cerasome-forming lipid, and the vesicular size of a cerasome is basically controllable by applying conventional methodologies for preparing monodispersed liposomes.

In this article, we review the design and preparation of cerasomes, as well as their morphological characterization. Additionally, the potential of the cerasome as a new family of artificial cell membranes is described from the viewpoints of surface modification versatility, hierarchical integration as a multicellular model and its functions as a cell-friendly drug carrier and molecular device.

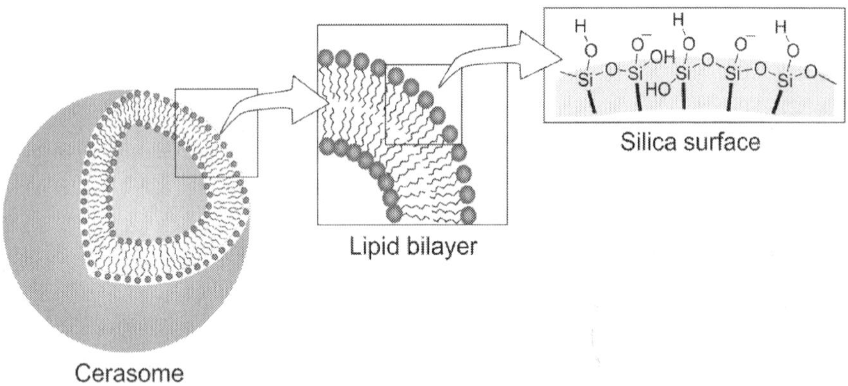

Fig. 1. Schematic drawing of a cerasome.

2. Design and preparation of cerasomes

The basic idea for designing a bilayer-forming lipid has been referred to as the concept of critical packing parameters for lipid assemblies (Israelachivili et al., 1976). Additionally, we considered the importance of a connector unit, which can form intermolecular hydrogen bonds to enhance morphological stability of the lipid assembly between the hydrophobic alkyl chains and the hydrophilic regions within a lipid molecule (Brockerhoff, 1977). We previously revealed the effect of a connector unit by systematic investigations of so-called peptide lipids, which have an amino acid or an oligopeptide moiety between the hydrophobic tail and the hydrophilic head (Murakami & Kikuchi, 1991). Our design of the cerasome-forming lipids takes these points into account, as well as the simplicity of synthesis. In addition, the silanol group as a head moiety is protected by ethoxy groups to store the synthesized lipid stably. The general molecular structure of a cerasome-forming lipid is shown in Fig. 2. Upon hydrolysis of the triethoxysilyl group, the lipid is converted into an amphiphilic structure to form a lipid bilayer in aqueous media. Condensation among the silanol groups of the relatively hydrophobic membrane surface proceeds to develop a silica-like inorganic framework, or a siloxane network, resulting in a cerasome.

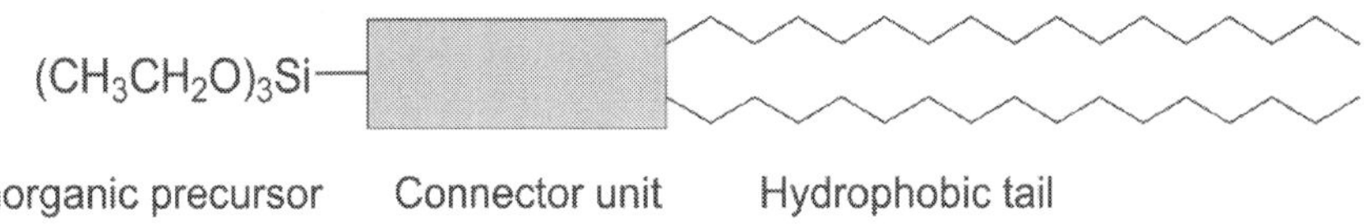

Fig. 2. General molecular structure of a cerasome-forming lipid.

Cerasome-forming lipids prepared along this design concept are shown in Fig. 3. First, we synthesized a cerasome-forming lipid (**1**) by simple condensation reactions between the three molecular components: dihexadecyamine, succinic anhydride and 3-aminopropyltriethoxylsilane (Katagiri et al., 1999). Cerasome-forming lipids with a simple molecular structure having one urea group (**2**) or one amide group (**3**) in the connector unit were also prepared (Hashizume et al., 2003). The cationic cerasome-forming lipids (**4**, **5**) with a similar molecular framework of the typical peptide lipid, composed of the hydrophobic double-chain segment, quaternary ammonium head and an amino acid residue interposed between them, were developed by replacing the methyl group of the trimethylammonium head to form a 3-triethoxysilylpropyl group (Katagiri et al., 2002a; Sasaki et al., 2006). A cerasome-forming lipid with two triethoxysilyl heads (**6**) was designed to tune the siloxane network on the cerasome surface (Hashizume et al., 2004). To provide biodegradability to the cerasome, a phospholipid with a triethoxysilyl head (**7**) was also designed and synthesized.
The preparation procedure for cerasomes with a multiwalled vesicular structure is basically analogous to that of the liposomes formed with phospholipids. In general, we can adopt two kinds of preparation methods. One is the direct dispersion of the cerasome-forming lipid in aqueous media by vortex-mixing (Katagiri et al., 2007). The procedure is very simple technically; however, we should pay attention to the reaction conditions, especially the effect of pH (Ariga et al., 2000; Katagiri et al., 2001). As for the water-insoluble lipids, such as lipids (**1-3**), hydrolysis of the triethoxysilyl head group of the proamphiphile gradually proceeds to give a corresponding amphiphilic molecule. This lipid readily forms a self-assembly of the liposome-like bilayer membrane in aqueous media. In addition, condensation among the silanol groups on the relatively hydrophobic membrane surface proceeds spontaneously to develop a siloxane network. However, if the hydrolysis and subsequent condensation is much faster prior to the self-assembly, formation of the bilayer structure may be disturbed. Therefore, control of the reaction rate in the sol–gel process, especially the hydrolysis, seems to be important to cerasome formation.
For example, lipid (**1**) does not change to the corresponding amphiphilic form after prolonged vortex-mixing in aqueous media under a neutral pH condition and remains as oil droplets, primarily because of the extremely slow hydrolysis of the head group. On the other hand, a translucent solution characteristic of a liposomal dispersion is obtained under moderate acidic conditions at pH 3, where hydrolysis of the ethoxysilyl groups is gently preceded by mild acid catalysis. Under stronger acidic conditions at pH 1, however, a stable

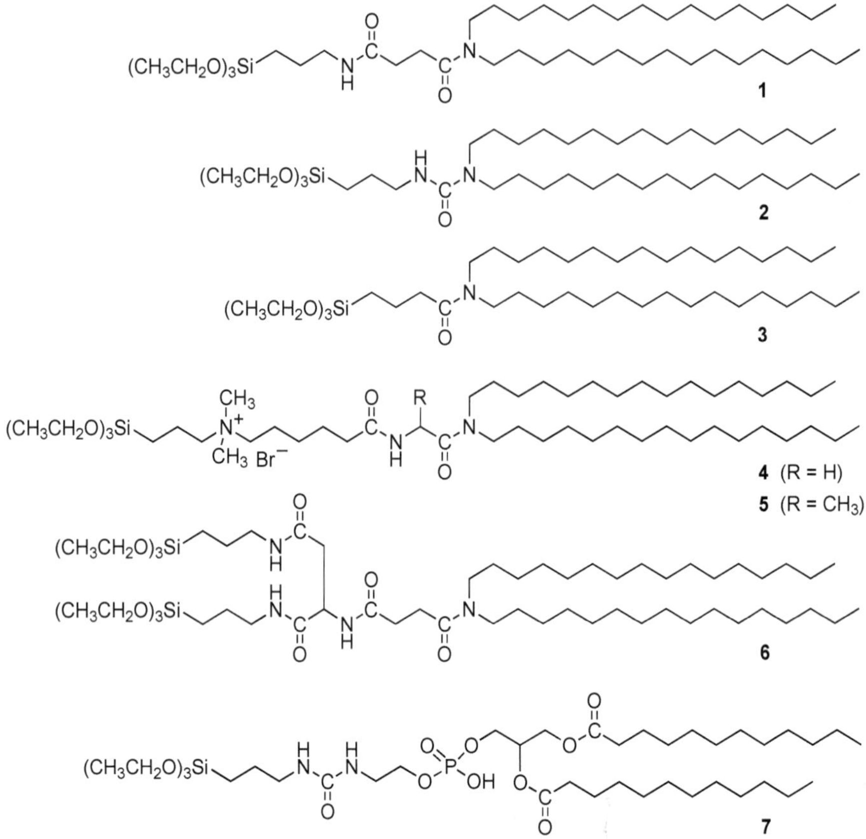

Fig. 3. Structural formulae of cerasome-forming lipids.

dispersion is not obtained, and precipitation is observed immediately. In this case, the hydrolysis and subsequent condensation reaction are so fast that the formation of the vesicular structure is prevented. At pH 12, the resulting solution is translucent, but oil droplets remain. Thus, the hydrolysis seems to proceed heterogeneously under basic conditions. The behaviors observed under the different pH conditions can be explained on the basis of a generally accepted mechanism for hydrolysis of alkoxysilane compounds in the sol–gel process, as follows. Under acidic conditions, hydrolysis of the triethoxysilyl group continues equally for each of the proamphiphile molecules in a one-by-one manner. This process provides a suitable condition for the preparation of the lipid bilayer assembly. On the other hand, under basic conditions, particular molecules are preferentially hydrolyzed, while the other molecules remain as unreacted species. This process leads to heterogeneous hydrolysis, and various reaction stages of the lipid are observed. Thus, basic conditions seem to be unsuitable for the preparation of cerasomes. In practice, the hydrolysis behavior of cerasome-forming lipids can be monitored by ^{1}H NMR spectroscopy.

Regarding the cerasome-forming lipids with good water solubility, such as lipids (**4**) and (**5**), the direct dispersion method was adopted for its ease and utility.

The second procedure of cerasome preparation is the ethanol sol injection method (Katagiri et al., 2003). In this method, the hydrolysis of cerasome-forming lipids is performed by incubating an acidic ethanol solution of the lipids for an appropriate time. The sol thus obtained is injected into water, and the solution is incubated for an additional 24 h. This method is useful for cerasome-forming lipids with poor water solubility.

In general, the size of the multiwalled cerasomes is in the range of sub-micrometers. Upon sonication of the aqueous dispersion of the cerasome, the multiwalled vesicles convert into the corresponding single-walled vesicles with a diameter less than 100 nm (Katagiri et al., 2007; Sasaki et al., 2006). For sonication conditions, the use of a probe-type sonicator at 30 W power above the phase transition temperature of the lipids for 3 min is generally recommended. The vesicular size can be evaluated by dynamic light scattering (DLS) measurement. Cell-sized cerasomes with a diameter larger than 1 μm can also be prepared by employing the preparation method of giant liposomes (Luisi & Walde, 1999).

3. Morphological characterization of cerasomes

3.1 Aggregate morphology

The aggregate structures of cerasomes can be evaluated by means of various microscopic measurements, such as transmission electron microscopy (TEM), scanning electron microscopy (SEM), atomic force microscopy (AFM) and optical microscopy. For TEM measurements of cerasomes, we can use three kinds of imaging techniques (Kikuchi & Yasuhara, in press). First, negative staining with heavy metal ions is a simple and convenient technique. For example, a negatively-stained TEM image of a cerasome formed with lipid (**4**), using the direct dispersion method, is shown in Fig. 4 (a). An internal view of

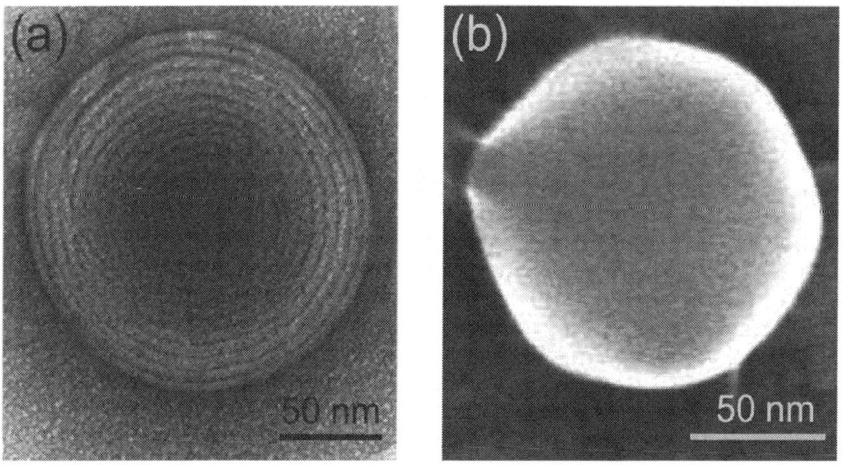

Fig. 4. Microscopic images of multiwalled cerasomes: a negatively stained TEM image of a cerasome formed with lipid (**4**) (a) and a SEM image of a cerasome formed with lipid (**2**) (b).

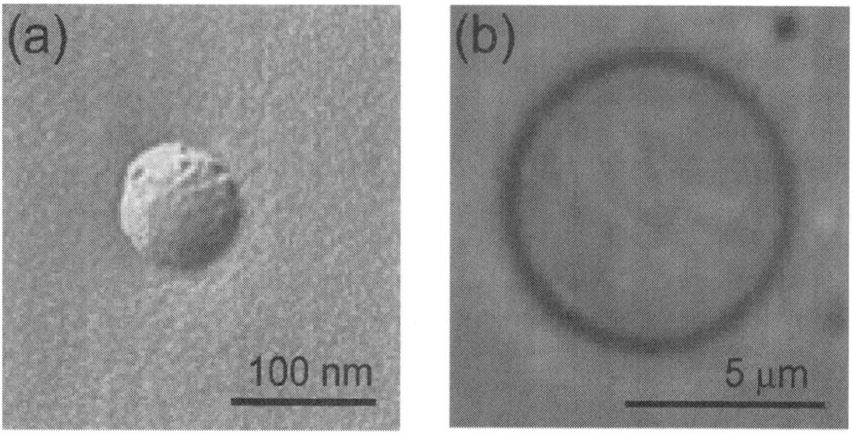

Fig. 5. Microscopic images of single-walled cerasomes: a freeze-fracture TEM image of a small cerasome formed with lipid (**5**) (a) and a phase contrast image of a giant cerasome formed with lipid (**5**) (b).

the multiwalled vesicles with a bilayer thickness of about 5 nm was clearly confirmed. A similar image was obtained by cryogenic TEM without a staining agent. On the other hand, freeze-fracture TEM imaging can provide information on the vesicular surface structure. Figure 5 (a) shows a surface image of a single-walled cerasome formed with lipid (**5**), as observed by freeze-fracture TEM.

In general, SEM is a challenging technique for imaging conventional liposomes formed with phospholipids because of the poor structural integrity of the samples. However, cerasomes can be visualized by SEM because of their high morphological stability. An SEM image of a multiwalled cerasome formed with lipid (**2**), using the ethanol sol injection method, is shown in Fig. 4 (b). The enhanced morphological stability of the cerasome also allows clear AFM imaging, as described later. For micrometer-sized giant cerasomes, optical microscopy is a powerful tool to provide dynamic imaging. Figure 5 (b) shows a phase contrast image of a giant cerasome formed with lipid (**5**). By using an appropriate fluorescent probe, we can visualize the lipid layer of a cerasome and its inner aqueous phase, separately.

3.2 Surface siloxane network

One of the important characteristics of the cerasomes is the presence of a surface siloxane network. This inorganic framework provides the cerasome much higher morphological stability compared with that of a conventional liposome.

The formation of siloxane bonds on the surface of a cerasome formed with lipid (**1**) was evaluated by Fourier transform infrared spectroscopy (Katagiri et al., 2007). Stretching bands assigned to the Si-O-Si and Si-OH groups were observed around 1100 and 950 cm^{-1}, respectively. The former peak intensity was much weaker than the latter in the cerasome in the aqueous dispersion state. Thus, it is suggested that the cerasome had a silica-like surface with a siloxane framework, but the degree of polymerization was not particularly high. The detectable species of lipid oligomers in the cerasome as evaluated by matrix assisted laser desorption ionization time-of-flight mass spectrometry (MALDI-TOF-MS) spectra are listed in Table 1. Trimethylsilylation was performed for the aqueous dispersion samples of a cerasome prepared after 10 h. While the monomer, dimer and trimer species were also detected in the sample as prepared, oligomers with higher molecular weights such as tetramers and pentamers were also detected in the sample during the prolonged incubation. This implies that the siloxane network grew as the incubation time increased. From cryoscopic measurements, the number-average molecular weight was determined to be 1300 for the aqueous dispersion of the cerasome incubated for 10 h. This value corresponds to the molecular weight of the dimer species. On the other hand, the size of the cerasome did not change appreciably after the allotted incubation time, as confirmed by TEM and DLS measurements. Accordingly, the siloxane network was not so highly developed on the cerasome surface. These observations were also supported by a computer-aided molecular model study, since the length of the Si-O-Si bond was much shorter than the calculated diameter of the cross-section of the dialkyl tail.

Species	Molecular weight	
	Observed [a]	Calcd
Monomer	901.7	900.7
Dimer	1640.4	1641.0
Trimer (cyclic)	ud	2217.9
Trimer (linear)	2380.3	2380.3
Tetramer (cyclic or branched)	2957.3	2957.3
Tetramer (linear)	3117.4	3119.6
Pentamer (cyclic or branched)	3695.3	3696.7
Pentamer (linear)	ud	3859.0

[a] Evaluated by MALDI-TOF-MS spectra after incubation for 10 h. ud: undetectable.

Table 1. Detectable species of lipid oligomers for a cerasome formed with lipid (**1**)

Surfactant solubilization is a useful method to evaluate morphological stability of liposomes in aqueous media. Thus, the resistance of a cerasome formed with lipid (**1**) against a nonionic surfactant, Triton X-100 (TX-100), was evaluated from the light scattering intensity of the vesicles (Katagiri et al., 2007). A liposomal membrane formed with 1,2-dimyristoyl-*sn*-glycero-3-phosphocholine (DMPC) was used as a reference. When three equivalents of TX-100 were added to the DMPC liposome, the light scattering intensity was drastically decreased, indicating a collapse of the vesicles. In contrast to the DMPC liposome, the cerasome exhibited a remarkable morphological resistance toward TX-100, and the light scattering intensity of the cerasome incubated for 24 h did not change, even in the presence of 36 equivalents of TX-100. Such surprising morphological stability of the cerasome was also confirmed by the DLS measurements. Morphological stability of such a cerasome seems to be superior to that of an excellent example of the polymerized liposomes recently developed (Mueller & O'Brien, 2002). It is noteworthy that the resistance of the cerasome toward TX-100 was insufficient immediately after preparation. Thus, it is clear that the morphological stability of the cerasome comes from development of the siloxane network on the vesicular surface. As for the cationic cerasomes prepared from lipids (**4**) or (**5**), the resistance against TX-100 was comparable to that of a conventional liposome, even after prolonged incubation. However, cationic cerasomes have an extremely high morphological stability against other kinds of surfactants, such as cetyltrimethylammonium bromide (CTAB), which completely dissolves DMPC liposomes (Sasaki et al., 2004). Accordingly, we can control the morphological stability of the vesicles through modification of the molecular design of the cerasome-forming lipids.

3.3 Phase transition and phase separation behavior

Phase transition parameters for the cerasomes were evaluated by differential scanning calorimetry (DSC). The enthalpy change from the gel to liquid-crystalline state (ΔH) and the temperature at the peak maximum (T_m) for the aqueous dispersion of a cerasome prepared from lipid (**1**) were 47.5 kJ mol^{-1} and 10.5 °C, respectively. Upon sonication of the cerasome with a probe-type sonicator for 10 min at 30 W, the ΔH value decreased to 11.5 kJ mol^{-1}, whereas the T_m value did not change. For a cerasome formed with lipid (**4**) in the aqueous dispersion state, the ΔH and T_m values were 33.3 kJ mol^{-1} and 25.7 °C, respectively. These phase transition parameters are comparable to those for peptide lipids previously reported (Murakami & Kikuchi, 1991). Upon sonication of the cerasome prepared from lipid (**4**) with a probe-type sonicator for 10 min at 30 W, the endothermic peak for the phase transition apparently disappeared. We have previously clarified that the transformation of the multiwalled vesicle to the corresponding single-walled vesicle is reflected in the decrease of both the ΔH and T_m values (Murakami & Kikuchi, 1991). Additionally, ΔH is more sensitive than T_m to such morphological changes. Since it is well known that the multiwalled vesicles formed with conventional liposomes generally transform to single-walled vesicles under the sonication conditions employed in this study, cerasome (**1**) is more tolerant towards morphological changes than the liposome-forming lipids. Formation of the siloxane network on the vesicular surface can prevent such morphological transformations.

Cerasomes enhance the creation of lipid domains in the vesicle (Hashizume et al., 2006a). For example, a cerasome prepared from the mixture of lipid (**1**) and 1,2-dipalmitoyl-*sn*-glycero-3-phosphatidylcholine (DPPC) formed a phase-separated lipid domain, as evaluated by DSC. That is, the aqueous dispersion of the homogeneous mixture of these lipids showed two phase transition peaks originating from the individual lipids. Similar phase separation behavior was observed in the cerasome formed with lipid (**1**), and the peptide lipid replaced the triethoxysilylpropyl group of lipid (**5**) as a methyl group. Such marked phase separation was not detected for the bilayer vesicle formed with DPPC and the peptide lipid. These results are mainly attributable to the polymerizable nature of the cerasome-forming lipid.

4. Surface modification of cerasomes

As mentioned, the surface of a cerasome is covered with a number of small siloxane oligomers. Since a cerasome exhibits analogous reactivity to the inorganic silica surface, we can modify a cerasome surface to give various unique organic-inorganic hybrid vesicles (Fig. 6).

4.1 Tuning of the siloxane network

Development of the siloxane network on a cerasome surface can be tuned when the cerasome is prepared by the ethanol sol injection method in the presence of

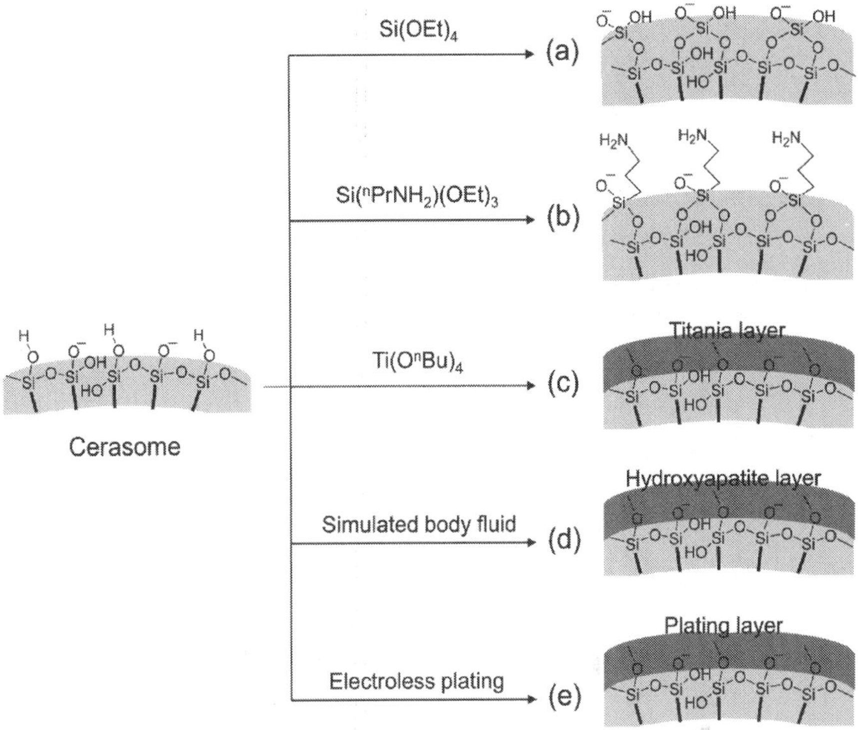

Fig. 6. Modification of the cerasome surface: development of a siloxane network (a), introduction of an organic functional group (b), coating with titania (c), hydroxyapatite (d) and a metallic nanolayer (e).

tetraethoxysilane (TEOS) (Katagiri et al., 2003). As such, when the sol prepared from lipid (**1**) with TEOS after 12 h incubation was injected into an aqueous solution under various pH conditions, the monodispersed and stable aggregates of the cerasome were formed. The hydrodynamic diameter and polydispersity index evaluated from the DLS measurements were 250–270 nm and 0.05– 0.13, respectively. Formation of the cerasomes with a diameter of 150–300 nm was observed for all the samples with and without a surface modification by TEOS, as confirmed by TEM. The values were in well agreement with those obtained from the DLS measurements.

Differences in the development of the siloxane network can be evaluated from a pH dependence of the zeta-potential of the cerasomes. For the cerasome without a surface modification, the zeta-potentials were in a range of +10 to -70 mV. The isoelectric point of the cerasome appeared at 4.3. Thus, the present cerasome possessed large negative charges under neutral and basic conditions, reflecting deprotonation of the silanol groups on the cerasome surface. For the cerasome modified with TEOS, a lower shift of the isoelectric point to 3.2 was observed. It has been reported that the isoelectric point of the typical silica particles derived from the sol-gel method lies in the range of 2–3, and the zeta-potentials for the particles are ranged from +20 to -80 mV in the analogous pH region (Nishimori et al., 1996). These results indicate that the surface electrical state of the cerasome modified with TEOS resembled that of the silica particles rather than that of the cerasome without surface modification. Thus, lipid (**1**) and TEOS were effectively co-polymerized to form the cerasome with a well-developed siloxane network.

4.2 Coating with functional layers

Surface modification of a cerasome with functional amino groups is readily achieved in a similar manner by replacing TEOS with 3-aminopropyltriethoxysilane (APS) (Katagiri et al., 2003). For a cerasome formed with lipid (**1**) in the presence of APS, the hydrodynamic diameter and polydispersity index were 210–220 nm and 0.19–0.25, respectively. The isoelectric point evaluated from the pH dependence of the zeta-potential was shifted to 10.0 for the APS-modified cerasome. In the pH range lower than 10, the zeta-potential of the cerasome increased with a decrease of pH to reach +100 mV at pH 6. The value is considerably higher than the corresponding maximal value of the cerasome derived from lipid (**1**) alone. Such a difference is attributable to an effective introduction of the amino group of APS on the former cerasome surface. Thus, in the physiological pH region, the cerasome prepared from lipid (**1**) without modification was present as a polyanionic vesicular particle, whereas the cerasome modified with APS was polycationic. Additionally, it may be possible to control the isoelectric point of the cerasome to a desired value by changing the molar ratio of lipid (**1**) and APS. Accordingly, we can prepare functionalized cerasomes modified with various alkoxysilane compounds by adopting this technique.

Using the ethanol sol injection method for cerasome preparation in the presence of titanium alkoxide, we can create a titania-coated cerasome (Hashizume et al., 2006b). Specifically, the cerasome-forming lipid (**1**) and titanium tetrabutoxide, $Ti(O^nBu)_4$, were incubated in acidic aqueous ethanol in the presence of acetylacetone as a co-catalyst. The sol was injected into the aqueous media and followed photo-irradiation to produce a cerasome with a diameter of c.a. 150 nm. The zeta-potential of the titania-coated cerasome changed from +30 to -40 mV, depending on the medium pH, and the isoelectric point was 4.8, which is comparable to that of colloidal titania, ranging between 5-7. The photocatalytic activity of the titania-coated cerasome was confirmed by photolysis of methylene blue in aqueous media by means of electronic absorption spectroscopy.

Biomimetic mineralization of supramolecular scaffolds consisting of biomolecules or their analogues has received much attention with regard to the creation of novel biomaterials. Likewise, we applied biomimetic deposition of hydroxyapatite (HAp) onto cerasomes (Hashizume et al., 2010). When a cerasome formed with lipid (**1**) was immersed into a solution having 1.5 times higher ion concentration than that of simulated body fluid (SBF), the cerasome induced heterogeneous nucleation of HAp, as evaluated by means of SEM, energy-dispersive X-ray spectroscopy and X-ray diffraction. The HAp deposition was further accelerated when dicarboxylic and monocarboxylic acid groups were displayed on the cerasome surface. These carboxylic acid groups were expected to enhance calcium ion binding to the cerasome surface, causing an increase of HAp nucleation sites. At lower surface concentrations on the cerasome surface, the dicarboxylic acid group is apparently more effective for HAp deposition than the monocarboxylic acid group. The HAp-coated cerasome is useful as a biocompatible material having unique properties deriving from the lipid bilayer structure of the cerasome.

The other system that highlights advantages of cerasomes is an asymmetric bilayer coating of monodispersed colloidal silica particles (Katagiri et al., 2004a). The particles were first coated with a cerasome-forming lipid and then coated with a bilayer-forming lipid to form an asymmetric lipid bilayer structure, which is usually seen in biological systems, but difficult to reconstitute by conventional techniques.

4.3 Coating with metallic nanolayers

Novel liposomal membranes having a metallic surface, so called metallosomes, are prepared by electroless plating of cerasomes (Gu et al., 2008). The electroless plating of a cerasome formed with lipid (**5**) was performed by first binding palladium tetrachloride ions ($PdCl_4^{2-}$) onto the cationic membrane surface through electrostatic interactions, then subsequently reducing this precursor catalyst to Pd(0) and finally depositing a layer of metal onto the cerasome surface using an appropriate plating bath. While the metallosome coated with an ultrathin Ni layer was successfully prepared by electroless Ni plating of the cerasome, it was not possible to derive the Ni-coated vesicle formed with the corresponding peptide lipid under similar plating conditions. Such results reflect the difference in the morphological stability of these vesicles. The characterization of the Ni-metallosomes was performed using various physical measurements, such as SEM, TEM, energy-dispersive X-ray spectroscopy, electron energy-loss spectroscopy and TEM tomography. The Ni layer thickness was controllable on the nanometer scale by changing the plating time. The gel to liquid-crystalline phase transition behavior of the Ni-metallosomes was observed by DSC, indicating that the metallosomes maintained the nature of the lipid bilayer membrane. Ni-metallosomes with various sizes were prepared from the corresponding cerasomes in a diameter range of 50-5000 nm. Metallosomes with an Au layer were also successfully obtained by electroless Ni/Au substitution plating of Ni-metallosomes.

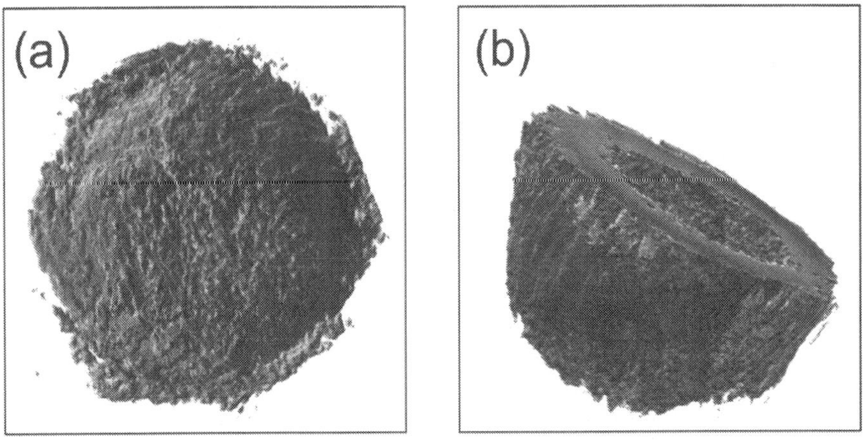

Fig. 7. Three-dimensional reconstitution of TEM images of a magnetic cerasome formed with lipid (**2**): the whole image (a) and the sliced image (b).

A magnetic cerasome, an artificial cell membrane having ultrathin magnetic metallic layers on the surface, was prepared through electroless plating of a magnetic metal alloy onto a cerasome (Minamida et al., 2008). Figure 7 shows three-dimensional images of a magnetic cerasome derived from lipid (**2**), as observed by TEM tomography. High morphological stability in the cerasome was important for constructing the magnetic lipid vesicle, and insertion of an alkylated metal ligand into the cerasome was essential for the magnetic metal alloy deposition on the cerasome surface. The magnetic property was evaluated by means of vibrating sample magnetometry. The magnetic field–magnetism hysteresis loop for the magnetic cerasome at different temperatures revealed that the magnetic cerasomes exhibited ferromagnetism, reflecting the nature of the plated magnetic metal alloy. Additionally, fluorescence microscopic observations revealed that the magnetic cerasomes were collected reversibly on the slide glass surface and manipulated by an external magnetic field.

5. Hierarchical integration of cerasomes

5.1 Three-dimensional integration on a substrate

Lipid bilayer vesicles with an inner aqueous compartment have been extensively employed as biomembrane models. Thus, it would be important to develop a new methodology to form hierarchically integrated vesicular assemblies, since the multicellular bodies in biological systems can create highly organized architectures and exhibit more functions than unicellular bodies can. Three-dimensional integration of the cerasomes on a substrate is successfully achieved by employing a layer-by-layer assembling method. As such, an anionic cerasome formed with lipid (**1**) was assembled on a substrate covered with oppositely charged polycations (Katagiri et al., 2002b). AFM images of the anionic cerasome layer and the cationic polymer layer are shown in Fig. 8 (a). The integration process was monitored by measuring the absorption mass changes on a quartz crystal microbalance. A similar three-dimensional assembly was created with an APS-modified cationic cerasome derived from lipid (**1**) and an anionic polymer on a substrate (Katagiri et al., 2004b). The alternate layer-by-layer assembly of two types of vesicles was obtained by employing the combination of an anionic cerasome formed with lipid (**1**) and a cationic cerasome formed with lipid (**4**) as shown in Fig. 8 (b) (Katagiri et al., 2002a). Notably, three-dimensional integration of lipid vesicles on a substrate can be achieved by use of morphologically stable cerasomes, but not by conventional bilayer-forming lipids.

5.2 Integration on DNA templates

In general, the interactions of ionic lipid vesicles with oppositely charged polymers induce morphological changes of the vesicles. However, the vesicular structure of cerasomes is much more stable than that of conventional liposomes. Thus, we can expect to create multicellular models by employing multipoint electrostatic interactions of the cerasomes with ionic polymers in aqueous media. In fact, we observed that cationic cerasomes formed with lipid (**5**) assembled on the DNA templates, as shown in Fig. 9 (Matsui et al., 2007; Hashizume et al., 2008). Under similar conditions, cationic peptide lipid in which the triethoxysilylpropyl group of lipid (**5**) was replaced by a methyl group, could not maintain the vesicular shape to support fusion of the vesicles.

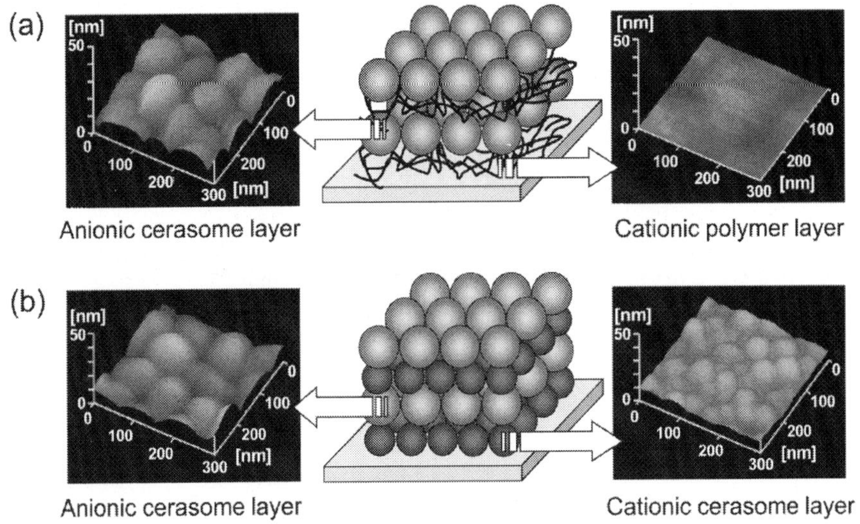

Fig. 8. AFM images of three-dimensional self-assemblies of cerasomes on a mica substrate: layer-by-layer assembly of an anionic cerasome (**1**) with a cationic polymer (a) and a cationic cerasome (**4**) (b).

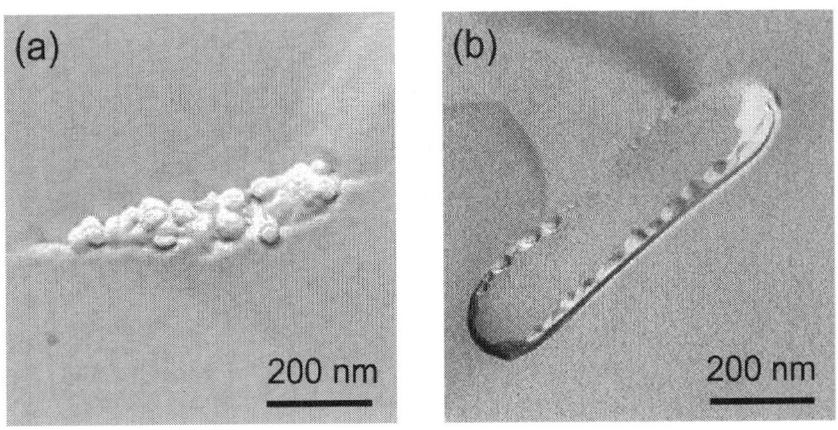

Fig. 9. Freeze-fracture TEM images of the self-assemblies of cationic cerasomes on DNA templates: assemblies of a cationic cerasome (**5**) on double-stranded DNA (a) and plasmid DNA (b).

6. Functionalization of Cerasomes

6.1 Potent drug carriers

Since the discovery of lipofection (Felgner et al., 1987), cationic lipids have been widely used as transfection agents in gene delivery (Behr, 1993; Kabanov & Kabanov, 1995; Mintzer & Simanek, 2009). They form cationic liposomes, to which anionic DNAs are electrostatically bound, to form complexes (or lipoplexes) that are taken in the cells via endocytosis. This is, however, an oversimplified picture. Liposomes are by no means rigid or robust. They are potentially fusible with cell membranes and therefore, toxic. They also easily undergo DNA-induced fusion to give larger particles that have lower endocytosis susceptibility and poorer vascular mobility. Additionally, serum components can interfere with fragile liposome-DNA complexes. Size instability, cytotoxicity and serum incompatibility, which are actually interrelated, are thus major problems in the current lipofection technology.

Recently, we developed an excellent transfection system using a cationic cerasome as a gene carrier (Matsui et al., 2006; Sasaki et al., 2006). We found that the cerasome formed with lipid (5) was infusible. The monomeric cerasome complex of plasmid DNA in a viral size (~70 nm) indeed exhibited a remarkable transfection performance, such as high activity, minimized toxicity and serum-compatibility, toward uterine HeLa and hepatic HepG2 cells (Fig. 10). This was in marked contrast to the non-silylated reference lipid, which forms fused, huge particles with significantly lower activity, by a factor of 10^2-10^3 and exhibited more pronounced toxicity. A couple of potential generalities of the present cerasome strategies with respect to nucleic acids to be delivered and cationic lipids as carriers are worth mentioning. The cerasome-plasmid complexation is strong and efficient, even at a stoichiometric lipid/nucleotide ratio. In this context, the cerasome could also be used as a size-regulated carrier for diverse types of functional nucleic acids, such as aptamers and siRNAs (Matsui et al., 2007). On the other hand, cerasomes encapsulating [70]fullerene also act as good carriers, exhibiting efficient photodynamic activity in HeLa cells (Ikeda et al., 2009).

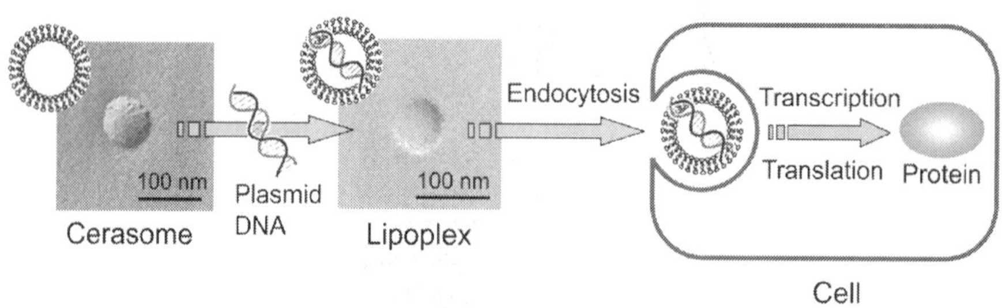

Fig. 10. Schematic representation of the transfection of a lipoplex formed with a cationic cerasome (5) and a plasmid DNA: images of the cerasome and its lipoplex were taken by freeze-fracture TEM.

6.2 Molecular devices for information processing

Signal transduction using molecules as information carriers is ingeniously designed in biological systems. Receptors and enzymes play leading roles for such information processing; however, biomembranes are also essential to provide a platform for the performance of these functional biomolecules. On these grounds, we have developed a biomimetic signal transduction system as a molecular device on artificial cell membranes (Kikuchi et al., 1999; Tian et al., 2005). When a molecular communication system was constructed on a cerasome formed with lipid (**4**), its signal transduction efficiency was much more effective than that created on the corresponding peptide lipid vesicle (Sasaki et al., 2004). The system contained a synthetic steroidal receptor and NADH-dependent lactate dehydrogenase, both embedded in the membrane through noncovalent interactions, as schematically shown in Fig. 11. A biologically important molecule, pyridoxal 5′-phosphate, acted as an input signal and was specifically recognized by the artificial receptor to form a signal-receptor complex on the membrane surface. The information from the molecular recognition was then transmitted to the enzyme by a copper(II) ion, as a mediator, which increased the enzymatic activity. We found that the efficiency of the molecular information processing in the cerasome was much higher than that in the peptide lipid vesicle. The former advantage comes from an enhanced phase separation of the steroidal receptor in the cerasome than in the peptide lipid membrane, which promotes the formation of a ternary complex of the receptor, signal and mediator species. Energy transfer is another important phenomenon in molecular information processing. Indeed, efficient fluorescence energy transfer between cyanine dyes was achieved with a cerasome formed with lipid (**5**) (Dai et al., 2009).

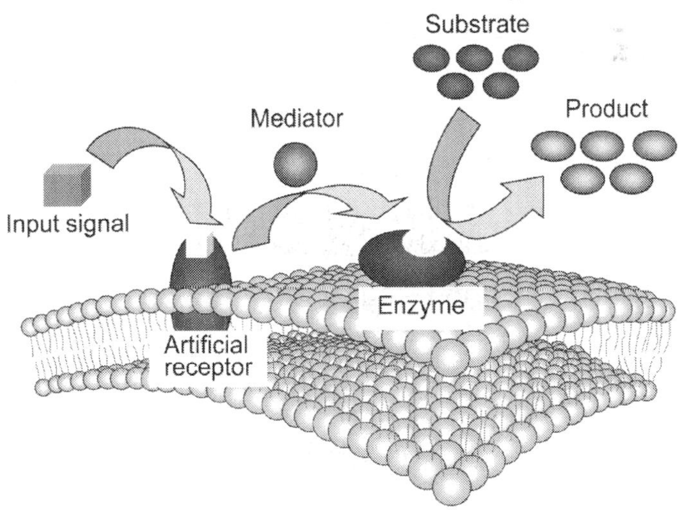

Fig. 11. Schematic representation of molecular information processing on a cerasome.

7. Conclusion

One of the useful guideposts in the creation of intelligent biomimetic materials is the hybridization of the functional building blocks of biological and artificial molecular components (Kikuchi et al., 2004). Cerasomes have been developed as a nanohybrid of membrane-forming lipids and ceramics along this line. Specifically, cerasomes behave as biomembrane models, as well as phospholipid liposomes and synthetic organic lipid vesicles. Owing to the enhanced morphological stability of the cerasome siloxane network on the vesicular surface, the hybrid performs as a superior vesicle in various applications as compared with conventional lipid vesicles. Moreover, cerasomes combine the structural and chemical characteristics of silica particles. Therefore, cerasomes have potential for application in a wide variety of novel functional fields, in which conventional lipid vesicles cannot be employed.

8. References

Ariga, K.; Katagiri, K. & Kikuchi, J. (2000). Preparation condition of a novel organic-inorganic hybrid vesicle "cerasome". *Kobunshi Ronbunshu*, 57, 4, 251-253, 0386-2186

Behr, J. P. (1993). Synthetic gene-transfer vectors. *Acc. Chem. Res.*, 26, 5, 274-278, 0001-4842

Brockerhoff, H. (1977). Molecular design of membrane lipids, In: *Bioorganic Chemistry*, Tamelen, E. E., (Ed), Vol. 3, 1-20, Academic Press, 0-12-714303-3, New York

Cölfen, H. & Mann, S. (2003). Higher-order organization by mesoscale self-assembly and transformation of hybrid nanostructures. *Angew. Chem. Int. Ed.*, 42, 21, 2350-2365, 1443-7851

Dabbs, D. M. & Aksay, I. A. (2000). Self-assembled ceramics produced by complex-fluid templation. *Annu. Rev. Phys. Chem.*, 51, 601-622, 0066-426X

Dai, Z.-F.; Tian, W.-J.; Yue, X.-L.; Zheng, Z.-Z.; Qi, J.-J.; Tamai, N. & Kikuchi, J. (2009). Efficient fluorescence resonance energy transfer in highly stable liposomal nanohybrid cerasome. *Chem. Commun.*, 15, 2032-2034, 1359-7345

Felgner, P. L.; Dadek, T. R; Holm, M.; Roman, R.; Chan, H. W.; Wenz, M.; Northrop, J. P.; Ringold, G. M. & Danielsen, M. (1987). Lipofection: A highly efficient, lipid-mediated DNA-transfection procedure. *Proc. Nat. Acad. Sci. U.S.A.*, 84, 21, 7413-7417, 0027-8424

Feng, P.; Bu, X.; Stucky, G. D. & Pine, D. J. (2000). Monolithic mesoporous silica templated by microemulsion liquid crystals. *J. Am. Chem. Soc.*, 122, 5, 994-995, 0002-7863

Gu, F.; Hashizume, M.; Okada, S.; Sasaki, Y.; Kikuchi, J. & Imori, T. (2008). Metallosome: An artificial cell membrane with ultrathin metallic surface derived from a cationic cerasome through electroless plating. *J. Ceram. Soc. Jpn.*, 116, 3, 400-405, 1882-0743

Hashizume, M.; Kawanami, S.; Iwamoto, S.; Isomoto, T. & Kikuchi, J. (2003). Stable vesicular nanoparticle "cerasome" as an organic-inorganic hybrid formed with organoalkoxysilane lipids having a hydrogen-bonding unit. *Thin Solid Films*, 438-439, 20-26, 0040-6090

Hashizume, M.; Inoue, H.; Katagiri, K.; Ikeda, A. & Kikuchi, J. (2004). Cerasome as an organic-inorganic vesicular nanohybrid. Characterization of cerasome-forming lipids having a single or a dual trialkoxysilyl head. *J. Sol-Gel Sci. Technol.*, 31, 1-3, 99-102, 9028-0707

Hashizume, M.; Saeki, I.; Otsuki, M. & Kikuchi, J. (2006a). Incorporation of lipid domains in cerasome, a morphologically-stable organic-inorganic vesicular nanohybrid. *J. Sol-Gel Sci. Technol.*, 40, 2-3, 227-232, 0928-0707

Hashizume, M.; Yamada, M.; Katagiri, K.; Tsuji, M. & Kikuchi, J. (2006b). Facile functionalization of lipid bilayer vesicles by titania: the use of cerasome-forming lipid for surface and core modification. *Bioconjugate Chem.*, 17, 4, 1099-1104, 1043-1802

Hashizume, M.; Sasaki, Y.; Terashima, T.; Komatsu, T. & Kikuchi, J. (2008). Creation of organized assembly of cerasomes on DNA templates. *Kobunshi Ronbunshu*, 65, 6, 421-426, 0386-2186

Hashizume, M.; Horii, H.; Kikuchi, J.; Kamitakahara, M.; Ohtsuki, C. & Tanihara, M. (2010). Effects of surface carboxylic acid groups of cerasomes, morphologically stable vesicles having a silica surface, on biomimetic deposition of hydroxyapatite in body fluid conditions. *J. Mater. Sci: Mater. Med.*, 21, 1, 11-19, 0957-4530

Hubert, D. H. W.; Jung, M.; Frederik, P. M.; Bomans, P. H. H.; Meuldijkm J. & German, A. L. (2000). Vesicle-directed growth of silica. *Adv. Mater.*, 12, 17, 1286-1290, 0935-9648

Huo, Q.; Margolese, D. I. & Stucky, G. D. (1996). Surfactant control of phases in the synthesis of mesoporous silica-based materials. *Chem. Mater.*, 8, 5, 1147-1160, 0897-4756

Ikeda, A.; Nagano, M.; Akiyama, M.; Matsumoto, M.; Ito, S.; Mukai, M.; Hashizume, M.; Kikuchi, J.; Katagiri, K.; Ogawa, T. & Takeya, T. (2009). Photodynamic activity of C_{70} caged within surface-cross-linked liposome. *Chem. Asian J.*, 4, 1, 199-205, 1861-4728

Inagaki, S.; Guan, S.; Fukushima, Y.; Ohsuna, T. & Terasaki, O. (1999). Novel mesoporous materials with a uniform distribution of organic groups and inorganic oxide in their frameworks. *J. Am. Chem. Soc.*, 121, 41, 9611-9614, 0002-7863

Israelachivili, J. N.; Mitchell, D. J. & Ninham, B. W. (1976). Theory of self-assembly of hydrocarbon amphiphiles into micelles and bilayers. *J. Chem. Soc. Faraday Trans. 2*, 72, 9, 1525-1568, 0300-9238

Kabanov, A. V. & Kabanov, V. A. (1995). DNA complexes with polycations for the delivery of genetic material into cells. *Bioconjugate Chem.*, 6, 1, 7-20, 1043-1802

Katagiri, K.; Ariga, K. & Kikuchi, J. (1999). Preparation of organic-inorganic hybrid vesicle "cerasome" derived from artificial lipid with alkoxysilyl head. *Chem. Lett.*, 7, 661-662, 0366-7022

Katagiri, K.; Ariga, K. & Kikuchi, J. (2001). Novel class of organic-inorganic hybrid vesicle "cerasome" derived from various amphiphiles with alkoxysilyl head. *Stud. Surface Sci. Catal.*, 132, 599-602, 0167-2991

Katagiri, K.; Hamasaki, R.; Ariga, K. & Kikuchi, J. (2002a). Layered paving of vesicular nanoparticles formed with cerasome as a bioinspired organic-inorganic hybrid. *J. Am. Chem. Soc.*, 124, 27, 7892-7893, 0002-7863

Katagiri, K.; Hamasaki, R.; Ariga, K. & Kikuchi, J. (2002b). Layer-by-layer self-assembling of liposomal nanohybrid "cerasome" on substrates. *Langmuir*, 18, 17, 6709-6711, 0743-7463

Katagiri, K.; Hamasaki, R.; Ariga, K. & Kikuchi, J. (2003). Preparation and surface modification of novel vesicular nano-particle "cerasome" with liposomal bilayer and silicate surface. *J. Sol-Gel Sci. Technol.*, 26, 1-3, 393-396, 0928-0707

Katagiri, K.; Hashizume, M.; Kikuchi, J.; Taketani, Y. & Murakami, M. (2004a). Creation of asymmetric bilayer membrane on monodispersed colloidal silica particles. *Colloids Surf. B*, 38, 1-3, 149-153, 0927-7765

Katagiri, K.; Hamasaki, R.; Hashizume, M.; Ariga, K. & Kikuchi, J. (2004b). Size-selective organization of silica and silica-like particles on solid interfaces through layer-by-layer assembly. *J. Sol-Gel Sci. Technol.*, 31, 1-3, 59-62, 0928-0707

Katagiri, K.; Hashizume, M.; Ariga, K.; Terashima, T. & Kikuchi, J. (2007). Preparation and characterization of a novel organic-inorganic nanohybrid "cerasome" formed with a liposomal membrane and silicate surface. *Chem. Eur. J.*, 13, 18, 5272-5281, 0947-6539

Kikuchi, J.; Ariga, K. & Ikeda, K. (1999). Signal transduction mediated by artificial cell-surface receptors. Activation of lactate dehydrogenase triggered by molecular recognition and phase separation of bile acid derivatives embedded in a synthetic bilayer membrane. *Chem. Commun.*, 6, 547-548, 1359-7354

Kikuchi, J.; Ikeda, A. & Hashizume, M. (2004). Biomimetic materials, In: *Encyclopedia of Biomaterials and Biomedical Engineering*, Vol. 1, Wnek, G. E. & Bowlin, G. L., (Eds.), 96-102, Marcel Dekker, 0-8247-5498-0, New York

Kikuchi, J. & Yasuhara, K. (in press) Microscopy & micro/nano imaging techniques: TEM, In: *Supramolecular Chemistry: From Molecules to Nanomaterials*, Vol. 1, Steed, J. W. & Gale, P. A., (Eds.), John Wiley & Sons, in press, Chichester

Krämer, E.; Förster, S.; Göltner, C. & Antonietti, M. (1998). Synthesis of nanoporous silica with new pore morphologies by templating the assemblies of ionic block copolymers. *Langmuir*, 14, 8, 2027-2031, 0743-7463

Kresge, C. T.; Leonowicz, M. E.; Roth, W. J.; Vartuli, J. C. & Beck, J. S. (1992). Ordered mesoporous molecular sieves synthesized by a liquid-crystal template mechanism. *Nature*, 359, 6397, 710-712, 0028-0836

Kunitake, T. (1992). Synthetic bilayer membranes: molecular design, self-organization, and application. *Angew. Chem. Int. Ed. Engl.*, 31, 6, 709-726, 0570-0833

Luisi, P. L. & Walde P. (1999). *Giant Vesicles*, John Wiley & Sons, 0471-97986-4, Chichester

Mackenzie, J. D. (1994). Structure and properties of ormosils. *J. Sol-Gel Sci. Technol.*, 2, 1-3, 81-86, 9028-0707

Matsui, K.; Sando, S.; Sera, T.; Aoyama, Y.; Sasaki, Y.; Komatsu, T.; Terashima, T. & Kikuchi, J. (2006). Cerasome as an infusible, cell-friendly, and serum-compatible transfection agent in a viral size. *J. Am. Chem. Soc.*, 128, 10, 3114-3115, 0002-7863

Matsui, K.; Sasaki, Y.; Komatsu, T.; Mukai, M.; Kikuchi, J. & Aoyama, Y. (2007). RNAi gene silencing using cerasome as a vial-size siRNA-carrier free from fusion and cross-linking. *Bioorg. Med. Chem. Lett.*, 17, 14, 3935-3938, 0960-894X

Melosh, N. A.; Lipic, P.; Bates, F. S.; Wudl, F.; Stucky, G. D.; Fredrickson, G. H. & Chmelka, B. F. (1999). Molecular and mesoscopic structures of transparent block copolymer-silica monoliths. *Macromolecules*, 32, 13, 4332-4342, 0024-9297

Minamida, D.; Okada, S.; Hashizume, M.; Sasaki, Y.; Kikuchi, J.; Hosoito, N. & Imori, T. (2008). Creation of magnetic cerasomes through electroless plating and their manipulation using external magnetic fields. *J. Sol-Gel Sci. Technol.*, 48, 1-2, 95-101, 0928-0707

Mintzer, M. A. & Simanek, E. E. (2009). Nonviral vectors for gene delivery. *Chem. Rev.*, 109, 2, 259-302, 0009-2665

Moreau, J. J. E.; Vellutini, L.; Man, M. W. C. ; Bied, C. ; Bantignies, J. L. ; Dieudonné, P. & Sauvajol, J.-L. (2001). Self-organized hybrid silica with long-range ordered lamellar structure. *J. Am. Chem. Soc.*, 123, 32, 7957-7958, 0002-7863

Mueller, A. & O'Brien, D. F. (2002). Supramolecular materials via polymerization of mesophases of hydrated amphiphiles. *Chem. Rev.*, 102, 3, 727-757, 0009-2665

Murakami, Y. & Kikuchi, J. (1991). Supramolecular assemblies formed with synthetic peptide lipids. Functional models of biomembranes and enzymes, In: *Bioorganic Chemistry Frontiers*, Vol. 2, Dugas, H. (Ed.), 73-113, Springer, 3-540-53365-6, Berlin

Nishimori, H.; Tatsumisago, M. & Minami, T. (1996). Influence of size of dispersed silica particles on preparation of thick silica films by using electrophoretic sol-gel deposition, *Bull. Chem. Soc. Jpn.*, 69, 3, 815- 818, 0009-2673

Ono, Y.; Nakashima, K.; Sano, M.; Kanekiyo, Y.; Inoue, K.; Hojo, J. & Shinkai, S. (1998). Organic gels are useful as a template for the preparation of hollow fiber silica. *Chem. Commun.*, 14, 1477-1478, 1359-7345

Ozin, G. A. (2000). Panoscopic materials: synthesis over 'all' length scales. *Chem. Commun.*, 6, 419-432, 1359-7345

Ruiz-Hitzky, E.; Letaïef, S. & Prévot, V. (2002). Novel organic-inorganic mesophases: Self-templating synthesis and intratubular swelling. *Adv. Mater.*, 14, 6, 439-443, 0935-9648

Ryoo, R.; Ko, C. H.; Kruk, M.; Antochshuk, V. & Jaroniec, M. (2000). , Block-copolymer-templated ordered mesoporous silica: Array of uniform mesopores or mesopore-micropore network? *J. Phys. Chem. B*, 104, 48, 11465-11471, 1520-6106

Sakata, K. & Kunitake, T. (1990). A multilayered film of an ultrathin siloxane network. *J. Chem. Soc. Chem. Commun.* 1990, 6, 504-505, 0022-4936

Sakka, S. (Ed.) (2005). *Handbook of Sol-Gel Science and Technology*, Vol. 1, Kluwer Academic, 1-4020-7966-4, Boston

Sanchez, C.; Soler-Illia, G. J. de A. A.; Ribot, F.; Lalot, T.; Mayer, C. R. & Cabuil, V. (2001). Designed hybrid organic-inorganic nanocomposites from functional nanobuilding blocks. *Chem. Mater.*, 13, 10, 3061-3083, 1897-4756

Sasaki, Y.; Yamada, M.; Terashima, T.; Wang, J.-F.; Hashizume, M.; Fan, S.-D. & Kikuchi, J. (2004). Construction of intermolecular communication system on "cerasome" as an organic-inorganic nanohybrid. *Kobunshi Ronbunshu*, 61, 10, 541-546, 0386-2186

Sasaki, Y.; Matsui, K.; Aoyama, Y. & Kikuchi, J. (2006). Cerasome as an infusible and cell-friendly gene carrier: Synthesis of cerasome-forming lipids and transfection using cerasome. *Nat. Protocols*, 1, 3, 1227-1234, 1754-2189

Schmidt, H. (1994). Inorganic-organic composites by sol-gel techniques. *J. Sol-Gel Sci. Technol.*, 1, 3, 217-231, 9028-0707

Schottner, G. (2001). Hybrid sol-gel-derived polymers: applications of multifunctional materials. *Chem. Mater.*, 13, 10, 3422-3435, 1897-4756

Scott, B. J.; Wirnsberger, G. & Stucky, G. D. (2001). Mesoporous and mesostructured materials for optical applications. *Chem. Mater.*, 13, 10, 3140-3150, 1897-4756

Shimojima, A.; Sugahara, Y. & Kuroda, K. (1997). Inorganic-organic layered materials derived via the hydrolysis and polycondensation of trialkoxy(alkyl)silanes. *Bull. Chem. Soc. Jpn.*, 70, 11, 2847-2853, 0009-2673

Sims, S. D.; Walsh, D. & Mann, S. (1998). Morphosynthesis of macroporous silica frameworks in bicontinuous microemulsions. *Adv. Mater.*, 10, 2, 151-154, 0935-9648

Tian, W.-J.; Sasaki, Y.; Fan, S.-D. & Kikuchi, J. (2005). Switching of enzymatic activity through functional connection of molecular recognition on lipid bilayer membranes. *Supramol. Chem.*, 17, 1-2, 113-119, 1061-0278

Torchilin, V. P. & Weissig, V. (2003). *Liposomes*, 2nd ed., Oxford Univ. Press, 0-19-963654-0, Oxford

Ulman, A. (1996). Formation and structure of self-assembled monolayers. *Chem. Rev.*, 96, 4, 1533-1554, 0009-2665

van Bommel, K. J. C.; Friggeri, A. & Shinkai, S. (2003). Organic templates for the generation of inorganic materials. *Angew. Chem. Int. Ed.*, 42, 9, 980-999, 1443-7851

Yanagisawa, T.; Shimizu, T.; Kuroda, K. & Kato, C. (1990). The preparation of alkyltrimethylammonium-kanemite complexes and their conversion to microporous materials. *Bull. Chem. Soc. Jpn.*, 63, 4, 988-992, 0009-2673

Zhang, Q.; Ariga, K.; Okabe, A. & Aida, T. (2004). A condensable amphiphile with a cleavable tail as a "lizard" template for the sol−gel synthesis of functionalized mesoporous silica. *J. Am. Chem. Soc.*, 126, 4, 988-989, 0002-7863

12

Biomimetic Model Membrane Systems Serve as Increasingly Valuable *in Vitro* Tools

Mary T. Le, Jennifer K. Litzenberger and Elmar J. Prenner
University of Calgary
Canada

1. Introduction

Biological membranes contain a multitude of lipids, proteins, and carbohydrates unique for any given cell or organism, and are a critical component of many biological processes. Animal and cell cultures have been used to understand these biological processes at the membrane level and more traditionally, to assess toxicity. However, the complex composition does not allow understanding of the detailed role of each membrane component, such as individual lipid species. This insight can be obtained from using simplified model systems, which include various kinds of vesicles (unilamellar or multilamellar), micelles, monolayers at an air-water interface, planar lipid bilayers/black lipid membranes, bicelles (bilayered micelles) and supported bilayers. All systems allow detailed control of composition and experimental conditions, and have been used to mimic various different membrane types, such as mammalian and bacterial.

Using various physicochemical techniques including nuclear magnetic resonance (NMR), differential scanning calorimetry (DSC), isothermal calorimetry (ITC), electron spin resonance, fluorescence spectroscopy, and X-ray diffraction, it is possible to investigate the mechanisms of membrane toxicity through differential changes in acyl chain melting temperature, membrane fluidity, and permeability of these different membrane models upon ligand binding. Moreover, the effects of ions (Na^+, K^+, Li^+, Ca^{2+}, Mg^{2+}, Ba^{2+}), toxic heavy metals (Hg^{2+}, Cd^{2+}) and a variety of drugs (e.g. Ellipticine for tumors and H1N1 virus or cyclosporine A to prevent graft rejection) have been evaluated on mammalian systems. For bacterial model membranes, the effects of antimicrobial peptides, antibiotics, the interaction of proteins with model membranes, and the insertion or reconstitution of membrane proteins into such systems have also been investigated.

When interpreting the results, it is important to note that some models may be better representatives of the natural membrane than others, and consequently, some results more relevant than others. Factors to consider include - but are not limited to - lipid composition, membrane curvature, or ionic strength of the solution, which all impart certain characteristics on the membrane model, influencing the results. Thus, while a single-component lipid model can be informative, it is important to consider its applications and limitations.

Overall, this chapter will provide insight as to the different lipid models used to mimic mammalian and bacterial membranes and how they have been found to be effective and useful research tools. Future development of these membrane models to more closely mimic the composition and complexity of the natural membrane will provide further insight into the mechanisms of membrane processes in biological systems.

1.1 Membranes

As lipids are small amphiphilic molecules, there are three aspects that define the physical characteristics of a lipid: the polar headgroup, the hydrophobic acyl chains and the interface between them. There are several different lipid headgroup classes, each with unique chemical properties. Some biological headgroups are negatively charged and exhibit charge-charge repulsions, which result in larger effective cross-sectional areas (Cullis *et al.*, 1986). However, the charge, and thus the area, is subject to the experimental conditions. Changes in the pH of the solution can impart or eliminate charges from the lipid based on the specific pKa values of the headgroup. The presence of mono- or divalent cations can serve to shield or neutralize the charge-charge repulsions, thus decreasing their effective cross-sectional area and consequently altering the properties of the lipid (Tate *et al.*, 1991).
Unlike the polar headgroups, which can be altered by the environment, the behavior of the hydrophobic acyl chains is mainly based on their chemical structure. Acyl chains are typically 14 to 22 carbons long and can be fully saturated, mono-unsaturated, or poly-unsaturated. Length and degree of saturation play a major role in lipid packing and the behaviour of the membrane. Fully saturated lipids pack more tightly than lipids with unsaturated acyl chains, changing the fluidity, transition temperature, and the lateral membrane pressure profile. Longer chains also have greater van der Waals interactions that stabilize membranes (Birdi, 1988). In contrast, the increased cross-sectional area of unsaturated lipids enhances membrane fluidity (de Kruijff, 1997).
Membranes are known to play an important role in many crucial biological functions, be it as the cellular membrane or as barrier of intracellular compartments. The fluid mosaic model of biological membranes (Singer and Nicolson, 1972) was groundbreaking in the understanding of membrane dynamics and organization, and the main concept of free diffusion of lipid and protein molecules within a dynamic fluid bilayer is still relevant. Current research supports the fact that several proteins are sensitive to the presence of specific lipids, with some experiencing an increase in activity while others require the presence of certain lipids for proper membrane insertion or multimeric stability (van der Does *et al.*, 2000; van Dalen *et al.*, 2002; van den Brink-van der Laan *et al.*, 2004).
However, one of the main emphases of the fluid mosaic model was that proteins and lipids were free to diffuse within the membrane, distributed randomly throughout with no regions of distinct composition. Research now supports the existence of lipid domains, distinct regions of specific lipid composition within the fluid bilayer (Rietveld and Simons, 1998; Zerrouk *et al.*, 2008). These domains possess unique physical properties and could be vital for many cell processes such as signal transduction, cell adhesion, and the function of several membrane proteins (Simons and Ikonen, 1997; Harder *et al.*, 1998).

1.2 The mammalian membrane

Mammalian membranes are primarily composed of phosphatidylcholine (PC), sphingomyelin (SM), phosphatidylserine (PS), phosphatidylethanolamine (PE), and cholesterol (Chol) lipid species in various ratios depending on cell type. The human erythrocyte membrane, one of the best characterized systems, is composed of 19.5% (w/w) of water, 39.5% of proteins, 35.1% of lipids, and 5.8% of carbohydrates (Yawata, 2003).

Lipids are asymmetrically distributed in the bilayer, in which 65-75% of PC and more than 85% of SM are found in the outer leaflet whereas 80-85% of PE and more than 96% of PS are found on the inner one (Zachowski, 1993). At physiological pH, SM, PC and PE are neutrally charged, PS is negatively charged and Chol is uncharged altogether. SM consists of a phosphocholine moiety ester-linked to the 1-hydroxy group of ceramide.

The zwitterionic PC makes up a large component of mammalian lipid model systems and therefore the membrane surface will primarily have a neutral charge. PE, another zwitterionic lipid species, can form the non-lamellar inverted hexagonal phase, affecting lipid-packing properties for membrane fusion or liposome budding. Negatively charged phospholipids like PS affect membrane functioning as the charge is influenced by pH and divalent ions like Ca^{2+} and Mg^{2+} (Vandijck et al., 1978). Moreover, PS has been shown to be an important lipid species in apoptotic processes in the presence of Hg^{2+}, for example (Eisele *et al.*, 2006).

It is important to mimic the fluidity properties of the biological membrane in mammalian model systems by varying the hydrophobic acyl chain in terms of length and saturation (e.g. palmitic acid versus oleic acid). Thus, egg PC, extracted from egg yolk, has also been used as it provides the required variety. Chol content in mammalian biomimetics may play an important role in modulating membrane fluidity and lipid raft formation (Simons and Toomre, 2000). Hence, by varying the composition of the lipid mixtures, these models will better mimic the heterogeneous nature of mammalian membranes.

1.3 The bacterial membrane

Based on the structure of their cell wall, bacteria are generally divided into two broad classes: Gram positive and Gram negative. The former includes those bacteria containing a single cell membrane surrounded by a thick layer of peptidoglycan, while the latter includes those with a thin layer of peptidoglycan surrounded by a second membrane (Dowhan, 1997). *E. coli* is a Gram negative bacterium, consisting of both an outer and an inner membrane. While the outer membrane is dominated by lipopolysaccharides, the inner membrane is composed of phospholipids PE, phosphatidylglycerol (PG), and cardiolipin (CL). PE is the most abundant species, making up 70-80% of the lipid portion of the inner membrane, while PG occupies 15-20% and CL roughly 5%, with these proportions varying depending on the mitotic state of and environmental stress imposed on the bacterium (Dowhan, 1997; Cronan, 2003). The different phospholipids impart unique physical properties on the membrane, which also facilitate bacterial adaptation to changing conditions. As mentioned, PE is a zwitterionic head group with both a positive and negative charge in neutral balance. The cross-sectional area of the headgroup is small compared to that of the acyl chains, and thus, while the conical-shaped PE lipids are part of a bilayer in the *E. coli* inner membrane, they also serve to create curvature stress. It has been shown that PE is an essential component in membrane protein assembly and enzyme function (Dowhan, 1997), and the non-lamellar propensity of some PEs may be an important factor in lipid-protein interactions in the membrane.

The second most abundant phospholipid, PG, has an anionic headgroup at physiological pH and corresponding charge-charge repulsions affect the physical properties of the bilayer. Like PE, PG has been shown to be required for important cellular functions, such as protein translocation across the *E. coli* membrane (Kusters *et al.*, 1991).

CL, also known as diphosphatidylglycerol, is the dimeric form of PG. CL has an anionic headgroup at physiological pH, but could potentially carry two negative charges under certain conditions (pK1=2.8, pK2>7.5) (Kates *et al.*, 1993). It is unique with four instead of two acyl chains, which in bacteria are typically fully saturated and mono-unsaturated chains with 14, 16, or 18 carbons (Mileykovskaya *et al.*, 2005). The much larger cross-sectional area of the acyl chains compared to the headgroup promotes non-lamellar phase transitions (Lewis and McElhaney, 2009). This tendency to form transient, non-bilayer domains in the membrane is significant for many cellular processes (Rietvald *et al.*, 1994).

In *E. coli* phospholipids, 43% of the acyl chains are fully saturated palmitic acid (C16:0), while the remaining 57% are monounsaturated palmitoleic (C16:1) and oleic (C18:1) acids at 33 and 24%, respectively (Ingraham *et al.*, 1983). This lipid variety may allow for the formation of different polymorphic phases (Hui and Sen, 1989) and lipid domains within the membrane. It has been shown that the specific lipid headgroup and acyl chain composition is responsible for characteristic packing and phase transition behaviours in a lipid monolayer compression system (Kaganer *et al.*, 1999).

1.4 The importance of lipid model systems

Manipulating the lipid content, salt concentration, pH, and other factors of the model systems allows for a greater understanding of the interactions within the membrane (de Kruijff, 1997). The native biological membrane can be mimicked by using natural or synthetic lipids if the lipid composition of the cell type or organism is known. For example, lipids were extracted from erythrocyte membranes and purified by thin layer chromatography before being incorporated into model systems (Keller *et al.*, 1998). Different models have advantages to assess particular interactions. Lipid monolayers enable the study of interactions at the surface of a cell membrane whereas supported lipid bilayers and bicelles allow for the investigation of toxicant interactions with lipid headgroups and other moieties. Vesicles encapsulated with a fluorophore and planar lipid bilayers can also be used to look at metal and drug permeability. Generally, lipid model systems usually lack proteins, making them less fluid than biological membranes (Suwalsky *et al.*, 2000). However, numerous studies have employed single, binary and ternary lipid mixtures in protein-free models to study ion, heavy metal, drug and peptide interactions.

2. Applications of mammalian membrane models

2.1 Essential ions

Various ions such as Ca^{2+}, Zn^{2+} and Mg^{2+} are important in membrane-associated biological processes. Ca^{2+} is involved in resting and action potentials (Akerman and Nicholls, 1983); Zn^{2+} is a nutritionally required element that is central to enzyme function and membrane structure (Bettger and O'Dell, 1981); and Mg^{2+} plays an important role in regulating ion channels (Mubagwa *et al.*, 2007). Hence, the study of essential ions with different biomimetic systems can give insight to their role with the biological membrane.

2.1.1 Essential ions: vesicles

Vesicles can be unilamellar, small (SUVs) or large (LUVs), as well as multilamellar (MLVs) and are most often used to mimic biological membranes since they enclose an aqueous compartment. In conjunction with various physicochemical techniques, these model systems have been used to study ion interactions with lipid bilayers as a function of ion type and concentration, overall ionic strength and lipid structure (head group, acyl chains) as discussed below for simple and more complex matrices.

Dimyristoylphosphatidic acid (DMPA) MLVs have been used in DSC experiments to investigate Ca^{2+} binding which resulted in an increase of T_m from 50-65°C with a decrease in transition enthalpy (Blume, 1985). Furthermore, dipalmitoyl-PC (DPPC) and dioleoyl-PC (DOPC) systems were used for X-ray diffraction and force measurement studies on Ca^{2+} and Mg^{2+} binding (Lis *et al.*, 1981) that showed stronger Ca^{2+} binding at concentrations of 10 and 30 mM. The testing of additional divalent ions resulted in the following order of ion binding to DPPC bilayers: $Ba^{2+} < Mg^{2+} \simeq Co^{2+} < Ca^{2+} \simeq Cd^{2+} \simeq Mn^{2+}$, whereas for DOPC bilayers, $Mg^{2+} < Co^{2+} \simeq Ca^{2+}$. Subsequently, PC lipid species with varied acyl chain composition such as dilauroyl-PC (DLPC), dimyristoyl-PC (DMPC) and distearoyl-PC (DSPC) were compared. In 30 mM $CaCl_2$, the order of binding was determined to be DOPC < DLPC < DMPC $\simeq$ DSPC $\simeq$ DPPC in which Ca^{2+} bound better to longer and saturated acyl chains (Lis *et al.*, 1981). Furthermore, in the presence of 30 mM $CaCl_2$, egg PC bilayers were observed to undergo phase separation when subjected to osmotic stress (Lis *et al.*, 1981). This phenomenon was attributed to the differences in the acyl chains and was further confirmed with 1:1 mixtures of DOPC/DLPC as well as DMPC/DLPC and DOPC/DMPC to a smaller extent. The binary mixtures were shown to be in one phase in pure water and two distinct lamellar phases in 30 mM $CaCl_2$ using X-ray diffraction (Lis *et al.*, 1981).

Single-lipid containing MLVs, composed of DMPC or dimyristoyl-PE (DMPE), were used to study Zn^{2+}-membrane interactions (Suwalsky *et al.*, 1996). Zn^{2+} was shown to interact with DMPE and DMPC bilayers using X-ray diffraction at a concentration as low as 10^{-5} µM. 1,6-diphenyl-1,3,5-hexatriene (DPH) steady state fluorescence anisotropy and Laurdan general polarization values were also observed to increase in the presence of Zn^{2+} in a concentration-dependent manner, indicating a less fluid bilayer.

Effects of Ca^{2+} on binary lipid models of various negatively charged phospholipid MLVs with PC have been investigated using freeze-fracture electron microscopy, ITC and DSC (Vandijck *et al.*, 1978; Blume, 1985; Sinn *et al.*, 2006). Although PG, PS and PA all contain one negative charge, they were shown to exhibit distinct mixing behaviors in the presence of Ca^{2+} (Vandijck *et al.*, 1978). In DMPC/dimyristoyl-PG (DMPG) mixtures, excess Ca^{2+} neutralized the negative charge and shifted the phase transition peak to higher temperatures. For DMPC/dipalmitoyl-PG (DPPG), similar results were seen with a shift in the transition peak and, moreover, a lateral phase separation occurred upon the addition of two carbons to the PG acyl chains (Vandijck *et al.*, 1978). An increase in T_m was also observed for binary mixtures of DMPA/DMPC when Ca^{2+} was added (Blume, 1985).

In DMPC/dimyristoyl-PS (DMPS) systems, increasing concentrations of the PS lipids resulted in a mixture of two types of structures - vesicles and stacked lamellae/cylinders. Interestingly, in DMPC/DMPA matrices, gel phase immiscibility was observed in the presence of Ca^{2+} independent of the PC/PA molar ratio. Ca^{2+} interactions were strongest with PA followed by PS and then PG-containing model systems, showing that in addition to the negative charge, the size of the lipid headgroup also plays an important role (Vandijck *et al.*, 1978).

2.1.2 Essential ions: monolayers

Another frequently used model system is the lipid monolayer at the air-water interface, which allows for the study of surface processes e.g. lipid-ion interactions. Parameters such as lipid composition, subphase, pH and temperature can be controlled in order to better mimic biological conditions. Extracted animal cephalin, consisting primarily of PE and PS, has been used in monolayer model systems to study the effect of Ca^{2+} (Suzuki and

Matsushita, 1968). At a concentration of 10^{-3} M, Ca^{2+} expanded the monolayer on the water subphase. The same research group also extended this study by covering monovalent (Na^{+} and Li^{+}), divalent (Ca^{2+} and Mn^{2+}) and trivalent (Fe^{3+} and In^{3+}) ions (Suzuki and Matsushita, 1969). Monovalent and divalent ions expanded the monolayer whereas the trivalent ions had a condensing effect. It has been proposed that the condensing effect by the trivalent metal ions is due to the bridging of phospholipid molecules and the cavities that result from the movement of fatty acyl chains (Suzuki and Matsushita, 1969).

Hexadecane/water emulsions containing DMPC or egg PC monolayers have also been used to investigate Ca^{2+}, Mn^{2+}, Cu^{2+} and Ni^{2+} binding to phospholipid molecules (Meshkov *et al.*, 1998). For DMPC monolayers, the ion binding constants (L mol^{-1}) at 25°C are 87, 21, 6, and 5.3 for Ca^{2+}, Mn^{2+}, Cu^{2+} and Ni^{2+} respectively. Interestingly, Cu^{2+} and Ni^{2+} had higher affinities for DMPC compared to egg lecithin monolayers (Meshkov *et al.*, 1998).

2.2 Heavy metals and neurotoxic cations

The toxic heavy metals mercury and cadmium are naturally mobilized from the earth's crust into the global environment, affecting the general population in many ways (Gailer, 2007). Cd^{2+} is an established carcinogen whereas chronic exposure to Hg^{2+} is linked to cardiovascular disease (Kostka, 1991; Huff *et al.*, 2007). It is important to study molecular interactions at the membrane to understand how these metals are involved in toxicity.

2.2.1 Heavy metals and neurotoxic cations: unilamellar vesicles

Binary lipid mixtures composed of DPPC/bovine brain PS (60:40) have been used to examine the effect of not only Ca^{2+} and Mg^{2+} but also Zn^{2+}, Cd^{2+} and Hg^{2+} using fluorescence spectroscopy (Bevan *et al.*, 1983). Phase transition temperatures (T_m) of the vesicles were determined using the fluorescence polarization of *trans*-parinaric acid methyl ester in which the free carboxyl group can interact with the divalent ions. Permeability studies were performed by encapsulating carboxyfluorescein and monitoring the increase of fluorescence due to dye release over time. 1.0 mM Ca^{2+} and Mg^{2+} as well as 0.1 mM Zn^{2+}, Cd^{2+} and Hg^{2+} were shown to increase the T_m of DPPC/PS vesicles. It was concluded that the ion-lipid interactions were a result of the PS molecules as there was little to no change in the T_m of pure DPPC vesicles (Bevan *et al.*, 1983). The permeability studies showed that the very same divalent cations that produced the greatest change in the T_m of the vesicles (Cd^{2+} and Zn^{2+}) were also the ones that altered the permeability of the vesicles and associated dye release (Bevan *et al.*, 1983).

SUVs made of PS or PS/DPPC were used to study the effects of neurotoxic cations such as Al^{3+} and Mn^{2+} in addition to Cd^{2+} (Deleers *et al.*, 1986). Membrane fusion was studied with PS vesicles by resonance energy transfer between N-(7-nitrobenz-2-oxa-1,3-diazol-4-yl)-PE (NBD-PE) and N-(lissamine rhodamine B-sulfonyl)-PE. Carboxyfluorescein-encapsulated PS vesicles were used to follow dye leakage, and fluorescence polarization of DPH in DPPC/PS (8:2) vesicles allowed for the monitoring of membrane rigidification (Deleers *et al.*, 1986). Fusion, leakage and rigidity increases in lipid models were seen in the presence of Al^{3+}, Cd^{2+} and Ca^{2+}. Although both Al^{3+} and Cd^{2+} decreased fluidity, seven-fold lower concentrations of Al^{3+} were seen to increase DPH polarization compared to Cd^{2+}. At 25 μM of Al^{3+}, a concentration inhibiting choline transport in erythrocytes (King *et al.*, 1983), membrane effects were indeed observed in the model system. This correlation between biological and model systems supports the relevance of the latter.

The permeability of ternary lipid model systems was utilized to study the effects of toxicant-membrane interactions. Vesicles containing egg lecithin, diacetyl phosphate and Chol in the molar ratio of 1.0 : 0.1 : 1.0 were incubated with methylmercuric chloride and mercuric chloride to measure the leakage of a glucose marker over time (Nakada *et al.*, 1978). As the Chol content was decreased in the model system, the amount of leakage increased with mercurial concentrations of 0.1 μM. Several divalent cations such as Ba^{2+}, Cd^{2+}, Co^{2+}, Cu^{2+}, Mn^{2+}, Pb^{2+}, and Zn^{2+} did not affect the permeability of egg lecithin/diacetyl phosphate/Chol vesicles (1.0 : 0.1 : 0.5), demonstrating that membrane leakage was specific for the two mercurial compounds (Nakada *et al.*, 1978).

Four-component lipid vesicles consisting of 35% 1-palmitoyl-2-oleoyl-PC (POPC) / 35% Chol / 15% 1-palmitoyl-2-oleoyl-PE (POPE) / 15% 1-palmitoyl-2-oleoyl-PS (POPS) have been used to investigate Hg^{2+} and Cd^{2+} binding affinity (Le *et al.*, 2009). As all the lipids had palmitic and oleic acyl chains, differences in metal affinity could be attributed to the nature of the headgroup. Using Phen Green ™ SK as a fluorescence probe, it was shown that Hg^{2+} preferentially binds to PS headgroups followed by PC and PE. In contrast, Cd^{2+} strongly prefers PE, followed by PC and PS.

2.2.1.1 Heavy metals and neurotoxic cations: multilamellar vesicles

A number of studies have used single component MLVs to investigate the effect of heavy metal interactions at the membrane surface to provide insight into the individual role of specific lipid classes. MLVs (DMPC and DMPE) were used with X-ray diffraction and LUVs (DMPC) with fluorescence spectroscopy to study the molecular mechanism of Hg^{2+} and Cd^{2+} interactions with the membrane (Suwalsky *et al.*, 2000; Suwalsky *et al.*, 2004). In addition, isolated resealed human erythrocyte membranes were analyzed by fluorescence spectroscopy, and perturbations of erythrocytes in the absence and presence of Hg^{2+} and Cd^{2+} were observed by scanning electron microscopy. Human erythrocytes incubated with 1 mM $HgCl_2$ exhibited both echinocyte and stomatocyte formation (Suwalsky *et al.*, 2000) whereas 1 mM $CdCl_2$ only induced echinocytes (Suwalsky *et al.*, 2004). According to the bilayer couple hypothesis, the shape induced in erythrocytes in the presence of heavy metals is due to the expansion of both monolayers in the membrane (Sheetz and Singer, 1974). Stomatocytes are formed when heavy metals interact with the inner monolayer and echinocytes upon interaction with the outer membrane surface. It was concluded that both Hg^{2+} and Cd^{2+} bind to the outer leaflet since echinocyte formation was most dominant, a result confirmed by X-ray diffraction. DMPC and DMPE MLVs, representing the outer and inner monolayer, generally showed a decrease in lipid reflection intensities in the presence of 10^{-5} - 10^{-1} M of Hg^{2+} and Cd^{2+}. A greater effect was observed with DMPC MLVs. The presence of Hg^{2+} and Cd^{2+} results in molecular disorder in the bilayer, affecting both the polar and acyl chain regions (Suwalsky *et al.*, 2000; Suwalsky *et al.*, 2004).

The effect of $HgCl_2$ at the membrane surface was investigated using DPH steady state fluorescence anisotropy to look at lipid acyl chain packing and Laurdan fluorescence spectral shifts via general polarization to observe interactions occurring in the phospholipid glycerol backbone (Suwalsky *et al.*, 2000; Suwalsky *et al.*, 2004). Hg^{2+} increased the DPH fluorescence anisotropy and Laurdan general polarization in erythrocyte membranes at 37°C and in DMPC LUVs at 18°C and 37°C (Suwalsky *et al.*, 2000). At 18°C, Cd^{2+} induced disorder in the DMPC bilayer whereas at 37°C the opposite effect was observed. At the higher temperature, the bilayer is in a more fluid state facilitating Cd^{2+}-phosphate interactions that result in an ordered state (Suwalsky *et al.*, 2004).

Cd-membrane interactions have been studied using single-lipid MLVs composed of DM- and DP-species of PC, -PS, -PA, -PG, and -PE as well as binary DMPE/egg PC (1:1) mixtures (Girault *et al.*, 1998). The physicochemical techniques used include ^{113}Cd-NMR to describe Cd^{2+} interactions at the membrane surface, DPH fluorescence polarization to look at changes in the acyl chain region and ^{31}P-NMR to monitor the mobility of the phosphate headgroup (Girault *et al.*, 1998).

Using ^{113}Cd-NMR, Cd binding to lipids resulted in a decrease of the Cd (II)-free isotropic signal. Because of the slow exchange between the free and bound cadmium, lipid/water coefficients {K_{lw}=(water vol./lipid vol.) x ([Cd II]$_{bound}$/[Cd(II)]$_{free}$)} at the lamellar gel (and fluid phase) were calculated to be: K_{lw} DMPC ~ K_{lw} egg PE ~ 2 $\pm$ 2 , K_{lw} DMPA = 392 $\pm$ 20 (505 $\pm$ 25), K_{lw} DMPG = 428 $\pm$ 21 (352 +17), and K_{lw} DMPS = 544 $\pm$ 27 (672 $\pm$ 34) (Girault *et al.*, 1998). Cd-lipid binding was observed to involve electrostatic interactions and more specifically, the phosphate group (Girault *et al.*, 1998). Fluorescence polarization experiments showed that the T_m increased for DPPG, DPPS, and bovine brain PS MLV systems in the presence of Cd (II) at R_i = [lipid]/[Cd] = 2. However, the gel-to-fluid phase transitions for DPPA, DPPS and DMPC/egg PC MLVs were suppressed with excess Cd (R_i=0.5). Salt concentrations of 0.8 and 1.8 M were used to reverse Cd-lipid interactions. Cd (II) affinities for negatively charged headgroups were determined as follows: PS>>PA>PG, due to the formation of $CdCl_n$ species (Girault *et al.*, 1998). Moreover, isotropic ^{31}P-NMR peaks, indicating non-lamellar phase formation, were observed for PG and the hexagonal phase was observed for egg PE lipid systems in the presence of Cd (II) at 24°C, suggesting that the membrane has been reorganized. Hexagonal phase formation of egg PE has important toxicological implications as this lipid phase is involved in fusion and transport processes (Girault *et al.*, 1998).

Fluorescence quenching studies have used MLVs of single and two-component lipid mixtures to investigate Hg-lipid interactions. Egg PC and bovine brain PS extracts were used in the following membrane models: 100% PC, 100% PS, 25% PS / 75% PC, and 50% PS / 50% PC (Boudou *et al.*, 1982). Pyrene fluorescence labels were used to assess the accessibility of the bilayer core for mercury compounds, as the ratio of monomer and excimer emission peaks was used to determine the fluidity. At pH 9.5, CH_3HgCl quenched pyrene better than $HgCl_2$ with increasing PS concentration whereas $HgCl_2$ quenching occurred at a pH of 5.0 (Boudou *et al.*, 1982). In addition to the lipid composition and the charge of the polar headgroup, pH was determined to be an important factor affecting both the nature of the membrane and the species of mercury present (Boudou *et al.*, 1982).

MLVs of DPPC, egg PC, DMPA, bovine PS, DMPS, DPPG and binary mixtures of egg PC/DMPE (1:1) and DPPC/Stearoylamine (SA) (1:1) and fluorescence polarization were used to study the effects of $HgCl_2$ (Delnomdedieu *et al.*, 1989). Phase transitions of model systems containing bovine PS, DMPS or DMPE were abolished with 0.5-1 mM of Hg (II), which was attributed to interactions with the primary amine groups. The charge of the phospholipids was not involved since all three systems took this into account i.e. neutral (DMPE), negative (bovine PS, DMPS) or positive (DPPC/SA). In contrast, the T_m of DPPC/PS (60:40) vesicles in the presence of Hg (II) were interpreted as a charge interaction (Bevan *et al.*, 1983).

In a follow up study, ^{199}Hg-NMR was used to look at $HgCl_2$ binding to MLVs of PE, PS and egg PC (Delnomdedieu *et al.*, 1992). Although not truly representative of the biological membrane, the single-lipid model systems used confirmed previous results that the amine group is a common binding site in PE and PS lipids (Delnomdedieu *et al.*, 1992). xxx

The same authors used PS MLVs to study the effects of $HgCl_2$ and $Hg(NO_3)_2$. According to the chemical speciation diagram for mercuric chloride at pH 5.8-6.0 and pCl 3.0, the $HgCl_2$ species is present. From the ^{199}Hg-NMR study, the dissociation of the $HgCl_2$ provides Hg^{2+} for PE and PS binding and the two Cl^- ions compete for binding with the Hg^{2+}. $Hg(NO_3)_2$ dissociation in water avoids Cl^- competition in order to observe Hg-lipid binding on its own (Delnomdedieu and Allis, 1993). DPH fluorescence polarization results indicated that the phase transition was abolished and fluidity decreased in the presence of 0.05-4.75 mM $HgCl_2$ and 0.066-0.6 mM $Hg(NO_3)_2$. Increasing concentrations of NaCl were also shown to affect the ability of Hg (II) to interact with lipid binding sites. 10 mM NaCl prevented membrane perturbations of 0.5 mM $HgCl_2$ at pH 5.5 but only partially suppressed it at pH 7.1. Chloride ions do not compete with lipid binding sites when the amino group is deprotonated at neutral pH. The study by Delnomdedieu et al. is one of the very few that utilize both model systems and extracted erythrocyte membranes to look at Hg (II) interactions (Delnomdedieu and Allis, 1993). Data from the model systems were consistent with those from sonicated rat erythrocyte ghosts, showing that single-lipid MLVs can be useful in DPH fluorescence polarization experiments. The presence of Chol and proteins in the biological membrane did not offset the fluidity changes of the lipid bilayer induced by Hg (II) (Delnomdedieu and Allis, 1993). Fluidity will subsequently affect permeability and potentially the osmotic fragility of erythrocytes.

2.2.2 Heavy metals and neurotoxic cations: micelles

Both natural and synthetic lipids can be used to make micelles, with the latter being more widely used. Girault et al. used micelles and ^{31}P-NMR to study Hg (II) binding to lipid headgroups (Girault *et al.*, 1995; Girault *et al.*, 1996). Micelles (15 mM lipid) were prepared by Triton X-100 addition (10% w/v) to multilamellar vesicles. ^{31}P-NMR spectra were obtained for single lipid systems (PE, PS and PC) and binary lipid systems (PE/PC or PE+PC and PS/PC or PS+PC). Mixed micelles (phospholipid 1/phospholipid 2, 15 mM each) were prepared by mixing and stirring both lipid aliquots in chloroform, which was then evaporated, dispersed in acetate buffer and solubilized with Triton X-100. In the second method (phospholipid 1+phospholipid 2 micelles), each lipid was separately prepared in the same manner as the phospholipid 1/phospholipid 2, before being mixed to obtain 15 mM of each lipid. In the absence of Hg, the chemical shift values for PE, PS and PC were +0.30, +0.15 and -0.40 ppm respectively. However, in the presence of $HgCl_2$, peak areas decreased for all lipids with stronger effects for PE and PS compared to PC. Interestingly, a +0.30 ppm upfield shift, indicative of Hg-lipid phosphate interactions, was observed for PS in the presence of $HgCl_2$ but no chemical shifts occurred for PC and PE (James, 1975). PE and PC micelles show no change in the chemical shift because it is speculated that the distance between the phosphate and Hg binding moiety (amine group) is greater compared to PS due to different headgroup structure (Girault *et al.*, 1995; Girault *et al.*, 1996). Furthermore, binary micelles (PE/PC or PE+PC and PS/PC or PS+PC) showed a reduction in ^{31}P-NMR peak areas when $HgCl_2$ was added and MLVs (PS/PC and PE/PC) showed a decrease in chemical shift anisotropy values, again exemplifying Hg (II) specificity for PE and PS lipid headgroups, independent of the type of model system used (Girault *et al.*, 1995; Girault *et al.*, 1996).

A PE/PS lipid model system would allow the observed effect of Hg (II) binding to two different lipid headgroups. Unfortunately, this system could not be used because of the overlap of signal using ^{31}P-NMR. The use of more complex lipid systems is limited by the capabilities of the physicochemical technique employed. Nonetheless, ^{31}P-NMR was able to determine that approximately 85% of $HgCl_2$ bound to phospholipids within 15 minutes, strongly suggesting that this metal adsorption to the lipid portion also occurs on the surface of biological membranes. Girault et al. also used egg yolk PC and DPPC micelles to show choline-specific binding by $HgCl_2$ (Girault *et al.*, 1996). This interaction was observed to be independent of acyl chain composition and more importantly, the Hg (II) affinity for PC is much less than for PE and PS. Delnomdedieu et al. were unable to detect any interactions between Hg (II) and the PC lipid headgroup using ^{199}Hg-NMR because of the higher concentrations of Hg (II) needed which may have masked the decrease in PC signal (Delnomdedieu *et al.*, 1992; Girault *et al.*, 1996).

In addition, natural membranes have also been used to produce micelle systems. Brush-border membranes isolated from pig jejunum epithelial cells were solubilized with Triton X-100 to form micelle models and were used to study the effect of zinc and cadmium ions on membrane structure (Tacnet *et al.*, 1991). ^{31}P-NMR spectra of the micelles in the absence and presence of Zn^{2+} and Cd^{2+} showed both interacting with negatively charged PI and PS but they have different effects on enzymatic phospholipid degradation: Zn^{2+} was observed to prevent lipid hydrolysis whereas Cd^{2+} greatly altered the lipid structure.

2.2.3 Heavy metals and neurotoxic cations: monolayers

Monolayers using animal cephalin have been used to study the effects of Hg^{2+} and Cd^{2+} (Suzuki and Matsushita, 1969). With as little as 10^{-7} M for Hg^{2+} and 10^{-8} M for Cd^{2+}, these heavy metals were not only observed to expand the monolayer but $C_{1/2}$ values calculated (the metal ion concentration giving half of the maximum pressure change) showed a linear correlation between logarithms of $C_{1/2}$ values and logarithms of the acute lethal doses of the metal chlorides in rabbits or rats (Suzuki and Matsushita, 1969).

Single component lipid monolayers of DPPG, DPPC, lyso-PC, and SM have also been utilized to observe interactions of Hg ions with membrane phospholipids (Broniatowski *et al.*, 2010). In the presence of 500 μM $HgCl_2$ in the aqueous subphase, mercury ions were observed to interact more strongly to SM and lyso-PC monolayers. Although DPPC, lyso-PC and SM share the choline headgroup, different lipid backbone and side chain architecture also plays an important role in lipid-metal interactions.

Fatty acids such as stearic acid, octadecylamine, octadecanol, and octadecane-1-thiol monolayers have also been used to study Hg^{2+} binding at the membrane surface (Broniatowski and Dynarowicz-Latka, 2009). Hg^{2+} not only interacted with the -SH group but also with -COOH and $-NH_2$ groups which can be found in proteins and membrane lipids. Moreover, behenic acid (C22:0) monolayers have been used to study heavy metals (Dupres *et al.*, 2003). Cd^{2+} concentrations were varied from 10^{-7} to 10^{-2} M and experiments were carried out at three different subphase pHs: 5.5, 7.5 and 10.5. Pressure-area isotherms revealed that the packing density of the monolayer increased upon Cd^{2+} interaction.

2.2.4 Heavy metals and neurotoxic cations: black lipid membranes (BLMs)

The toxicant must cross cell membranes if it is to be distributed throughout the organism i.e. within erythrocytes circulating in the blood, storage cells in the target organs etc. (Boudou *et al.*, 1982). This process is dependent on membrane composition and surface charge, the ion size and speciation, and the external and internal environment in terms of pH and temperature (Boudou *et al.*, 1982). Hence, permeability studies provide insight on how toxicants exert membrane toxicity.

BLMs have been useful to study metal transport. Diphytanoyl-PC in decane (20 mg/mL) has been used to investigate Cd^{2+} and Tl^{+} permeability through the lipid membrane (Gutknecht, 1983). Permeability coefficients for the metal ions were Cd^{2+} (<1.1 x 10^{-11} cm/s) > Tl^{+} (1.8 x 10^{-11} cm/s) > Hg^{2+} (<3.8 x 10^{-11} cm/s) (Gutknecht, 1983). For neutral complexes, the permeability coefficient order was $HgCl_2$ (1.3 x 10^{-2} cm/s) > TlCl (1.1 x 10^{-6} cm/s) > $CdCl_2$ (4.1 x 10^{-8} cm/s) (Gutknecht, 1981; Gutknecht, 1983). The low permeabilities of $CdCd_2$ and TlCl are attributed to the more polar and ionic nature of these metals in comparison to $HgCl_2$ which is more nonpolar and covalent (Gutknecht, 1981).

Binary egg lecithin/Chol (1:1) BLMs have been used to study the diffusion of Hg^{2+}, the effects of chloride concentration and pH (Gutknecht, 1981). The ^{203}Hg tracer and conductance measurements were used to determine membrane permeabilities for the different Hg forms. For example, $HgCl_2$ is highly permeant with a permeability coefficient of approximately 10^{-2} cm·sec^{-1} which is 20 times higher than water and a million times more than Na^{+}, K^{+} and Cl^{-} (Gutknecht, 1981). The lecithin/Chol bilayer in a 1:1 ratio is a suitable model for erythrocyte membranes which shows how easily Hg^{2+} can cross the membrane, where it can subsequently lead to toxic events.

Membrane solutions containing egg PC, PS, PC/Chol or PC/PS mixtures (2% w/w of each component in n-decane) were used to study the $HgCl_2$ and CH_3HgCl transport through BLMs (Bienvenue *et al.*, 1984). It was shown that both mercury compounds cross the membrane in their neutral forms in which pH and salt play an important role. The same lipid model systems were used to monitor quenching interactions between mercury and pyrene that showed the importance of charge (Boudou *et al.*, 1982). The fluorophore pyrene embedded in PS-containing lipid systems was quenched by Hg^{2+} (Boudou *et al.*, 1982).

Initially, mercurial compounds are attracted by the charges in the membrane but then neutralization occurs, facilitating the transport of mercury compounds such as $HgCl_2$ and CH_3HgCl across the membrane (Bienvenue *et al.*, 1984). At pH 9.5 and low chloride concentrations, $HgCl_2$ is in the $Hg(OH)_2$ form whereas the chloride form is the main species found at pH 5.0 with small amounts of $HgOH^{+}$, $HgCl^{+}$, $HgCl_4^{2-}$, and $HgCl^{3-}$ (Hahne and Kroontje, 1973; Shin and Krenkel, 1976). CH_3HgCl is in the chloride form at pH 5.0 and CH_3HgOH at pH 9.5 with small quantities of CH_3Hg^{+} found at both pH values (Shin and Krenkel, 1976). In the PC/Chol BLM, diffusion decreased by 89% with $HgCl_2$ and 36% with CH_3HgCl when the pH was changed from 5.0 to 9.5 (Bienvenue *et al.*, 1984).

It was also hypothesized that translocation through the bilayer is limited by interactions at the membrane-solution interface after adsorption takes place (Bienvenue *et al.*, 1984). Diffusion of the mercurial compounds was observed to be PC < PC/Chol < PC/PS for $HgCl_2$ and PC/PS < PC < PC/Chol for CH_3HgCl. Chol, which usually decreases the permeability of the lipid bilayer, was shown to increase the permeability in this study (Bienvenue *et al.*, 1984). The presence of PS slightly increases the diffusion for $HgCl_2$ but not for CH_3HgCl. Increasing concentrations of NaCl decreased the transport of $HgCl_2$. Overall, neutrally charged $HgCl_2$ and CH_3HgCl were shown to cross the lipid bilayer and that the permeability of both mercury compounds was dependent on pH and chloride conditions (Bienvenue *et al.*, 1984).

The various lipid model systems have provided further insight as to how metals exert toxicity. Lipid-metal interactions are pH- and salt-dependent, affecting both the nature of the lipid and metal speciation. This is followed by the transport across the membrane where metals can subsequently interact with other intracellular components resulting in permeability changes, leakage etc.

2.3 Drugs

Research has focused on the determination of the physiological activity and how drugs influence the cell membrane e.g. transport, distribution, accumulation etc. In certain diseases, cell lipid composition may be altered. Examples shown below illustrate how biomimetic lipid systems can help in the design of better drugs.

2.3.1 Drugs: vesicles

Ellipticine [5,11-dimethyl-6H-pyrido(4,3-b)-carbazole] and its derivatives have been studied as potential cancer chemotherapy agents by using liposome model systems (Terce *et al.*, 1982; Terce *et al.*, 1983). MLVs of DMPG and DMPG/DPPC (8 μM and 5 μM) and SUVs of DPPG or DPPC were used as membrane models in addition to the natural *Micrococcus luteus* membrane (18% dimannosyldiglyceride, 65% cardiolipin, 12% PG and 5% phosphatidylinositol) to study the effects of Ellipticine (Terce *et al.*, 1982). UV spectra revealed that the drug stays in the hydrophobic environment and not in the aqueous medium. Ellipticine not only interacted with PG in a 1:1 ratio but at a pH of 10, the drug was not released from the lipid phase, emphasizing the importance of both electrostatic and hydrophobic interactions. In a subsequent study, PS/PC vesicles were used in electrophoretic mobility measurements at a 4:1 and permeability assays at 1:1 ratio to observe the effects of Ellipticine and its derivatives: amphiphilic 9-methoxyellipticine and dipolar 9-amino- and 9-hydroxyellipticine compounds. Electrophoretic measurements revealed that the drug-derivatives neutralized the surface charge almost completely, indicative of drug interactions with the membrane surface. Once the electrostatic barrier is lowered, the drugs can exert cytotoxic effects, leading to increased permeability. The fluorescence of 6-carboxyfluorescein was used to monitor dye leakage from liposomes and both 9-methoxyellipticine and 9-hydroxyellipticine increased dye leakage, although stronger effects were observed with the former. Maximum leakage was observed for 2×10^{-5} M 9-methoxyellipticine with liposome and resealed ghost models (Terce *et al.*, 1983).

2.3.2 Drugs: monolayers

Interactions of cyclosporine A (CsA) with the membrane have been investigated using binary mixtures of PC and Chol in monolayers (Soderlund *et al.*, 1999). CsA is a hydrophobic drug that is used to prevent graft rejections after organ transplants. Monolayers were prepared in circular wells drilled in Teflon and CsA penetration was indicated by surface pressure changes using the Wilhelmy plate method. The effect of CsA on the lateral distribution of the fluorescence probe 1-palmitoyl-2-(N-4-nitrobenz-2-oxa-1,3-diazol) aminocaproyl-PC (NBD-PC) in lipid monolayers was also studied using fluorescence microscopy. These experiments showed rapid insertion of CsA into egg PC and egg PC/Chol (1:1) monolayers as indicated by the increase in surface pressure. These changes, compared to the initial surface pressure, showed biphasic interactions of CsA with both types of monolayers. But Söderlund et al. showed that the morphology of lipid domains was dependent on the composition. NBD-PC is a useful fluorescent probe as it partitions into the boundaries between fluid and gel regions, imaged as light and dark areas in the fluorescence microscope (Soderlund *et al.*, 1999). Dark areas contain very small amounts of NBD-PC. CsA was observed to change NBD-PC distribution in DPPC/β-Chol (88:10) mixtures compared to DPPC monolayers (Soderlund *et al.*, 1999).

DPPC monolayers have also been used to mimic the surfactant layer lining the surface of the lung alveoli in order to study the interactions with gelatin based nanoparticles for the purposes of drug delivery (Lai *et al.*, 2010). Using Brewster angle microscopy, the nanoparticles were shown to change the shape and reduce the size of the DPPC domains, thus these propensities need to be considered for potential pulmonary drug vehicles.

2.4 Antimicrobial peptides

Increased bacterial resistance to antibiotics has encouraged the investigation of other antibacterial approaches for biomedical research, including antimicrobial peptides (AMPs). They are generally short, amphiphilic structures containing 12-100 residues with several of those residues being positively charged (Jenssen *et al.*, 2006). AMPs decrease bacterial viability through several mechanisms, including altering gene expression, inhibiting nuclease activity, and by disrupting the bacterial membrane (Hui and Sen, 1989; Epand and Vogel, 1999; Jenssen *et al.*, 2006). AMPs do not interact with specific membrane receptors, but directly with the negatively charged bacterial membrane in many different ways e.g. by creating pores or regional disintegration, by acting as detergents or by disruption of the membrane potential (Epand and Vogel, 1999; Lohner and Prenner, 1999; Bechinger and Lohner, 2006). Among the most common methods to study the effects of membrane-disrupting antimicrobial peptides are dye leakage assays from bacterial membrane mimetic systems.

2.4.1 Antimicrobial peptides: vesicle controls

Vesicles are widely used models to investigate the structure of membrane-bound antimicrobial peptides (Mani *et al.*, 2006; Chongsiriwatana *et al.*, 2008; Sevcsik *et al.*, 2008; Tang and Hong, 2009). In particular, zwitterionic systems such as POPC LUVs have been used as a control mammalian system in the study of indolicidin and tritrpticin along with its derivatives (Andrushchenko *et al.*, 2008). ITC titrations of lipid suspension into peptide solutions revealed a stronger peptide binding affinity for POPE/POPG and *E. coli* membrane systems compared to the mammalian one.

Binary mixtures of egg PC/Chol (10:1) in SUVs have served as useful controls in the study of melittin diastereomers (Oren and Shai, 1997). LUVs of POPC/Chol (1:1) and POPE/POPG (3:1) mimic erythrocyte and bacterial membranes and have been used to study protegrin-1 (PG-1) (Mani *et al.*, 2006). This peptide is a disulfide-linked, β-hairpin antimicrobial peptide that is isolated from pig leukocytes (Kokryakov *et al.*, 1993). ^{1}H solid state NMR showed that PG-1 interacts with lipid acyl chains and headgroups in the bacteria-mimetic POPE/POPG (3:1) indicating peptide insertion in contrast to POPC/Chol (1:1) bilayers (Mani *et al.*, 2006). Furthermore, ^{19}F spin diffusion experiments indicated that PG-1 assembles into $(NCCN)_n$ multimers suggesting a β-barrel structure which is surrounding a water pore in the bacterial mimetic membrane. However, the N and C strands of PG-1 organize into tetramers, suggesting that β-sheets form at the mammalian erythrocyte membrane surface.

More complex three- and four-component mixtures have also been used i.e. POPC/POPE/Chol (65:25:10) in the absence and presence of 10% POPS prepared by freeze-thaw cycles and extrusion to study the effects of c[D-Pen^{2},D-Pen^{5}] enkephalin (DPDPE) and biphalin and to show how electrostatic interactions impact peptide permeability in the membrane (Romanowski *et al.*, 2002). DPDPE is a zwitterionic, cyclic enkephalin analogue whereas biphalin is a cationic, dimeric peptide. For the permeability assay, the sample of liposome encapsulated peptides were dialyzed and the amount of peptide released into the buffer was determined by a fluorescence assay, which measured the reaction product from the peptide amino group with fluorescamine (ex380/em475) (Romanowski *et al.*, 2002). Partition coefficients were obtained using equilibrium dialysis experiments and the fluorescence measurements of the peptide Tyr and Trp residues (Romanowski *et al.*, 1997). Interestingly, increased surface charge by addition of POPS showed increased biphalin binding but reduced translocation of the peptide across the bilayer. Conversely, only a small decrease in permeability was observed for DPDPE with increased negative charge. These results show how the negative charges in the biological membrane can affect peptide membrane transport processes and must be taken into account when designing peptide drugs (Romanowski *et al.*, 2002).

2.4.2 Antimicrobial peptides: monolayer controls

Monolayers have become important tools to investigate antimicrobial peptide interactions with the lipid membrane (Maget-Dana, 1999). Single lipids such as DPPC and DPPG have been used in monolayers (20 μL of a 0.5 g/L) to see if peptide interactions occurred (Lad *et al.*, 2007). Melittin is a non-specific membrane peptide whereas magainin II and cecropin P1 are known to specifically interact with prokaryotic cell membranes. Surface pressure-area isotherms of the lipid monolayers were obtained in the absence of the various peptides. The barriers were then fixed in position to obtain the desired surface pressure and the peptide solution was then introduced into the subphase through a custom-made metal tube incorporated below the buffer surface. A greater increase in surface pressure indicated binding between the lipid headgroup and the cationic peptide. The melittin, and the antimicrobial peptides magainin II and cecropin P1 (0.7 μM) were shown to interact more with DPPG over DPPC monolayers (Lad *et al.*, 2007).

Mixtures of POPC/Chol have also been used to test synthetic peptides Phd1-3, which span the carboxy-terminal region of human β-defensins HBD 1-3 (Krishnakumari and Nagaraj, 2008). The peptide analogues have a single disulfide bridge and have exhibited antibacterial activity. No significant increase in pressure in POPC/Chol (7:3) was observed for all three peptides in contrast to POPC/POPG (7:3) indicating no interaction with the mammalian model (Krishnakumari *et al.*, 2006).

3. Applications of bacterial membrane models

As previously discussed, different lipid composition can alter the physical and chemical characteristics of the membrane. The changes in behaviour exhibited in the different model systems provide information on the mechanism of action exhibited by these peptides upon interaction with natural bacterial membranes. Illustrated below are several examples of biomimetic systems used to study bacterial membranes, with a focus on antimicrobial peptides and the membrane protein EmrE. While these examples are by no means an exhaustive list of the systems used, they serve to illustrate how different lipid compositions can be used.

3.1.1 Antimicrobial peptides: vesicles

Using a simplified model system to represent the bacterial cell facilitates the study and thus the understanding of the complicated molecular interactions involved in antimicrobial activity. Vesicles have been widely used to study the effect of lipid composition on the ability of AMPs to disrupt the membrane. Dye leakage assays take advantage of the encapsulation properties of vesicles and have been extensively used for testing the activity of AMPs on model membranes. Biomimetic vesicles are loaded with a fluorescent dye, such as calcein, and assayed for AMP-induced leakage (Kendall and MacDonald, 1982; Patel *et al.*, 2009). Differences in AMP activity in response to different mimetics can be assayed by the extent of dye release.

One of the interesting aspects is the understanding of the mechanism through which AMPs differentiate between target and host membranes, thereby avoiding or minimizing host toxicity. A major factor is the increased abundance of anionic lipids in bacterial membranes compared to eukaryotes, giving the cell an overall negative charge providing a natural electrostatic target for the cationic AMPs. A calcein leakage assay was used to study the effects of lipid charge on the activity of magainin, a widely characterized AMP (Matsuzaki *et al.*, 1989) whereby magainin induced significant leakage in negatively charged PS vesicles, compared to neutral PC vesicles or positive 9:1 (mol/mol) PC/SA. The negatively charged bacterial lipid PG behaved in a similar manner to the PS, emphasizing the importance of an electrostatic interaction with the positively charged AMP (Matsuzaki *et al.*, 1989; Lohner and Prenner, 1999).

A more accurate representation of the *E. coli* membrane was provided by using a headgroup ratio of 75:20:5 POPE/DPPG/CL in SUVs and LUVs (Glukhov *et al.*, 2005) to study the differential targeting of novel cationic AMPs to bacterial versus mammalian membranes. They found that the initial attraction between the positive AMP and negatively charged bacterial membranes was an important component of bacterial/mammalian selectivity. DSC has been used to elucidate the impact of the peptide interactions on the physical properties of the membrane, specifically the effect of AMP binding on the lipid phase transitions from gel to liquid crystalline (Prenner *et al.*, 1999). Using PC, PE, and PG vesicles, it was found that gramicidin S reduced the temperature and increased the cooperativity of the main phase transition of PG, but had moderate effects on the phase behaviour of PC, and practically no effect on PE (Prenner *et al.*, 1999). From these results, it follows that AMPs interact differently with the various lipid species, and that specific lipid interactions may be important for activity.

Along with the negative charge of the membranes, there are other components that could enable AMP differentiation between host and target membranes. In the presence of gramicidin S, a strong antimicrobial peptide, vesicles containing (4:1 mol/mol) PC/Chol showed less dye leakage than PC vesicles alone (Prenner *et al.*, 2001). Vesicles composed of 3:1 POPE/POPG were used to monitor the effect of zwitterionic phospholipids and sterols on membrane destabilization by the synthetic AMP pleurocidin-amide (Mason *et al.*, 2007). These authors also found that the presence of sterols can reduce AMP destabilization of a membrane, even if the membrane has anionic character. This decreased activity in Chol-containing vesicles could be a possible mechanism for the selectivity of antimicrobial peptides, explaining why AMPs are highly selective towards bacterial membranes, which do not contain sterols (Mason *et al.*, 2007).

There are several other factors that are involved in the lipid-protein interaction in the membrane, including the properties of the AMPs themselves. In 2001, Zhang et al. studied whether AMPs with varying structures and activities had similar mechanisms of action for inducing membrane leakage, as well as lipid redistribution and peptide translocation (Zhang *et al.*, 2001). They measured AMP-induced lipid flip-flop in unilamellar PG/PC (1:1) vesicles (in 10 mM Tris-HCl, 150 mM NaCl, and 1 mM NaEDTA, pH 7.5) asymmetrically labeled with 0.5 mol% C_6-NBD-PC in the inner leaflet. Calcein release was tested as a measure of membrane leakiness, and also taken as a control to ensure that the lipid flip flop observed was not simply due to bilayer disruption. Peptide translocation was measured using chymotrypsin-entrapped LUVs of 50% egg PC, 45% egg PG, and 5% dansyl-PE (in 150 mM NaCl, 20 mM HEPES, pH 7.4). It was determined that lipid flip-flop, membrane leakiness, and peptide translocation could not individually be related to AMP structure or charge, concluding that many factors must be involved in AMP activity which have a varying impact on membranes (Zhang *et al.*, 2001). In a detailed investigation, it was shown that the ability of gramicidin S to differentiate between mammalian and bacterial membranes depended on many peptide parameters as well, such as solubility, beta-sheet content, self-aggregation propensity, hydrophobicity and amphiphilicity (Prenner *et al.*, 2005).

These examples illustrate how changing the properties of the model system can illuminate the interactions involved. Not all lipid systems used as bacterial models reflect the natural composition of a bacterial membrane, yet these models have been used to provide valuable information in regards to the behaviour and influence of AMPs on the membrane. Synthetic polydiacetylene (PDA) has been used in combination with lipids in bacterial membrane mimetics because of its colorimetric properties (Kolusheva *et al.*, 2000). PDA monomers are similar in structure to lipids, and vesicles exhibit colorimetric blue-red transitions when exposed to several environmental perturbations, including changes in surface pressure. When mixed with PDA, lipids tend to form bilayers in interspersed, segregated phases, creating a convenient model system of the lipid bilayer. Kolushiva et al. used 3:1:6 PE/PG/PDA and 3:1:6 PE/CL/PDA vesicles to create a simple screening assay to study the interaction of AMPs with the membrane (Kolusheva *et al.*, 2000). Using colorimetric analyses, the insertion of AMPs into the membrane was found to depend on bilayer composition, with higher insertion into the PG-containing system, consistent with observed biological data for levels of antimicrobial activity.

3.1.2 Antimicrobial peptides: monolayer

Although vesicles are a useful membrane mimetic for studying antimicrobial activity, other mimetic systems have provided valuable data, including monolayers. An increase in the surface pressure of a lipid monolayer at the air-water interface has been used as an indicator for AMP insertion and a method to study the probability of membrane disruption as the mechanism of action for different AMPs. In a fairly accurate representation of the headgroup ratio of *E. coli* phospholipids, Zhang et al. created a 78 : 4.7 : 14.4 PE/egg PG/CL mimic of the *E. coli* inner membrane, and studied the interaction of several natural and synthetic AMPs with the mixture as well as the individual monolayer constituents (Zhang *et al.*, 2001). Increasing peptide concentration resulted in a sigmoidal increase in the surface pressure of the mixture, indicating peptide insertion which is likely a cooperative event. As expected, the AMPs interacted more strongly with anionic monolayers, especially egg PG. Most of their AMPs had minimal interaction with zwitterionic lipids, however a few exceptions indicated that electrostatic interactions are not the only attraction between cationic AMPs and negatively charged bacterial membranes.

Planar lipid films have also been used combined with Brewster angle microscopy (BAM) to image the interaction of several AMPs with monolayers (Volinski *et al.*, 2006). While two AMPs were immiscible in 1:1 ratios of peptide:DMPC, valinomycin showed phase-separation in the monolayer. BAM was used to image valinomycin-induced changes to the lateral film architecture in 1:1 DMPC/PDA. Further characterization using fluorescent NBD-PE and confocal microscopy also revealed significant changes to the DMPC-PDA membrane mimetic film (0.2 : 0.8 : 9 NBD-PE/DMPC/PDA) upon peptide addition since some AMPs preferentially formed distinct domains within the phospholipid portion of the mixed monolayer. Thus, phospholipid-PDA systems could be used, especially in conjunction with BAM, to elucidate surface phenomena of lipid-AMP interactions (Volinski *et al.*, 2006).

3.1.3 Antimicrobial peptides: supported bilayer

Understanding the mechanism through which AMPs disrupt the membrane requires insight into the orientation of the peptide within the lipid bilayer, which can be obtained by using supported lipid bilayers. These are two layers of lipids deposited as a bilayer onto a solid support, such as a glass slide, silica beads, or muscovite. An advantage of supported bilayers is their long-term durability and the ability for high definition imaging techniques due to their stable orientation (Henzler Wildman *et al.*, 2003; Davis *et al.*, 2009). Characterization methods include atomic force microscopy, solid-state NMR, and several fluorescence microscopy techniques (Henzler Wildman *et al.*, 2003).

Oriented lipid bilayers on glass plates were used to study the structure and mechanism of membrane disruption of LL-37, a human antimicrobial peptide that may be important in treating cystic fibrosis (Henzler Wildman *et al.*, 2003). Solid-state NMR was used to compare the orientation of LL-37 in zwitterionic DMPC and anionic DMPG to get insight into the potential mechanism of action. Although LL-37 showed no difference in surface orientation between the two systems, the cationic peptide exhibited greater disruption towards anionic bilayers. Moreover, when the two zwitterionic matrices POPC and POPE were compared LL-37 was more disruptive towards the smaller PE.

Comparisons between PC/PG and the more *E. coli*-like PE/PG systems were made using binary 4:1 (mol:mol) mixtures, whereby PE/PG behaved more like *E. coli* lipid extract. The role of acyl chain saturation was determined using monounsaturated and fully saturated PC and PG lipids, with an increase in membrane disruption in the less fluid, fully saturated bilayer. No effects of ionic strength or pH on LL-37 were observed. Combined with DSC results, these data suggest that LL-37 adopts the toroidal-pore model of membrane disruption (Henzler Wildman *et al.*, 2003).

3.2 Membrane proteins

The investigation of membrane protein insertion or orientation in model systems involves many experimental difficulties due to their hydrophobic nature, already severely limiting their purification. Thus, much less is known about membrane protein structure and function, or even the basic question such as their orientation within a membrane.

There are, however, a few proteins that have been purified and studied more extensively. For these membrane proteins, various lipid and detergent systems have been used to provide a hydrophobic environment to study their structure and function. For example, the structure and organization of the transmembrane retinal proteins rhodopsin and bacteriorhodopsin, as well as the conformation and activity of *E. coli* multidrug resistance protein EmrE, have been studied in several membrane mimetics (see below). However, as previously discussed, lipid composition may alter the physical characteristics of a membrane and affect how membrane proteins behave.

3.2.1 Membrane proteins: liposomes

SUVs have been used to study folding and ligand binding of membrane proteins. Native lipid vesicles have been used to investigate the refolding mechanisms of the well-studied *Halobacterium* retinal protein bacteriorhodopsin by circular dichroism and absorption spectroscopy (Popot *et al.*, 1987). Denatured by SDS before renaturing into lipid vesicles, a two-stage refolding mechanism of bacteriorhodopsin was determined since stable transmembrane helices are formed first before structural rearrangement results in the proper tertiary structure (Popot *et al.*, 1987). Later fluorescence spectroscopy studies using DPPC vesicles, and micelles composed of DMPC and the detergent CHAPS or DMPC/DHPC (di-7:0-PC) show that bacteriorhodopsin forms two intermediate folding stages followed by two-step retinal binding to form native bacteriorhodopsin (Booth, 2000).

The rate of protein folding and insertion is affected by membrane characteristics, particularly the lateral pressure profile of the bilayer. As some lipid species prefer to form non-bilayer structures, their presence increases the lateral chain pressure. Using PC liposomes and increasing amounts of non-bilayer PE, a decrease in the rate of bacteriorhodopsin folding/insertion was found corresponding to the increase in lateral chain pressure (Curran *et al.*, 1999). Similarly, longer acyl chains and thus increased chain pressure decreased the rate of bacteriorhodopsin folding (Booth *et al.*, 1997). Hence systematical alteration of liposome composition allows for the assessment of the effects of each lipid.

SUVs have also been used to assay binding affinity and conformation of the integral membrane protein EmrE, a multidrug resistance transporter found in *E. coli* (Federkeil *et al.*, 2003; Sikora and Turner, 2005). Although EmrE solubilized into SUVs composed of *E. coli* lipid extracts is the best mimic of its natural membrane, detergents such as sodium-dodecyl-sulfate (SDS) and N-dodecyl-β-D-maltoside (DM) have been used as well as membrane mimetics. Fluorescence spectroscopy and circular dichroism were utilized to monitor the conformation of EmrE in different detergents and organic mimetic systems such as SDS, ethanol, and urea (Federkeil *et al.*, 2003). Trp fluorescence spectra of EmrE in such systems were compared to EmrE in SUVs composed of *E. coli* polar extract, whereby the DM systems had similar spectral properties to the bacterial lipid vesicles. While the secondary structure was similar for all systems, the tertiary structure of EmrE depended more on the environment based on the mobility and exposure of Trps (Federkeil *et al.*, 2003).

Moreover, ITC experiments of ligand binding to EmrE solubilized in *E. coli* extract SUVs or in either SDS or DM micelles were performed to determine the binding constant and stoichiometry for several ligands (Sikora and Turner, 2005). Both SUVs and micelles showed weak and non-specific binding of EmrE for its ligands. In addition, while multimerization is important for its ligand/proton anti-transport, these results suggest that EmrE monomers bind the ligand in a 1:1 ratio (Bay *et al.*, 2010).

3.2.2 Membrane proteins: monolayers

One of the major concerns of studying membrane proteins in monolayers has been protein denaturation due to the lack of a second, outer leaflet. However, it has been shown that under certain conditions, some proteins indeed maintain their native secondary structure and activity in these systems. Parameters such as initial surface pressure, compression speed and temperature influence protein stability in monolayers, and some proteins are more susceptible to denaturation than others (Boucher *et al.*, 2007). Infrared spectroscopy showed that the retinal membrane protein bacteriorhodopsin maintained its native secondary structure under varying experimental conditions (see above), while the related rhodopsin was more susceptible to denaturation (Lavoie *et al.*, 1999). However, upon spreading at higher initial surface pressure rhodopsin maintained its structural integrity. These are only a few examples of model systems used to study membrane proteins but they demonstrate how properly selected membrane biomimetics and experimental conditions allow the elucidation of the biophysical characteristics of lipid-membrane protein interactions.

4. Conclusion

Lipid models have enabled e.g. the study of lipid-lipid and lipid-protein interactions by mimicking the composition, curvature, electrostatic potential or permeability properties of biological membranes. Their continuous improvement in terms of complexity will further increase their suitability to reveal the structure and function of biological membranes and the multitude of processes and interactions involved. Thus, such systems provide an important tool for a more detailed understanding of structure and function of biomembranes and their interactions with biomolecules and drugs.

5. References

Akerman, K. E. O., and Nicholls, D. G. (1983). Ca^{2+} transport and the regulation of transmitter release in isolated nerve endings. *Trends Biochem. Sci.* 8, 63-64, 0968-0004.

Andrushchenko, V. V., Aarabi, M. H., Nguyen, L. T., Prenner, E. J., and Vogel, H. J. (2008). Thermodynamics of the interactions of tryptophan-rich cathelicidin antimicrobial peptides with model and natural membranes. *Biochim. Biophys. Acta* 1778, 1004-1014, 0006-3002.

Bay, D. C., Budiman, R. A., Nieh, M.-P., and Turner, R. J. (2010). Multimeric forms of small multidrug resistance protein EmrE in anionic detergent. *Biochim. Biophys. Acta* 1798, 526-535, 0006-3002.

Bechinger, B., and Lohner, K. (2006). Detergent-like actions of linear amphipathic cationic antimicrobial peptides. *Biochim. Biophys. Acta.* 1758, 1529-1539, 0006-3002.

Bettger, W. J., and O'Dell, B. L. (1981). A critical physiological role of zinc in the structure and function of biomembranes. *Life Sci.* 28, 1425-1438, 0024-3205.

Bevan, D. R., Worrell, W. J., and Barfield, K. D. (1983). The Interaction of Ca^{2+}, Mg^{2+}, Zn^{2+}, Cd^{2+}, and Hg^{2+} with Phospholipid Bilayer Vesicles. *Colloids and Surfaces* 6, 365-376,

Bienvenue, E., Boudou, A., Desmazes, J. P., Gavach, C., Georgescauld, D., Sandeaux, J., Sandeaux, R., and Seta, P. (1984). Transport of mercury compounds across bimolecular lipid membranes: effect of lipid composition, pH and chloride concentration. *Chem. Biol. Interact.* 48, 91-101, 0009-2797.

Birdi, K. S. (1988). *Lipid and Biopolymer Monolayers at Liquid Interfaces.* Plenum Press, 0306428709 9780306428708, New York.

Blume, A. (1985). Calorimetry of lipid model membranes. *Thermochimica Acta* 85, 469-472,

Booth, P. J. (2000). Unravelling the folding of bacteriorhodopsin. *Biochim. Biophys. Acta* 30, 4-14, 0006-3002.

Booth, P. J., Riley, M. L., Flitsch, S. L., Templer, R. H., Farooq, A., Curran, A. R., Chadborn, N., and Wright, P. (1997). Evidence that bilayer bending rigidity affects membrane protein folding. *Biochemistry* 36, 197-203, 0006-2960.

Boucher, J., Trudel, E., Methot, M., Desmeules, P., and Salesse, C. (2007). Organization, structure and activity of proteins in monolayers. *Colloids Surf. B Biointerfaces* 58, 73-90, 0927-7765.

Boudou, A., Desmazes, J. P., and Georgescauld, D. (1982). Fluorescence quenching study of mercury compounds and liposome interactions - effect of charged lipid and pH. *Ecotoxicol. Environ. Saf.* 6, 379-387, 0147-6513.

Broniatowski, M., and Dynarowicz-Latka, P. (2009). Search for the molecular mechanism of mercury toxicity. Study of the mercury (II)-surfactant complex formation in Langmuir monolayers. *J. Phys. Chem. B* 113, 4275-4283, 0022-3654.

Broniatowski, M., Flasinski, M., Dynarowicz-Latka, P., and Majewski, J. (2010). Grazing incidence diffraction and X-ray reflectivity studies of the interactions of inorganic mercury salts with membrane lipids in Langmuir monolayers at the air-water interface. *J. Phys. Chem.* 114, 9474-9484
0022-3654.

Chongsiriwatana, N. P., Patch, J. A., Czyzewski, A. M., Dohm, M. T., Ivankin, A., Gidalevitz, D., Zuckermann, R. N., and Barron, A. E. (2008). Peptoids that mimic the structure, function and mechansim of helical antimicrobial peptides. *Proc. Natl. Acad. Sci. U.S.A.* 105, 2794-2799, 0027-8424.

Cronan, J. E. (2003). Bacterial membrane lipids: where do we stand? .*Annu. Rev. Microbiol.* 57, 203-224, 0066-4227.

Cullis, P. R., Hope, M. J., and Tilcock, C. P. S. (1986). Lipid polymorphism and the roles of lipids in membranes. *Chem. Phys. Lipids* 40, 127-144, 0009-3084.

Curran, A. R., Templer, R. H., and Booth, P. J. (1999). Modulation of folding and assembly of the membrane protein bacteriorhodopsin by intermolecular forces within the lipid bilayer. *Biochemistry* 38, 9328-9336, 0006-2960.

Davis, R. W., Arango, D. C., Jones, H. D. T., Van Benthem, M. H., Haaland, D. M., Brozik, S. M., and Sinclair, M. B. (2009). Antimicrobial peptide interactions with silica bead supported bilayers and *E. coli*: burofin II, magainin II, and arenicin. *J. Pept. Sci.* 15, 511-522, 1075-2617.

de Kruijff, B. (1997). Lipid polymorphism and biomembrane function. *Curr. Opin. Chem. Biol.* 1, 564-569, 1367-5931.

Deleers, M., Servais, J. P., and Wulfert, E. (1986). Neurotoxic cations induce membrane rigidification and membrane fusion at micromolar concentrations. *Biochim. Biophys. Acta* 855, 271-276, 0006-3002.

Delnomdedieu, M., and Allis, J. W. (1993). Interaction of inorganic mercury salts with model and red cell membranes: importance of lipid-binding sites. *Chem. Biol. Interact.* 88, 71-87, 0009-2797.

Delnomdedieu, M., Boudou, A., Desmazes, J. P., and Georgescauld, D. (1989). Interaction of mercury chloride with the primary amine group of model membranes containing phosphatidylserine and phosphatidylethanolamine. *Biochim. Biophys. Acta* 986, 191-199, 0006-3002.

Delnomdedieu, M., Boudou, A., Georgescauld, D., and Dufourc, E. J. (1992). Specific interactions of mercury chloride with membranes and other ligands as revealed by mercury-NMR. *Chem. Biol. Interact.* 81, 243-269, 0009-2797.

Dowhan, D. (1997). Molecular basis for membrane phospholipid diversity: why are there so many lipids? *Annu. Rev. Biochem.* 66, 199-232, 0066-4154.

Dupres, V., Cantin, S., Benhabib, F., Perrot, F., Fontaine, P., Goldmann, M., Daillant, J., and Konovalov, O. (2003). Superlatttice formation of fatty acid monolayers on a divalent ion subphase: Role of chain length, temperature, and subphase concentration. *Langmuir* 19, 10808-10815, 0743-7463.

Eisele, K., Lang, P. A., Kempe, D. S., Klarl, B. A., Niemoller, O., Wieder, T., Huber, S. M., Duranton, C., and Lang, F. (2006). Stimulation of erythrocyte phosphatidylserine exposure by mercury ions. *Toxicol. Appl. Pharmacol.* 210, 116-122, 0041-008X.

Epand, R. M., and Vogel, H. J. (1999). Diversity of antimicrobial peptides and their mechanisms of action. *Biochim. Biophys. Acta* 1462, 11-28, 0006-3002.

Federkeil, S. L., Winstone, T. L., Jickling, G., and Turner, R. J. (2003). Examination of EmrE conformational differences in various membrane mimetic environments. *Biochem. Cell Biol.* 81, 61-70, 0829-8211.

Gailer, J. (2007). Arsenic-selenium and mercury-selenium bonds in biology. *Coord. Chem. Rev.* 251, 234-254, 0010-8545.

Girault, L., Boudou, A., and Dufourc, E. J. (1998). ^{113}Cd-, ^{31}P-NMR and fluorescence polarization studies of cadmium (II) interactions with phospholipids in model membranes. *Biochim. Biophys. Acta* 1414, 140-154, 0006-3002.

Girault, L., Lemaire, P., Boudou, A., Debouzy, J. C., and Dufourc, E. J. (1996). Interactions of inorganic mercury with phospholipid micelles and model membranes. A ^{31}P-NMR study. *Eur. Biophys. J.* 24, 413-421, 0175-7571.

Girault, L., Lemaire, P., Boudou, A., and Dufourc, E. J. (1995). Inorganic mercury interactions with lipid ocmponents of biological membranes: ^{31}P-NMR study of Hg(II) binding to headgroups of micellar phospholipids. *Water Air Soil Pollut.* 80, 95-98, 0049-6979.

Glukhov, E., Stark, M., Burrows, L. L., and Deber, C. M. (2005). Basis for selectivity of cationic antimicrobial peptides for bacterial *versus* mammalian membranes. *J. Biol. Chem.* 280, 33960-33967, 0021-9258.

Gutknecht, J. (1981). Inorganic mercury (Hg^{2+}) transport through lipid bilayer membranes. *J. Membr. Biol.* 61, 61-66, 0022-2631.

Gutknecht, J. (1983). Cadmium and thallous ion permeabilities through lipid bilayer membranes. *Biochim. Biophys. Acta* 735, 185-188, 0006-3002.

Hahne, H. C. H., and Kroontje, W. (1973). The simultaneous effect of pH and chloride concentrations upon mercury as a pollutant. *Soil Sci. Soc. Am. J.* 37, 838-843, 0361-5995.

Harder, T., Scheiffele, P., Verka, P., and Simons, K. (1998). Lipid domain stucture of the plasma membrane revealed by patching of membrane components. *J. Cell Biol.* 141, 929-942, 0021-9525.

Henzler Wildman, K. A., Lee, D.-K., and Ramamoorthy, A. (2003). Mechanism of lipid bilayer disruption by the human antimicrobial peptide, LL-37. *Biochemistry* 42, 6545-6558, 0006-2960.

Huff, J., Lunn, R. M., Waalkes, M. P., Tomatis, L., and Infante, P. F. (2007). Cadmium-induced cancers in animals and in humans. *Int J Occup Environ Health* 13, 202-212, 1077-3525.

Hui, S. W., and Sen, A. (1989). Effects of lipid packing on polymorphic phase behavior and membrane properties. *Proc. Natl. Acad. Sci. U.S.A.* 86, 5825-5829, 0027-8424.

James, T. L. (1975). *Nuclear magnetic resonance in biochemistry*. Academic Press, 0123809509 9780123809506, New York.

Jenssen, H., Hamill, P., and Hancock, R. E. W. (2006). Peptide antimicrobial agents. *Clin. Microbiol. Rev.* 19, 491-511, 0893-8512.

Kaganer, V. M., Möhwald, H., and Dutta, P. (1999). Structure and phase transitions in Langmuir monolayers. *Reviews of Modern Physics* 71, 779-819, 0034-6861.

Kates, M., Syz, J.-Y., Gosser, D., and Haines, T. H. (1993). pH-dissociation characteristics of cardiolipin and its 2'-deoxy analogue. *Lipids* 28, 877-882, 0024-4201.

Keller, S. L., Pitcher III, W. H., Huestis, W. H., and McConnell, H. M. (1998). Red blood cell lipids form immiscible liquids. *Phys. Rev. Lett.* 81, 5019-5022, 0031-9007

Kendall, D. A., and MacDonald, R. C. (1982). A fluorescence assay to monitor vesicle fusion and lysis. *J. Biol. Chem.* 257, 13892-13895, 0021-9258.

King, R. G., Sharp, J. A., and Boura, A. L. A. (1983). The effects of Al^{3+}, Cd^{2+} and Mn^{2+} on human erythrocyte choline transport. *Biochem. Pharmacol.* 32, 3611-3617, 0006-2952.

Kokryakov, V. N., Harwing, S. S. L., Panyutich, E. A., Shevchenko, A. A., Aleshina, G. M., Shamova, O. V., Korneva, H. A., and Lehrer, R. I. (1993). Protegrins: leukocyte antimicrobial peptides that combine features of corticostatic defensins and tachyplesins. *FEBS Lett.* 327, 231-236, 0014-5793.

Kolusheva, S., Boyer, L., and Jelinek, R. (2000). A colorimetric assay for rapid screening of antimicrobial peptides. *Nat. Biotechnol.* 18, 225-227, 1087-0156.

Kostka, B. (1991). Toxicity of mercury compounds as a possible risk factor for cardiovascular diseases. *Br J Ind Med* 48, 845-845, 0007-1072.

Krishnakumari, V., and Nagaraj, R. (2008). Interaction of antibacterial peptides spanning the carboxy-terminal region of human B-defensins 1-3 with phospholipids at the air-water interface and inner membrane of *E. coli*. *Peptides* 29, 7-14, 0196-9781.

Krishnakumari, V., Singh, S., and Nagaraj, R. (2006). Antibacterial activities of synthetic peptides corresponding to the carboxy-terminal region of human beta-defensins 1-3. *Peptides* 27, 2607-2613, 0196-9781.

Kusters, R., Dowhan, W., and de Kruijff, B. (1991). Negatively charged phospholipids restore prePho E translocation across phosphatidylglycerol-depleted *Escherichia coli* inner membranes. *J. Biol. Chem.* 266, 8659-8662, 0021-9258.

Lad, M. D., Birembaut, F., Clifton, L. A., Frazier, R. A., and Webster, J. R. P. (2007). Antimicrobial peptide-lipid binding interactions and binding selectivity. *Biophys. J.* 92, 3575-3586, 0006-3495.

Lai, P., Nathoo, S., Ku, T., Gill, S., Azarmi, S., Roa, W., and Lobenberg, R. (2010). Real-time imaging of interactions between dipalmitoylphosphatidylcholine monolayers and gelatin based nanoparticles using Brewster angle microscopy. *J Biomed Nanotechnol* 6, 145-152, 1550-7033.

Lavoie, H., Gallant, J., Grandbois, M., Blaudez, D., Desbat, B., Boucher, F., and Salesse, C. (1999). The behavior of membrane proteins in monolayers at the gas-water interface: comparison between photosystem II, rhodopsin and bacteriorhodopsin.

Mater Sci Eng C Biomim Mater Sens Syst 10, 147-154, Not currently indexed for MEDLINE.

Le, M. T., Gailer, J., and Prenner, E. J. (2009). Hg^{2+} and Cd^{2+} interact differently with biomimetic erythrocyte membranes. *Biometals* 22, 261-274, 0966-0844.

Lewis, R. N. A. H., and McElhaney, R. N. (2009). The physicochemical properties of cardiolipin bilayers and cardiolipin-containing lipid membranes. *Biochim. Biophys. Acta* 1788, 2069-2079, 0006-3002.

Lis, L. J., Lis, W. T., Parsegian, V. A., and Rand, R. P. (1981). Adsorption of divalent cations to a variety of phosphatidylcholine bilayers. *Biochemistry* 20, 1771-1777, 0006-2960.

Lohner, K., and Prenner, E. J. (1999). Differential scanning calorimetry and X-ray diffraction studies of the specificity of the interaction of antimicrobial peptides with membrane-mimetic systems. *Biochim. Biophys. Acta.* 1462, 141-156, 0006-3002.

Maget-Dana, R. (1999). The monolayer technique: a potent tool for studying the interfacial properties of antimicrobial and membrane-lytic peptides and their interactions with lipid membranes. *Biochim. Biophys. Acta* 1462, 109-140, 0006-3002.

Mani, R., Cady, S. D., Tang, M., Waring, A. J., Lehrer, R. I., and Hong, M. (2006). Membrane-dependent oligomeric structure and pore formation of ß-hairpin antimicrobial peptide in lipid bilayers from solid-state NMR. *Proc. Natl. Acad. Sci. U.S.A.* 103, 16242-16247, 0027-8424.

Mason, A. J., Marquette, A., and Bechinger, B. (2007). Zwitterionic phospholipids and sterols modulate antimicrobial peptide-induced membrane destabilization. *Biophys. J.* 93, 4289-4299, 0006-3495.

Matsuzaki, K., Harada, M., Handa, T., Funakoshi, S., Fujii, N., Yajima, H., and Miyajima, K. (1989). Magainin 1-induced leakage of entrapped calcein out of negatively-charged lipid vesicles. *Biochim. Biophys. Acta* 981, 130-134, 0006-3002.

Meshkov, B. B., Tsybyshev, V. P., and Livshits, V. A. (1998). The interaction of double-charged metal ions with monolayers and bilayers of phospholipids. *Russian Chemical Bulletin* 47, 2490-2495,

Mileykovskaya, E., Zhang, M., and Dowhan, W. (2005). Cardiolipin in energy transducing membranes - Review. *Biochemistry Mosc.* 70, 191-196, 0006-2979.

Mubagwa, K., Gwanyanya, A., Zakharov, S., and Macianskiene, R. (2007). Regulation of cation channels in cardiac and smooth muscle cells by intracellular magnesium. *Arch. Biochem. Biophys.* 458, 73-89, 0003-9861.

Nakada, S., Inoue, K., Nojima, S., and Imura, N. (1978). Change in permeability of liposomes caused by methylmercury and inorganic mercury. *Chem. Biol. Interact.* 22, 15-23, 0009-2797.

Oren, Z., and Shai, Y. (1997). Selective lysis of bacteria but not mammalian cells by diastereomers of melittin: structure-function study. *Biochemistry* 36, 1826-1835, 0006-2960.

Patel, H., Tscheka, C., and Heerklotz, H. (2009). Characterizing vesicle leakage by fluorescence lifetime measurements. *Soft Matter* 5, 2849-2851, 1744-683X.

Popot, J.-L., Gerchman, S.-E., and Engelman, D. M. (1987). Refolding of Bacteriorhodopsin in lipid bilayers: a thermodynamically controlled two-stage process. *J. Mol. Biol.* 198, 655-676, 0022-2836.

Prenner, E. J., Kiricsi, M., Jelokhani-Niaraki, M., Lewis, R. N. A. H., Hodges, R. S., and McElhaney, R. N. (2005). Structure-activity relationships of diastereomeric lysine ring size analogs of the antimicrobial peptide gramicidin S - Mechanism of action and discrimination between bacterial and animal cell membranes. *J. Biol. Chem.* 280, 2002-2011, 0021-9258.

Prenner, E. J., Lewis, R. N. A. H., Jelokhani-Niaraki, M., Hodges, R. S., and McElhaney, R. N. (2001). Cholesterol attenuates the interaction of the antimicrobial peptide gramicidin S with phospholipid bilayer membranes. *Biochim. Biophys. Acta* 1510, 83-92, 0006-3002.

Prenner, E. J., Lewis, R. N. A. H., Kondejewski, L. H., Hodges, R. S., and McElhaney, R. N. (1999). Differential scanning calorimetric study of the effect of the antimicrobial peptide gramicidin S on the thermotropic phase behavior of phosphatidylcholine, phosphatidylethanolamine and phosphatidylglycerol lipid bilayer membranes. *Biochim. Biophys. Acta* 1417, 211-223, 0006-3002.

Rietvald, A. G., Chupin, V. V., Koorengevel, M. C., Wienk, H. L., Dowhand, W., and de Kruijff, B. (1994). Regulation of lipid polymorphism is essential for the viability of phosphatidylethanolamine-deficient *Escherichia coli* cells. *J. Biol. Chem.* 269, 28670-28675, 0021-9258.

Rietveld, A., and Simons, K. (1998). The differential miscibility of lipids as the basis for the formation of functional membrane rafts. *Biochim. Biophys. Acta* 1376, 467-479, 0006-3002.

Romanowski, M., Zhu, X., Kim, K., Hruby, V. J., and O'Brien, D. F. (2002). Interaction of enkephalin peptides with anionic model membranes. *Biochim. Biophys. Acta* 1558, 45-53, 0006-3002.

Romanowski, M., Zhu, X., Ramaswami, V., Misicka, A., Lipkowski, A. W., Hruby, V. J., and O'Brien, D. F. (1997). Interaction of a highly potent dimeric enkephalin analog, biphalin, with model membranes. *Biochim. Biophys. Acta* 1329, 245-258, 0006-3002.

Sevcsik, E., Pabst, G., Richter, W., Danner, S., Amenitsch, H., and Lohner, K. (2008). Interaction of LL-37 with model membrane systems of different complexity:Influence of the lipid matrix. *Biophys. J.* 94, 4688-4699, 0006-3495.

Sheetz, M. P., and Singer, S. J. (1974). Biological membranes as bilayer couples. A molecular mechanism of drug-erythrocyte interactions. *Proc. Natl. Acad. Sci. U.S.A.* 71, 4457-4461, 0027-8424.

Shin, E. B., and Krenkel, P. A. (1976). Mercury uptake by fish and biomethylation mechanisms. *J Water Pollut Control Fed* 48, 473-501, 0043-1303.

Sikora, C. W., and Turner, R. J. (2005). Investigation of ligand binding to the multidrug resistance protein EmrE by isothermal titration calorimetry. *Biophys. J.* 88, 475-482, 0006-3495.

Simons, K., and Ikonen, E. (1997). Functional rafts in cell membranes. *Nature* 387, 569-572, 0028-0836.

Simons, K., and Toomre, D. (2000). Lipid rafts and signal transduction. *Nat. Rev. Mol. Cell Biol.* 1, 31-39, 1471-0072

Singer, S. J., and Nicolson, G. L. (1972). The fluid mosaic model of the structure of cell membranes. *Science* 175, 720-731, 0193-4511.

Sinn, C. G., Antonietti, M., and Dimova, R. (2006). Binding of calcium to phosphatidylcholine-phosphatidylserine membranes. *Colloids Surf A Physicochem Eng Asp* 282-283, 410-419, 0927-7757.

Soderlund, T., Lehtonen, J. Y. A., and Kinnunen, P. K. J. (1999). The interactions of Cyclosporin A with phospholipid membranes: Effect of cholesterol. *Mol. Pharmacol.* 55, 32-38, 0026-895X.

Suwalsky, M., Ungerer, B., Aguilar, F., and Sotomayor, C. P. (1996). Interaction of Zn^{2+} ions with phospholipid multilayers. *Intern. J. Polymeric Mater.* 34, 225-232,

Suwalsky, M., Ungerer, B., Villena, F., Cuevas, F., and Sotomayor, C. P. (2000). $HgCl_2$ disrupts the structure of the human erythrocyte membrane and model phospholipid bilayers. *J. Inorg. Biochem.* 81, 267-273, 0162-0134.

Suwalsky, M., Villena, F., Norris, B., Cuevas, F., and Sotomayor, C. P. (2004). Cadmium-induced changes in the membrane of human erythrocytes and molecular models. *J. Inorg. Biochem.* 98, 1061-1066, 0162-0134.

Suzuki, Y., and Matsushita, H. (1968). Interaction of metal ions and phospholipid monolayer as a biological membrane model. *Ind. Health* 6, 128-133, 0019-8366.

Suzuki, Y., and Matsushita, H. (1969). Interaction of metal ions with phospholipid monolayer and their acute toxicity. *Ind. Health* 7, 143-154, 0019-8366.

Tacnet, F., Ripoche, P., Roux, M., and Neumann, J. M. (1991). ^{31}P-NMR study of pig intestinal brush-border membrane structure - effect of zinc and cadmium ions. *Eur. Biophys. J.* 19, 317-322, 0175-7571.

Tang, M., and Hong, M. (2009). Structure and mechanism of beta-hairpin antimicrobial peptides in lipid bilayers from solid-state NMR spectroscopy. *Mol Biosyst* 5, 317-322, 1742-206X

Tate, M. W., Eikenberry, E. F., Turner, D. C., Shyamsunder, E., and Gruner, S. M. (1991). Nonbilayer phases of membrane lipids. *Chem. Phys. Lipids* 57, 147-164, 0009-3084.

Terce, F., Tocanne, J.-F., and Laneelle, G. (1982). Interactions of Ellipticine with model or natural membranes: A spectrophotometric study. *Eur. J. Biochem.* 125, 203-207, 0014-2956.

Terce, F., Tocanne, J. F., and Laneelle, G. (1983). Ellipticine-induced alteration of model and natural membranes. *Biochem. Pharmacol.* 32, 2189-2194, 0006-2952.

van Dalen, A., Hegger, S., Killian, J. A., and de Kruijff, B. (2002). Influence of lipids on membrane assembly and stability of the potassium channel KcsA. *FEBS Lett.* 525, 33-38, 0014-5793.

van den Brink-van der Laan, E., Killian, J. A., and de Kruijff, B. (2004). Nonbilayer lipids affect peripheral and integral membrane proteins via changes in the lateral pressure profile. *Biochim. Biophys. Acta* 1666, 275-288, 0006-3002.

van der Does, C., Swaving, J., van Klompenburg, W., and Driessen, A. J. (2000). Non-bilayer lipids stimulate the activity of the reconstituted bacterial protein translocase. *J. Biol. Chem.* 275, 2472-2478, 0021-9258.

Vandijck, P. W. M., de Kruijff, B., Verkleij, A. J., Vandeenen, L. L. M., and Degier, J. (1978). Comparative studies on effects of pH and Ca^{2+} on bilayers of various negatively charged phospholipids and their mixtures with phosphatidylcholine. *Biochim. Biophys. Acta* 512, 84-96, 0006-3002.

Volinski, R., Kolusheva, S., Berman, A., and Jelinek, R. (2006). Investigations of antimicrobial peptides in planar film systems. *Biochim. Biophys. Acta* 1758, 1393-1407, 0006-3002.

Yawata, Y. (2003). *Cell Membrane: The Red Blood Cell as a Model.* Wiley, 3527304630 9783527304639 3527601538 9783527601530.

Zachowski, A. (1993). Phospholipids in animal eukaryotic membranes - transverse asymmetry and movement. *Biochem. J.* 294, 1-14, 0264-6021.

Zerrouk, Z., Alexandre, S., Lafontaine, C., Norris, V., and Valleton, J.-M. (2008). Inner membrane lipids of *Escherichia coli* form domains. *Colloids Surf B Biointerfaces* 63, 306-310, 0927-7765.

Zhang, L., Rozek, A., and Hancock, R. E. W. (2001). Interaction of cationic antimicrobial peptides with model membranes. *J. Biol. Chem.* 276, 35814-35722, 0021-9258.

13

Biomimetic Membranes as a Tool to Study Competitive Ion-Exchange Processes on Biologically Active Sites

Beata Paczosa-Bator[1], Jan Migdalski[1] and Andrzej Lewenstam[1,2]
[1]Faculty of Material Science and Ceramics, AGH University of Science and Technology, PL-30059 Cracow
[2]Centre for Process Analytical Chemistry and Sensor Technology 'ProSens', Process Chemistry Centre, Åbo Akademi University, FIN-20500 Åbo-Turku,
[1]Poland
[2]Finland

1. Introduction

The change in membrane potential with time is of fundamental importance in cell biology. From the biological point of view we are interested in the mechanism of voltage dependent channel block and related ionic antagonism that happens on the ion-binding sites forming channel necks (Migdalski at al., 2003; Paczosa at al., 2004; Paczosa-Bator at al., 2006). We argue that by applying biomimetic approach, the processes invisible in routine membrane research could be "amplified" and exposed for further scientific exploration. In our case, this argument refers to electrical potential transients and/or local concentration redistributions provoked a competitive calcium/magnesium or potassium/sodium/lithium ions exchange on the biological sites. Voltage-activation of the N-methyl-d-aspartate (NMDA) receptor channel, allowing for calcium ion influx by relieving the block by magnesium ion (Nowak at al., 1984; McBain at al., 1994), or monovalent ion effects such as potassium-sodium/ lithium/TEA(tetraethylammonium) in the case of potassium and sodium channels (Hille, 1992) is used to illustrate the value of biomimetic methodology.

From the electrochemical point of view, our strategy means an interest in the time-dependent (dynamic) characteristics of a membrane potential resulting from competitive ion-exchange processes. The membranes used in our studies are in electrochemistry known as the electroactive parts of ion-selective sensors sensitive for magnesium, calcium, potassium, sodium and lithium, which are the ions of our interest.

To bridge mentioned above biological and electrochemical interests we use biomimetic membranes. The novelty of our approach is in applying conductive polymers (CPs) as with purposely dispersed bioactive sites. This allows observation of a competitive (antagonistic) ion exchange and its coupling with a membrane potential formation process on biologically active sites (BL). The sites in focus of our research, adenosinotriphosphate (ATP), adenosinodiphosphate (ADP), heparin (Hep) and two amino acids - asparagine (Asn) and glutamine (Gln), competitively bind calcium, magnesium, lithium, sodium and potassium ions and thus play an important role in ion-dependent biological membrane processes (Saris

at al., 2000). In particular, ATP takes part in active membrane potential formation, Hep in the anticoagulation process (Desai, 2004) and Asn and Gln in the voltage-ligand gated influx on calcium ions via the NMDA channels (McBain & Mayer, 1994).
The following methodology is accepted for applying CPs as biomimetic membranes. In order to obtain the membranes (CP-BL-Y, where Y = K^+, Na^+, Li^+, Ca^{2+}, Mg^{2+}), first ATP, ADP, Hep, Asn or Gln are introduced into the CP matrix during electropolymerization. Next, the calcium, magnesium, lithium, sodium or potassium potentiometric sensitivity is induced by soaking in an alkaline solution of one of these ions until close-to-Nernstian sensitivity for the films is obtained. The films are then used to monitor the equilibration processes induced by the change in bulk concentration of magnesium/calcium or lithium/potassium/sodium ions or stimulation with external electrical signal (Paczosa-Bator at al., 2009). The resulting transitory potential response is recorded and characteristic potential transients observed are theoretically interpreted.

2. Conducting polymers used and their properties

It is well known that conducting polymers (CPs) such as poly(pyrrole) (PPy), poly(N-methylpyrrole) (PMPy) or poly(3,4-ethylenedioxythiophene) (PEDOT) in the oxidation process during electrodeposition are easily doped with small inorganic anions and in consequence exhibit anionic open-circuit sensitivity.
Cationic sensitivity can be observed if the CP films are doped with cations during reduction. This happens when the CP film is doped with bulky immobile anions, for instance naphthalenesulphonate, indigo carmine or methylene blue (Gao at al., 1994; Bobacka et al., 1994). The ionic sensitivity induced in this way is dependent on the redox status of the polymer film and is rather nonselective (Lewenstam at al., 1994).
As we shown, the cationic sensitivity may be enhanced and stabilized with use of bulky, metal-complexing ligands from the group of metallochromic indicators as dopants. This happens because the bulky dopants retain in the polymer film their complexing properties known from water chemistry and the selective cationic sensitivity results from the complex formation inside CP films (Migdalski et al., 1996).
This provides the unique possibility of forming CP films doped with bulky and biologically active anions such as adenosinotriphosphate (ATP), adenosinodiphosphate (ADP), heparin (Hep) or amino acids - asparagine (Asn) and glutamine (Gln). These films may be used as biomimetic membranes to inspect processes important for membrane potential formation or membrane transport (Paczosa-Bator at al., 2007).
Our observations have shown that the conducting polymer designed for biomimetic membranes should have smooth surface morphology (a. Paczosa-Bator at al., 2006). It is well known that the morphology of conducting polymer films depends on many experimental parameters, such as substrate used, electrodeposition method, kind of monomer and doping anions, kind of solvent, pH and post deposition treatment of the film. Depending on the further application of conducting polymer layers, different surface morphology (rough or smooth) and different structure are required (Niu at al., 2001; Unsworth at al., 1992; Maddison & Unsworth 1989).

3. Materials and methods

The electrosynthesis of conducting polymer membranes on GC and ITO electrodes was carried out using an Autolab general Purpose System (AUT20.Fra2-Autolab, Eco Chemie,

B.V., Utrecht, The Netherlands) connected to a conventional, three-electrode cell. The working electrode was a glassy carbon (GC) disk with an area of 0.07 cm^2 or conducting glass pieces with an area of about 1 cm^2 (ITO, Lohja Electronics, Lohja, Finland, used for the FTIR, EDAX, XPS and LA-ICP-MS experiments). The reference electrode was an Ag/AgCl/3M KCl electrode connected to the cell via a bridge filled with supporting electrolyte solution, and a glassy carbon (GC) rod was used as the auxiliary electrode. The solutions used for polymerization contained selected monomer and an electrolyte that provided the doping ion. Electropolymerization was performed in solutions saturated with argon at room temperature.

The potentials were measured using a 16-channel mV-meter (Lawson Labs, Inc., Malvern, PA). The reference electrode was an Ag/AgCl/3M KCl electrode. All experiments were performed at room temperature.

The X-ray photoelectron spectroscopy (XPS) analysis was performed with a Physical Electronics Quantum 2000 XPS-spectrometer equipped with a monochromatized Al-X-ray source. The Energy Dispersive Analysis of X-ray (EDAX) measurements were performed using a Scanning Electron Microscope, SEM model LEO 1530 from LEO Electron Microscopy Ltd, which was connected to an Image and X-ray analysis system - model Vantage from ThermoNoran. The LA-ICP-MS measurements were performed using a model 6100 Elan DRC Plus of ICP-MS from Perkin Elmer SCIEX (Waltham, USA) and UP-213 of Laser Ablation from "New wave Research" Merchantek Products (Fremont, USA). The Fourier Transform Infrared (FTIR) spectra were recorded with a Bruker IFS 66/S instrument. The Atomic Force Microscopy (AFM) images were recorded with a NanoScope IIIa microscope (Digital Instruments Inc., Santa Barbara, CA), equipped with the extender electronics module enabling phase imaging in tapping mode. For numerical calculations Mathcad 2001 Professional by MathSoft, Inc. Canada, was used.

4. Procedures of CP-BL-Me electrode preparation

4.1 Conducting polymer films - deposition

The electrodeposition of the poly(pyrrole), poly(N-methylpyrrole) or poly(3,4-ethylenedioxytiophene) films was carried out from solution that contained dopant and selected monomer. The monomer concentration was equal to 0.1M for pyrrole and N-methylpyrrole or 0.01 M for 3,4-ethylenedioxythiophene. Dopant concentration was equal to 0.1M for ATP, ADP, Gln or Asn. PEDOT, PMPy and PPy were electrodeposited onto the working electrode potentiostatically, under constant potential or dynamically with potential cycling. In the last case the scan rate was equal to 20 $mV \cdot s^{-1}$. Deposition time or number of cycles was selected to obtain desired charge density.

CP films doped with ATP and ADP were deposited potentiostatically under +0.9 V or +1.02 V (PEDOT), +0.66, 0.68 or +0.70 V (PPy) as well as +0.8 V (PMPy) (vs. Ag/AgCl/3M KCl) or dynamically by scanning the potential in the range 0 - (+0.9) V or 0 - (+1.02) V (PEDOT films) and 0 - (+0.70) V (PPy films) (vs. Ag/AgCl/3M KCl). The charge density was equal to 510 - 750 $mC \cdot cm^{-2}$.

PPy-Asn(Gln) films were grown on the working electrode at a potential of +1.00 V (vs. Ag/AgCl/3M KCl) and charge density of 240 $mC \cdot cm^{-2}$ was used.

The growth of heparin-doped poly(pyrrole) and poly(3,4-ethylenedioxythiophene) was performed using solutions containing 40 $mg \cdot ml^{-1}$ of heparin and 0.1 M pyrrole or 0.01M 3,4-ethylenedioxythiophene. Dynamic growth was performed by scanning the potential between 0 and +0.80 V (PPy) or 0 and +0.92 V (PEDOT) (vs. Ag/AgCl/3M KCl) and potentiostatic growth was achieved by holding a potential at +0.80 V (PPy) and +0.92 V or +0.96 V (PEDOT) (vs. Ag/AgCl/3M KCl) for different times in order to obtain charge density 480 - 840 mC·cm^{-2}.

4.2 The process of making CP-BL membranes cation-sensitive

After synthesis, the polymer membranes were washed with deionized water and then the electrodes were soaked and stored in a alkaline mixture of 0.1 M YCl_n and $Y(OH)_n$ were Y was a main cation. Only conditioning in the alkaline solution was effective. The cation complexes with BL were formed after CP-BL film deprotonation in alkaline solutions (protons were substituted with other cations) as shown on Fig. 1. As a rule, a cationic response with a linear range within the K^+, Na^+, Li^+ activities from 10^{-1} M to 10^{-4} M and Ca^{2+}, Mg^{2+} activities from 10^{-1} M to 10^{-5} M with a close-to-Nernstian slope was observed for the CP-BL films usually after 1 week of soaking.

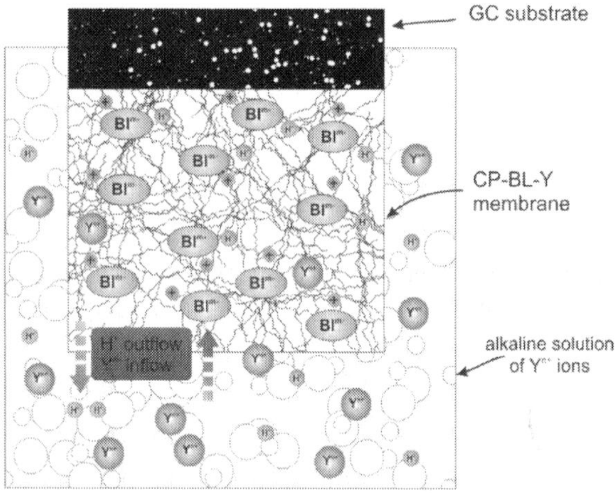

Fig. 1. Ion-exchange processes during conditioning of CP-BL membrane in alkaline solution.

5. Results and discussion

5.1 Electrodeposition and its influence on potentiometric response

The short response time of the CP-BL membranes is highly desirable to study the transient membrane potential changes during equilibration processes. As we have shown for CP-ATP membranes, the response time is strongly dependent on the film morphology. The AFM and potentiometric study conducted in parallel have exemplified the strong influence of the film preparation conditions on its further potentiometric response.

Generally, CP-BL films made under dynamic conditions are close to two dimensional structures i.e. they are flat and compact, while the potentiostatic deposition leads to three-dimensionally morphology of the films. Fig. 2 presents the exemplary AFM phase contrast images of the PPy-ATP membranes taken after film deposition under different conditions: potentiostatic under +0.66 V (a), +0.68 V (b), +0.70 V (c) and dynamic (0- (+0.7) V) (d). The size of each image is equal to 3 μm × 3 μm and the thickness of all compared films was equal to 2 μm.

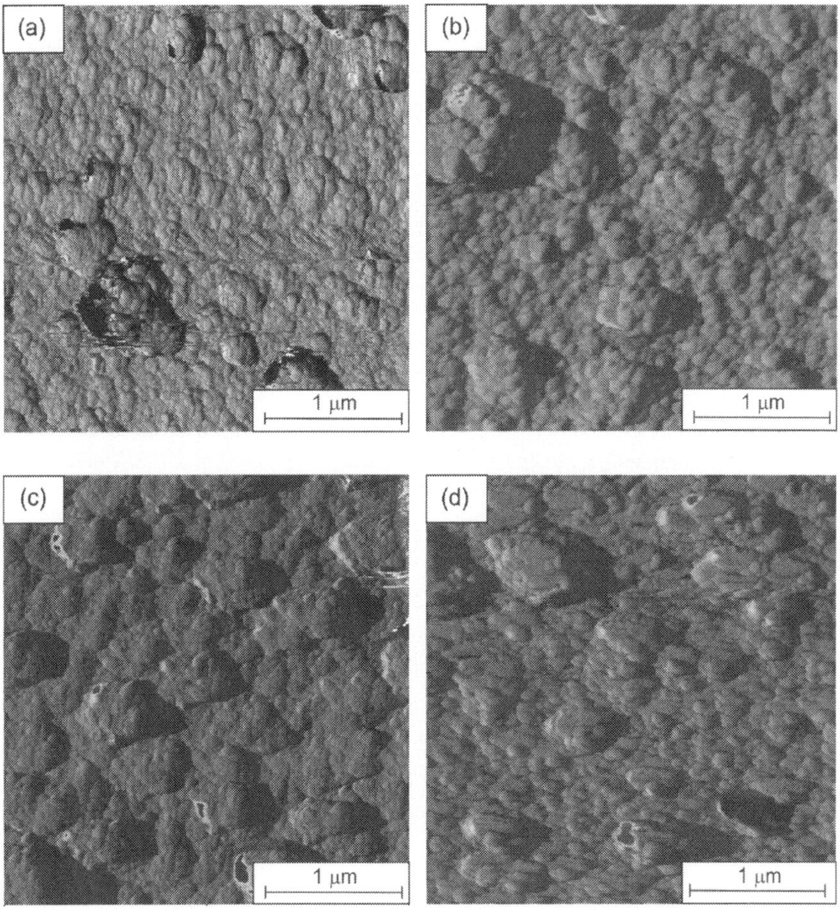

Fig. 2. AFM phase contrast images of the PPy-ATP layers prepared by electropolymerization under different conditions: potentiostatic under (a) +0.66 V, (b) +0.68 V, (c) +0.70 V and (d) dynamic with potential cycling between 0 and +0.70 V. The size of each image is 3 μm x 3 μm.

As shown in Fig. 2(b) and 2(c), the PPy layers prepared potentiostatically under +0.68 V and +0.70 V exhibit quite rough surface (large RMS roughness (S_q) and ten-point height (S_z)) with relatively high effective surface area (S_{dr}), see Table 1. In contrast, the membrane prepared by potential cycling were smoother (smaller S_q and S_z) as well as have smaller effective surface area Fig. 2(d). The membranes prepared by potentiostatic method but under the lowest potential +0.66 V (Fig. 2(a)) show the smoothest surface and the densest structure (the smallest value of RMS and the highest value of skewness (S_{sk})). The films prepared under higher potentials have a less compact structure with more porous surface (smaller value of skewness (S_{sk})), resulting from rapid film growth, and have a less glossy appearance.

Method and potential of electrodeposition	Potentiostatic +0.66	Potentiostatic +0.68	Potentiostatic +0,70	Dynamic 0 - (+0,70)
Scan size, μm × μm	3×3	3×3	3×3	3×3
S_q, nm	70.4	78.1	81.1	72.7
S_z, nm	426	481	500	423
S_{sk}, -	3.16	2.03	1.64	1.32
S_{dr}, %	28.7	36.6	38.1	30.2

Table 1. Roughness analysis of AFM images shown in Fig. 2: S_q (RMS roughness) and S_z (average of 5 minima and 5 maxima); S_{sk} (skewness); S_{dr} (effective surface area).

A comparison of the responses time of CP-BL membranes prepared by different methods (namely, potentiostatically and dynamically) proves that the surface of the polymer films greatly influence this parameter. After 2 weeks of conditioning, the films prepared by potential cycling and under potentiostatic conditions with the smallest potential, (which showed the most smooth surface among all films studied), were characterized by the shortest response time ($t_{90} \approx$ 7-10 s), in contrast to the films obtained potentiostatically with +0.68 and +0.70 V ($t_{90} \approx$ 70-95 s). After 4 months of soaking the response time of all studied electrodes have become similar ($t_{90} \approx$ 5-8 s). PPy-ATP membranes with more compact structure required longer conditioning to induce the theoretical cationic response (in comparison with porous PEDOT-ATP membranes that show value of skewness close to 0 or negative as we showed in b. Paczosa-Bator at al., 2006). PPy-BL membranes exhibit also longer response time in comparison with PEDOT-BL. Exemplary potentiometric response of calcium sensitive PEDOT-ATP membranes taken after 2 weeks of conditioning in alkaline calcium solution is shown on Fig. 3. It is evident that different parameters of electropolymerization, and subsequent soaking, influence the potentiometric response of CP-BL films.

The thickness of CP-BL membranes also influence their potentiometric sensitivity. For example, calibration curves recorded for PEDOT-ATP membranes with different thickness taken after 1 month of soaking with alkaline calcium solution are shown on Fig. 4. As can be seen, from Fig. 4, thinner membranes showed narrow linear range (only from 10^{-5} to 10^{-3} M) and thicker membranes need longer time of conditioning in order to induce cationic response (even 2 months). The obtained results have shown that optimal thickness of membranes deposited under potentiostatic conditions was 2 μm but for the membranes prepared by potential cycling the optimal thickness was between 2 - 4 μm.

Generally the best cationic response with linear and the close-to-Nernstian slope value in the range 10^{-1} M - 10^{-4} M (for monovalent cations) or 10^{-1} M - 10^{-5} M (for divalent cations) was observed for membranes obtained dynamically with thickness 2-4 μm.

Freshly deposited and unsoaked CP-BL electrodes did not respond to studied ions (potassium, sodium, lithium, calcium and magnesium). In order to induce potentiometric sensitivity, the CP-BL membranes were conditioned in the alkaline solution containing chosen cations.

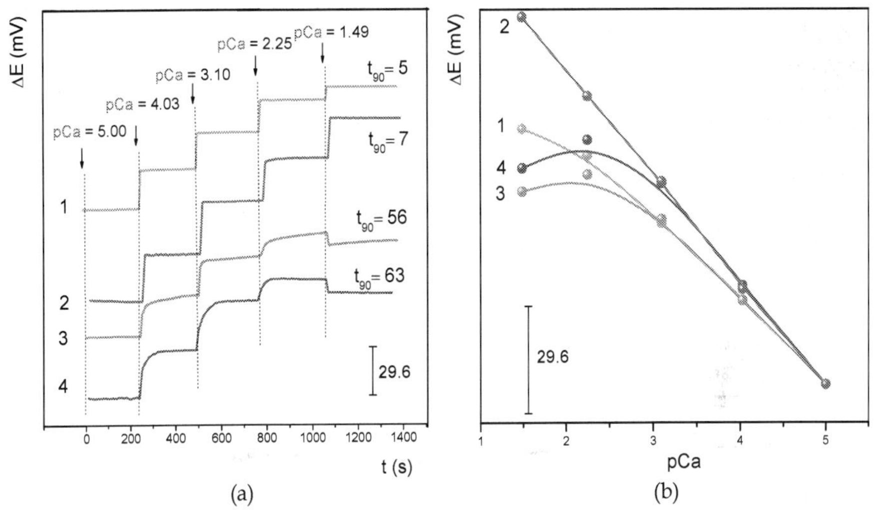

Fig. 3. Comparison of the potentiometric responses of the PEDOT-ATP electrodes performed after two weeks of soaking with alkaline calcium solution for membranes deposited under different conditions: dynamically by cyclic the potential between (1) 0 and +0.90 V, (2) 0 and +1.02 V and potentiostatically under (3) +0.90, (4) +1.02 V.

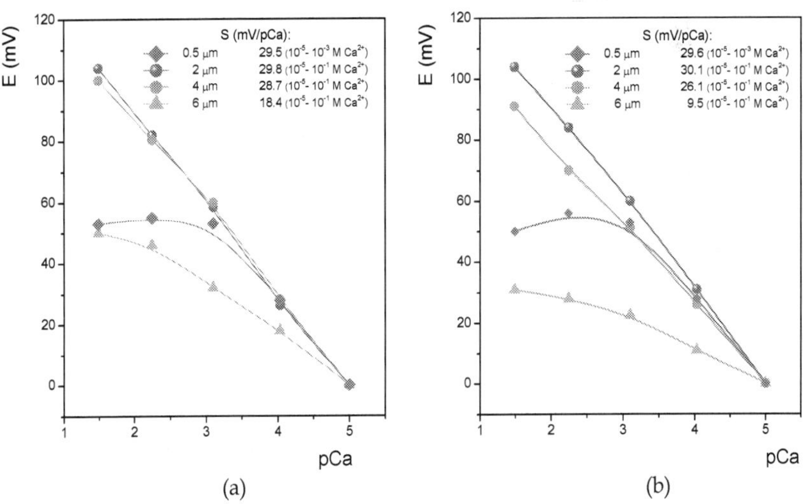

Fig. 4. Comparison of the potentiometric responses of the PEDOT-ATP films with different thickness and deposited under different conditions. Deposition conditions: (a) dynamically by cyclic the potential between 0 and +0.90 V, (b) potentiostatically under +0.90 V. Calibrations with $CaCl_2$ were performed after 1 month of soaking with alkaline calcium solution.

The response of CP-BL membranes was tested in chloride salts of different cations. Usually, after 1-2 weeks of soaking in alkaline solution of sodium, potassium, lithium, calcium or magnesium ions CP-BL membranes exhibit close to theoretical slope value. Fig. 5 presents the influence of soaking period on cationic sensitivity of the PPy-ATP membranes conditioning in different main ions solutions. Similar behaviour was observed for the all CP-BL membranes.

Induced cationic sensitivity was very stable even after using considerably long period of soaking (6-8 months). For example, the slope values for PPy-heparin and PEDOT-ATP films prepared potentiostatically at low potential, adequately +0.66 V and +0.90 V were equal to 29.24±1.01 mV/pMg and 28.56±1.12 mV/pCa during 8 months of PPy-heparin membranes conditioning and 58.92±0.62 mV/pK, 57.58±0.92 mV/pLi and 59.12±0.42 mV/pNa during 6 months of PEDOT-ATP films soaking. It should be noted that all measurements were performed for the same thickness of films (2 μm).

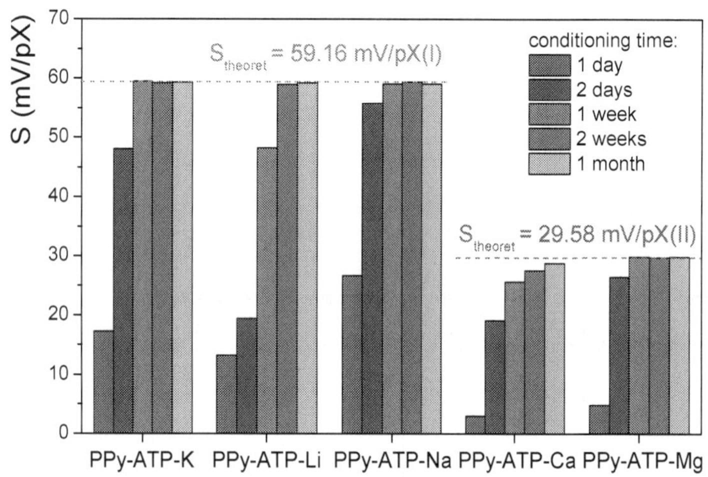

Fig. 5. Influence of soaking period on cationic sensitivity of PPy-ATP membranes (S is the obtained slope value).

5.2 Influence of soaking (conditioning) on the surface morphology of biomimetic membranes

In order to study possible topographic changes during soaking of the CP-BL membranes, AFM topography images were registered for freshly deposited films as well as after different period of soaking in alkaline solution.

Fig. 6 shows exemplary AFM images recorded for PPy-heparin membranes prior to and after soaking in alkaline magnesium solution for one week and one month. These images provide evidence that the conditioning process greatly influences the surface topography. The roughness parameters S_q and S_z clearly show that the films become smoother after conditioning (Table 2). Simultaneously, the effective surface area of the films decreases, most considerably between 1 week and 1 month of soaking (see Fig. 6 and Table 2). The phase contrast images nicely reveal the structural boundaries not so clearly visible in the topographs. They demonstrate that the peaks or spheroidal growths observed before conditioning disappear as a result of conditioning. The skewness (S_{sk}) values confirm this change, changing from positive (Fig. 6a) to negative (Figs. 6b,c) values during conditioning. The surface hence changes from that dominated by peaks (Fig. 6a) to a Gaussian (Fig. 6b) or even porous (Fig. 6c) surface (Table 2).

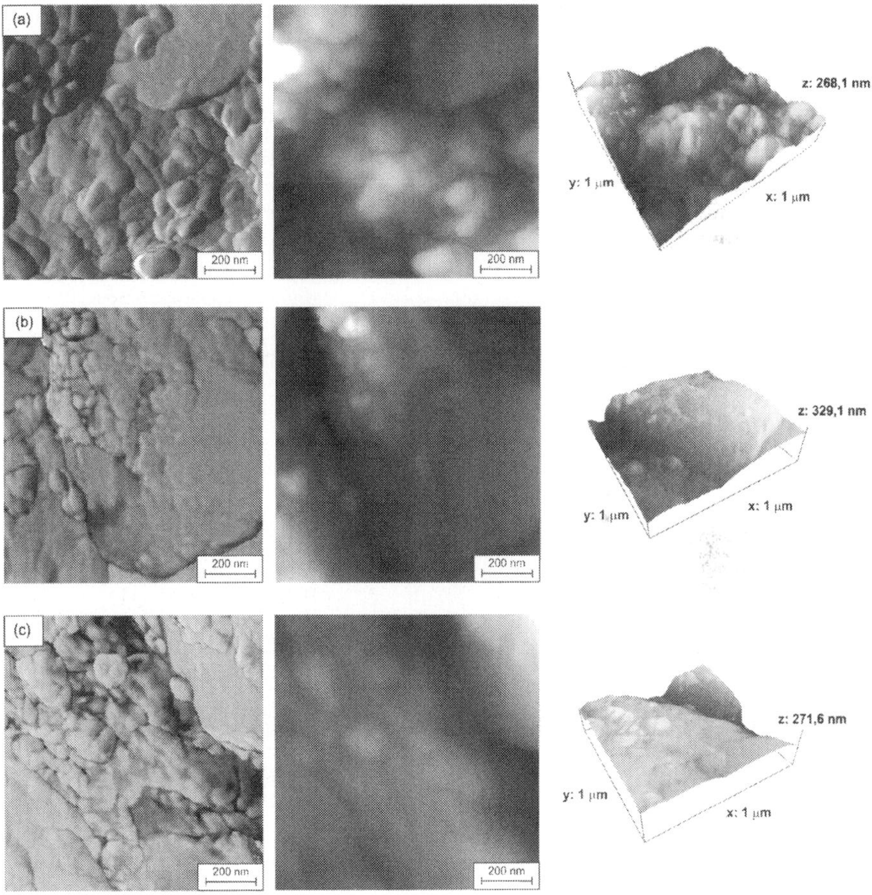

Fig. 6. AFM phase contrast topography and three-dimensional images of PPy membranes prepared potentiostatically at +0.80 V: (a) before conditioning and after conditioning in alkaline magnesium solution for 1 week (b) and 1 month (c).
The size of each image is 1 µm × 1 µm.

A long time soaking does not result in any "mechanical disintegration" of the films due to overoxidation, but makes the polymer surface smoother. At the same time the response time became shorter (see paragraph 4.1.). In consequence, a long time of soaking results in CP-BL films showing very similar potentiometric responses, irrespective on deposition method used.

Time of post-deposition conditioning	-	1 week	1 month
Scan size, µm × µm	1×1	1×1	1×1
S_q, nm	68.1	59.4	42.7
S_z, nm	165	135	120
S_{sk}, -	1.66	-0.75	-1.35
S_{dr}, %	25.1	19.11	8.1

Table 2. Roughness analysis of AFM images shown in Fig. 6.

5.3 Chemical characterization of polymer films

The elemental analysis of CP-BL membranes was performed using four different methods: Fourier transform infrared spectroscopy for membranes doped with amino acids, X-ray photoelectron spectroscopy and energy dispersive analysis of X-ray for CP-BL films sensitive towards divalent ions and laser ablation inductively coupled plasma mass spectrometry for CP-BL films sensitive towards monovalent ions to assess qualitatively the deposition process and influence of soaking on the composition of these membranes.
For the chemical and morphological analysis two kinds of samples were prepared namely: CP-BL without soaking and CP-BL after 2 weeks of soaking in the solution of main ions.

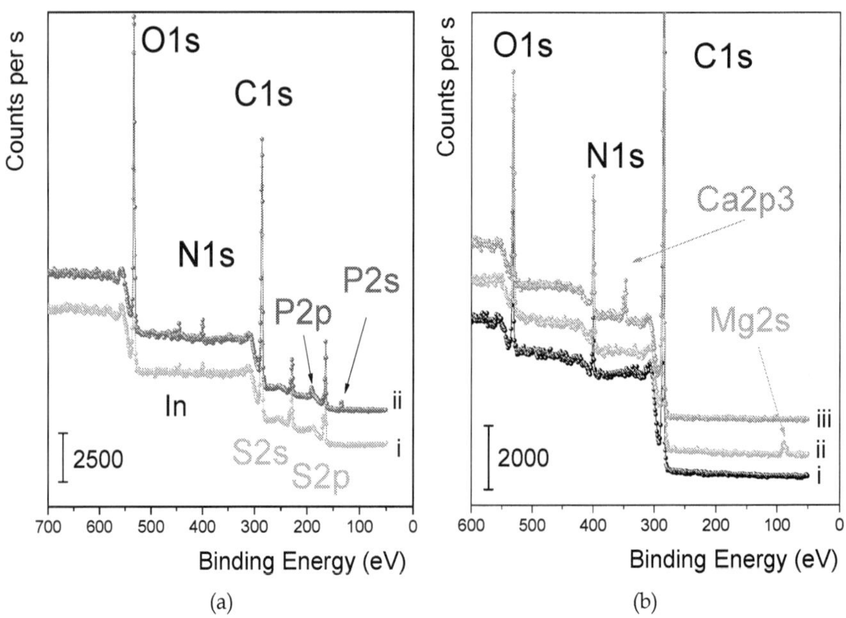

Fig. 7. The exemplary XPS spectra recorded for (a) PEDOT-heparin (i curve) and PEDOT-ATP (ii curve) membranes and (b) PPy-Asn membranes: i) freshly deposited and unsoaked, ii) after conditioning in alkaline magnesium solution, iii) after conditioning in alkaline calcium solution.

The presence of the phosphorus signal in the case of CP-ATP films in the XPS and LA-ICP-MS spectra as shown in Fig. 7a (ii curve) and Fig. 8b proves that counter-ions dope the films formed during electrodeposition (in the case of PEDOT membranes, ATP presence additionally proves nitrogen peak originating from this counter-ion. The heparin in the polymer matrix was identified by presence of nitrogen peak (in the case of PEDOT membranes) or sulfur peak (in the case of PPy membranes) as shown on Fig. 7a (i curve) and Fig. 8a. On the FTIR spectra of the PPy-amino acid films, a large absorbance band in the NIR region caused by the oxidized state of PPy was observed. The spectra of the poly(pyrrole) films showed a C=O stretching - vibration peak at 1651 cm^{-1}, O-H at 1260 cm^{-1}, O-C=O near 800 cm^{-1} and 725 cm^{-1} assigned for Gln or Asn.

The EDAX and XPS analysis of CP-BL films showed that after the conditioning process also calcium or magnesium peaks had appeared on the spectrum (as show exemplary for PPy-Asn membranes on Fig. 7b and PEDOT-Heparin membranes on Fig. 8a).

The LA-ICP-MS measurements for the CP-BL sample sensitive toward monovalent ions proved that after the conditioning desired cations were present in the membranes, e.g. after conditioning in alkaline lithium solution the potentiometric sensitivity towards these ions had been induced and the LA-ICP-MS spectrum showed a lithium signal (which was not observed before the conditioning process) as presented in Fig. 8b. The same behaviour was observed for potassium and sodium ions.

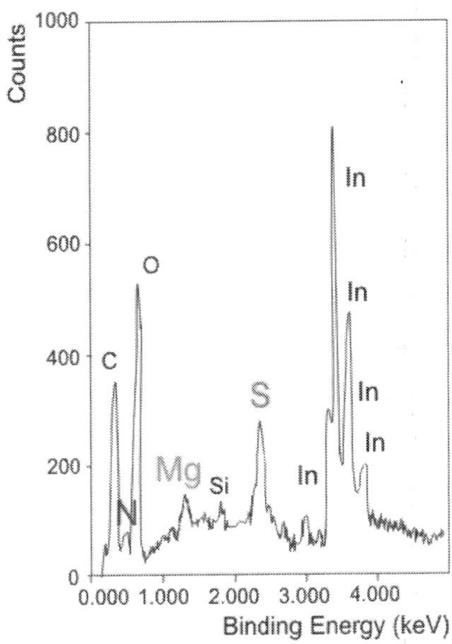

(a)

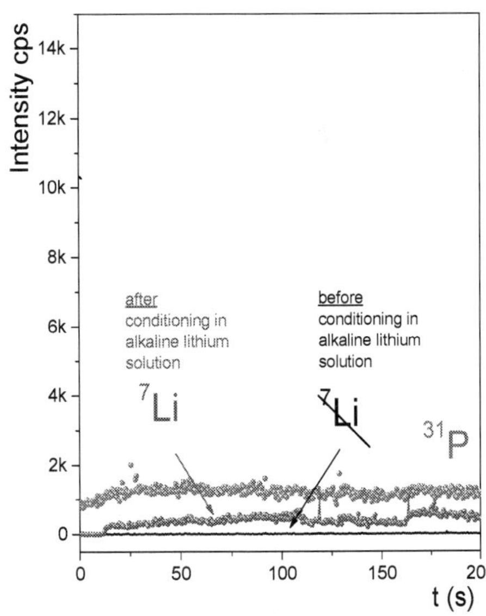

(b)

Fig. 8. The exemplary EDAX spectrum of PPy-Heparin-Mg membrane (a) and LA-ICP-MS spectra recorded for PMPy-ATP films before and after conditioning in alkaline lithium solution (b).

5.4 Influence of interfering cations on biomimetic CP-BL membranes

After inducing a proper sensitivity the influence of other ions on biomimetic membranes potential was studied by adding the interfering ions to the solution of main ions. As expected, in the case of membranes sensitive towards monovalent cations, strong interferences of divalent cations were observed. Divalent cations-sensitive membranes were insensitive towards sodium, potassium or lithium ions, but strong interferences form cations forming a stronger complex with BL (e.g. Zn(II) or Cu(II)) were observed (as exemplary shown on Fig. 9). Importantly, the selectivity coefficient values for the membranes sensitive to divalent cations $K_{Mg,Ca}$ and $K_{Ca,Mg}$ as well as sensitive to monovalent cations $K_{Na,Li}$, $K_{Na,K}$, $K_{Li,K}$ were close to 1. This manifestation of similar thermodynamic properties of ions (in the groups studied), and makes any dissimilarity on the response attributed to the kinetic properties of these ions in the membrane systems studied.

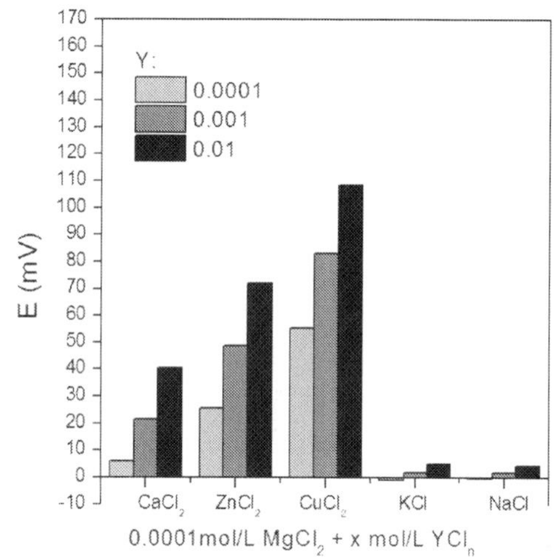

Fig. 9. The exemplary potential-response of PPy-Heparin membrane sensitive towards magnesium ions at interfering ions presence.

6. Ion competition and transient open-circuit response

In spite of similar sensitivity and selectivity of both groups of polymer films (namely, CP-BL-Ca(Mg) or CP-BL-K(Li)(Na)) towards divalent ions (calcium and magnesium) ions or monovalent ions (sodium, potassium and lithium), the transitory potential provoked by the changes in bulk concentrations of these groups of ions was strikingly different.

The representative plots for the measurements made for monovalent and divalent ion-sensitive membranes are shown on Fig. 10, for example PMPy-ATP-Na, PMPy-ATP-K and PPy-Asn-Ca(Mg) electrodes.

As can be seen from Fig. 10, potential-time (E-t) response strongly depends on the kind of ion that was involved in the competitive ion-exchange equilibration process. Lithium ion-exchange with sodium-rich CP-ATP-Na membranes results in a monotonic response (Fig. 10a), while if potassium ions are engaged in the ion exchange, instead of lithium, a non-monotonic (overshoot-type) response is observed (Fig. 10b). If sodium-rich membrane is

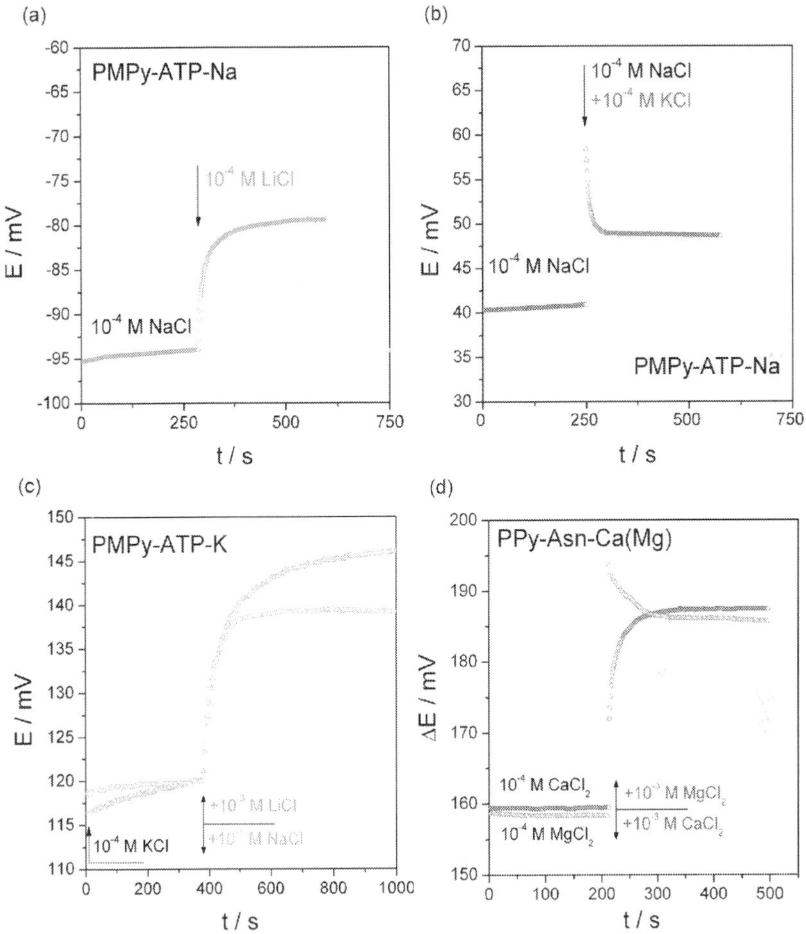

Fig. 10. Potential-time behaviour of sodium (a-b), potassium (c) sensitive PMPy-ATP and calcium and magnesium (d) PPy-Asn films observed after increase of a bulk concentration of: (a) Li^+, (b) K^+, (c) Li^+ (triangles), Na^+ (circles), (d) Ca^{2+} (triangles), Mg^{2+} (circles) ions.

converted to a potassium-rich one, then both a lithium and sodium response, as expected, is monotonic (Fig. 10c). A similar pattern is observed for CP-ATP-Mg membrane (Fig. 10d). Changes in bulk concentrations of magnesium ion are always associated with monotonic potential changes, while changes in concentration of calcium ions are associated with overshoot-type responses. These characteristic differences between potassium, sodium and lithium, as well as magnesium and calcium can be called "ionic antagonism". Interestingly, and most probably not coincidentally, the same pairs of ions, i.e. Ca^{2+}-Mg^{2+}, Na^+/Li^+-K^+, are indeed considered as antagonistic in real biological membrane systems, and specialized voltage and/or ligand-gated ion channels engaging these ions, e.g. NMDA.

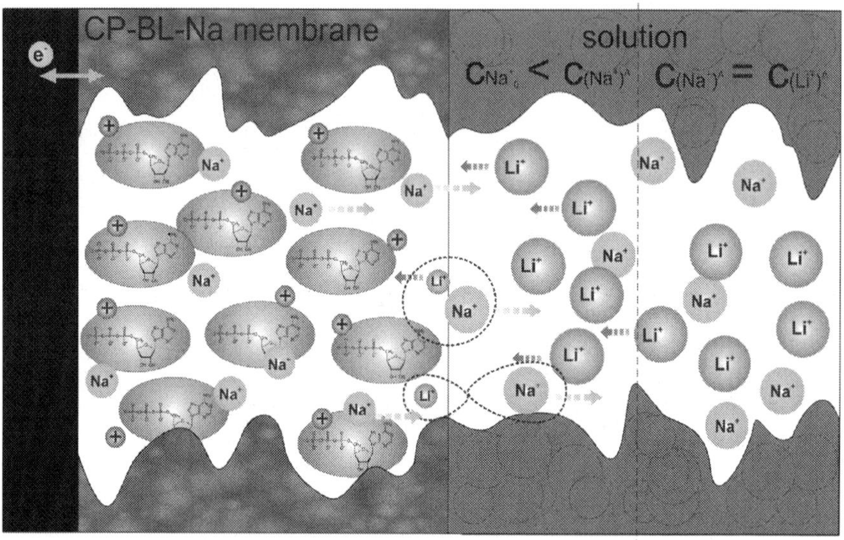

(a)

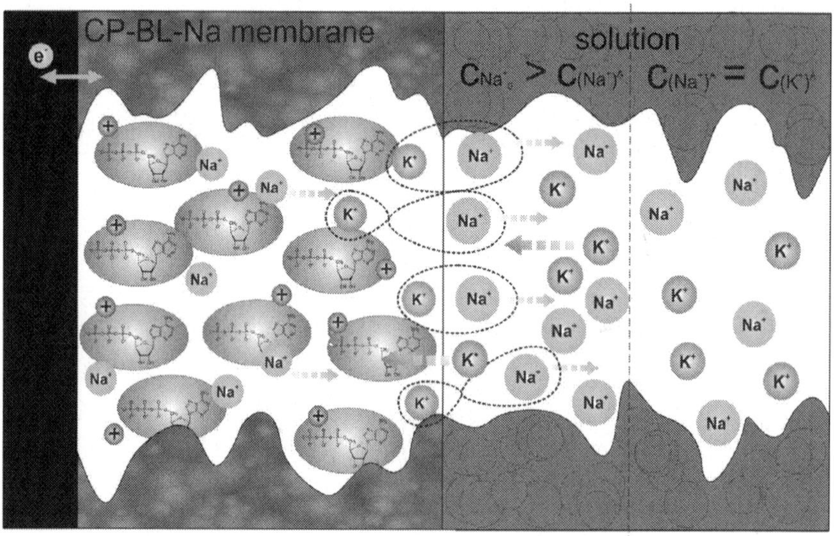

(b)

Fig. 11. The simplified view of ion-exchange processes on CP-ATP-Na electrode in the mixed solution of primary (Na^+) and interfering ions after (a) lithium and (b) potassium concentration change.

As stated above, when discussing the selectivity of the membranes used, conventional interpretation based on thermodynamic equilibrium does not allow predicting any striking difference in membrane responses. This fact lends credence to kinetic aspects in signal formation. A different rate in the transport of ions to and from the bioactive sites contributes to the effects observed. In other words, ion-exchange at the interface between bathing solution and membrane containing the sites and the ion transport are the source of the "antagonism" observed (Paczosa-Bator at al., 2007). The hypothesis is that faster ions (Ca and K characterized by the mobility 6.17 and 7.62 10^{-8} $m^2 \cdot s^{-1} \cdot V^{-1}$ respectively (Fraústo da & Williams, 2001) coming from the solution bulk and substituting via ion exchange slower ions from the film sites (Mg, Na and Li characterized by the mobility 5.49. 5.19 and 4.01 10^{-8} $m^2 \cdot s^{-1} \cdot V^{-1}$ respectively (Fraústo da & Williams, 2001)) which allow for local accumulation of slower ions in the vicinity of membrane interface. And vice-versa if slower ions come from the solution to the film containing faster ions a deficit of this ion can be observed near to membrane surface. This mechanism is schematically illustrated for Na^+-K^+ and Na^+-Li^+ ions pair in Fig. 11.

7. Ion competition during stimulation with external electrical signal

As shown in Fig. 10, the changes in bulk concentration of ions result in characteristic changes of potential vs. time, and are attributed, as shown in Fig. 11, to local redistributions of ions in the vicinity of the membrane-solution interface. It is of great interest to convert the problem and ask whether one could observe any manifestation of this process in the experiment where the membrane ion redistribution is provoked by external electric signal, potential impulse. In this respect, in the absence of a method for direct visualization of the ionic concentration changes in the vicinity of membrane interface, a chrono-amperometric method was used. In this method, the external potential (+5/-5 and +10/-10 mV from the open-circuit potential) was applied to provoke ion fluxes to and from the membrane, and the fluxes are characterized by (ionic) current changes over time. It would be expected that after stimulation with external electrical signal faster ions (potassium or calcium) would produce currents that come to a base-line faster than in the case with ions of lower mobility (sodium/lithium or magnesium). The current response of the PMPy-ATP-Na electrode with time was measured in solutions of chloride salt of sodium, lithium and potassium with concentration equal to 10^{-4} M under different values of potential. In Fig. 12, the current-time (I-t) responses for sodium sensitive PMPy-ATP membrane are shown. The plots indeed prove the interrelation between the size of ions (resp. mobility of ions) and the I-t signal measured.

For the faster potassium ion (resp. calcium ion), after bigger initial cathodic or anodic current values a fast current drop was observed, while for slower sodium and lithium (resp. magnesium) ions the initial current were smaller and followed by slower current drop. This amperometric behaviour can be attributed to different mobility "antagonistic" ions. It can be concluded that transient response of the biomimetic membrane observed both in the open circuit and as well as under potential stimulation is dictated by different mobility of the ions. The kinetic difference is thus a prerequisite of the "ionic antagonism".

8. Theoretical interpretation and implications

The change in membrane potential over time provoked by bulk concentration changes is attributed to local redistributions of ions at the membrane-solution interface and ion transport to and from this interface. If the membrane potential is changed by an external

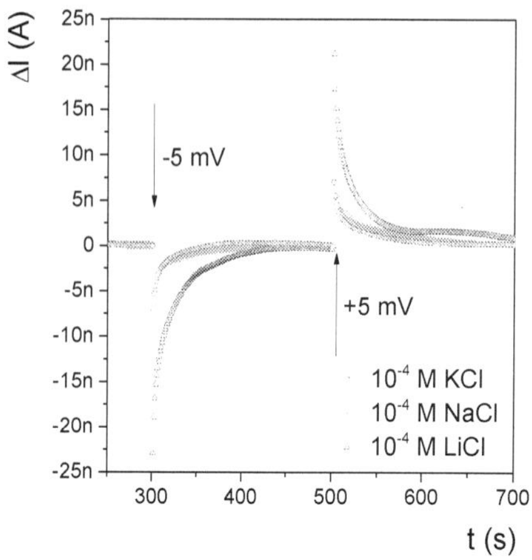

(a)

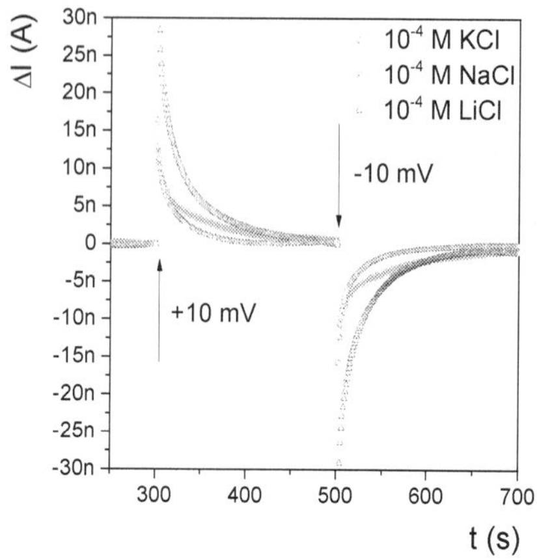

(b)

Fig. 12. The current (I) - time (t) response of PMPy-ATP-Na electrode recorded in chloride salt of the main and interfering ions under different value of potential (a) first -5 mV then +5 mV (b) + first +10 mV then -10 mV.

source resulting ionic fluxes could be observed and the ionic currents depend on the physicochemical properties of the ions engaged. These observations allow development of a general interpretation of E-t response for this biomimetic system using the Nernst-Planck-Poisson model (NPP) (Sokalski & Lewenstam, 2001; Sokalski at al., 2003; Bobacka at al., 2008) or simpler diffusion-layer model (DLM) (Lewenstam at al., 1987; Paczosa-Bator at al., 2007). The time-dependent potential profiles observed experimentally are in excellent agreement with these predicted formally. According to the DLM model, the electrode response depends on the different hydration energy (and mobility) of ions involved in ion-exchange processes. The lower hydration energy of calcium ions (as well as potassium or sodium ions) makes the transport of these ions to and into the membrane faster in comparison to magnesium or lithium, with resulting redistribution of the surface concentration of ions (see Fig. 11). The influx, or outflow, of slower ions determines the speed of the ion-exchange process. This is why, after a change of the e.g. Mg^{2+} ion concentration in the solution bulk, deficiency of e.g. Ca^{2+} ions in the vicinity of the CP-BL-Ca membrane surface vs. bulk is predicted and accordingly a monotonic response type is observed (Fig. 13a). In contrast, after the change of bulk Ca^{2+} ion concentration, the local excess of Mg^{2+} ions at the surface of the CP-BL-Mg membrane is predicted and an overshoot-type response is observed (as shown on Fig. 13b).

Both theoretical models (NPP and DLM) support a fundamental idea of the biomimetic membrane concept presented and show that when a biologically active site is allowed for a competitive ion-exchange the extent of the competition is regulated by the electric potential "applied" to this site and the transport of ions to and from the site. Different E-t patterns have to be observed for faster ions in comparison to slower which is known as "ionic antagonism". Our study shows that a local e.g. magnesium ion concentration increase is

expected when positive vs. equilibrium (rest) potential is applied. In other words it means that magnesium ions leave the coordinating sites and smaller calcium ion is admitted. This is exactly what happens at the neck of magnesium blocked NMDA channel where this ion is attracted by Asn and Gln. When excited by action potential the channel gets unblocked and allows faster calcium ions to pass through (Nowak at al., 1984; Vargas-Caballero & Robinson, 2004). Obviously, deficiency of magnesium in external compartments can facilitate calcium influx and modulation of intracellular calcium concentration. Interestingly, this mechanism and magnesium-calcium antagonism in relation to NMDA receptor channel were recently considered as one possible reason for inflammatory response and metabolic syndrome (Rayssiguier at al., 2006; Mazur at al., 2007). The importance of the effects of Ca^{2+}, Mg^{2+} and ATP and other phosphorylated species on cardiac action potentials was recently as well emphasized (Michailova & McCulloch, 2008). A similar case of a competitive ion mechanism can be in interaction of the exogenous lithium ion with negatively-charged inositol phospholipids which is considered to be relevant in treatment of bipolar disorders (Atack at al., 1995; Gibbons at al., 2008).
Presented here potential-dependent local concentration redistribution of ions at the membrane binding sites undoubtedly adds a new dimension in interpretation of above effects. We address these issues in our present research.

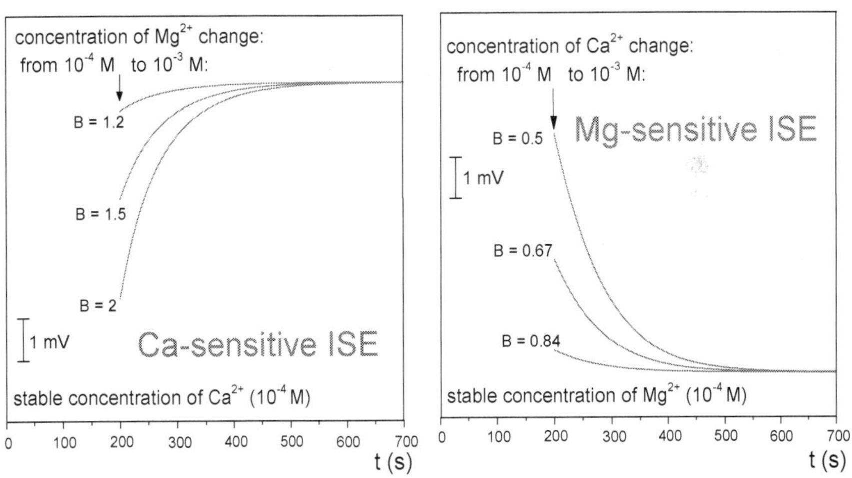

(a) (b)

Fig. 13. The time - dependent response of calcium (a) and magnesium (b) sensitive electrode, calculated on the ground DLM model for various B parameter ($B = \overline{U}_{N^{2+}} / \overline{U}_{Y^{2+}}$ where $\overline{U}_{N^{2+}}, \overline{U}_{Y^{2+}}$ represent the mobilities of ions in the membrane phase and $K_{Y,N} = 1$):
(a) represents response after increase Mg^{2+} activity in the solution of mix magnesium and calcium ions for B = 1.2, 1.5 and 2,
(b) potential response after increase Ca^{2+} activity in the solution of mix magnesium and calcium ions for B = 0.5, 0.67 and 0.84.

9. Conclusion

The biomimetic membrane methodology allows visualization and inspection of the competitive and voltage-dependent ion exchange on biologically active sites. By using selected and relevant to real ionic sites of biological membranes and their channels (e.g. ATP, Asn, Gln) it is possible to access the ionic redistribution on the sites in the function of the bulk concentration of ions, external potential and time. In other words, the concept presented provides a tool to study the role of ions and the influence of ion supplementation, ion deficiencies, and ion antagonism on membrane potential. It as well can be a tool for investigating the bias between voltage effects (long-term potentiation (LTP), cardiac arrhythmias, and low-frequency signals in brain) on ionic local (at/on site) or transmembrane redistributions.

10. Acknowledgements

This work is supported by the National Centre for Research and Development (NCBiR). Grant No. DWM/232/MATERA/2006 and KBN Grant R15 005 03.

11. References

Atack. J.R.; Broughton. H.B. & Pollack. S.J. (1995) Inositol monophosphatase - a putative target for Li^+ in the treatment of bipolar disorder. *Trends Neurosci*, Vol. 18, No. 8, (343-349), ISSN 0166-2236

Bobacka. J.; Gao. Z.; Ivaska. A. & Lewenstam A. (1994) Mechanism of ionic and redox sensitivity of p-type conducting polymers. Part 2. Experimental study of polypyrrole. *J. Electroanal. Chem.*, Vol. 368, No. 1-2, (33-41), ISSN 0022-0728

Bobacka. J.; Ivaska. A. & Lewenstam. A. (2008) Potentiometric ion sensors. *Chem. Rev.*, Vol. 108, No. 2, (329-351) ISSN 0009-2665

Desai. U.R. (2004) New antithrombin-based anticoagulants. *Med. Res. Rev.*, Vol. 24, No. 2, (151-181), ISSN: 0198-6325

Fraústo da Silva. JJR. & Williams. RJP. (2001). *The Biological Chemistry of the Elements*, Oxford University Press Inc., ISBN 0198508476, New York USA

Gao. Z.; Bobacka. J.; Lewenstam. A. & Ivaska. A. (1994) Electrochemical behaviour of polypyrrole film polymerized in indigo carmine solution. *Electrochim. Acta*, Vol. 39, No. 5, 755-762, ISSN 0013-4686

Gibbons. C.E.; Maldonado-Pérez. D.; Shah. A.N.; Riccardi. D. & Ward. D.T. (2008) Calcium-sensing receptor antagonism or lithium treatment ameliorates aminoglycoside-induced cell death in renal epithelial cells. *Biochim. Biophys. Acta*, Vol. 1782, No. 3, (188-195), ISSN 0005-2736

Hille. B. (1992) Selective permability: saturation and binging. In: *Ionic Channels of excitable membranes*, 471-502, Sinauer Associates Inc., ISBN 0878933239, Massachusetts USA

Lewenstam. A.; Hulanicki. A. & Sokalski. T. (1987) Response mechanism of solid state ion selective electrodes in the presence of interfering ions. *Anal. Chem.*, Vol. 59, No. 11, (1539- 1544), ISSN 0003-2700

Lewenstam. A.; Bobacka. J. & Ivaska. A. (1994) Mechanism of ionic and redox sensitivity of p-type conducting polymers. Part I. Theory. *J. Electroanal. Chem.*, Vol. 368, No. 1-2, (23-31), ISSN 0022-0728

Maddison. D.S. & Unsworth. J. (1989) Optimization of synthesis conditions of polypyrrole from aqueous solutions. *Synth. Met.*, Vol. 30, No. 1, (47-55), ISSN 0379-6779

Mazur. A.; Maier. J.A.M.; Rock. E.; Gueux. E.; Nowacki. W. & Rayssiguier. Y. (2007) Magnesium and the inflammatory response: Potential physiopathological implications. *Archiv. Biochem. Biophys.*, Vol. 458, No. 1, (48-56), ISSN 0003-9861

McBain. C.J. & Mayer. M.L. (1994) N-methyl-D-aspartic acid receptor structure and function. *Physiol. Rev.*, Vol. 74, No. 3, (723-760), ISSN 0031-9333

Michailova. A. & McCulloch. A.D. (2008) Effects of Mg^{2+}, pH and PCr on cardiac excitation-metabolic coupling. *Magnesium Research*, Vol. 21, No. 1, (16-28), ISSN 0953-1424

Migdalski. J.; Blaz. T. & Lewenstam. A. (1996) Conducting polymer-based ion-selective electrodes. *Anal. Chem. Acta*, Vol. 322, No. 3, (141-149), ISSN 0003-2670

Migdalski. J.; Blaz. T., Paczosa. B.; Lewenstam A. (2003) Magnesium and calcium-dependent membrane potential of poly(pyrrole) films doped with adenosine triphosphate. *Microchim. Acta*. Vol. 143, No. 2-3, (177-185), ISSN 0026-3672

Niu. L.; Kvarnström C.; Fröberg K. & Ivaska A. (2001) Electrochemically controlled surface morphology and crystallinity in poly(3,4-ethylenedioxythiophene) films. *Synth. Met.*, Vol. 122, No. 2, (425-429), ISSN 0379-6779

Nowak. L.; Bregestovski. P.; Ascher. P.; Herbet. A. & Prochiantz. A. (1984) Magnesium gates glutamate-activated channels in mouse central neurons. *Nature*, Vol. 307, No. 5950, (462-465), ISSN 0028-0836

Paczosa. B., Blaz. T., Migdalski. J. & Lewenstam, A. (2004) Conducting polymer films as model biological membranes. Electrochemical and ion-exchange properties of PPy and PEDOT films doped with heparin. *Polish J. Chem.* Vol. 78. No. 9. (1543-1552). ISSN 0137-5083.

Paczosa-Bator. B.; Migdalski. J. & Lewenstam. A. (2006) (a) Conducting polymer films as model biological membranes. Electrochemical and ion-exchange properties of poly(pyrrole) films doped with asparagine and glutamine. *Electrochim. Acta*, Vol. 51, No. 11, (2173-2181), ISSN 0013-4686

Paczosa-Bator. B.; Peltonen. J.; Bobacka. J. & Lewenstam A. (2006) (b).Influence of morphology and topography on potentiometric response of magnesium and calcium sensitive PEDOT films doped with adenosinetriphosphate (ATP). *Anal. Chim. Acta*, Vol. 555, No. 1, (118-127), ISSN 0003-2670

Paczosa-Bator. B., Blaz. T., Migdalski. J. & Lewenstam. A. (2007) Conducting polymers in modelling transient potential of biological membranes. *Bioelectrochemistry*, Vol. 71, No. 1, (66-74), ISSN 1567-5394

Paczosa-Bator. B.; Stepien. M., Maj-Zurawska. M & Lewenstam A. (2009). Biomimetic study of the Ca^{2+}-Mg^{2+} and K^{+}-Li^{+} antagonism on biologically active sites - new methodology to study potential dependent ion exchange. *Magnesium Research*, Vol. 22, No. 1, (10-20), ISSN 0953-1424

Rayssiguier. Y.; Gueux. E.; Nowacki. W.; Rock. E. & Mazur. A. (2006) High fructose consumption combined with low dietary magnesium intake may increase the incidence of the metabolic syndrome by inducing inflammation. *Magnesium Research*, Vol. 19, No. 4, (237-243), ISSN 0953-1424

Saris. N.E.; Mervaala. E.; Karppanen. H.; Khawaja. J.A. & Lewenstam. A. (2000). *Clin. Chim. Acta*, Vol. 294, No. 1-2, (1-26), ISSN 0009-8981

Sokalski. T. & Lewenstam. A. (2001)Application of Nernst-Planck and Poisson equations for interpretation of liquid-junction and membrane potentials in real-time and space domains. *Electrochem. Comm.*, Vol. 3, No. 3, (107-112), ISSN 1388-2481

Sokalski. T.; Lingenfelter. P. & Lewenstam. A. (2003) Numerical solution of the coupled Nernst-Planck and Poisson equations for liquid-junction and ion-selective membrane potentials. *J. Phys. Chem. B*, Vol. 107, No. 11, (2443-2452), ISSN 1089-5647

Unsworth. J.; Innis. P.C.; Lunn. B.A. & Norton G.P. (1992) The influence of electrolyte pH on the surface morphology of polypyrrole. *Synth. Met.*, Vol. 53, No. 3, (59-69) ISSN 0379-6779

Vargas-Caballero. M. & Robinson. H.P.C. (2004) Fast and slow voltage-dependent dynamics of magnesium block in the NMDA receptor: The asymmetric trapping block model. *J. Neuroscience*, Vol. 24, No. 27, (6171-6180), ISSN 0270-6474

14

Mechanism of Co-salen Biomimetic Catalysis Bleaching of Bamboo Pulp

Yan-Di Jia and Xue-Fei Zhou
Kunming University of Science & Technology
China

1. Introduction

Biomimetics have enzymatically and chemically the catalytic performance and the advantage to reduce pollution (Xie, 1999), and thus have been introduced into the pulping and bleaching field (Huynh, 1986; Cui & Dolphin, 1994). Co-salen can be easily synthesized with high yield. It was shown, in our studies, that Co-salen biomimetic pretreatment improved the bleachability of pulp with a small loss of carbohydrate, increased the brightness of 5.3 % ISO compared to the control when bamboo kraft pulp was bleached with total chlorine free (TCF) sequence. In this work, structural changes in residual lignin isolated and their effects on the bleached pulp were elucidated to provide fundamental basis for the biomimetic catalytic bleaching.

2. Important

Besides being environmentally more benign, catalytic oxidation of organic compounds based on the use of terminal oxidants such as molecular oxygen and hydrogen peroxide is less wasteful from the economical points of view, and is now an important reaction in both research laboratories and industry. Metal salen compounds have been investigated as catalysts in several different reactions, for example epoxidation, epoxide ring opening, carbonyl addition, cycloaddition and oxidation of sulphides to sulphoxides. Earlier work on the Co-salen catalyzed oxidation of phenols with oxygen has been extended to include substrates that serve as models for lignin subunits to provide fundamental basis for the improvement in pulp bleaching industry.

Our laboratory has been investigating the process parameters of Co-salen catalyzed bleaching of bamboo pulp. The mechanism for the oxidation of residual lignin of pulp using Co-salen as catalyst is largely unstudied. In the present study, we studied the structural changes in residual lignin isolated of bamboo pulp across the Co-salen catalytic treatment in the presence of molecular oxygen and hydrogen peroxide using pyridine as axial ligand with GPC, FTIR, ^{1}H-NMR, ^{31}P-NMR and element analysis. It was found that the methoxyl group, phenolic hydroxyl group, aliphatic hydroxyl group, guaiacyl and syringyl were reduced; the content of carbonyl group increased; the aromatic ring was opened, the linkages of β-O-4, β-1, β-5 and β-β were cleaved; the molecular weight of residual lignin decreased. The chromophore of the bleached pulp with Co-salen biomimetic pretreatment was reduced and its crystallinity increased. The experimental formulas(C_9) of the residual lignin of the oxygen delignified bamboo pulp before and after biomimetic treatment were also obtained.

3. Experimental

3.1 Material

Co-salen was synthesized following the procedure of published literature (Liu et al., 1991; Liu et al., 2002).

Oxygen delignified kraft pulp of bamboo (OKP) used was prepared in our laboratory with the property as follows: kappa number 9.1, viscosity 1043 ml/g, brightness 39.5 % ISO.

3.2 Experimental methods

3.2.1 Co-salen treatment of OKP

The treatment was carried out in a 1 L stainless steel tank. Reaction tank was tempered at 90 °C for 5 h by contant-temperature water bath. Oxygen flow was directed into the tank at the pressure of 0.2 MPa. The charge of chemicals (o.d.p.), 0.03% Co-salen, 1:1 pyridine/Co-salen (molar ratio), 3% NaOH, 1.5% H_2O_2, was used at 5 %pulp consistency.

3.2.2 Bleaching of OKP with TCF sequence

OKP was bleached with the sequence of Co-salen pretreatment (Co), alkali extraction with addition of H_2O_2 (Ep), peracetic acid (Pa) and hydrogen peroxide (P) bleaching. Control trial was also performed instead of any chemicals with distilled water at pretreatment stage.

3.2.3 Isolation of residual lignin in pulp, oxygen delignified and Co-salen pretreated pulp

The pulps acetone-preextracted were extracted with 0.1 M HCl in dioxane/water (82 : 18) under nitrogen positive pressure and subsequently worked up according to established procedures (Shi & He, 2003).

3.2.4 Acetylation of lignin samples

Lignin samples were acetylated with pyridine-acetic anhydride solution (1 : 2, v : v) for ^{1}H-NMR analysis.

3.3 Analytical methods

3.3.1 Molecular weight of lignin samples

Molecular weight of lignin samples were determined with Waters 515 Gel Permeation Chromatography (GPC).

3.3.2 Elemental analysis

Analysis of C, H, N in lignin samples was performed on Vario EL Organic Elemental Analyser. Content of O was as calculated from that of C, H, N.

3.3.3 FTIR analysis

Bruker Tensor 27 FT-IR Spectroscopy was used at 400-4000 cm^{-1}.

3.3.4 NMR analysis

The analytical techniques of ^{1}H-NMR and ^{31}P-NMR are employed for the determination of residual lignin structural features on Bruker DRX 500 NMR Spectroscopy.

3.4 Methoxyl content of lignin samples

Vieböck method was used for the determination of methoxyl content of lignin samples (Shi & He, 2003).

3.5 C_9 experimental formula of lignin samples

C_9 experimental formula of lignin samples was obtained based on the elemental and methoxyl analysis according to the formula $C_xH_yO_z(OCH_3)_n$ provided by Vazquez et al (Vazquez et al., 1997).

4. Results and discussion

4.1 Elemental and methoxyl analysis of isolated residual lignins before and after Co-salen biomimetic treatment

The data are listed in Table 1 on elemental composition, methoxyl content and experimental formula of residual lignins isolated from pulps obtained during Co-salen biomimetic treatment. Content in methoxyl was reduced possibly due to the cleavage of methyl aryl ether. Molecular weight of structural uint (C_9) was also increased due to the increase in oxygen element content which resulted from the catalytic oxidation of aryl ring and side chain by Co-salen.

Samples	C/%	H/%	O/%	N/%	OCH_3/%	Experimental formulas (C_9)	Unit molecular weight
Untreated	59.03	6.455	33.74	0.780	17.67	$C_9H_{9.82}O_{3.18}(OCH_3)_{1.18}$	205.3
Treated	55.84	6.423	37.34	0.396	12.85	$C_9H_{11.00}O_{4.08}(OCH_3)_{0.88}$	211.5

Table 1. Results of elemental and methoxyl analysis of isolated residual lignins before and after Co-salen biomimetic treatment

4.2 Molecular weight analysis of isolated residual lignins before and after Co-salen biomimetic treatment

Molecular weight (Mn, Mw) and polydispersity of residual lignin was all decreased across the oxidation degradation in Co-salen biomimetic treatment according to the data obtained by GPC (Table 2).

Samples	RT/min	Mn	Mw	Polydispersity
Untreated	7.2	4813	5418	1.12
Treated	7.2	4759	5199	1.09

Table 2. Molecular weight of isolated residual lignins before and after Co-salen biomimetic treatment

4.3 FTIR analysis of isolated residual lignins before and after Co-salen biomimetic treatment

AS seen in Table 3, the band of ~ 3430 cm^{-1} was assigned to hydroxyl, it was reduced according to the relative intensity, which was just because of the oxidation reaction in which obvious increase in carbonyl (1640 cm^{-1}) was observed. This increase can enhance the

No.	Assignment (Jiang, 2009)	Wavenumber /cm^{-1}		Rel. intensity	
		Untreated	Treated	Untreated	Treated
1	OH stretching vibration	3425	3432	0.555	0.485
2	CH asymmetrical stretching vibration in CH_3, CH_2, CH	2924	2923	0.198	0.191
3	CH symmetrical stretching vibration in CH_3, CH_2, CH	2853	2852	0.016	0.036
4	C=O stretching vibration in β-C=O, COOH, ester	1721	1720	0.086	0.072
5	C=O stretching vibration in α-C=O, conjugated C=O	1640	1630	0.030	0.210
6	Benzene skeleton vibration	1600	1603	0.240	0.015
7	Benzene skeleton vibration	1509	1508	0.092	0.060
8	CH deformation vibration in CH_3, CH_2	1462	1462	0.140	0.101
9	Benzene skeleton vibration	1422	1422	0.047	0.033
10	CH deformation vibration in benzene ring	1380	1381	0.012	0.018
11	C-O stretching vibration in syringyl ring	1326	1327	0.030	0.016
12	C-O stretching vibration in guaiacyl ring	1267	1266	0.013	0.010
13	C-O stretching vibration in syringyl ring	1216	1217	0.056	0.038
14	C-H stretching vibration in syringyl ring	1121	1125	0.015	0.018
15	C-O bending vibration in secondary alcohol, ether	1085	1084	0.018	0.364
16	C-O bending vibration in primary alcohol, ether	1051	1052	0.529	0.027
17	C-H bending vibration in benzene ring	898	899	0.023	0.006

Table 3. Results of FTIR analysis of isolated residual lignins before and after Co-salen biomimetic treatment

reactivity of residual lignin in pulp. The decrease in relative intensity of 2924, 1462 cm^{-1} indicated that aliphatic side chains were oxidized, in the mean time aryl rings were also seriously degraded as seen the observed significant weakening of signals at 1600, 1509, 1422 cm^{-1}. Syringyl structures (1326, 1216 cm^{-1}) was preferentially degraded, and guaiacyl ones (1267 cm^{-1}) basically did not change in reaction.

4.4 NMR analysis of isolated residual lignins before and after Co-salen biomimetic treatment

4.4.1 ^{1}H-NMR analysis

The results of ^{1}H-NMR analysis on residual lignins isolated from pulps in Co-salen biomimetic treatment were shown in Table 4. It was found that syringyl units were significantly reduced, guaiacyl units changed little, which was in agreement with the results obtained by FTIR, and p-OH benzene ones were increased. Demethylation occured as reaction proceeding leading to the decrese of methoxyl in residual lignin. The decrease in phenolic hydroxyl may be related to the etherification. In accordance with the FTIR analysis the decrease in aliphatic hydroxyl was due to the oxidation, in which H atom of COOH, CHO present in residual lignin was found to be obviously increased based on the ^{1}H-NMR data (Table 4). In addition H atom at 5.7-6.17, 3.03-3.54 ppm was reduced, which indicated that the structures with the linkages of β-O-4, β-1, β-5, β-β were partially cleaved.

No.	δ/ppm	Assignment (Shi & He, 2003)	H/%		H/C_9	
			Untreated	Treated	Untreated	Treated
1	8.01-11.50	H in COOH, CHO	1.01	6.21	0.20	1.23
	7.50-8.01	H in aromatic nucleus of p-OH benzene	1.64	2.78	0.32	0.55
2	6.97-7.50	H in aromatic nucleus of guaiacyl	6.07	5.72	1.19	1.13
	6.17-6.97	H in aromatic nucleus of syringyl	5.06	3.76	0.99	0.74
3	5.70-6.17	$H_α$ in side chain (β-O-4, β-1); $H_β$ (conjugated between α and β)	3.16	2.29	0.62	0.45
4	5.20-5.70	$H_α$ in phenyl coumaran	1.90	2.45	0.37	0.48
	4.40-5.20	$H_α$ (β-β); $H_β$ (β-O-4); $H_γ$ (cinnamyl alcohol)	4.55	5.88	0.89	1.16
5	4.14-4.40	$H_γ$ (β-1, β-5, β-O-4, β-β)	2.91	3.10	0.59	0.60
	3.54-4.14	H in CH_3O	11.25	10.13	2.21	2.00
	3.03-3.54	$H_β$ (β-1, β-5, β-β)	7.96	6.37	1.56	1.26
6	2.20-3.03	Aromatic OH	13.65	13.07	2.68	2.48
7	1.47-2.20	Aliphatic OH	22.00	21.41	4.31	4.23

Table 4. Results of ^{1}H-NMR analysis of isolated residual lignins before and after Co-salen biomimetic treatment

4.4.2 ^{31}P-NMR analysis

No.	δ/ppm	Assignment (Granata & Argyropoulos, 1995)	mmol · g^{-1} Untreated	Treated
1	149.8-145.2	Aliphatic OH	1.12	1.08
2	144.5-143.6	Condensed aromatic OH	0.34	0.23
3	143.6-142.3	Syringyl aromatic OH	0.14	0.08
4	140.1-138.5	Guaiacyl aromatic OH	0.20	0.13
5	138.5-137.0	p-aromatic OH	0.15	0.11
6	136.5~133.6	COOH	0.48	0.51

Table 5. Results of ^{31}P-NMR analysis of isolated residual lignins before and after Co-salen biomimetic treatment

The data obtained by ^{31}P-NMR (Table 5) also showed that aliphatic and phenolic hydroxyls present in residual lignin were reduced, and carboxyls increased after Co-salen biomimetic bleaching of oxygen delignified bamboo pulp, where the change of syringyl-type phenolics was more obvious than other functional groups as listed in Table 5. Especially condensed-type phenolic structures were significantly degraded, which may improved the removal of residual lignin from the pulp.

4.5 FTIR analysis of resultant bleached pulp compared to the control sample

The signals at 1237, 1059, 1032, 987 cm^{-1} in FTIR spectra were assigned to carbonyl group present in cellulose, hemicellulose and lignin. The relative intensity of these signals were weakened compared to the control sample as shown in Table 6, which indicated that Co-salen biomimetic pretreatment may reduced chromophores produced during the bleaching process. In addition the crystallinity of bleached pulp was also increased when oxygen delignified pulp of bamboo was pretreated by Co-salen biomimetic system.

5. Conclusion

During Co-salen biomimetic pretreatment of oxygen delignified bamboo pulp, ary rings were opened, the functional groups of methoxyl, phenolic and aliphatic hydroxyl reduced. Carbonyls were increased due to the oxidation of aliphatic hydroxyls. Structural units of guaiacyl and syringyl-type present in residual lignin were degraded. Structural linkages were cleaved including β-O-4, β-1, β-5 and β-β. Molecular weight of residual lignin was decreased as reaction proceeding, oppositely that of C_9-structural uint was increased due to the increase in oxygen element content according to the C_9-experimental formulas obtained in this study. Besides the structural changes occured in residual lignin mentioned above, Co-salen biomimetic pretreatment may reduce chromophores and increase crystallinity of resultant bleached pulp of bamboo.

No.	Assignment (Stenius & Vuorinen, 1999)	Wavenumber / cm^{-1} Control	Bleached pulp	Rel. intensity Control	Bleached pulp
1	CH asymmetrical stretching vibration in CH_3, CH_2, CH in cellulose	2899	2901	0.141	0.121
2	CH_2 shear vibration in cellulose	1433	1432	0.054	0.055
3	CH bending vibration in cellulose and hemicellulose	1375	1376	0.120	0.116
4	C=O stretching vibration in lignin	1237	1238	0.008	0.001
5	C=O stretching vibration in cellulose and hemicellulose	1059	1059	0.423	0.386
6	C=O stretching vibration in cellulose, hemicellulose and lignin	1032	1032	0.029	0.026
7	C=O stretching vibration in cellulose and hemicellulose	987	988	0.022	0.012
8	C_1 deformation vibration in polysaccharide	896	896	0.060	0.049
9	Crystallinity index (Shi & He, 2003) $O'KI$ = A 1433cm^{-1}/ A 896cm^{-1} $N{\cdot}O'KI$ = A 1375cm^{-1}/ A 2899cm^{-1}			0.783 0.849	0.903 0.949

Table 6. Results of FTIR analysis of resultant bleached pulp when oxygen delignified bamboo pulp was treated with the sequence CoEpPaP

6. Acknowledgements

The authors are grateful to the National Natural Science Foundation of China (No.20766002) and the Foundation of Research Center for Analysis and Measurement (Kunming University of Science and Technology) of China, for the financial support.

7. References

Cui, F.; Dolphin, D. (1994). The biomimetic oxidation of β-1, β-O-4, β-5, and biphenyl lignin model compounds by synthetic iron porphyrins. *Bioorganic&Medicinal Chemistry*, 2, 7, 735-742, ISSN 0968-0896

Granata, A. & Argyropoulos, D. S. (1995). 2-chloro-4,4,5,5-tetramethyl-1,3,2-dioxaphospholane, a reagent for the accurate determination of the unconcondensed and condensed phenolic moieties in lignins. *Journal of. Agricultural & Food Chemistry*, 43, 6, 1538-1544, ISSN 0021-8561

Huynh, V. B. (1986). Biomimetic oxidation of lignin model compounds by simple inorganic complexes. *Biochemical & Biophysical Research Communications*, 139, 3, 1104-1110, ISSN 0006-291X

Jiang, T. D. (2009). *Lignin*, Chemical Industrial Press, ISBN 978-7-122-03796-1, Beijing

Liu, J.; Shanguan, G. Q. & Li, J. (1991). Synthesis and oxygen-carrying effect of [Co II(salen)] complex. *Journal of Jining Medical University*, 14, 4, 19-20, ISSN 1000-9760

Liu, Z. C.; Liu, F.; Lu, Y.; Xie, M. X. & Zhang, Y. Q. (2002). Studies on characters and synthesis of metal-salen complexes. *Journal of Leshan Teachers College*, 17, 4, 30-33, ISSN 1009-8666

Shi, S. L. & He, F. W. (2003). *Analysis & Detection of Pulp & Paper*, China Light Industry Press, ISBN 7-5019-3920-9/TS.2332, Beijing

Stenius, P. & Vuorinen, T (1999). Direct Characterization of Chemical Properties of Fibers, In: *Analytical Methods in Wood Chemistry, Pulping and Papermaking*, Sjöström, E. & Alén, R., (Ed.), 149-191, Springer-Verlag, ISBN 3-540-63102-X, Berlin, Heidelberg, New York

Vazquez, G.; Antorrena, G.; Gonzalez, J. & Freire, S. (1997). FTIR, ^{1}H and ^{13}C NMR characterization of acetosolv-solubilized pine and eucalyptus lignins. *Holzforschung*, 51, 2, 158-166, ISSN 0018-3830

Xie, R. G. (1999). Mimic enzyme catalysis and green chemistry. *Chemical Research & Application*, 11, (4), 344-349, ISSN 1004-1656

15

Bioinspired Strategies for Hard Tissue Regeneration

Anne George and Chun-Chieh Huang
Brodie Tooth Development Genetics & Regenerative Medicine Research Laboratory,
Department of Oral Biology,
University of Illinois at Chicago,
Department of Oral Biology,
Chicago, IL 60612,
USA

1. Introduction

Synthesis of biomaterials has seen tremendous growth in the past decade and protein templates have emerged as a high utility scaffold to facilitate cell-matrix interactions. The development of new biomaterials play a central role in modern regenerative medicine and tissue engineering. Protein-engineered biomaterials have recently received much attention. The diversity of peptide modules available throughout the proteome broadens the horizon that protein engineered biomaterials can achieve (1). The current challenges for developing protein-based scaffolds for tissue engineering lies in the fabrication of three-dimensional hierarchical materials that mimic the structural complexity of the natural ECM. The natural ECM is a hierarchically structured composite material that is able to furnish several cues for cellular proliferation and differentiation (2, 3). Complex protein-engineered scaffolds can be synthesized by designing scaffolds that self-assemble into specific hierarchical structures.

Molecular self-assembly presents a very attractive strategy to construct nanoscale materials at multiple length scales due to its simplicity in application (4-6). Self assembly can be defined as the spontaneous organization of individual entities such as molecules under thermodynamic equilibrium conditions into coherent, well-defined and stable arrangements without human interventions. In nature, peptides and proteins have the ability to self-organize hierarchically and precisely into well-defined two or three dimensional structures. The building blocks that can undergo the self-assembly process undergo stepwise aggregation through the formation of the hydrogen bonds, electrostatic interactions, hydrophobic interactions, van der Waals interactions and π- stackings (7-10). It is the collective strengths of these weak interactions that form the basis for fabrication of very supramolecular architectures and bioinspired nanomaterials with chemical complimentarity and structural compatibility (7, 9, 11).

In nature we find myriad examples of peptides and proteins that fold with great precision into three dimensional structures. Researchers have identified different protein domains for various end use applications in tissue engineering. Manipulation of the protein domains can be used to control the material properties of the hydrogel. Tailor-made protein scaffolds should provide mechanical properties similar to the extracellular matrix. Further, self-

assembling protein scaffolds are capable of presenting multiple cell-interactive components in spatially resolved networks via supramolecular self-assembly. Self-assembled materials provide several advantages: namely they can be multifunctional, possess high multifunctionality and control over the nanoscale positioning of ligands and other biomolecular features. Self-assembling based peptide materials can be used for regenerative medicine and drug-delivery technologies as they are found to be minimally immunogenic, inherently biocompatible and biodegradable. Thus, protein based scaffolds would be highly beneficial to guide spatially-and temporally-complex multicellular processes of tissue regeneration.
Peptide and protein based biomaterials have emerged as a new class of biomaterials that possesses unique and often superior properties when compared to conventional materials and are widely used for regenerative and reparative medicine (2, 12-14) . The main application of peptide-based biopolymers for tissue engineering is an injectable scaffold. Such hydrogels can serve as a three-dimensional artificial extracellular matrix to provide embedded cells with structural integrity and functionality for tissue repair and regeneration. There are many protein domains and peptide motifs available for tissue engineering applications particularly for hard tissue regeneration. However, peptide-based biomaterials have limitations such as short shelf-life and thermal instability.

2. Hydrogels

Hydrogels are hydrophilic polymers that can retain a significant amount of water while maintaining a distinct three-dimensional structure (15, 16). Based on the nature of the crosslinking, hydrogels can be categorized as chemical or physical gels. The structure and properties of the primary chains as well as the crosslinking density, contribute to the overall properties of chemical hydrogels. Physical gels are networks held together by molecular entanglement or secondary molecular interactions. These interactions can be disrupted by changes in the environment, such as temperature, pH, ionic strength, presence of specific solutes and stress; consequently, the formation of physical hydrogels may be reversible(16). The fact that properties of a peptide domain can be imposed on the whole hybrid hydrogel suggests that the supramolecular organization of hybrid materials is driven mainly by the biorecognition of peptide segments (17).

3. Rheological properties

The mechanical properties of the peptide hydrogels are important for determining their suitability in various tissue engineering applications. As protein-based scaffolds in tissue engineering are used as a structural component to support cell growth, it is therefore important that they possess sufficient mechanical strength. Cellular responses to ligand-presenting materials are strongly influenced by the material's stiffness. In order to elucidate a relationship between the molecular structure of a polypeptide and its rheological properties it is necessary to determine G' the elastic modulus which indicates the solid-like component of a viscoelastic hydrogel and the viscous modulus G'' represents the liquid-like component (13). To maintain the hydrogel in a solid-like state it is necessary to have G' larger than G''(13). Therefore, modifying substrate stiffness influences cell morphology, proliferation and differentiation and is an important factor in tailoring matrices for regenerative medicine.

4. Hard tissue regeneration

Bone and dentin are biological composites of organic and inorganic phases have a microstructure that provides an unusual combination of toughness and fracture resistance. Cartilage is composed of specialized cells called chondrocytes that produce a large amount of extracellular matrix composed of Type II collagen, proteoglycans and elastin fibers. The rapidly emerging field of tissue engineering holds great promise for the generation of functional bone and cartilage tissues. To this end molecular self-assembly presents a very attractive strategy to construct nanoscale materials for hard tissue engineering. This free energy-driven process spontaneously organizes molecules into ordered structures at multiple-length scales.

Molecular Biology techniques can be employed to synthesize protein domains and peptide motifs to create responsive protein for tissue engineering bone, dentin and cartilage. A critical requirement for materials designed to interact with cell receptors is the organization of multiple ligands on the surface of a scaffold in order to engage the receptors more effectively. Structures forming α-helices and β-sheets have been used to mediate self-assembly into hydrogels of peptides. In this review we review these processes on a few peptides that possess self-assembling properties and their use in hard tissue engineering.

5. Genetically engineered polypeptides in hard tissue engineering

(a) Self-Assembly of Elastin: Elastin is the major extracellular matrix protein which is responsible for the properties of extensibility and elastic recoil of many tissues such as the large arterial blood-vessels, lung parenchyma and skin (18). Elastin is synthesized as a monomer, tropoelastin, which is subsequently assembled into a stable, polymeric structure in the extracellular matrix (19). This self-assembly property of full-length tropoelastin can also be mimicked by smaller polypeptides.

Elastin-like polypeptides (ELPs) have the ability to undergo organized self-assembly into network structures through a process of temperature-induced phase separation or coacervation (20) . Elastin-like polypeptides are derived from a repeating motif within a hydrophobic domain of mammalian tropoelastin: the most common motif has the sequence $(VPGXG)_m$, where X can be any amino acid other than proline, and m is the number of repeats (1). There are many other variants of ELPs that range from other pentapeptides with the repeat sequence KGGVG (21) or LGGVG (22) to heptapeptides with the sequence LGAGGAG and nonapeptides with the sequence LGAGGAGVL. All of these elastin analogues appear to exhibit elastin-like properties.

Wright et al. and Nagapudi et al.(23, 24) have synthesized self-assembling elastin-mimetic triblock polypeptides. The copolymers composed of a plastic domain VPAG as the end blocks and an elastomeric domain VPGVG as the middle block. The single substitution of an alanine residue for a glycine residue in the third amino acid position of the repeating sequence converts the blocks mechanical behavior from elastic to plastic. This change is caused by the structural change from the Pro-Gly type II β-turn structure to the Pro-Ala type I β-turn structure (23). For ELPs the important biophysical characterization is the determination of the inverse temperature transition behavior and is usually represented by the lower critical solution temperature (LCST) or transition temperature (T_t). Rheological measurements of an aqueous triblock copolymer solution as a function of temperature showed that the copolymers would be well-suited for biomedical applications.

Fabrication of these covalently cross-linked aggregates of ELPs into membrane-like matrices has been exploited for cartilage tissue engineering. Betre et al. have demonstrated that chondrocytes can be encapsulated in the gel-like material formed by aggregated ELPs (25, 26). These chondrocytes maintained their characteristic morphology and synthesized phenotypic markers such as collagen type II and sulphated glycosaminoglycans.

A critical requirement for materials designed to interact with cell receptors is the organization of multiple ligands on the surface of a scaffold in order to engage the receptors more effectively. Kaufmann et al. have demonstrated a new approach for the preparation of bioactive elastin-mimetic hydrogels (27). Osteoblast adhesion was dependent on the ligand type, ligand density and the use of a spacer. Nettles et al. have used ELP as an injectable peptide into osteochondral defects and demonstrated cell infiltration and cartilage matrix synthesis in critically sized defects (28).

(b) Self-assembly of Leucine Zipper-based triblock proteins: The DNA binding leucine zipper proteins contain a self-assembling leucine zipper domain. Leucine zippers are a structural motif commonly found in transcription factors. The leucine zipper domain is a reversible self-assembly domain (29-31). Hydrophobic forces drive the assembly of the coiled-coil bundles as the hydrophobic planes along the length of the α-helices are buried. The leucine zipper domains are composed of a repeating heptad motif designated *abcdefg* where *a* and *d* are hydrophobic amino acids (leucine is preferred at position d) and *e* and *g* are charged amino acids (glutamic acid is common). The repeating domain has an α-helix structure and easily forms inter-and intra-chain coiled coil dimers due to the hydrophobic interaction between the *a* and *d* residues, which are positioned on a single face of the helix. The charged e and g residues positioned on the opposite phase of the helix impart pH-sensitivity to the coiled-coil dimers. Upon elevation of the pH, temperature or ionic strength, the leucine zipper domains reversibly dissociate and create a viscous polymeric solution (13). The reversible assembly makes the leucine zipper domain to facilitate the formation of physical crosslinks in hydrogel structures. The motif's name reflects the predominance of leucine residues at the *a* and *d* positions. Hydrogels are usually based on physical or chemical crosslink's of hydrophilic gelators to form a three-dimensional network (32). It is able to immobilize and entrap large amounts of water resulting in tissue-mimicking environment.

Petka et al. have demonstrated that genetically synthesized triblock copolymers consisting of leucine zipper helix endblocks and water-soluble polyelectrolyte midblock will self-assemble into pH and temperature-sensitive hydrogels upon dimerization of the leucine zipper coils (29). Wang et al. described the use of leucine zipper domains in a hybrid synthetic polymer-protein material (17). The hybrid material undergoes a volume change in response to temperature change as leucine zipper coiled coils dissociate at high temperature (15, 33).

In order to exploit the use of leucine zipper polypeptides in hard tissue engineering, Gajjeraman et al. have designed a leucine zipper polypeptide with motifs from the hydroxyapatite nucleating domain and cell-adhesive motifs from dentin matrix protein 1 (DMP1) (34). Although, DMP1 was initially isolated from the dentin matrix and was thought to be unique to dentin and named accordingly, it has now been found to be present in all mineralized tissues of the vertebrate system (35, 36). The C-terminal polypeptide of DMP1 contains the HAP nucleating domain as well as an RGD motif for cell-adhesion which makes it a highly desirable polypeptide for *in-vivo* applications requiring calcified tissue formation (36).

In this system a modular design was used to genetically engineer de *novo* self-assembled chimeric protein hydrogels comprising leucine zipper motifs flanked by the C-terminal domain of DMP1. Results from this study showed that the leucine zipper hydrogel exhibited both osteoconductive and osteoinductive properties. Recently Huang et al. (unpublished data) have introduced several cysteine residues in the leucine zipper construct to enable the formation of intermolecular disulphide bonds which would effectively crosslink the nanofibers into a high molecular weight polymer (Fig 1). Cryo SEM showed that the introduction of cysteines was effective in promoting nanofiber networks. Integration of RGD domains in this construct facilitated cell attachment and proliferation (Fig 3). Thus, integration of biological self-organization and cell-attachment components are important to synthesize complex materials that exhibit order from the molecular to the macroscopic scale. Such hydrogels from self-assembled peptides have a potential to serve as synthetic extracellular matrices.

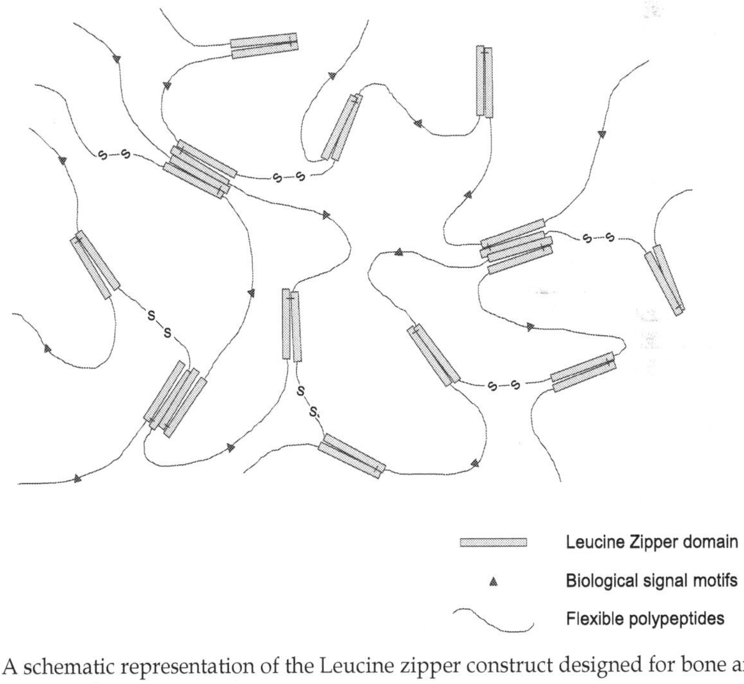

Fig. 1. A schematic representation of the Leucine zipper construct designed for bone and dentin regeneration.

(c) Self-Assembling peptide MDG1 (Mineral Directing Gelator): In a recent study Gungormus et al. described the synthesis of an *in situ* forming self-assembling peptide hydrogel that is capable of directing the mineralization of calcium phosphate (37). The peptide construct MDG1 is a 27 residue peptide designed to undergo triggered intra-molecular folding and subsequent self-assembly to form a fibrillar network resulting in a mechanically rigid gel. This peptide folds in a solution containing calcium chloride and beta-glycerophosphate and in pH buffered water at low ionic strength the peptide remains

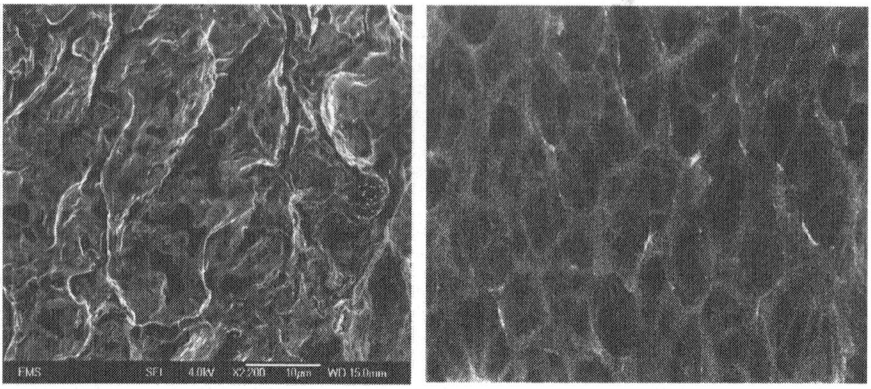

Fig. 2. SEM image of the self-assembled leucine zipper hydrogel

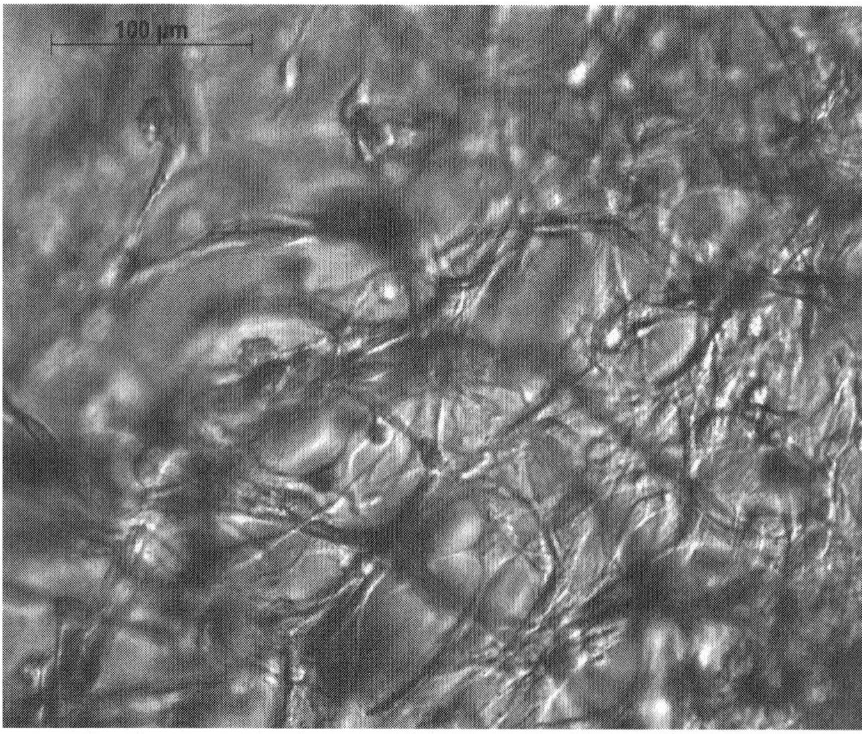

Fig. 3. Attachment and spreading of the human mesenchymal stem cells on the leucine zipper hydrogel at 2 days.

unfolded. The N-terminal twenty residues of MDG1 are designed to adopt an amphiphilic β-hairpin when the peptide folds. The N-terminal portion contains 2 β-strands connected by a four residue sequence (-V^{D}PPT-) known to adopt a type II′ β-turn (38). The β-strands are composed of alternating hydrophobic and hydrophilic residues that give the hairpin its amphiphilic character in the folded state. The complete N-terminal peptide has been reported in the literature as MAX8 and contains the sequence VKVKVKVKV^{D}PPTKVEVKVKV-$CONH_2$ (39) . The C-terminal seven residues of MDG1 contain the sequence MLPHHGA and this sequence directs mineralization. The C-terminal peptide slows the mineralization rate and accelerates the transformation of amorphous calcium phosphate into crystalline octacalcium phosphate during mineralization. Hydrogels for mineralization were formed by the addition of calcium chloride solution containing alkaline phosphatase directly in the cassette. At the end of 2 hrs of gelation the cassette was immersed in a bath that contained a buffered solution of beta-glycerophosphate and calcium chloride. Such a system enabled controlled mineralization of the scaffold as the calcification process occurred when the β-GP diffused into the cassette and was cleaved by the enzyme. Characterization of the mineral deposits within the hydrogel showed that they were highly crystalline and elongated resembling biological apatite. Further, this scaffold supported the viability of cementoblasts and was able to produce a calcified matrix.

(d) Self-Assembly of β-sheet fibrillizing peptides: β-sheet fibrillizing peptides have received particular attention recently as scaffolds for tissue engineering due to their ability to form hydrogels (40-43). β-sheets are well known for their ability to assemble into long fibrous structures. The basic motif present in most β-sheets consists of alternating hydrophobic, hydrophilic residues. As a consequence of this alternating pattern, they give rise to a hydrophobic and hydrophilic face when assembled into a sheet. RAD16 peptide which is derived from the self-assembling sequences of laminin is a β-sheet fibril forming peptide that is capable of presenting bioactive ligands on their surface (44-46). Q11 a peptide containing the sequence (QQKFQFQFEQQ) was designed to present ligands such as RGDS or IKVAV at their N-termini (47). The RGDS sequence found in fibronectin, laminin, vitronectin and many other extracellular matrix proteins is an integrin binding peptide and is neutrally charged and hydrophilic (48). The peptide IKVAV is a cryptic sequence found at the carboxy-terminal end of the α1 chain of laminin is known to be a modulator of neuronal cell attachment and growth (49). This peptide is positively charged and comparatively hydrophobic. Stiffness of Q11 gels was dependent on peptide concentration with storage moduli ranging from 1 to 10kPa for gels having peptide concentrations between 5 and 30mM respectively. Jung et al. have recently shown that the co-assembling hydrogel based on Q11 peptides with the RGD containing ligand influenced HUVEC attachment, spreading and growth (47).

Pochan and Schneider have demonstrated that short amphiphilic peptides that fold into β-hairpin structures will self-assemble into injectable hydrogels that can be used for tissue engineering (42, 43, 50-52). Haines-Butterick et al. used β-hairpin molecules with a lower net positive charge to homogenously encapsulate the mesenchymal stem cells within the hydrogel network (53). In the presence of growth factors these cells could be coaxed into an osteoblast lineage.

(e) Self-assembly of chemically synthesized Peptide Amphiphiles: Peptide amphiphiles (PAs) are a class of molecules that combine the structural features of amphiphilic surfactants with the functions of bioactive peptides and are known to self- assemble into a variety of nanostructures (54). The peptide amphiphiles are obtained chemically using an automated peptide synthesizer and consist of an alkyl tail connected to a short peptide sequence. The peptide sequence always ends in a hydrophilic head group, giving the PA its amphiphilic character. Stupp et al. have synthesized peptide amphiphiles that consist of 4 key structural domains (55). Domain 1 consists of a hydrophobic region typically consisting of a long alkyl tail. Domain 2 consists of a short peptide sequence capable of forming intermolecular hydrogen bonding, typically in the form of β-sheets. Domain 3 contains charged amino acids for enhanced solubility in water and for the formation of networks. Domain 4 is used for the presentation of bioactive signals for interaction with cells or proteins(56). The self-assembly of PAs in water is due to hydrophobic interactions of the alkyl tails, hydrogen bonding among the middle peptide segments and electrostatic repulsion between the charged amino acids. The PAs developed by Stupp and coworkers self-assemble into high-aspect-ratio nanofibers under specific solution conditions (57, 58) . Molecular packing within a cylindrical geometry allows for the presentation of biological signals at very high density on the fiber surface. Control of PA nanostructures and their subsequent gelation could be controlled through the molecular forces that contribute to the self-assembly process. Thus, molecularly designed peptide amphiphile materials are capable of self-assembling into well-defined nanofibers.

The chemistry on the surface of the PA nanofibers can be customized to create templates for mineralization. Hartgerink et al. designed PA templates with phosphoserines to aid hydroxyapatite deposition (55). Interestingly, the crystallographic c-axis of hydroxyapatite aligned with the long axis of PA nanofibers, mimicking the crystallographic orientation of hydroxyapatite crystals in bone with respect to the long axis of collagen fibers. Recently, Mata et. al reported on the *in vivo* osteogenic potential of self-assembling Pas (59). Results from this study demonstrated that a combination of functionalized PAs i.e RGDS-PA along with S (P)-PA (phosphorylated serine) self-assembling gel promoted bone formation in a rat femoral critical-sized defect within 4 weeks. The newly formed bone was comparable to animals treated with a clinically used allogenic bone matrix. Thus, self-assembling nanofibrous PA matrices could promote formation of biomimetic bone crystals.

Shah et al. designed a coassembly system of PA molecules containing epitopes to transforming growth factor beta-1, that were designed to form nanofibers for cartilage regeneration (60). *In-vitro* studies indicated that these materials were able to support the survival and promoted the chondrogenic differentiation of human mesenchymal stem cells. These studies demonstrated the potential of a completely synthetic bioactive biomaterial as a therapy to promote cartilage regeneration.

Varying the design of the molecular structures of PAs as well as manipulation of their self-assembly environment can be exploited to control the self-assembly process and generate novel materials for hard tissue regeneration and repair.

6. Conclusions

Thus, molecular self-assembly can be used as a toolbox to produce functional materials. The rapidly emerging field of tissue engineering holds great promise for the regeneration and repair of hard tissues. There have been a number of successful approaches to tissue engineer bone and cartilage with the use of natural biomaterial scaffolds; however, there are many challenges ahead with these natural scaffolds. Biomaterials for the future could be envisaged to behave dynamically in their environment and facilitate repair and regeneration within a shorter time-frame.

7. Acknowledgements

We like to acknowledge support for these studies from the Brodie Endowment Fund and National Institute of Dental and Craniofacial Research, National Institute of Health Grant DE 11657.

8. References

[1] Banta S, Wheeldon, IR, Blenner, M Protein engineering in the development of functional hydrogels. Annu Rev Biomed Eng 12:167-186.

[2] Sengupta D, Heilshorn, SC Protein-engineered biomaterials: highly tunable tissue engineering scaffolds. Tissue Eng Part B Rev 16:285-293.

[3] Romano NH, Sengupta, D, Chung, C, Heilshorn, SC Protein-engineered biomaterials: Nanoscale mimics of the extracellular matrix. Biochim Biophys Acta.

[4] Palmer LC, Stupp, SI (2008) Molecular self-assembly into one-dimensional nanostructures. Acc Chem Res 41:1674-1684.

[5] Palmer LC, Velichko, YS, de la Cruz, MO, Stupp, SI (2007) Supramolecular self-assembly codes for functional structures. Philos Transact A Math Phys Eng Sci 365:1417-1433.

[6] Scheibel T, Parthasarathy, R, Sawicki, G, Lin, XM, Jaeger, H, Lindquist, SL (2003) Conducting nanowires built by controlled self-assembly of amyloid fibers and selective metal deposition. Proc Natl Acad Sci U S A 100:4527-4532.

[7] Zhang S (2002) Emerging biological materials through molecular self-assembly. Biotechnol Adv 20:321-339.

[8] Zhao X, Zhang, S (2007) Designer self-assembling peptide materials. Macromol Biosci 7:13-22.

[9] Zhang S (2003) Fabrication of novel biomaterials through molecular self-assembly. Nat Biotechnol 21:1171-1178.

[10] Ulijn RV, Smith, AM (2008) Designing peptide based nanomaterials. Chem Soc Rev 37:664-675.

[11] Zhang S, Marini, DM, Hwang, W, Santoso, S (2002) Design of nanostructured biological materials through self-assembly of peptides and proteins. Curr Opin Chem Biol 6:865-871.

[12] Lutolf MP, Hubbell, JA (2005) Synthetic biomaterials as instructive extracellular microenvironments for morphogenesis in tissue engineering. Nat Biotechnol 23:47-55.

[13] Chow D, Nunalee, ML, Lim, DW, Simnick, AJ, Chilkoti, A (2008) Peptide-based Biopolymers in Biomedicine and Biotechnology. Mater Sci Eng R Rep 62:125-155.

[14] Langer R, Tirrell, DA (2004) Designing materials for biology and medicine. Nature 428:487-492.

[15] Kopecek J (2007) Hydrogel biomaterials: a smart future? Biomaterials 28:5185-5192.

[16] Kopecek J, Yang, J (2009) Peptide-directed self-assembly of hydrogels. Acta Biomater 5:805-816.

[17] Wang C, Stewart, RJ, Kopecek, J (1999) Hybrid hydrogels assembled from synthetic polymers and coiled-coil protein domains. Nature 397:417-420.

[18] Keeley FW, Bellingham, CM, Woodhouse, KA (2002) Elastin as a self-organizing biomaterial: use of recombinantly expressed human elastin polypeptides as a

model for investigations of structure and self-assembly of elastin. Philos Trans R Soc Lond B Biol Sci 357:185-189.
[19] Mecham RP, Broekelmann, T, Davis, EC, Gibson, MA, Brown-Augsburger, P (1995) Elastic fibre assembly: macromolecular interactions. Ciba Found Symp 192:172-181; discussion 181-174.
[20] Cirulis JT, Keeley, FW Kinetics and morphology of self-assembly of an elastin-like polypeptide based on the alternating domain arrangement of human tropoelastin. Biochemistry 49:5726-5733.
[21] Martino M, Tamburro, AM (2001) Chemical synthesis of cross-linked poly(KGGVG), an elastin-like biopolymer. Biopolymers 59:29-37.
[22] Martino M, Coviello, A, Tamburro, AM (2000) Synthesis and structural characterization of poly(LGGVG), an elastin-like polypeptide. Int J Biol Macromol 27:59-64.
[23] Wright ER, Conticello, VP (2002) Self-assembly of block copolymers derived from elastin-mimetic polypeptide sequences. Adv Drug Deliv Rev 54:1057-1073.
[24] Nagapudi K, Brinkman, WT, Thomas, BS, Park, JO, Srinivasarao, M, Wright, E, Conticello, VP, Chaikof, EL (2005) Viscoelastic and mechanical behavior of recombinant protein elastomers. Biomaterials 26:4695-4706.
[25] Betre H, Ong, SR, Guilak, F, Chilkoti, A, Fermor, B, Setton, LA (2006) Chondrocytic differentiation of human adipose-derived adult stem cells in elastin-like polypeptide. Biomaterials 27:91-99.
[26] Betre H, Setton, LA, Meyer, DE, Chilkoti, A (2002) Characterization of a genetically engineered elastin-like polypeptide for cartilaginous tissue repair. Biomacromolecules 3:910-916.
[27] Kaufmann D, Fiedler, A, Junger, A, Auernheimer, J, Kessler, H, Weberskirch, R (2008) Chemical conjugation of linear and cyclic RGD moieties to a recombinant elastin-mimetic polypeptide--a versatile approach towards bioactive protein hydrogels. Macromol Biosci 8:577-588.
[28] Nettles DL, Kitaoka, K, Hanson, NA, Flahiff, CM, Mata, BA, Hsu, EW, Chilkoti, A, Setton, LA (2008) In situ crosslinking elastin-like polypeptide gels for application to articular cartilage repair in a goat osteochondral defect model. Tissue Eng Part A 14:1133-1140.
[29] Petka WA, Harden, JL, McGrath, KP, Wirtz, D, Tirrell, DA (1998) Reversible hydrogels from self-assembling artificial proteins. Science 281:389-392.
[30] Stevens MM, Allen, S, Davies, MC, Roberts, CJ, Sakata, JK, Tendler, SJ, Tirrell, DA, Williams, PM (2005) Molecular level investigations of the inter- and intramolecular interactions of pH-responsive artificial triblock proteins. Biomacromolecules 6:1266-1271.
[31] Shen W, Zhang, K, Kornfield, JA, Tirrell, DA (2006) Tuning the erosion rate of artificial protein hydrogels through control of network topology. Nat Mater 5:153-158.
[32] Boztas AO, Guiseppi-Elie, A (2009) Immobilization and release of the redox mediator ferrocene monocarboxylic acid from within cross-linked p(HEMA-co-PEGMA-co-HMMA) hydrogels. Biomacromolecules 10:2135-2143.
[33] Kopecek J (2009) Hydrogels from Soft Contact Lenses and Implants to Self-Assembled Nanomaterials. J Polym Sci A Polym Chem 47:5929-5946.

[34] Gajjeraman S, He, G, Narayanan, K, George, A (2008) Biological assemblies provide novel templates for the synthesis of hierarchical structures and facilitate cell adhesion. Adv Funct Mater 18:3972-3980.
[35] George A, Sabsay, B, Simonian, PA, Veis, A (1993) Characterization of a novel dentin matrix acidic phosphoprotein. Implications for induction of biomineralization. J Biol Chem 268:12624-12630.
[36] George A, Veis, A (2008) Phosphorylated proteins and control over apatite nucleation, crystal growth, and inhibition. Chem Rev 108:4670-4693.
[37] Gungormus M, Branco, M, Fong, H, Schneider, JP, Tamerler, C, Sarikaya, M Self assembled bi-functional peptide hydrogels with biomineralization-directing peptides. Biomaterials 31:7266-7274.
[38] Pantoja-Uceda D, Santiveri, CM, Jimenez, MA (2006) De novo design of monomeric beta-hairpin and beta-sheet peptides. Methods Mol Biol 340:27-51.
[39] Branco MC, Nettesheim, F, Pochan, DJ, Schneider, JP, Wagner, NJ (2009) Fast dynamics of semiflexible chain networks of self-assembled peptides. Biomacromolecules 10:1374-1380.
[40] Horii A, Wang, X, Gelain, F, Zhang, S (2007) Biological designer self-assembling peptide nanofiber scaffolds significantly enhance osteoblast proliferation, differentiation and 3-D migration. PLoS One 2:e190.
[41] Kretsinger JK, Haines, LA, Ozbas, B, Pochan, DJ, Schneider, JP (2005) Cytocompatibility of self-assembled beta-hairpin peptide hydrogel surfaces. Biomaterials 26:5177-5186.
[42] Pochan DJ, Schneider, JP, Kretsinger, J, Ozbas, B, Rajagopal, K, Haines, L (2003) Thermally reversible hydrogels via intramolecular folding and consequent self-assembly of a de novo designed peptide. J Am Chem Soc 125:11802-11803.
[43] Schneider JP, Pochan, DJ, Ozbas, B, Rajagopal, K, Pakstis, L, Kretsinger, J (2002) Responsive hydrogels from the intramolecular folding and self-assembly of a designed peptide. J Am Chem Soc 124:15030-15037.
[44] Gelain F, Bottai, D, Vescovi, A, Zhang, S (2006) Designer self-assembling peptide nanofiber scaffolds for adult mouse neural stem cell 3-dimensional cultures. PLoS One 1:e119.
[45] Kasai S, Urushibata, S, Hozumi, K, Yokoyama, F, Ichikawa, N, Kadoya, Y, Nishi, N, Watanabe, N, Yamada, Y, Nomizu, M (2007) Identification of multiple amyloidogenic sequences in laminin-1. Biochemistry 46:3966-3974.
[46] Kasai S, Ohga, Y, Mochizuki, M, Nishi, N, Kadoya, Y, Nomizu, M (2004) Multifunctional peptide fibrils for biomedical materials. Biopolymers 76:27-33.
[47] Jung JP, Nagaraj, AK, Fox, EK, Rudra, JS, Devgun, JM, Collier, JH (2009) Co-assembling peptides as defined matrices for endothelial cells. Biomaterials 30:2400-2410.
[48] Ruoslahti E, Pierschbacher, MD (1987) New perspectives in cell adhesion: RGD and integrins. Science 238:491-497.
[49] Adams DN, Kao, EY, Hypolite, CL, Distefano, MD, Hu, WS, Letourneau, PC (2005) Growth cones turn and migrate up an immobilized gradient of the laminin IKVAV peptide. J Neurobiol 62:134-147.
[50] Nagarkar RP, Hule, RA, Pochan, DJ, Schneider, JP (2008) De novo design of strand-swapped beta-hairpin hydrogels. J Am Chem Soc 130:4466-4474.

[51] Ozbas B, Rajagopal, K, Schneider, JP, Pochan, DJ (2004) Semiflexible chain networks formed via self-assembly of beta-hairpin molecules. Phys Rev Lett 93:268106.
[52] Rajagopal K, Lamm, MS, Haines-Butterick, LA, Pochan, DJ, Schneider, JP (2009) Tuning the pH responsiveness of beta-hairpin peptide folding, self-assembly, and hydrogel material formation. Biomacromolecules 10:2619-2625.
[53] Haines-Butterick L, Rajagopal, K, Branco, M, Salick, D, Rughani, R, Pilarz, M, Lamm, MS, Pochan, DJ, Schneider, JP (2007) Controlling hydrogelation kinetics by peptide design for three-dimensional encapsulation and injectable delivery of cells. Proc Natl Acad Sci U S A 104:7791-7796.
[54] Silva GA, Czeisler, C, Niece, KL, Beniash, E, Harrington, DA, Kessler, JA, Stupp, SI (2004) Selective differentiation of neural progenitor cells by high-epitope density nanofibers. Science 303:1352-1355.
[55] Hartgerink JD, Beniash, E, Stupp, SI (2001) Self-assembly and mineralization of peptide-amphiphile nanofibers. Science 294:1684-1688.
[56] Hung AM, Stupp, SI (2007) Simultaneous self-assembly, orientation, and patterning of peptide-amphiphile nanofibers by soft lithography. Nano Lett 7:1165-1171.
[57] Pashuck ET, Cui, H, Stupp, SI Tuning supramolecular rigidity of peptide fibers through molecular structure. J Am Chem Soc 132:6041-6046.
[58] Cui H, Webber, MJ, Stupp, SI Self-assembly of peptide amphiphiles: from molecules to nanostructures to biomaterials. Biopolymers 94:1-18.
[59] Mata A, Geng, Y, Henrikson, KJ, Aparicio, C, Stock, SR, Satcher, RL, Stupp, SI Bone regeneration mediated by biomimetic mineralization of a nanofiber matrix. Biomaterials 31:6004-6012.
[60] Shah RN, Shah, NA, Del Rosario Lim, MM, Hsieh, C, Nuber, G, Stupp, SI Supramolecular design of self-assembling nanofibers for cartilage regeneration. Proc Natl Acad Sci U S A 107:3293-3298.

16

Biomimetics in Bone Cell Mechanotransduction: Understanding Bone's Response to Mechanical Loading

Marnie M Saunders
The University of Akron
Akron, OH,
USA

1. Introduction

In biomimetics work, bone has often been cited as inspiration, ranging from the architectural influences in the Eiffel Tower to aerospace influences and adaptive strengthening of wing structures subjected to overload. However, the intricate complexity of bone itself means that there is still much to learn regarding how this composite can adapt so well to its loading environment. Moreover, many believe identifying and understanding these pathways and mechanisms holds the key to eradicating metabolic bone diseases such as osteoporosis and osteopetrosis. Specifically, as bone researchers, our goal is to understand how the bone cells which are responsible for the formation/destruction of bone coordinate their activities. In the laboratory, isolated cells (*in vitro*) and animal (*in vivo*) models are employed based upon unique advantages. *In vitro* systems have the advantage of isolating key factors to be studied but given their simplicity, their relevance to the *in vivo* world is questionable. *In vivo* systems have the advantage of clinical relevance and long-term study, but given their complexity, tweezing out the effects of the isolated loading events is difficult. Recently we have proposed using organ culture (*ex vivo*) bone models to study the effects of mechanical loading on bone cells. In these systems, whole bones are maintained in culture and the effects of an isolated load may be studied. The goal in essence is to study the bone cell response in a system that mimics the biological event. The intent is to increase the relevance of *in vitro* studies by maintaining and studying the response of the cells as they interact with each other (and other cell types) in a native, three-dimensional matrix with intact communication networks, a biomimetic system. However, these models also have disadvantages. Specifically, cut off from any blood supply, they are a dying organ and the question remains to be answered if they remain viable for a long enough period of time to be useful models for dissecting the response of bone cells to mechanical loading. This chapter will introduce the reader to the research area of bone mechanotransduction with a focus on engineering mechanics and address the validity of *ex vivo* systems as biomimetic models in comparison to *in vitro* and *in vivo* approaches. Finally we will look at the application of the organ culture approach and assess its usefulness in modeling the clinical procedure known as distraction osteogenesis.

When one thinks of bone and mechanics, the common images conjured up are of biomechanics tests. In bone biomechanics, mechanical testing principles and techniques are applied to, for instance, testing a bone under bending or torsion to determine material and structural properties, or the bone may be used as a holder to determine useful life of an implant or fracture fixation system. In bone biomechanics tests the bone is viewed largely as a static structure and the mechanical loading is used to determine an endpoint condition or value (strength, toughness, shear modulus, fatigue life). In contrast to biomechanics, in the field of bone mechanobiology it is recognized that bone is a highly dynamic structure which is subjected to mechanical forces/loading and that these loads are necessary, even critical, for bone growth, maintenance and function. Furthermore, bone metabolic diseases, such as osteoporosis, may be associated with the inability of the bone cells in the aging skeleton to sense and/or respond to mechanical loading levels that are sufficient to maintain bone quality in the younger skeleton. In bone mechanobiology, it is recognized that bone is a highly dynamic composite and mechanical loading is an input or impetus critical for normal bone quality and quantity and its maintenance. More specifically, since it is not the bone that responds to the mechanical loading but the bone cells that are responsible for the bone formation/destruction that respond to mechanical loading, mechanotransduction is a focused area of study in the bone mechanobiology field aimed at identifying and understanding the mechanisms and pathways by which bone cells sense and respond to mechanical stimulation in normal and abnormal (disease, implant introduction, spaceflight) loading environments.

Mechanotransduction work relies heavily on 'testing systems' that can provide load/stimulation to a cell, tissue, organ or animal model system. These testing systems provide an accurate and reproducible load/stimulation to the model and vary greatly in cost, function and flexibility. Given the engineering intent of this article, the testing platform will be explained in some depth. Commercial testing machines are uniaxial and biaxial with the latter comprising both torsional and rotational capabilities. While these systems can be quite expensive, they offer a degree of accuracy and precision under a variety of loading controls (displacement, load and strain) that is unparalleled. However, given the nature of extramurally funded research and the inclusion of engineers in the mechanobiology field, much of the mechanical testing system development is done in-house and a variety of single-purpose systems have evolved for these studies. While describing all these systems is not possible, and several excellent articles utilizing these systems are available to the interested reader (Rubin and Lanyon, 1984; Rubin and Lanyon, 1985; Turner, et al., 1991; Hillam and Skerry, 1995; Brown, 2000; Gross, et al., 2002), we will describe in some detail the development of a platform used in our lab and then utilize this system to explain the applications to the mechanotransduction work and the accompanying engineering strengths and limitations of the systems. It is important, given the multidisciplinary nature of the field that engineers involved in this research appreciate the limitations of the loading devices and communicate this to the biological scientists. The converse is also true, engineers need to be made aware of the biological limitations of the systems to better design and develop systems that accurately mimic the physiologic environment.

The initial platform designed in-house accommodated standard biomechanics tests including: bend testing of bones, compression testing of hard tissues, tension testing of soft tissues, and mini-implant evaluation and mechanotransduction tests, including: *in vivo* exercise loading and fluid shear and substrate deformation of bone cells. This device is a uniaxial system; torsional loading is made possible with the addition of a rack and pinion fixture. While most commercial systems are single axis (uniaxial) machines built on a fixed base, we opted for a movable base and found that an inexpensive way to create the two main components of the platform, the linear, vertical motion and the base frame was to purchase a slide and milling machine table. The milling machine table, given its routine use in machine shops offered a very cost-effective alternative to expensive stereotaxic platforms without compromising accuracy or precision. The slide and table are connected via aluminum plates. All connections are slotted with keyways to make assembly reproducible. To reinforce the machine for larger loads, side plates running the vertical length of the slide may be added (not shown in Figure 1). A range of transducers accommodate a variety of testing needs. Load cells range from 50 gm to 445 N; torque cell capacity is 176.5 Nmm (25 oz-in); and, displacement sensors accommodate 5 and 25 mm of travel (Saunders and Donahue, 2004). As is typical of biomechanical testing systems, machine deformation is largely unaccounted for, but assumed to be negligible given that machine stiffness is much greater than specimen stiffness (Currey, 2009).

While the system is highly flexible and cost-effective, it is extremely important to acknowledge the limitations of the in-house device. For instance, the device does not have feedback and as built can only be run under displacement control. While this does not negate the usefulness of this system for relatively rigid fracture (single load to failure) testing, it does affect highly elastic and viscoelastic materials and the fatigue (multiple loading cycles to failure at loading levels below that inducing fracture) of these materials. In the case of displacement control, the particular slide chosen is controlled by a servo motor that operates under a series of user-developed programs that control for variables such as displacement, velocity and acceleration. Again, while this does not greatly affect a bone fracture test, the device is not a convenient tool for applying a frequency driven waveform, such as a pure sinusoid. For these needs, user-defined programs are curve fit to characterize oscillatory waveforms that approximate within reason (< 5%) a desired sine wave. It also requires the adaptation of ASTM standard protocols requiring load control to a displacement control model. In the case of feedback, the simplest way of envisioning this concept is that feedback provides the machine with the information to understand or 'eyes' to 'see' the material/specimen that is being tested. For instance, feedback settings (such as rates, gains and loops) enable a machine (running under load control) to quickly adjust to changes in the material/test to maintain a constant load. It is not hard to appreciate how different this adjustment would be for the same constant load test on a steel bar in comparison to a rubber strip. And the need for this information becomes critical when testing highly elastic/viscoelastic (high degree of hysteresis) materials under fatigue to ensure that the load is efficiently reached and maintained. In the absence of such feedback, the overshooting/undershooting of the load can lead to very erroneous data. While this does not negate the utility of a system without feedback, it does put the responsibility with the operator to understand the limitations of the testing system and determine if reliable data can be obtained with a particular platform.

Once the basic platform is developed, as with biomechanics, mechanobiology research reduces to developing fixtures/models that accurately address the question at hand. In biomechanics this may be as simple as developing a compression platen that correctly distributes an even load across the surface of a scaffold (Figure 2), or a four-point bend fixture that concomitantly applies load to all four points of contact on a long bone, regardless of geometric symmetry. In mechanotransduction, this process is generally more

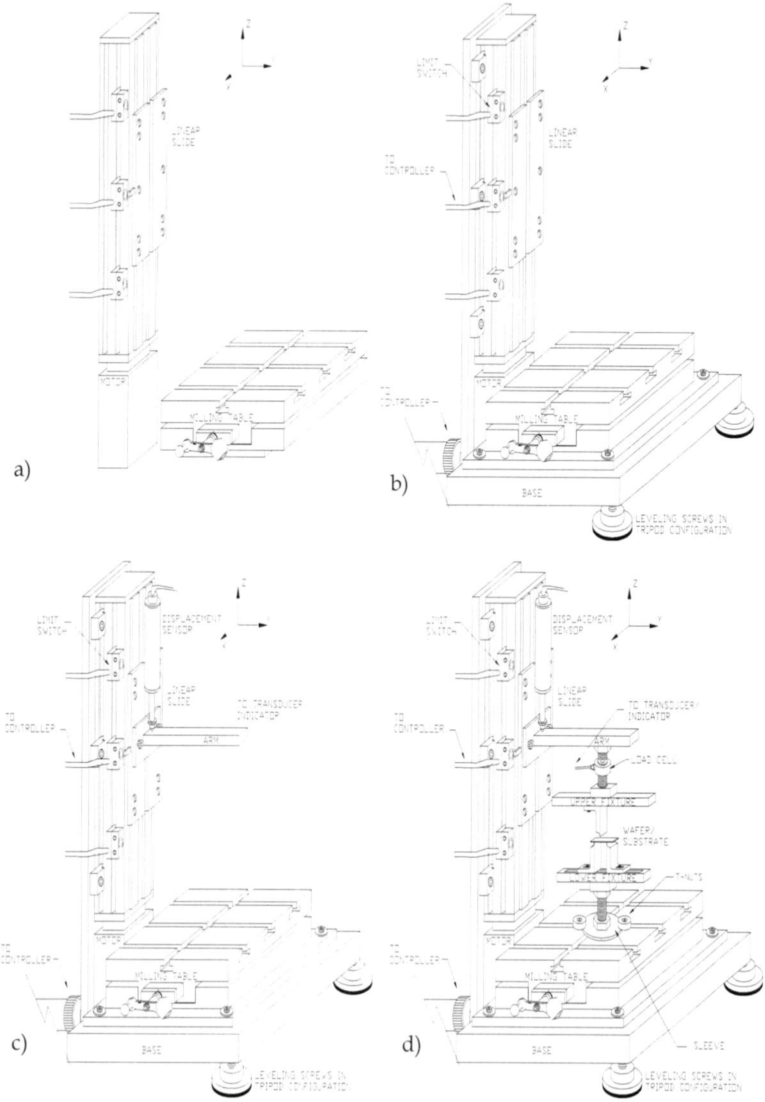

Fig. 1. (a) Small-scale loading machine designed around a commercially-available linear slide and milling machine table. (b) Aluminum plates were fabricated to connect the slide and table with keyways for easy and reproducible assembly. (c) An arm attached to the slide and t-slots in the milling machine table enables a variety of fixtures to be assembled in the platform, such as those shown for three-point bending (d).

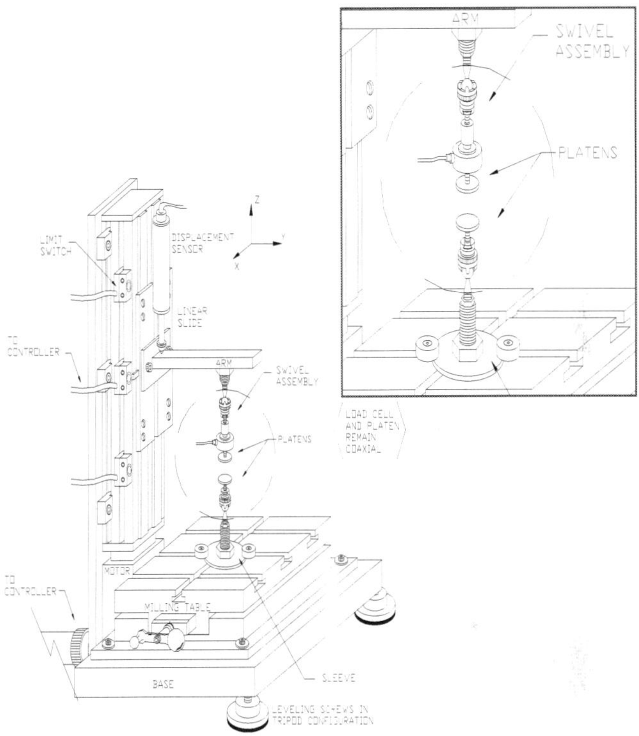

Fig. 2. Once a basic platform is developed, biomechanics work reduces to adequately developing fixtures and testing protocols to test the tissue. Here simple platens utilize a pair of swivel assemblies to ensure loading across the specimen faces regardless of parallelism.

involved and must consider not only the loading apparatus, but also the environment which needs to be held at physiologic conditions. For example, cells need to be tested in a hydrated environment while controlling for variables such as temperature, pH, osmolarity and medium content.

In mechanotransduction, researchers are interested in stimulating bone cells (directly and indirectly) to study the effects of the stimulation on factors such as message (mRNA) and protein production. These models vary greatly in the level of complexity but the two common types of mechanotransduction models are *in vitro* and *in vivo* systems. We will introduce the reader to the idea of mechanotransduction modeling by introducing the *in vitro* and *in vivo* systems and then we will focus on the development of a new approach - *ex vivo*, or biomimetic modeling using an organ culture system. Figure 3 illustrates these types of mechanotransduction systems.

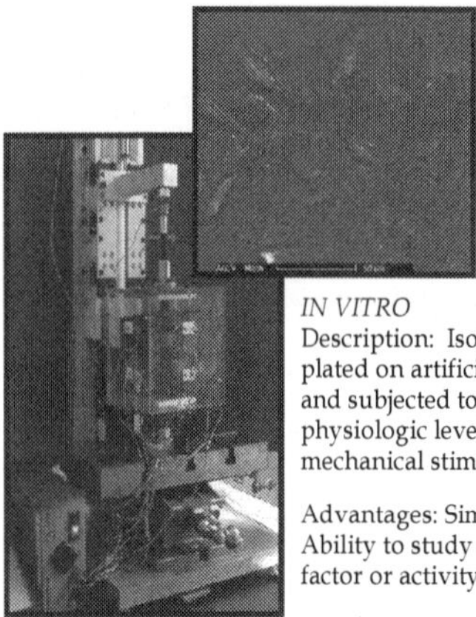

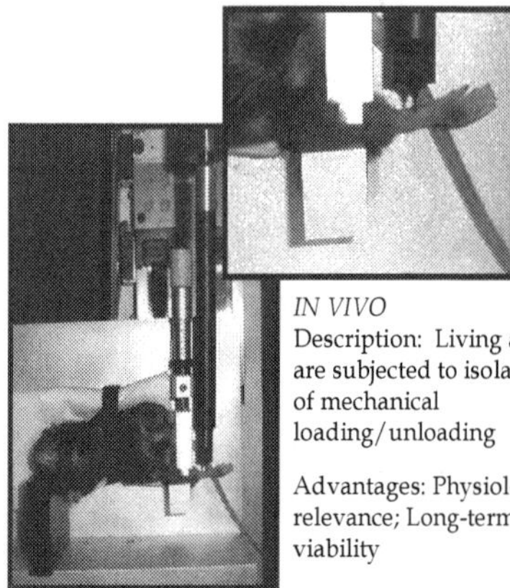

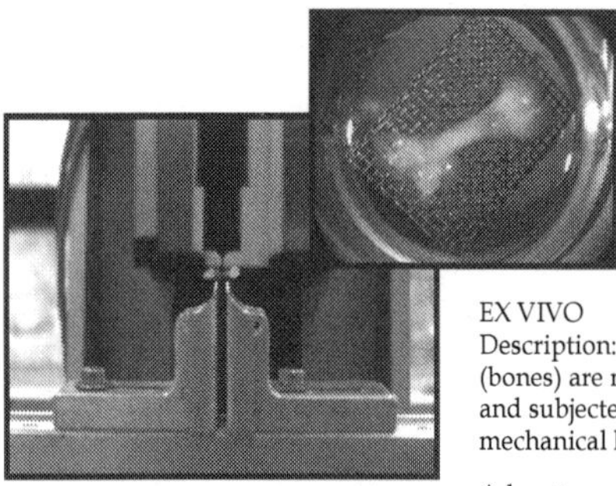

Fig. 3. Mechanotransduction research is commonly conducted with *in vitro* and *in vivo* systems. A third model, the organ culture, or *ex vivo* model may also prove beneficial to increase the physiologic relevance over *in vitro* systems while reducing the complexity of the *in vivo* models.

In *in vitro* mechanotransduction work, isolated cells are subjected to mechanical stimulation. As such, it is important that the stimulation/loading mode be physiologically relevant. That is, cells in the experimental system should be stimulated in a manner that corresponds to the living system. In recent years, one of the more physiologically acceptable modes of bone cell stimulation to emerge has been fluid shear (Piekarski and Munro, 1977; Reich, et al., 1990; Weinbaum, et al., 1994; Hung, et al., 1995; Hung, et al., 1996; Owan, et al., 1997). When one considers the unique environment of particularly the osteocyte, this loading mode becomes evident. That is, osteocytes are mature bone cells that share a common mesenchymal lineage with the osteoblast, the principal bone-forming cell in the body. In fact, the osteocyte is considered an 'aged' osteoblast that in the process of forming bone became walled off in the mineralizing tissue. As the bone-forming osteoblast becomes encased in the bone matrix and transitions to an osteocyte, it takes on a highly dendritic morphology accompanied by structural changes to accompany the reduced need for protein production. A cartoon of the osteocyte environment is shown in Figure 4.

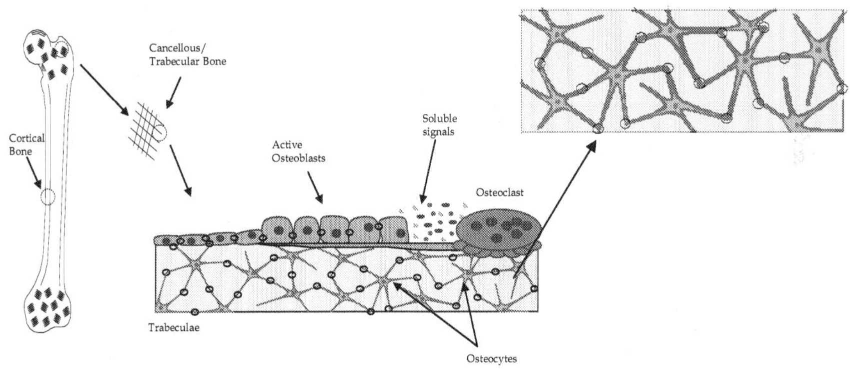

Fig. 4. Osteocytes are former osteoblasts that became encased in the bone mineral during bone formation. Within the matrix, the osteocytes are physically linked to each other via gap junctions in a fluid-bathed lacunocanalicular network. The gap junctions, which also exist between osteoblasts and themselves and osteoblasts and osteocytes (black circles) enable the cells to 'communicate' and share small molecules and ions.

The osteocytes are housed in lacunae, or lenticular shaped cavities that are connected via canaliculi, or little canals. The lacunocanalicular system enables the processes of neighboring osteocytes to physically link while the interstitial fluid found throughout the network bathes the cells and enables important metabolic regulation (Cowin, 1999; Wang, et al., 2004). Given the physical system, what is created is a network of fluid bathed bone cells in a mineralized matrix that is flexed upon loading. As such, the osteocyte is positioned to be a key player in bone mechanoregulation (Bonewald, 2007). During the repetitive loading and unloading of the tissue that occurs during walking, the shifts in the load cause corresponding shifts in pressure gradients that force the fluid from regions of higher pressure to lower pressure. With the rhythmic repetition of walking, the osteocytes are subjected to an oscillatory (not necessarily sinusoidal) fluid shear stress generated by the directional shift in interstitial fluid flow (Piekarski and Munro, 1977; Jacobs, et al., 1998).

One way to generate this loading mode is with the system shown in Figure 5. Here, a parallel plate flow chamber is used in conjunction with a loading platform to deliver physiologic levels of shear stress to cells in monolayer (2-25 dyne/cm^2) via medium-filled glass syringes (Frangos, et al., 1985; Frangos, et al., 1988; Jacobs, et al., 1998). The base of the syringe is anchored to the base of the loading platform while the syringe plunger is attached to the moving slide. Tubing attached to the syringe tip and connected to the inlet of the parallel plate chamber connects the chamber to the platform motion. The parallel plate flow

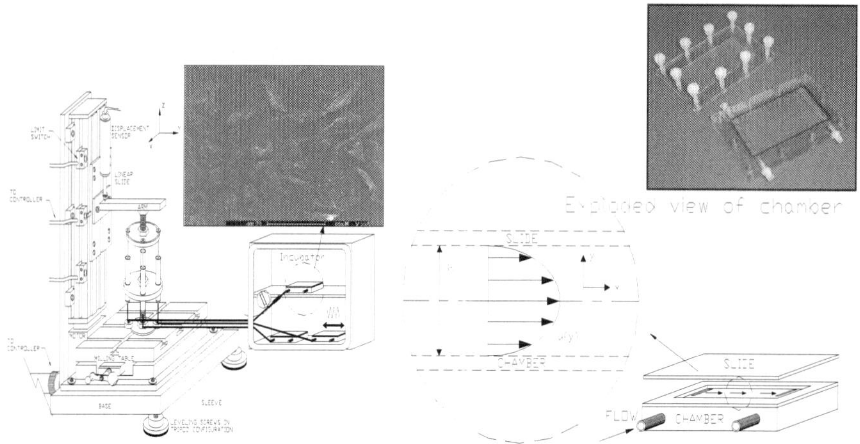

Fig. 5. (a) Syringe assembly used to subject bone cells in a parallel plate flow chamber to physiologic levels of fluid shear (modified from the setup of Jacobs, et al., 1998).

chamber is a polycarbonate chamber with recessed base and slits connected to the channels for the inlet and outlet flows. The cells are seeded on a glass microscope slide that when inverted on the plate forms the lid of the chamber and closes off the fixed volume of the flow chamber. A gasketed lid screwed to the top of the system holds the assembly together and prevents fluid leaks. This system has readily become an accepted method of fluid shear stimulation with fluid shear stress defined by the equation:

$$\tau_w = \left(\frac{6\mu Q}{bh^2} \right)$$

where μ is the viscosity of the fluid; Q is the flow rate; and, b and h represent chamber dimensions of base and height, respectively (Hung, et al., 1985). In *in vitro* stimulation studies, the cells are subjected to the isolated stimulation and depending upon the activity being studied, the cells, supernatant, or cells and supernatant may be collected and analyzed. For example, supernatant may be collected and analyzed for soluble factors released by the cells and the cells may be collected for mRNA analysis or used to normalize the volume of supernatant activity. Time courses are not uncommon and the effect of stimulation over a pre-defined time period may be assessed. It is important in the experimental design to determine the activity to be studied. Whereas soluble activity may be collected over a short duration, the study of mRNA requires a longer time course and sterility issues with the cell maintenance in culture post-flow, as well as flow system sterility are critical.

From an engineering perspective it is important to understand the limitations of this system. As often occurs, the parallel plate flow systems are considered highly characterized and bone scientists have proposed that chamber dimensions and flow properties that yield shear stresses on the order of 5-25 dyne/cm^2 are physiologic for bone cells. Attached as an Appendix is a derivation of the shear stress in the parallel plate flow chamber. What is important to note is that the derivation is based on the dimensions of the flow chamber without allowance for the cells, or how the flow at the cellular level might be affected by the cell size, cell adhesion, cell density, cell properties (membrane viscoelasticity), etc.. In addition, developing flow around the slits is not acknowledged and what is derived is an equation for the 'average' shear stress in the empty chamber of known dimensions. These slides hold relatively large volumes of cells and the average response (even when normalized to cell protein) does not yield particularly valuable insights into individual and small cell subpopulation responses.

Another concern when using these systems is to subject the appropriate bone cell type to the appropriate stimulus. For example, there are a number of studies that subject osteoblasts to fluid shear. While osteoblasts (primary and immortalized cell lines) have been readily available for several decades, the osteocytic cell model is much more difficult to primary harvest given the encasement in the mineralized matrix and the current standard immortalized line (MLO-Y4) is relatively new, by comparison to the osteoblast models (Kato, et al., 1997). As such, osteoblasts were subjected to fluid shear under the justification that they mimicked 'young' osteocytes. Although osteoblasts respond to fluid shear levels (You, et al., 2000) information from these types of studies may be very productive in the development of a mechanically loaded bioreactor where the justification of a desired response of the cell to an applied stimulus is less critical than obtaining the desired response, studies conducted to determine underlying mechanisms of osteoblast responsiveness to physiologic stimulation should strive to model an appropriate stimulus. The system illustrated in Figure 6 was developed to apply a physiologic (global level) substrate deformation to surface-residing osteoblasts. Again, the goal was not to determine the most stimulatory loading mode, but to stress the need for physiologically-appropriate systems which mimic the native loading environment (Saunders, et al., 2006).

For these studies, cells were seeded on tissue culture plastic (polystyrene) slides and subjected to three-point bending. The bending subjected the slides to a physiologic strain (maximum 3500 microstrain) verified with strain gauges placed on the underside of the slide. Direct cell strain was not quantified. In addition, an environmental chamber was developed from polycarbonate and heated with microheaters. The environmental chamber held a medium-filled reservoir that enabled the cells to be submerged during testing and pH and humidity were controlled. As shown in Figure 6, three-point bending was selected over four-point bending to maintain a combination of bending and shear throughout the field of loading. This was in contrast to the four-point bending scenario in which pure bending resulted between the inner two points of contact. Given the previous response of the osteoblasts to shear, three-point bending was used to subject cells to a physiologic environment of primary substrate deformation and secondary fluid shear. Strain gradient changed as a function of contact placement, but a linear relationship was assumed and verified with preliminary strain gauge testing on the substrate. Regardless of stimulus, the need to maintain cell hydration results in the presence of secondary fluid shear forces that can confound findings.

In vitro mechanotransduction systems have also incorporated co-culture models. In these systems it is acknowledged that the interaction between the various cells types is critical and devices to load the systems in a tandem model have been developed. Shown in Figure 7, is a device in which osteoblasts and osteocytes are co-cultured (Taylor, et al, 2007). The focus of this work was to study the mechanically-stimulated osteocytic effects on osteoblasts in physical contact with the osteocytes via gap junctions, but effectively isolated from the stimulation. In this system, osteocytes are grown on one side of a porous mesh and

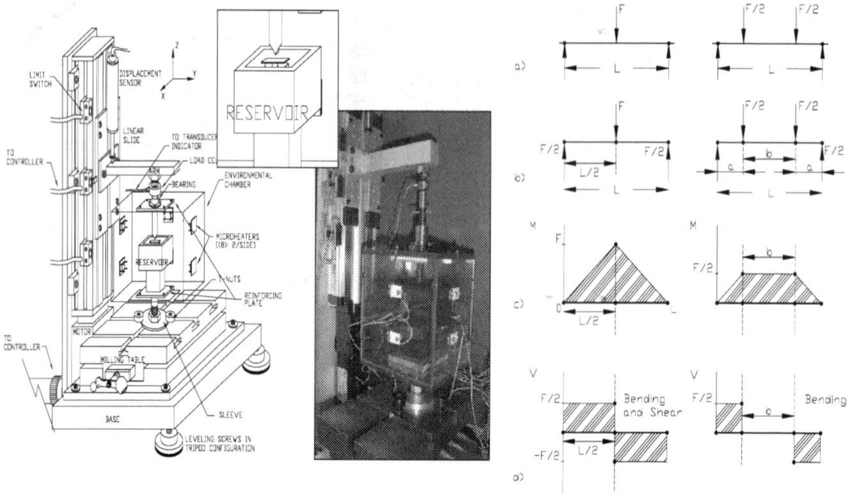

Fig. 6. Substrate deformation assembly used to subject osteoblasts to physiologic levels of bending (and secondary fluid shear). The environmental chamber was developed to maintain temperature; pH and humidity were also regulated. Cells in these systems are plated in monolayer on a synthetic substrate and subjected to stimulation.

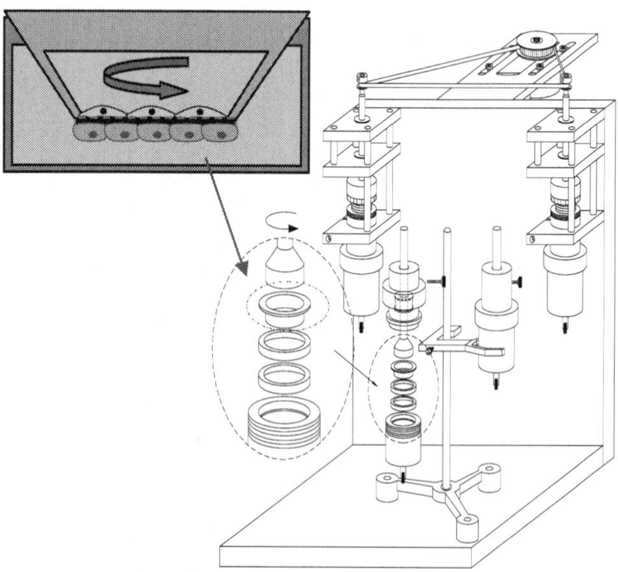

Fig. 7. Rotary stimulatory system to study osteocyte/osteoblast interactions via gap junctions. Stimulated systems are compared to controls placed in similar chambers (ring stand) without the load.

osteoblasts are grown on the other. The well containing the co-cultured mesh is placed in the loading device and a programmable motor enables a belt-driven assembly to apply fluid shear to the osteocytes in culture via a rotating disk. The cell density and the thickness of the mesh effectively ensures that the only physical contact the cell types have with each other is via the gap junction channels that grow through the porous mesh. The system is then utilized to study the indirect effect of mechanical stimulation (via fluid shear) on osteoblastic activity, as well as the importance of osteocytes (and gap junctions) in transducing a mechanical signal. These types of models are important not only for the basic science value of the findings, but because they represent a necessary trend toward increasing the physiologic complexity (and biomimicry) of the isolated *in vitro* environment. These are just three examples of *in vitro* stimulation systems. And while others exist (Ajubi, et al., 1996; Bottlang, et al., 1997; Ziambaras, et al., 1998; Brown, et al., 1998; Brown, 2000), they all have the same purpose. *In vitro* mechanotransduction models strive to understand the cellular pathways and mechanisms by which bone cells respond to mechanical stimulation. Advantages of these systems include their simplicity and the ability to isolate a particular factor for further study. Disadvantages include their simplicity which makes relevant comparisons to the physiologic models difficult, at best. There are also cellular concerns that should at least be acknowledged but are beyond the focus of this work. For example, it is not clear (and highly improbable) if the extrinsic load translates directly to an intrinsic load and the cell 'sees' the identical global load. Furthermore disparities within and between cell models (primary sources and immortalized lines) and the day to day changes that occur with cells further complicates comparisons. As such, results from cellular studies generally are presented with respect to a particular osteoblastic cell line or cell lines with emphasis on maintaining appropriate culture conditions and low passage numbers for immortalized cells or noting digestion numbers and passage numbers (generally not more than 3-4) for primary isolations (Sorkin, et al., 2004).

In *in vivo* models, living animals are subjected to loading environments under highly regulated conditions. In these systems, animals may be subjected to sub-physiologic (underload), physiologic or supra-physiologic (overload) loading environments and the isolated effects may be studied for an extended period of time. For example, these models include loading to simulate use and overuse and unloading to simulate weightlessness and bed rest/paralysis. For loading studies bones may be loaded by training the animals (generally rodents) to stand on their hindlimbs while increasing the weight on their backs. A common way to accomplish this is to train the animals in cages with a live floor to send an electric shock as negative reinforcement and food as positive reinforcement (Buhl, et al., 2001). Another method to apply load to *in vivo* models is to anesthetize the animals and put them in a device that loads the limbs in a desired manner (Turner, et al., 1991; Hillam and Skerry, 1995; Gross, et al., 2002). To this end, the in-house platform was used and a loading fixture developed that enabled the application of a concentrated, cantilevered load to rodent tibiae, Figure 8. In addition, the platform was designed to rotate such that the limb could be loaded in the anteroposterior or mediolateral orientation. For torsion and *in vivo* stimulation studies the movable base of the milling machine table makes it trivial to align the specimens in the loading machine for testing. Unlike standard commercial testing systems, the planar motion provided by the milling machine table of the in-house platform enables the attached fixtures to be dialed-in either front-to-back or side-to-side then locked down for testing. Advantages of *in vivo* systems include their physiologic relevance and the ability to study the outcome of the cellular stimulation (bone formation/resorption) over a longer period of time. Disadvantages include the physiologic complexity that makes it difficult to discern the direct response of the cell to the stimulation and the loss in sensitivity that has been observed in using these systems with repeated loading.

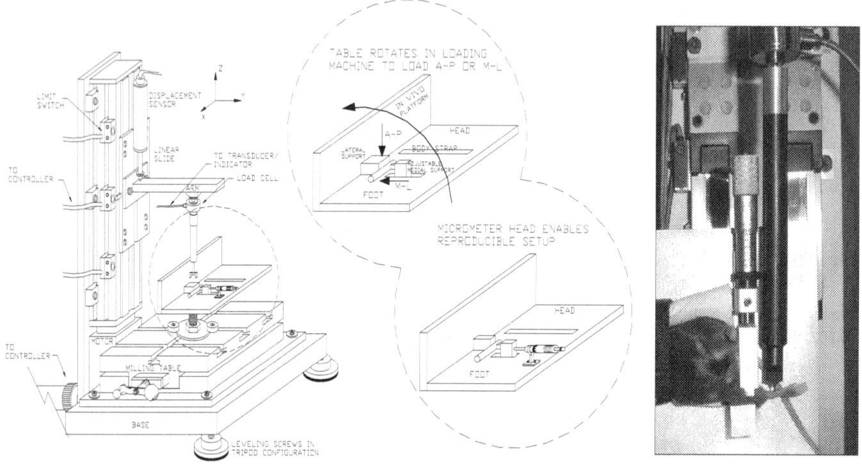

Fig. 8. Bending assembly for *in vivo* stimulation studies. The platform rotates to load rodent tibiae in the anteroposterior (A-P; front-to-back) or mediolateral (M-L; side-to-side) orientations. A cantilevered loading is produced in which the proximal end of the tibia is held in place and the distal end is cyclically stimulated (modified from the setup of Gross, et al., 2002).

As with any type of research model, there are advantages and disadvantages to using each system and it is important for the researcher to appreciate this such that they may utilize each system to their full advantage. It is also important to realize that it takes time for research models to be proven valid and acceptable in a given area, but there will always be inherent flaws in any model. For example, the use of osteoblastic cell lines in mechanotransduction is well accepted. However, the new investigator may be surprised to learn that in many cases the cells that are modeled as osteoblastic are not derived from the bone directly, but from bone cancers. For example the long-used ROS 17/2.8 immortalized cell line is, as its name implies a Rat Osteoblastic Sarcoma cell line derived from bone tumor since tumor cells do not undergo terminal differentiation, but continue to proliferate. Additional immortalized lines derived from tumorigenic sources include the rat UMR-106 and UMR-108 lines (Forrest, et al., 1985) and the human U-2 OS and MG-63 lines (Ponten and Saksela, 1967; Billiau, et al., 1977). Furthermore, it has been recognized that some nontumorigenic cell lines, such as the mouse MC3T3-E1 line loses its osteogenic properties with time in culture (Takahashi, et al. 2002). In addition, the ultimate goal will always be the use of these systems to address, regardless of origin, the human condition. Osteoclast (bone-resorbing cells) models that have been widely studied include the chick model; however, the chick osteoclast, in contrast to the human osteoclast, was originally thought not to possess the calcitonin receptor (Nicholson, et al., 1987) and later determined to possess detectable levels under dietary modification (Gay, 1991). While this is not to imply that these research models are irrelevant, the intent is to show that all models have limitations and perfect systems do not exist. The goal of developing a new model is to look at the strengths and limitations of the available systems and weigh the benefits of a new model against those of the accepted standards. With this in mind, we set out to develop an *ex vivo* (organ culture) model for bone mechanotransduction that we feel may fill a specific niche in the research field by providing a system that is biomimetic.

Organ culture models are not a new concept (Fell, 1972; Boyd, 2005). The earliest organ culture experiments date back to 1859 when Valpian attempted to maintain frog embryo tail fragments in water (Fell, 1972). In 1897 Born and Loeb used this approach to maintain small fragments of rabbit organs in serum. In 1912 McWhorter and Whipple successfully used the organ culture approach to maintain entire avian and mammalian embryos in blood plasma to study the development of chick blastoderms (Fell, 1972). A pioneer in the field of organ culture modeling, Dame Honor B Fell considered the first true organ culture to be the work of David Thompson (1914). Thompson used a hanging drop method to explant toes, feather germs, tongue tips, optic lenses and tail buds from embryonic chicks into plasma to study their development (Balls, 1976). Fell's research was critical to the use of organ culture in the musculoskeletal field (Fell, et al., 1976). She began her organ culture research in 1924 when she studied the development of undifferentiated limb buds of chick embryos. She found that when cartilaginous bone from the limb of 5-6 day old chick embryos were kept in culture, they continued to grow and develop histologically and anatomically. Later it was found that these bones gave essentially the same response to certain vitamins and hormones in culture as they did *in vivo*. Additional pivotal organ culture work in the bone field was conducted by Glucksmann who showed that bone could respond to mechanical stimulation. Glucksmann used a clever culture technique to show that bones grown in small culture dishes were, as they grew, subjected to stresses from the culture dish walls that resulted in ossified tissue aligning along directions of tensile stress (Glucksmann, 1942). Organ culture systems enjoy a wide use in research (Stepita-Klauco and Dolezalova, 1968; Barrett and Trump, 1978; Jubb, 1979; Merrilees and Scott, 1982; Weiss, et al., 1988; Wetzel and Salpeter, 1991; Ishizeki, et al., 1995; Merrick, et al., 1997; Voisard, et al., 1999; Takezawa, et al., 2000; Del Rizzo, et al., 2001; Swanson, et al., 2002; Lyubimov and Gotleib, 2004) but their presence in the bone field is much less prevalent. Historically the use of organ culture models in bone research has been as an experimental system to study the effects of resorptive agents on bone (Raisz, 1965; Raisz and Niemann, 1967; Reynolds, 1976; Murrills, 1996). To be useful for biomimetic mechanotransduction modeling, not only must the model retain its viability in culture, but it must be able to respond to mechanical stimulation with a response indicative of an osteogenic event. In addition, it is important to note that there are systems in which bone explants/rudiments are maintained quite successfully for significant periods of time (Jones, et al., 2003; Takai, et al., 2004; Davies, et al., 2006; Chan, et al., 2009). One such system, the 'Zetos' system is a clever perfusion chamber that enables trabecular cores (from bovine sources) to be kept viable for extended periods of time (Jones, et al., 2003; Davies, et al., 2006). While the value of this system is significant, our goal was to develop an organ culture model of an intact bone. In addition to incorporating both cortical and trabecular bone, the whole organ culture model aimed to preserve the integrity of the periosteum.

The major drawback with the use of the organ culture is that it is a dying tissue at the time of harvest and it remains to be determined if these systems can provide acceptable models of bone cell mechanotransduction pathways and mechanisms. Indeed, they have shown promise in short-term studies on the order of hours (Zaman, et al., 1992; Dallas, et al., 1993).

If proven acceptable, these systems could be used to study isolated loading effects that would increase the physiologic relevance over *in vitro* systems (adding biomimicry) while reducing the complexity of the *in vivo* systems (ie, eliminating systemic effects). For the concept of biomimetic mechanotransduction modeling to be validated it is necessary to show that the models remain viable in culture, continue to grow and respond to brief bouts of physiologic stimulation. Ideally it would also be advantageous to demonstrate that these models can simulate relevant clinical systems and provide an additional tool for bone scientists.

Our organ culture work initially employed a rodent long bone model. The femur was chosen for its routine subjection to repetitive loads (walking). Neonatal rodents given the increased porosity of this model over a fully calcified adult system were selected. Rodents were chosen to enable future molecular analysis and rats (Wistar), over mice, were chosen for convenience given the larger size of the bones. Work to date has used neonates ranging from 2-5 days old with much of the repetitive loading studies conducted in 5 day old models given their reduced fragility at this age. Bones were isolated using blunt finger dissection to preserve the periosteum and maintained in an incubator (5% CO_2) in BGJb medium supplemented with 15% fetal bovine serum and 2% penicillin/streptomycin as previously recommended (Meghji, et al., 1998; Garrett, 2003; Saunders, et al., 2010). The initial systems were maintained in standard organ culture medium and passive diffusion provided the only source of transport. Bones were cultured in 12 well culture dishes on stainless steel mesh inserts such that 2 ml of medium covered the bone shafts while exposing a small region of the cartilaginous ends to the air to maintain the bones at a liquid/gas interface. Medium was topped off daily to keep the bone shafts submerged and completely replaced every 3 days. Medium was warmed to 37 °C before adding to the cultures to avoid shocking the bones. In addition, with the exception of viability studies where control bones were taken immediately post-harvest (maximum viability), all other controls were taken at 24 hr for growth studies. The 24 hr period was necessary to allow the bones to equilibrate to the culture conditions. (Meghji, 1998) Furthermore, in all cases, the initial medium change was 24 hr post-harvest to remove any deleterious soluble effects of the harvest on the cultures. For example prostaglandin levels increase as a result of trauma (dissection) and prostaglandins have a direct effect on bone formation/resorption (Jee, et al., 1985; Imamura, et al., 1990; Klein-Nulend, et al., 1997; Hagino, et al., 2005).

It is important to keep in mind that the benefit of using the organ culture system is that the cells are stimulated in their native environment and the response of the cells at the tissue level may be quantified. However, the tissue level response is not instantaneous and the culture must stay viable long enough for the stimulation at the tissue level to be observed. Furthermore, much of the mechanotransduction field is concerned with understanding the response to physiologic levels of loading which incorporate modest magnitudes and short durations. That is, to be effective it is necessary to demonstrate that the organ culture model can respond to a brief physiologic bout of loading and can maintain viability during this period. Pilot studies (not shown) suggested that 1 wk was an appropriate culture time to anticipate a response in these systems, and as such, was used as a starting time point for the organ culture studies.

To assess the viability of the cultures, standard hematoxylin and eosin (H&E) and lactate dehydrogenase (LDH) staining were completed. H&E staining, as shown in Figure 9 is beneficial to show that there are osteocytes present in the lacunae. In Figure 9, the midshaft bone section, taken from a 2 day old neonate and maintained in culture for 2 wk indicates that in the midshaft of the femur, (sectioned between 5-10 microns thick) osteocytes are abundant in the lacunae. However, the H&E stain does not indicate if the cells are viable, it only verifies their presence in the matrix at the time of fixation. To quantify osteocyte viability, LDH staining was completed.

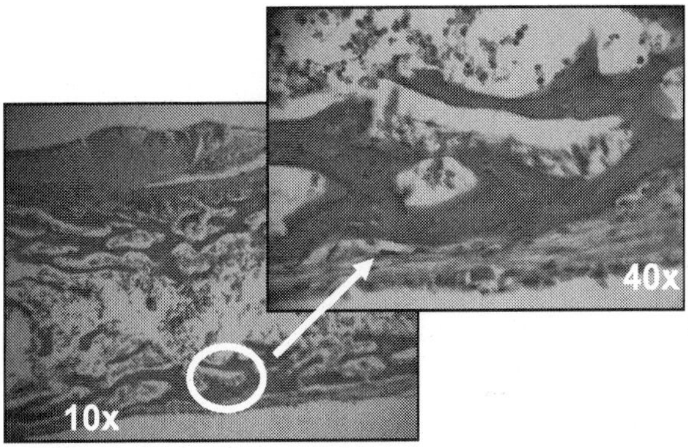

Fig. 9. H&E staining on femurs following 2wk of culture supported osteocyte viability as shown by the majority of lacunae showing osteocyte bodies.

Just as humans require energy to complete any function, cells require energy for all their normal activities. Lactate dehydrogenase is an enzyme involved in energy conversion and since only living cells require energy, cells staining positive for LDH are viable (alive) while cells not staining positive are non-viable (dead). In cryosectioned slices, matrix-embedded osteocytes were quantified for viability (Wong, et al., 1982). To determine viability as a function of time in culture, bone pairs were randomly analyzed with 1 femur stained immediately at the time of harvest and the contralateral control was stained following 1 or 2 wk in culture. The 2 wk time point was completed to assess the viability of the cultures passed the desired time point of 1 wk. All lacunae in a given section were counted and a minimum of 12 sections were counted for each time point. As shown in Figure 10, approximately 93% of the osteocytes were viable at the time of harvest while 70% of the osteocytes were viable at 1 wk and 42% were viable at the 2 wk time point (data not shown) (Saunders, et al., 2010). Given that no additional efforts were made to enhance viability (eg, perfusion or topical additives), the viability counts were adequate. Computational permeability modeling proposed by Botchwey and Beno supported these findings (Botchwey, et al., 2003a; Botchwey, et al., 2003b; Beno, et al., 2006). It is anticipated that these viability results could be improved. However, it must be kept in mind that the intent is to determine the usefulness of this culture model and as such, perfusion or topical additives should aid viability without being overly stimulatory to the culture. The objective is to be able to discern the effect of the isolated loading and the efforts to improve viability should not confound the effects of the loading.

To assess growth in culture, bones taken from 2 day old neonates were analyzed for changes in length, weight and mass distribution. Presented here are results during the 1 wk culture period. The control limb was analyzed 24 hr after harvest. For length comparisons, overall femur length, shaft length and shaft diameter were determined. Bones were digitally imaged at the corresponding time point and NIHImage software (ImageJ) was used to determine measurements. Three measurements for each location were determined and averaged. Femur length increased 10.3%; shaft length increased 6.3%; and, shaft diameter increased 6.5% in culture. All increases were statistically significant (Saunders, et al., 2010), Figure 11.

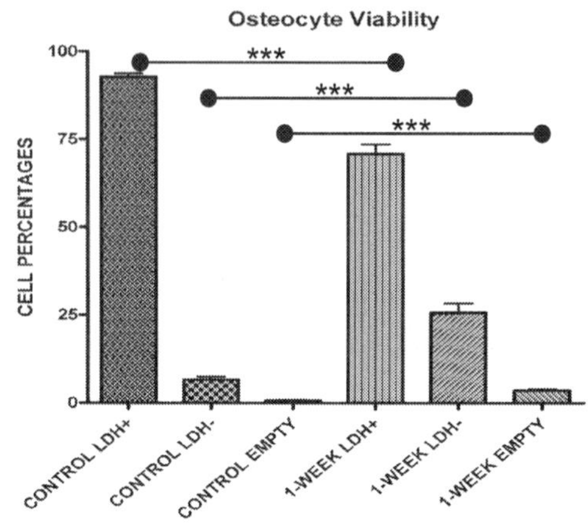

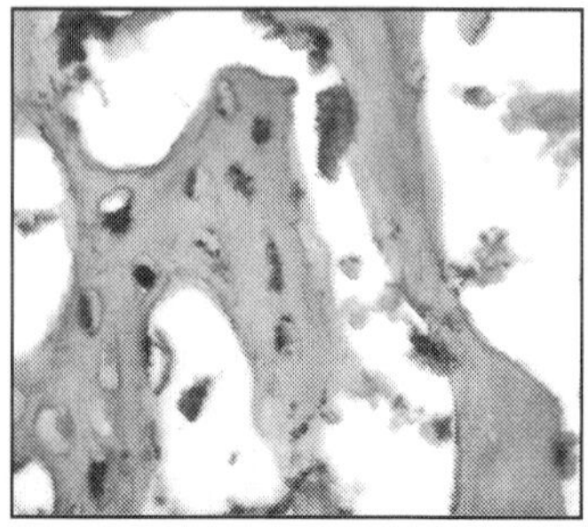

Fig. 10. Osteocyte viability was quantified with LDH stains and manual cell counts. Osteocyte viability at 1 wk of culture was 70 % as determined by the number of osteocytes staining positive for LDH.

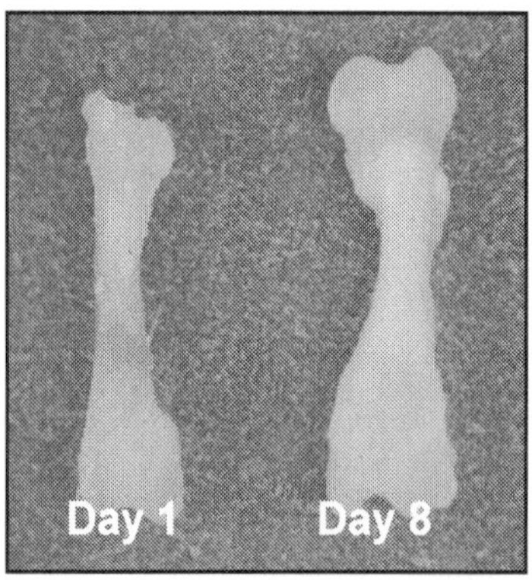

Fig. 11. Femur growth over the 1 wk culture period was significant.

Weight changes in culture were quantified using previously established techniques (Mikic, et al., 2002). Wet, dry and ash weights were obtained and represent, to a crude degree, the content of the bone. Wet weight, as the name implies represents the natural culture weight (including water content) of the bone and is obtained after removal of any free medium from the bone. Dry weight is obtained following defatting of the bones in acetone and thoroughly drying under low heat. Ash weight represents the mineral content and is obtained following burning the bones at high temperatures (600 °C) for an extended period of time (6 hr). For *ex vivo* models, ash weight is an important parameter to assess changes in bone mineral development as a function of culture period and environment. Weights continued to increase with the 1 wk culture period. Specifically, wet weight increased 85.2% in culture; dry weight increased 49.5%; and, ash weight increased 57.5%. All increases were statistically significant (Saunders, et al., 2010). The increases in wet weights revealed that the bulk of the weight in these cultures, not unexpectedly, was the result of tissue hydration and the cartilaginous material. However, the increases in the ash weights over the 1 wk culture period suggests that the bone was also increasing in mineralization, which is what would be desirable in a mechanotransduction system.

The distribution of the mass of bone reveals useful information about its strength and its ability to resist loading and deflections in given orientations. For example, the polar moment of inertia provides a measure of the ability of the specimen to resist torsion. To assess areal properties, bone shafts were embedded in polymethylmethacrylate (PMMA) bone cement and sectioned on a diamond saw following dehydration in alcohol and digitally imaged. Moments of inertia increased 40.9% and 34.9% in culture assuming an elliptical cross-section, Figure 12. Polar moment of inertia increased 37.7% while cortical area increased 16.6%. All areal changes were statistically significant.

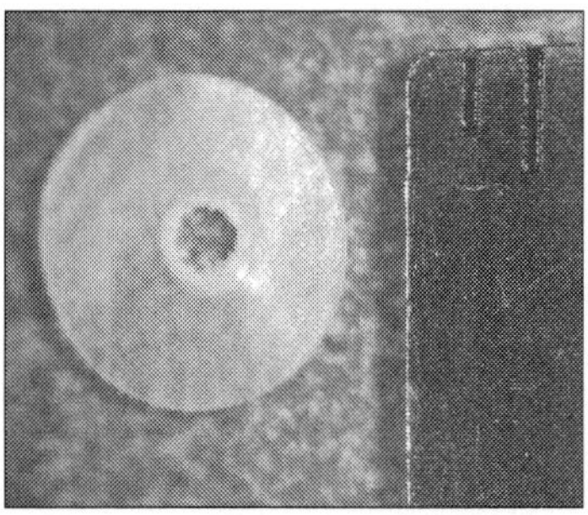

Fig. 12. Typical cross-section of neonatal femur. Ruler ticks represent 1.6 mm increments.

While these results taken together clearly show that the bones are viable over the 1 wk culture period and continue to grow, these measurements are rather rudimentary. To strengthen the premise that organ cultures may be used as biomimetic models of mechanotransduction, additional, more accurate techniques have also been employed. Whereas the LDH stain indicates cell, particularly osteocyte, viability, the overall organ viability was also assessed with micro computed tomography, or microCT. In microCT studies, femurs from 5-day old neonates were harvested and maintained in culture for 1 (n=9), 2 (n=9) or 4 wk (n=10) of culture while the contralateral control was analyzed 24 hr post-harvest. Bones were analyzed using a MicroCT-40 scanner (Scanco Medical, Basserdorf, Switzerland) using source settings of 55 kV, 145 μA and high resolution. A midshaft analysis was performed, producing 50, 2048 x 2048 2D axial slices in the midshaft of each bone (0.4 mm). Inertial, areal, volumetric and density measurements were determined. Cultured bones at 1, 2 and 4 wk were normalized to their contralateral controls and compared. Shown in Figure 13 are results for the 1, 2 and 4 wk culture comparisons. Overall, all properties were found to significantly increase over the 1 wk culture period ($p<0.001$) and normalized 2 and 4 wk comparisons are reported as percent decreases relative to the 1 wk observations. Specifically, polar moments of inertia (pMOI) decreased 23.4% ($p<0.05$) and 36.5% ($p<0.001$) over the 2 and 4 wk culture periods, respectively. Resistance to bending (assuming an elliptical cross-section) decreased 25.9% (Imax/Cmax) ($p<0.05$) and 24.0% (Imin/Cmin) ($p<0.05$) over the 2 wk culture period and 39.3% (Imax/Cmax) ($p<0.001$) and 38.6% (Imin/Cmin) ($p<0.001$) over the 4 wk culture period. Density decreased 41.6% ($p<0.05$) and 53.0% ($p<0.001$) over the 2 and 4 wk culture periods, respectively. These findings, not surprisingly, suggest that the organ culture models, as maintained here, are most effective if used for short term studies (≤ 1 wk) and that while the bones at 2 wk of culture are more dense and stronger than their counterparts at 24 hr post-harvest, their loss of viability is significant given the comparison to the 1 wk bones. Four week results indicate a relatively dead culture that in many cases was approximately equivalent to the 24 hr controls.

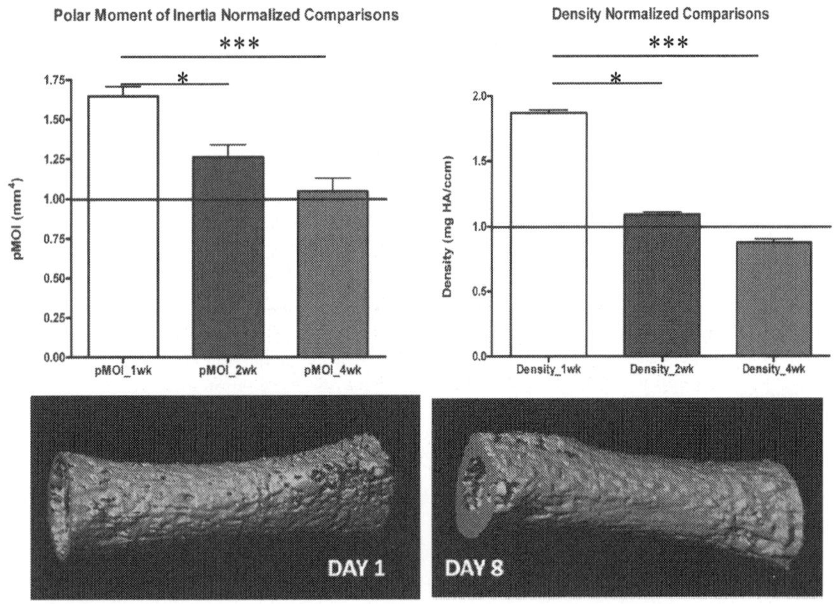

Fig. 13. Results from microCT analysis indicate significant increases in bone shaft quantity (moment of inertia) and quality (density) at 1 wk of culture that significantly degrades by 2 wk of culture.

Once it was determined that the bones could remain viable in culture for 1 wk and could continue to grow under the culture conditions, the bones were subjected to an isolated bout of stimulation and the response assessed. A major objective of the organ culture system is to show that it is capable of responding to a brief, isolated load. The reason for this from a research standpoint is to be able to utilize the model to study the immediate response to short-term loading; from a practical standpoint, given the consistency of the cultures it is unlikely that they would survive, i.e. keep their structural integrity, extended bouts of loading.

Gross' group has successfully developed *in vivo* models of mechanotransduction in which the rodent limbs are subjected to short durations of stimulation and the organ culture systems utilized similar loading durations (Gross, et al., 2002). To minimize contamination risk associated with a loading regime over multiple days, the bones were subjected to one bout of loading in which 350 cycles of loading were applied over 5 mins (1.17 Hz). In these experiments, the control bone was maintained in culture for 1 wk without load, while the treated limb was subjected to 350 cycles of loading at a maximum strain of 500 microstrain (minimum of 50 microstrain) 24 hr after harvest. Following stimulation via three-point bending, the bones were returned to culture for 1 wk. Following the 1 wk culture period the control and stimulated bones were mechanically loaded to failure and the structural effect of the loading was quantified. It was determined that the brief bout of loading resulted in a significant increase in stiffness (34.5%) (Saunders, et al., 2010). Failure load was increased 5.8% and displacement was decreased 11.2%. Taken as a whole, the mechanical testing results of an increasing trend in stiffness and failure load with a subsequent decreasing trend in failure displacement are indicative of an increase in strength with the stimulation, or an osteogenic response.

The initial objective of developing a biomimetic organ culture model of bone mechanotransduction has been completed. To date, it has been demonstrated that the neonatal bones may be maintained in culture for periods exceeding 1 wk and that these cultures remain viable, continue to grow and respond to a brief, isolated physiologic bout of stimulation with an increase in mechanical strength. While not an exhaustive analysis, the results of these studies suggest the biomimetic bone mechanotransduction system shows promise. Additional objectives would be to show that these models can be used in studies relating to mechanical load, similarly to *in vitro* and *in vivo* systems. For example, it would be beneficial to show that these systems can respond to topical additives and may be used in a similar way in which the *in vitro* models are used to topically affect a single protein, factor or activity and study the effect. In initial topical studies using the organ culture models, functional communication (gap junction function) was topically inhibited and the effect on mechanical strength during growth in culture was assessed.

Gap junctions are protein channels that enable neighboring cells to physically connect, Figure 14. These channels enable the cells to share molecules and small ions in their interior compartments with each other. As a result, these channels allow the cells to 'communicate'. Gap junctions are abundantly found in bone and osteocytes and osteoblasts are able to communicate with themselves (homotypic coupling) as well as with each other (heterotypic communication). As such, this communication network provides an ideal system of conduits by which cells can coordinate responses to mechanical stimulation (Saunders, et al., 2001; Saunders, et al., 2003). Functional communication may be inhibited with the topical inhibitor 18α-glycyrrhetinic acid (αGA). While inhibiting communication in *in vitro* studies has enabled isolated markers to be studied, *in vivo* models have been hampered by the embryonic lethal nature of the knock-out models (Ewart, et al., 1997). Utilizing the organ culture system, neonatal rat long bones were harvested from 5 day old Wistar rats, digitally photographed, weighed and cultured in standard growth medium supplemented with 30 μM αGA (in DMSO) for 96 hr then replaced with standard growth medium for the remainder of the wk; this process was repeated for an additional 96 hr for the 2 wk culture model. Topically treated femurs were normalized to intact controls. Additional control limbs were treated with an equal concentration of DMSO, normalized to intact controls and compared at 1 and 2 wk of culture. Preliminary results demonstrated that 96 hr in 30 μM αGA decreased mechanically-induced stiffness 10% following 1wk of culture and 20% following 2 wk of culture in comparison to contralateral controls (Figure 15) illustrating that the topical αGA is effective in inhibiting communication and that this communication contributes to organ culture development.

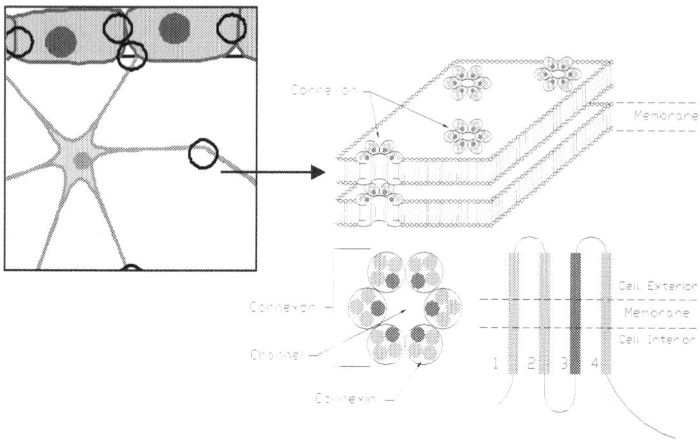

Fig. 14. (Left) Osteocytes communicate with osteoblasts and other osteocytes via gap junctions. (Right) Gap junctions are channels that physically link cell membranes and enable cells to exchange their intracellular contents. Gap junctions are protein channels formed from the union of connexons in adjacent membranes; connexons are comprised of six protein sub-units called connexins named for their molecular weight and abundant in bone cells.

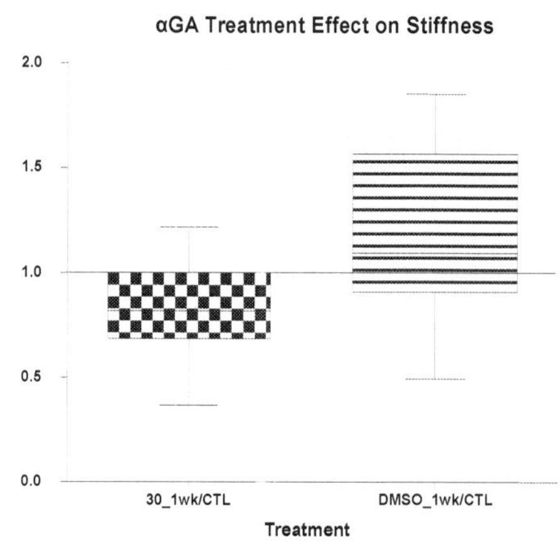

Fig. 15. Decrease in organ culture stiffness with addition of topical gap junction inhibitor.

In addition to being useful for topical studies, the biomimetic models also show promise in preliminary work simulating distraction osteogenesis. Distraction osteogenesis (DO) is a clinical procedure in which bones are subjected to distraction forces that induce new bone formation. While DO has successfully been used to correct orthopaedic and dental deficiencies, DO has also been used to treat mandibular hypoplasia in children associated with Goldenhar's, Nager's and Pierre Robin syndrome (Pruzansky, 1969; Murray, et al., 1979; Lauritzen, et al., 1985). In these cases, DO is performed to correct facial deformities of varying severity and symmetry which can have tremendous psychological benefit. Of more immediate concern, distraction of the mandible can also correct tongue-base airway obstruction and restore respiratory function in neonatal infants as young as 2 weeks of age (Sidman, et al., 20001). However, optimization of the distraction technique is not likely given that the mechanically-induced cellular response of bone has not been elucidated, and the vast majority of clinical applications of DO have been in adult patients. To develop successful loading strategies for DO, quantification of the cellular and tissue responses to loading is required. As such, research addressing the cellular response of bone to distraction in organ culture neonates may help to maximize clinical outcome by optimizing load parameters including magnitude, orientation and duration. A major advantage of the DO technique is that the cellular stimulation induced by distraction can result in sufficient osteogenesis independent of additional bone grafting, and as such offers a significant native improvement over techniques requiring avascular bone grafting. DO, popularized by Gavril Ilizarov in 1951 was originally applied to long bones, and most of the characterization of the approach has been studied in this model system. Considerably less characterization has been conducted in cranial models; the complicated geometry of the jaw in comparison to the femur has been a major factor contributing to this disparity. Thus, using only *in vivo* models with poorly defined distraction has failed to enable the isolated study of the effects of the mechanical loading on cellular response; model system development enabling this would be advantageous.

In essence, DO requires the creation of a pseudo growth plate. The bone is fractured and a distraction device spanning the fracture is used to apply mechanical forces across the fracture to create new bone to fill in the bone gaps. Generally DO involves three phases, the latency phase following an osteotomy/corticotomy where the bone is allowed to begin healing, an active distraction phase in which the bone is actively distracted at a rate generally not exceeding 1 mm/day and a consolidation phase in which the bone is no longer distracted and is allowed to strengthen before the distraction device is removed. In cases of mandibular distraction such as that which occurs in neonates as a result of airway obstruction, the latency phase is not necessary and the bone is pliable enough at this stage to be osteogenic without requiring the initial osteotomy/corticotomy. However, as previously noted, given that little is understood about the response of bone to distraction loading, the procedure often reduces to trial and error. Moreover, in cases of craniofacial deformity correction, symmetry is critical to achieve the desired aesthetics to within fractions of a millimeter. To begin to address DO in organ culture, femur models and linear distraction were utilized. Femurs harvested from 5 day old neonatal rats were subjected to distraction. For loading, a single purpose distraction device was developed given the need for greater accuracy than the in-house loading platform provided and utilized a micrometer head, Figure 16. Utilizing this device, initial studies were conducted in which bones were subjected to 2% strain via linear distraction for 2 hr at 24, 72 and 120 hr of culture. Strain was verified with optical techniques and bones were kept hydrated at all times throughout the loading period. While distraction is generally performed daily, these initial studies utilized loading every other day to minimize handling and the risk of contamination. At 1 wk the loaded bones were mechanically tested to failure and their no-load contralateral counterparts were used as controls.

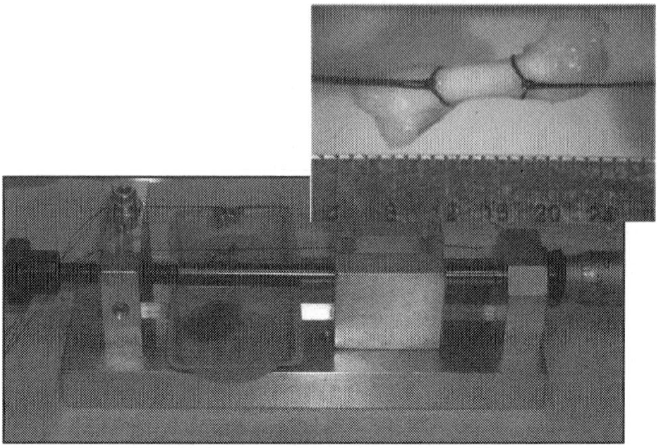

Fig. 16. In-house device used to apply distraction to organ cultures at 2 % bone shaft strain for 2 hr at 24, 72 and 120 hr of culture.

As shown in Figures 17 and 18, bones subjected to 3, 2 hr distraction loads resulted in a significant increase in failure load and stiffness at the 1 wk culture period. Given that the structural integrity of the bones was maintained during the multiple loading bouts and the loaded bones demonstrated an osteogenic response consistent with distraction, the biomimetic models may hold promise in elucidating the pathways and mechanisms by which the bone cells respond under mechanical distraction.

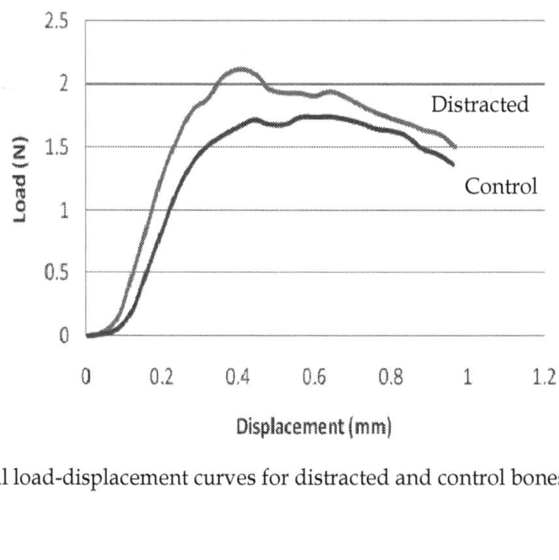

Fig. 17. Typical load-displacement curves for distracted and control bones.

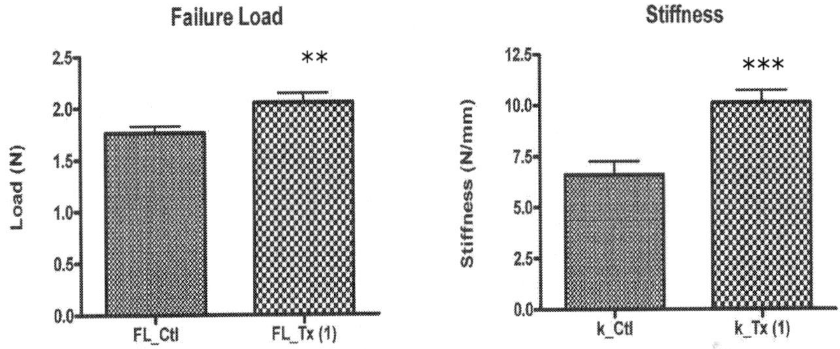

Fig. 18. Distraction in organ culture increased bone strength. Failure load (FL) and stiffness (k) were significantly increased in comparison to their no-load counterparts maintained in culture for 1 wk.

At this point, it has preliminarily been shown that organ culture systems may hold some potential as biomimetic models of bone cell mechanotransduction. Additional goals would be to expand the age of the organs beyond the neonatal stage. While the neonatal model has a higher chance of maintaining viability in culture given the increased porosity and decreased mineralization in comparison to adult bones, the neonatal system is somewhat limited in its usefulness. For instance, these models would not be appropriate for addressing issues related to osteoporosis. Where one could argue that osteoporosis is a disease indicative of increased porosity and bone destruction and would therefore likely have a reasonable life in culture, the control for an osteoporotic model would be an adult, normal bone. The adult bone would have an increased level of mineralization that would not be conducive to organ culture. Thus, it may prove helpful to investigate means to increase culture viability to enhance survival of mineralized, mature bones. Two obvious avenues of research would be to optimize culture conditions with topical additives and/or to develop active perfusion systems. Current efforts to develop the perfusion chambers are underway and chamber dimensions have been developed based upon laminar flow profile analysis, Figure 19. Solid modeling software and time dependent fluid flow analysis were utilized to develop a chamber that enabled fully developed laminar flow to reach the bone. Rapid prototyping techniques have been employed to fabricate the chambers and studies are ongoing to determine a flow profile that prolongs culture viability, without providing measurable stimulation to the bones.

Efforts are also underway to demonstrate that additional bone models are appropriate for organ culture studies. Given the need for models that can be used for craniofacial DO studies and the need to develop planar models of loading that more appropriately model clinical DO scenarios, studies examining the viability of mandibles in culture have also been initiated. Prior to applying load to mandibular models, it is necessary to characterize the development of the mandibles in organ culture. As shown in Figure 20, mandibles maintained in culture for 4 wk stain heavily for calcium content and display a resorption pattern consistent with tooth eruption. In addition, although bone is lost as a result of this possible eruption, the ash weight of mandibles at 4 wk of culture is significantly greater than that of controls taken at 24 hr, increasing 22% (data not shown). Current microCT studies

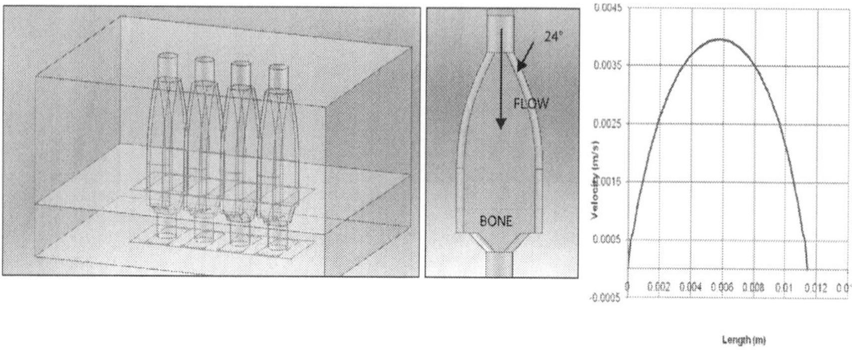

Fig. 19. 3D solid model of a perfusion chamber providing a laminar flow profile to organ culture in an effort to prolong culture viability and extend the biomimetic systems to include adult, mineralized bone models.

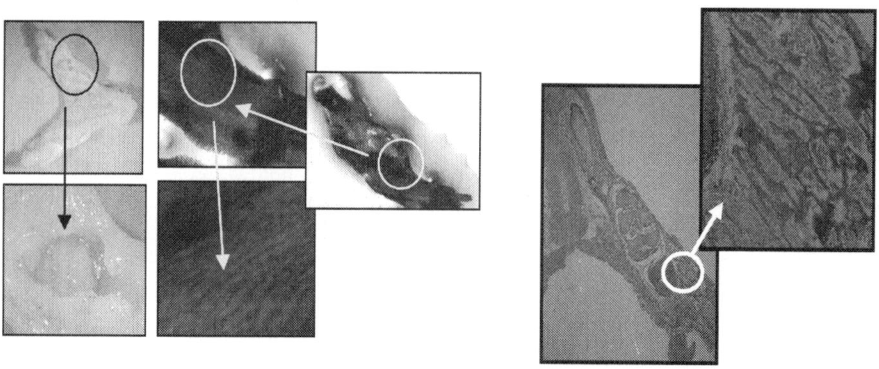

Fig. 20. (Left) Alizarin red staining at 4 wk in cultured demonstrated the presence of calcium and good bone quality and quantity. (Right) 10 micron H&E sections (decalcified) demonstrated the presence of healthy bone, tooth development and model viability (presence of cellular nuclei) at 4 wk of culture.

are underway to determine if tooth development in culture parallels that of age-matched controls to establish baseline culture properties prior to applying distraction. While only preliminary work has been initiated in this area, continued work will help to determine the validity of organ culture systems for biomimetic mechanotransduction modeling of craniofacial distraction osteogenesis. As this work progresses, new mechanical loading devices will need to be developed which will apply the appropriate vectors to the bone and will ultimately enable 2D and 3D distraction.

Bone, because of its unique ability to adapt to its environment will always be a target of biomimicry. Its innate modification to structural design to prevent failure is an extremely attractive property of bone that if emulated could have countless benefits to the public and private sectors. While biomimetics often cites bone as inspiration, our understanding of bone's ability to adapt to its environment is still in its nascency and biomimetic bone models may help elucidate the response of bone to mechanical stimulation. Understanding this response would have significant benefit to the medical field and could aid in the improved design and fixation of implant systems, functional tissue engineered bone constructs, bioreactor development and the eradication of metabolic bone diseases such as osteoporosis. As such, the focus of this work has been to introduce the reader to the field of bone mechanotransduction research by focusing on the engineering systems and models currently available. Furthermore, the objective was to introduce the reader to the concept of an organ culture, or *ex vivo* mechanotransduction system that we believe may be more biomimetic than *in vitro* models and less complex than *in vivo* models. Laying the groundwork for biomimetic models in bone mechanotransduction research, we demonstrated that neonatal, whole bone organ culture models remain viable, continue to grow and are osteogenic in response to mechanical stimulation. Furthermore, we demonstrated in a variety of preliminary studies that these models may prove useful in mechanistic studies requiring culture additives and are capable of simulating clinical procedures, such as distraction osteogenesis. Groundwork has been laid to develop perfusion chambers to prolong culture viability and the characterization of additional bone models in culture is underway to assess their future usefulness in mechanotransduction research. However, a major question that remains to be answered regarding the organ culture systems is to determine whether or not the pathways and mechanisms by which the bone cells respond are altered in the organ culture system. That is, does the bone respond along the same mechanisms and pathways to stimulation in culture that it would if maintained in the body, or do compensatory mechanisms/pathways take over such that the very nature of the response is altered by the use of the organ culture? In engineering terms, this would be equivalent to the concern as to whether or not the measurand affects the measurement. While only time will tell if the organ culture model will prove to be acceptable for biomimetic mechanotransduction studies, the initial work is promising.

Appendix: Derivation of fluid shear stress generated with a parallel plate flow configuration:

Starting with the Navier-Stokes equation assuming steady, incompressible and fully developed flow

$$\rho g_x - \frac{\delta P}{\delta x} + \mu\left(\frac{\delta^2 u}{\delta x^2} + \frac{\delta^2 u}{\delta y^2} + \frac{\delta^2 u}{\delta z^2}\right) = \rho\frac{\delta u}{\delta t}$$

$$\frac{\delta P}{\delta x} = \frac{dP}{dx}$$

$$\left(\frac{\delta^2 u}{\delta x^2} + \frac{\delta^2 u}{\delta y^2} + \frac{\delta^2 u}{\delta z^2}\right) = \frac{d^2 u}{dy^2}$$

$$\frac{\delta u}{\delta t} = 0$$

The Navier-Stokes equation becomes

$$\mu\left(\frac{d^2u}{dy^2}\right)=\frac{dP}{dx}=C=-K$$

$$\left(\frac{d^2u}{dy^2}\right)=\frac{-K}{\mu}$$

Integrating twice

$$u(y)=\frac{-Ky^2}{2\mu}+C_1y+C_2$$

And given the no slip condition at the boundaries

$$u=0;@\,y=\pm\frac{h}{2}$$

$$@\,y=\frac{h}{2};\quad 0=\frac{-K}{2\mu}\left(\frac{h^2}{4}\right)+C_1\frac{h}{2}+C_2$$

$$0=-K\left(\frac{h^2}{8\mu}\right)+C_1\frac{h}{2}+C_2$$

And

$$u=0;@\,y=-\frac{h}{2}$$

$$@\,y=-\frac{h}{2};\quad 0=\frac{-K}{2\mu}\left(\frac{h^2}{4}\right)+C_1\left(-\frac{h}{2}\right)+C_2$$

$$0=-K\left(\frac{h^2}{8\mu}\right)-C_1\frac{h}{2}+C_2$$

Adding equations to solve for C_2

$$-K\left(\frac{h^2}{8\mu}\right)+C_1\frac{h}{2}+C_2+\left(-K\left(\frac{h^2}{8\mu}\right)-C_1\frac{h}{2}+C_2\right)$$

$$C_2=K\left(\frac{h^2}{8\mu}\right)$$

Substituting to solve for C_1

$$0=\frac{-K}{2\mu}\left(\frac{h^2}{4}\right)+C_1\left(\frac{h}{2}\right)+K\left(\frac{h^2}{8\mu}\right)$$

$$0=C_1\left(\frac{h}{2}\right);\quad C_1=0$$

The equation takes the form

$$u(y) = \frac{-Ky^2}{2\mu} + \frac{Kh^2}{8\mu}$$

$$u(y) = \frac{K}{8\mu}(h^2 - 4y^2)$$

The volume flow rate (Q) may be determined by integrating the velocity (u) over the flow chamber's cross-sectional area

$$Q = \int_{\frac{-h}{2}}^{\frac{h}{2}} \frac{K}{8\mu}(h^2 - 4y^2)\,(bdy)$$

$$Q = \frac{bK}{8\mu} \int_{\frac{-h}{2}}^{\frac{h}{2}} (h^2 - 4y^2)\,dy$$

$$Q = \frac{bK}{8\mu} \left(h^2y - \frac{4}{3}y^3\right)\Big|_{\frac{-h}{2}}^{\frac{h}{2}}$$

$$Q = \frac{bK}{8\mu} \left[\frac{h^3}{2} - \frac{4h^3}{24} - \left[-\frac{h^3}{2} + \frac{4h^3}{24}\right]\right]$$

$$Q = \frac{bK}{8\mu} \left[\frac{2h^3}{2} - \frac{8h^3}{24}\right]$$

$$Q = \frac{bK}{8\mu} \left[\frac{2h^3}{3}\right]$$

$$Q = \frac{bh^3K}{12\mu}$$

Since wall shear stress is defined as

$$\tau_w = \mu \frac{du}{dy}\Big|_{y=\pm\frac{h}{2}}$$

$$\tau_w = \mu \frac{d}{dy}\left(\frac{K}{8\mu}(h^2 - 4y^2)\right)\Big|_{y=\pm\frac{h}{2}}$$

$$\tau_w = \frac{K}{8}\left(\frac{d}{dy}(h^2 - 4y^2)\right)\Big|_{y=\pm\frac{h}{2}}$$

$$\tau_w = \frac{K}{8}\left(0 - 2(4y)\right)\Big|_{y=\pm\frac{h}{2}}$$

$$\tau_w = \frac{K}{8}(-8y)\Big|_{y=\pm\frac{h}{2}}$$

$$\tau_w = (-Ky)|_{y=\pm\frac{h}{2}}$$

$$\tau_w = -K\frac{h}{2}$$

Upon substituting back

$$Q = \frac{bh^3K}{12\mu} = \frac{Kh}{2}\left(\frac{bh^2}{6\mu}\right) = \tau_w\left(\frac{bh^2}{6\mu}\right)$$

$$\tau_w = \left(\frac{6\mu Q}{bh^2}\right)$$

2. References

Ajubi NE, Klein-Nulend J, Nijweide PJ, Vrijheidlammers T, Albas MJ, Burger EH (1996) Pulsating fluid flow increases prostaglandin production by cultured chicken osteocytes: a cytoskeleton-dependent process. Biochem Biophy Res Commun 225:62-68.

Balls MM (1976) Organ culture in biomedical research: festschrift for Dame Honor Fell, London: Cambridge University Press.

Barrett LA, Trump BF (1978) Maintaining human aortas in long-term organ culture. Meth Cell Sci 4(13):861-862.

Beno T, Yoon Y, Cowin SC, Fritton SP (2006) Estimation of bone permeability using accurate microstructural measurements. J Biomech 39(13):2378-2387.

Billiau A, Edy VG, Heremans H, Van Damme J, Desmyter J, georgiades JA, De Somer P (1977) Human interferon: mass production in a newly established cell line, MG-63. Antimicrob Agents Chemother 12:11-15.

Bonewald LF (2007) Osteocytes as dynamic multifunctional cells. Ann NY Acad Sci 1116:281-290.

Botchwey EA, Dupree MA, Pollack SR, Levine EM, Laurencin CT (2003a) Tissue engineered bone: measurement of nutrient transport in three-dimensional matrices. J Biomed Mater Res, 67A(1): 357-367.

Botchwey EA, Pollack SR, El-Amin S, Levine EM, Tuan RS, Laurencin CT (2003b) Human osteoblast-like cells in three-dimensional culture with fluid flow. Biorheology 40:299-306.

Bottlang M, Simnacher M, Schmidt H, Brand RA, Claes L (1997) A cell strain system for small homogenous strain applications. Biomedizinische Technik 42:305-309.

Boyd JD (2005) Embryology in war-time Britain. Anat Rec 87(1):91-97.

Brown TD, Bottlang M, Pedersen DR, Banes AJ (1998) Loading paradigms - intentional and unintentional - for cell culture mechanostimulus. Amer J Med Sci 316:162-168.;1359-1364.

Brown TD (2000) Techniques for mechanical stimulation of cells *in vitro*: a review. J Biomech 33(1):3-14.

Buhl KM, Jacobs CR, Turner RT, Evans GL, Farrell PA, Donahue HJ (2001) Aged bone displays an increased responsiveness to low-intensity resistance exercise. J Appl Physiol 90

Chan ME, Lu XL, Huo B, Baik AD, Chiang V, Guldberg RE, Lu HH, Guo XE (2009) A trabecular bone explants model of osteocyte-osteoblast co-culture for bone mechanobiology. Cell Molec Bioeng 2(3):405-415.

Cowin SC (1999) Bone poroelasticity. J Biomech 32(3):217-238.

Currey JD (2009) Measurement of the mechanical properties of bone. A recent history, Clin Orthop Relat Res 467:1948-1954.

Dallas SL, Zaman G, Pead MJ, Lanyon LE (1993) Early strain-related changes in cultures embryonic chick tibiotarsi parallel those associated with adaptive modeling *in vivo*. J Bone Miner Res 8(3):251-259.

Davies CM, Jones DB, Stoddart MJ, Koller K, Smith E, Archer CW, Richards RG (2006) Mechanically loaded *ex vivo* bone culture system 'Zetos': systems and culture preparation. Eur Cell Mater 11:57-75.

Del Rizzo DF, Moon MC, Werner JP, Zahradka P (2001) A novel organ culture method to study intimal hyperplasia at the site of a coronary artery bypass. Ann Thorac Surg 71:1273-1279.

Ewart JL, Cohen MF, Meyer RA, Huang GY, Wessels A, Gourdie RG, Chin AJ, Park SMJ, Lazatin BO, Villabon S, Lo CW (1997) Heart and neural tube defects in transgenic mice overexpressing the Cx43 gap junction gene. Development 124:1281-1292.

Fell HB (1972) Tissue culture and its contribution to biology and medicine. J Exper Biol 57:1-13.

Fell HB, Balls M, Monnickendam MA (1976) Organ culture in biomedical research. Cambridge University Press, Cambridge.

Forrest SM, NG KW, Findlay DM, Michelangeli VP, Livesey SA, Partridge NC, Zajac JD, Martin TJ (1985) Characterizqation of an osteoblast-like clonal cell line which responds to both parathyroid hormone and calcitonin. Calcif Tissue Int 37:51-56.

Frangos JA, Eskin SG, McIntire LV, Ives CL (1985) Flow effects on prostacyclin production by cultured human endothelial cells. Science 227:1477-1479.

Frangos JA, McIntire LV, Eskin SG (1988) Shear stress induced stimulation of mammalian cell metabolism. Biotechnol Bioeng 32:1053-1060.

Garrett R (2003) Assessing bone formation using mouse calvarial organ cultures. In:Helfrich MH, Ralston SH (eds) Bone research protocols, chap 14, Humana Press, Totowa.

Gay CV (1991) Avian osteoclasts. Calcif Tissue Int 49:153-154.

Glucksmann A (1942) The role of mechanical stresses in bone formation *in vitro*. J Anat 76:231-239.

Gross TS, Srinivasan S, Liu CC, Clemens TL, Bain SD (2002) Non-invasive loading of the murine tibia: an *in vivo* model for the study of mechanotransduction. J Bone Miner Res 17(3):493-501.

Hagino H, Kuraoka M, Kameyama Y, Okano T, Teshima R (2005) Effect of a selective agonist for prostaglandin E receptor subtype EP4 (ONO-4819) on the cortical bone response to mechanical loading. Bone 36(3):444-453.

Hillam RA, Skerry TM (1995) Inhibition of bone resorption and stimulation of formation by mechanical loading of the modeling rat ulna *in vivo*. J Bone Miner Res 10(5):683-689.

Hung CT, Pollack SR, Reilly TM, Brighton CT (1995) Real-time calcium response of cultured bone cells to fluid flow. Clin Orthop Relat Res 313:256-269.

Hung CT, Allen FD, Pollack SR, Brighton CT (1996) Intracellular Ca2+ stores and extracellular Ca2+ are required in the real-time Ca2+ response of bone cells experiencing fluid flow. J Biomech 29:1411-1417.

Imamura K, Ozawa H, Hiraide T, Takahashi N, Shibasaki Y, Fukuhara T, Suda T (1990) Continuously applied compressive pressure induces bone resorption by a mechanism involving prostaglandin E2 synthesis. J Cell Physiol 144:222-228.

Ishizeki K, Takigawa M, Harada Y, Suzuki F, Nawa T (1995) Meckel's cartilage chondrocytes in organ culture synthesize bone-type proteins accompanying osteocytic phenotype expression. Anat Embryol 185:421-430.

Jacobs CR, Yellowley CE, Davis BR, Zhou Z, Donahue HJ (1998) Differential effect of steady versus oscillating flow on bone cells. J Biomech 31:969-976.

Jee WS, Ueno K, Deng YP, Woodbury DM (1985) The effects of prostaglandin E2 in growing rats: increased metaphyseal hard tissue and cortico-endosteal bone formation. Calcif Tissue Int 37:148-157.

Jones DB, Broeckmann E, Pohl T, Smith EL (2003) Development of a mechanical testing and loading system for trabecular bone studies for long term culture. Eur Cell Mater 5:48-60.

Jubb RW (1979) Effect of hyperoxia on articular tissues in organ culture. Ann Rheum Dis 38(3):279-286.

Kato Y, Windle JJ, Koop BA, Mundy GR, Bonewald LF (1997) Establishment of an osteocyte-like cell line, MLO-Y4. J Bone Miner Res 12:2014-2023.

Klein-Nulend J, Burger EH, Semeins CM, Raisz LG, Pilbeam CC (1997) Pulsating fluid flow stimulates prostaglandin release and inducible prostaglandin G/H synthase mRNA expression in primary mouse bone cells. J Bone Miner Res 12:45-51.

Lauritzen C, Munro IR, Ross RB (1985) Classification and treatment of hemifacial microsomia. Scand J Plast Reconstr Surg 19:33–39.

Lyubimov EV, Gotleib AI (2004) Smooth muscle cell growth monolayer and aortic organ culture is promoted by a nonheparin binding endothelial cell-derived soluble factors. Cardiovas Pathol 13(3):139-145.

Meghji S, Hill PA, Harris M (1998) Bone organ cultures. In:Henderson B, Arnett T (eds) Methods in bone biology, chap 4, Thomson Science, New York.

Merrick AF, Shewring LD, Cunningham SA, Gustafsson K, Fabre JW (1997) Organ culture of arteries for experimental studies of vascular endothelium in situ. Transpl Immunol 5(1):3-7.

Merrilees MJ, Scott L (1982) Organ culture of rat carotid artery: maintenance of morphological characteristics and of pattern of matrix synthesis. *In vitro* 18(11):900-910.

Mikic B, Battaglia TC, Taylor EA, Clark RT (2002) The effect of growth/differentiation factor-5 deficiency on femoral composition and mechanical behavior in mice. Bone 30(5):733-737.

Murray JE, Mulliken JB, Kaban LB, Belfer M (1979) Twenty-year experience in maxillocraniofacial surgery. An evaluation of early surgery and growth, function and body image. Ann Surg 190:320–331.

Murrills RJ (1996) *In vitro* bone resorption assays. In: Bilezekian JP, Raisz LG, Rodan GA (eds) Principles of bone biology, chap 90, Academic Press, San Diego.

Nicholson GC, Moseley JM, Sexton PM, Martin TJ (1987) Chicken osteoclasts do not possess calcitonin receptors. J Bone Miner Res 2(1):53-9.

Owan I, Burr DB, Turner CH, Qui J, Tu Y, Onyia JE, Duncan RL (1997) Mechanotransduction in bone: osteoblasts are more responsive to fluid forces than mechanical strain. Amer J Physiol Cell Physiol 273 (3 Pt 1), C810-C815.

Piekarski K, Munro M (1977) Transport mechanism operating between blood supply and osteocytes in long bones. Nature 269:80-82.

Ponten J, Saksela E (1967) Two established in vitro cell lines from human mesenchymal tumours. Int J Cancer 2:434-447.

Pruzansky S (1969) Not all dwarfed mandibles are alike. Birth Defects 1:120.

Raisz L (1965) Bone resorption in tissue culture. Factors influencing the response to parathyroid hormone. J Clin Inv 44:103-116.

Raisz L, Niemann I (1967) Early effects of PTH and thyrocalcitonin in bone organ culture. Nature 214:486-488.

Reich KM, Gay CV, Frangos JA (1990) Fluid shear stress as a mediator of osteoblast cyclic adenosine monophosphate production. J Cell Physiol 143:100-104.

Reynolds JJ (1976) Organ cultures of bone: studies on the physiology and pathology of resorption. In: Balls M, Monnickendam M (eds) Organ culture in biomedical research. Cambridge University Press, Cambridge, pp 355-366.

Rubin CT, Lanyon LE (1984) Regulation of bone formation by applied dynamic loads. J Bone Joint Surg 66A:397-402.

Rubin CT, Lanyon LE (1985) Regulation of bone mass by mechanical strain magnitude. Calcif Tissue Int 37:411-417.

Saunders MM, You J, Trosko JE, Yamasaki H, Donahue HJ, Jacobs CR (2001) Gap junctions and fluid flow in MC3T3-E1 cells. Am J Physiol Cell Physiol 281(6):1917-1925.

Saunders MM, You J, Zhou Z, Li Z, Yellowley CE, Kunze E, Jacobs CR, Donahue HJ (2003) Fluid-flow induced prostaglandin E2 response of osteoblastic ROS 17/2.8 cells is gap junction-mediated and independent of cytosolic calcium. Bone 32(4):350-356.

Saunders MM, Donahue HJ (2004) Development of a cost-effective loading machine for biomechanical evaluation of mouse transgenic models. Med Eng Phys 26:595-603.

Saunders MM, Taylor AF, Du C, Zhou Z, Pellegrini VD Jr, Donahue HJ (2006) Mechanical stimulation effects on functional end effectors in osteoblastic MG-63 cells. J Biomech 39(8):1419-1427.

Saunders MM, Simmerman LA, Reed GL, Sharkey NA, Taylor AF (2010) Biomimetic bone mechanotransduction modeling in neonatal rat femur organ cultures: Structural verification of proof of concept. Biomech Model Mechanobiol 9:539-550.

Sidman JD, Sampson D, Templeton B (2001) DO of the mandible for airway obstruction in children. Laryngoscope 111(7):1137-1146.

Sorkin AM, Dee KC, Knothe Tate ML (2004) "Culture shock" from the bone cell's perspective: emulating physiological conditions for mechanobiological investigations. Am J Cell Physiol Cell Physiol 287:C1527-C1536.

Stepita-Klauco M, Dolezalova H (1968) Organ culture of skeletal muscle subjected to intermittent activity. Biomed Lif Sci 24(9):971

Swanson N, Javed Q, Hogrefe K, Gershlick A (2002) Human internal artery organ culture model of coronary stenting: a novel investigation of smooth muscle cell response to drug-eluting stents. Clin Sci 103(4):347-353.

Takahashi M, Chernin MI, Yamamoto O, Tonzetich J, Kinsey CG, Novak JF (2002) Transformation of MC3T3-E1 cells following stress and transfection with pSV2neo plasmid. Anticancer Res 22(2A):585-598.

Takai E, Mauck RL, Hung CT, Guo XE (2004) Osteocyte viability and regulation of osteoblast function in a 3D trabecular bone explants under dynamic hydrostatic pressure. J Bone Miner Res 19(9):1403-1410.

Takezawa T, Inoue M, Aoki S, Sekiguchi M, Wada K, Anazawa H, Hanai N (2000) Concept of organ engineering: a reconstruction method of rat liver for *in vitro* culture. Tiss Eng 6(6):641-650.

Taylor AF, Saunders MM, Shingle D, Cimbala JM, Zhou Z, Donahue HJ (2007) Osteocytes communicate fluid flow-mediated effects to osteoblasts altering phenotype. Am J Physiol Cell Physiol 292:C545-C552.

Turner CH, Akhter MP, Raab DM, Kimmel DB, Recker RR (1991) A noninvasive *in vivo* model for studying strain adaptive bone remodeling. Bone 12:73-79.

Voisard R, v Eicken J, Baur R, Gschwend JE, Wendroth U, Kleinschmidt K, Hombach V, Hoher M (1999) A human arterial organ culture model of postangioplasty restenosis: results up to 56 days after ballooning. Atherosclerosis 144(1):123-134.

Wang L, Ciani C, Doty SB, Fritton SP (2004) Delineating bone's interstitial fluid pathway in vivo. Bone 34(3):499-509.

Weinbaum S, Cowin SC, Zheng YA (1994) A model for the excitation of osteocytes by mechanical loading induced bone fluid shear stresses. J Biomech 27:339-360.

Weiss A, Livne E, von der Mark K, Heinegard D, Silbermann M (1988) Growth and repair of cartilage: organ culture system utilizing chondroprogenitos cells of condylar cartilage in newborn mice. J Bone Miner Res 3(1):93-100.

Wetzel DM, Salpeter MM (1991) Fibrillation and accelerated A Ch R degradation in long-term muscle organ culture. Muscle Nerve 14(10):1003-1012.

Wong SY, Dunstan CR, Evans RA, Hills E (1982) The determination of bone viability: a histochemical method for identification of lactate dehydrogenase activity in osteocytes in fresh calcified and decalcified sections of human bone. Pathology 14(4):439-442.

You J, Yellowley CE, Donahue HJ, Zhang Y, Chen Q, Jacobs CR (2000) Substrate deformation levels associated with routine physical activity are less stimulatory to bone cells relative to loading-induced oscillatory fluid flow. J Biomech Eng 122:387-393.

Zaman G, Dallas SL, Lanyon LE (1992) Cultured embryonic bone shafts show osteogenic responses to mechanical loading. Calcif Tissue Int 51(2):132-136.

Ziambaras K, Lecanda F, Steinberg TH, Civitelli R (1998) Cyclic stretch enhances gap junctional communication between osteoblastic cells. J Bone Miner Res 13:218-228.

17

Novel Biomaterials with Parallel Aligned Pore Channels by Directed Ionotropic Gelation of Alginate: Mimicking the Anisotropic Structure of Bone Tissue

Florian Despang[1], Rosemarie Dittrich[2] and Michael Gelinsky[1]
[1]*Max Bergmann Center of Biomaterials and Institute for Materials Science, Technische Universität Dresden, 01062 Dresden*
[2] *Institut für Elektronik- und Sensormaterialien, TU Bergakademie Freiberg, 09596 Freiberg*
Germany

1. Introduction

Regenerative medicine intends to restore lost functionality by healing tissues defects. For this novel types of biodegradable implants have to be used that first foster healing and later take part in the natural remodelling cycle of the body. In this way, patient's cells can reconstruct and adapt the tissue according to the local situation and needs. Ideally, the implant should mimic the desired tissue. That means that the biomaterial should resemble the extracellular matrix (ECM) which is expressed by specific cells and acts as the biological scaffold of living tissues. The closer an artificial scaffold material mimics the pattern the easier it can be involved in the natural healing and remodelling processes, which is why more and more researchers try to establish biomimetic approaches for the development of tissue engineering scaffolds. Biological materials are seldom isotropic and for many tissue engineering applications distinct anisotropic materials are needed. E. g. compact bone exhibits a honeycomb-like structure with overlapping, cylindrical units (osteons) with the so-called Haversian canal in the centre. Scaffolds with parallel aligned pores, mimicking the osteon structure of compact bone can be synthesised by directed ionotropic gelation of the naturally occurring polysaccharide alginate. The parallel channels are formed *via* a sol-gel-process when di- or multivalent cations diffuse into the sol in broad front, forming an alginate hydrogel. The pore size and pore alignment of such gels is influenced by the starting materials (e.g. concentrations, additives like powders or polymers) and the preparation process (e.g. temperature, drying process). The phenomenon was discovered already in the 50th of the last century but the biomedical potential of alginate scaffolds with parallel aligned pores structured by ionotropic gelation has been explored for osteoblasts, stem cell based tissue engineering, axon guiding or co-culture of vascular and muscle cells only in the past few years.

2. Biomimetic approaches for biomaterials and Tissue Engineering (TE)

In natural tissues, cells are embedded in three dimensional, fibrous environments - the so called extracellular matrix (ECM). General task of the ECM is to act as a scaffold for cell adhesion, to provide certain mechanical stability and elasticity, to protect the cells and to facilitate the development of the proper cell morphology. In addition, ECM is the space of nutrient and oxygen supply, of intercellular communication and it is relevant for storage of water and soluble substances. Each ECM is perfectly adapted to the special needs of a distinct tissue and its dedicated cells.

When developing artificial tissues in terms of tissue engineering a biomaterial called scaffold has to take over the basic functions of the natural ECM, at least until the construct has been fully integrated and remodelled by the host tissue after implantation. It is obvious that it is difficult to design artificial materials which meet all the requirements described above. Therefore many researchers started to mimic the natural ECM with their scaffold material, either concerning chemical composition, micro- or nanostructure or special properties like anisotropy which is also an important feature of most tissues (Ma, 2008). Biomimetic strategies can include the utilisation of ECM components like natural biopolymers (e. g. collagen), material synthesis under physiological conditions (37°C, pH of 7.4, buffered aqueous solutions etc.) or the creation of structural features similar to those of extracellular matrices.

The better an artificial scaffold material mimics its biological model, the faster it will be integrated by the host tissue after implantation and the easier it will be included in the remodelling cycle, leading finally to a complete degradation and healing of the defect.

3. Bone tissue: a natural, highly anisotropic nanocomposite material

In humans (general in mammals), different types of bone exist or are formed intermediately during development or healing, mainly cortical (compact), spongy (trabecular) and woven bone (Weiner & Wagner, 1998). Their organisation is highly hierarchical, but at the lowest level all consist of the same nanocomposite, made of fibrillar collagen type I and the calcium phosphate phase hydroxyapatite (HAP). Collagen is produced by bone cells called osteoblasts, which also express the enzyme alkaline phosphatise (ALP), necessary for calcium phosphate mineral formation. A variety of non-collagenous proteins, also synthesised by osteoblasts, are responsible for control of the matrix formation and mineralisation processes, but the molecular mechanisms are not completely understood yet. With the exception of woven bone, collagen fibrils are deposited in an alternating, sheet-like manner and with a parallel fibre alignment (called "lamellae") into the free space, created by resorbing osteoclasts during bone remodelling. Lamellae form osteons in compact bone - always aligned parallel to the bone axis - and trabecules in spongy bone (Rho et al., 1998). These structure elements are responsible for the outstanding mechanical properties of bone tissue and its perfect adaptation to the local force distribution.

Compact bone has only pores with diameters in the micrometer range, filled either with blood capillaries (Haversian canals, located in the centre of the osteons) or osteocytes (*lacunae* - interconnected by the *canaliculi* pore system). In contrast, the trabecules in spongy bone form a highly open porous structure with pore widths of up to a few millimetres. Fig. 1 shows the hierarchical organisation of (cortical) bone tissue - from the macroscopic organ down to the nanometre scale.

4. Directed ionotropic gelation of alginate – a biomimetic method for generating anisotropic materials

Alginate is the structural saccharid of brown algae. Being a co-polymer, it consists of mannuronic (M) and guluronic acid (G) monosaccharide units, possessing identical

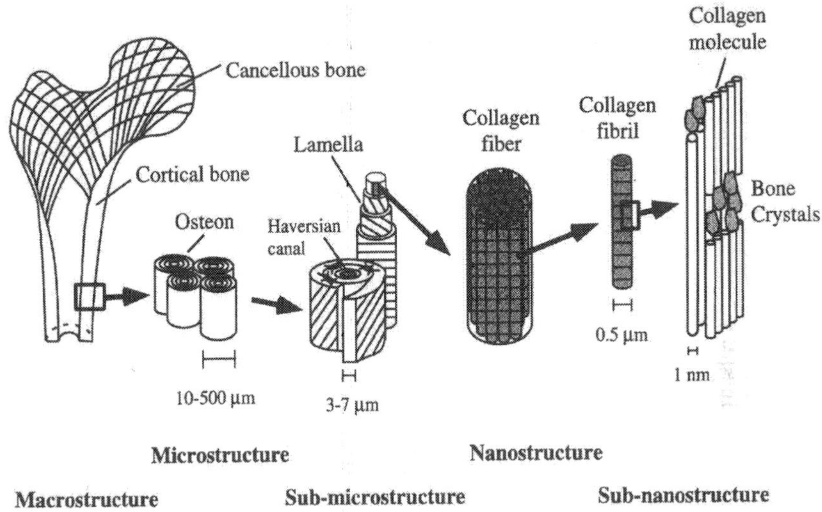

Fig. 1. Hierarchical organisation of cortical bone tissue from the centimetre to the nanometre scale (taken from Roh et al. (1998) with permission)

carboxylic and hydroxyl functional groups but differing in their configuration. These functional groups coordinate multivalent cations and build intermolecular complexes which results in the formation of a stable hydrogel. Straight MM-sequences do not exhibit sites for specific binding of cations (Braccini et al., 1999); the interaction takes place between GG-sequences leading to so-called egg-box motifs (Grant et al., 1973; Braccini & Perez, 2001). Alternating MG-sequences may also contribute but to a much lower extent (Donati et al., 2005). The composition of the alginates derived from different algae varies; the flexible stipes of algae, growing next to the sea surface, contain M-rich alginate whereas those exposed to strong flow exhibit high G-content (Zimmermann et al., 2007).

If an alginate sol gets into contact with gelling ions (electrolyte), the molecules gel immediately by covering the sol with a dense skin or membrane. Microbeads are produced by dropping small volumes into electrolyte solutions whereas the skin is trapping the sol which gets radially transformed into a gel by the diffusing ions. Anisotropic gels with channel-like pores develop when cations diffuse in broad front from one direction into an alginate sol whereas the saccharide molecules get arranged and complexed. Together with the gelation parallel aligned, channel-like pores are formed which can run through the whole length of the gel (Fig. 2).

4.1 Theoretical models for the phenomenon

The discoverer of the phenomenon, the German colloid scientist Heinrich Thiele, proposed the phase separation mechanism of droplet segregation. The gelation process

$$\text{Sol} + \text{Electrolyte (A)} \leftrightarrow \text{Gel} + \text{Electrolyte (B)} + \text{Water} \qquad (1)$$

is accompanied by dehydration. The finely distributed drops of water are trapped within the zone of sol-gel-transition. Further delivered water molecules will accumulate and are

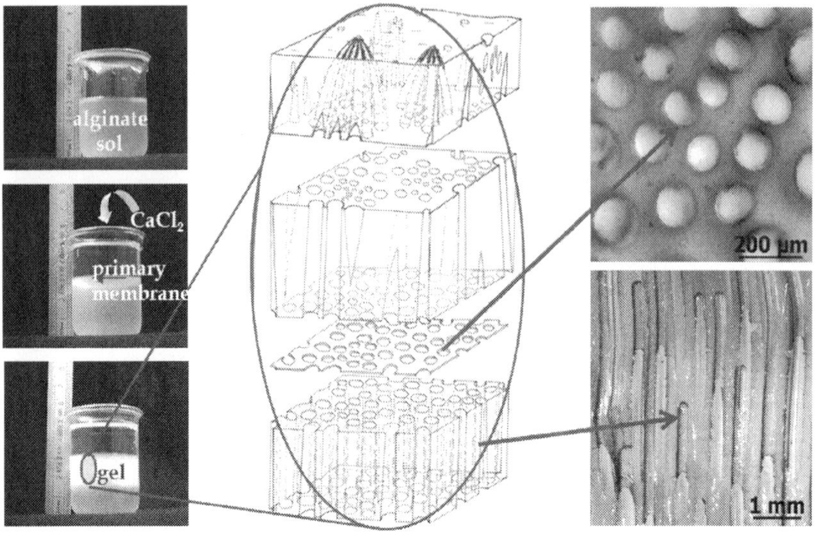

Fig. 2. Sketch of the process of ionotropic gelation of alginate. The scheme in the middle was adapted from Wenger (1998)

pushed by the gelation front towards the sol creating electrolyte containing and alginate free pore channels (Thiele & Hallich, 1957; Thiele, 1967b). Khairou and co-workers described the sol-gel-formation as diffusion controlled process which one step of primary membran formation and further growth of the anisotropic gel (Khairou et al., 2002).

In a series of 5 articles, Kohler and his group developed the theory of chemically fixed dissipative structure formation from the first idea (Kohler & Thumbs, 1995) until the summary of the work (Treml et al., 2003). Based on the observation, that there was a movement in the sol next to already gelled alginate visualized by tiny glass beads, they assumed a coupled mechanism of convection and diffusion. The alginate chains are subject to a conformational change during the complexation by the cations. If the sol exhibits an adequate viscosity, this contraction will induce a movement of the sol which resembles to pattern of the Rayleigh-Benard-Konvection. This pattern gets fixed by the sol-gel-transition. For a stable reaction, a sufficient mass transport is needed to ensure a certain contraction velocity of the alginate molecules. The mathematical description consists of the Navier-Stokes equation for the hydro-dynamical model (Kohler & Thumbs, 1995; Thumbs & Kohler, 1996), Fick's law for the diffusional macroscopic part (Treml & Kohler, 2000) and the results from random walk simulations of a phantom chain (Woelki & Kohler, 2003). The phenomenon of capillary creation due to the ionotropic gelation was postulated as chemically fixed dissipative formation, which is based on the concentration of the alginate sol and gel as well as the electrolyte, the diffusion coefficients of the reactants, the degree of polymerization, length and number of rigid segments of the alginate chain and the gelation rate constant (a fitting parameter obeying to boundary conditions) (Treml et al., 2003).

So far about growth but what about the initiation of the pores? Thiele and Hallich postulated periodic water droplets which segregate by the dehydration during gelation (Thiele & Hallich, 1957). The contraction of the alginate causes accumulations and lower concentrated areas as nucleation seeds (Purz, 1972). Lateral variations in chain mass fraction and composition were also considered which would laterally vary the contraction capacity (Thumbs & Kohler, 1996). The origin of first segregation and pore creation was tried to identify by Purz and coworkers by electron microscopy - interestingly not with alginate but cellulose xanthate (Purz, 1972; Purz et. al., 1985). The ionotropic gelation is not specific for alginate but can occur also with other polymers (e.g. pectin, cellulose) and even inorganic anisometric colloids (e. g. V_2O_5) get oriented by the flux of counter ions.

4.2 History of ionotropic gelation

The phenomenon of ionotropic gelation was discovered by Heinrich Thiele, professor at the chemical department of Kiel University, Germany. Initially he studied in- and organic anisometric colloids which were oriented by diffusing ions. He created the term ionotropy (*ionos* = ion, *trepein* = turn) (Thiele, 1964) as a special case of gelation (Higdon, 1958). The properties of the gels were birefringence, anisotropic swelling and reversible ion exchange. He was fascinated by the similarity between structures of biological origin and the artificially created anisotropic gels (Thiele & Andersen, 1953). In his pioneering work, Thiele intensively studied parameters which influence the structure formation and different methods to characterise the oriented colloids (Thiele, 1967b). He restlessly compared the structure of ionotropic gels with those of tissues or other biological specimens and found a variety of similarities (Thiele, 1954b; Thiele, 1967a). Based on this comparison, he predicted a model for the principle of biological structure formation - especially supported by studies on dissolution and re-constitution of an eye lens (Thiele et al., 1964). His last publication on ionotropic gelation was dealing with mineralisation of the gels especially with calcium phosphates (Thiele & Awad, 1969).
More than 25 years later, the phenomenon was theoretically investigated with a new vision on the mechanism (Kohler & Thumbs, 1995) as well as towards the kinetics of ionotropic gelation (Khairou et al., 2002) - and finally, the capillary formation could be described by a mathematical model (Treml et al., 2003). At the same time, the idea re-emerged to use the membranes, produced by ionotropic gelation, as filters with adjustable pore diameter. Not only the hydrogels could be utilised for this application (Thiele & Hallich, 1959; Moll, 1963), but also sintered ceramics, derived by structuring slurries of alginate mixed with ceramic powders like e.g. Al_2O_3 (Weber et al., 1997) or even with the mineral phase of bone, hydroxyapatite (HAP) (Dittrich et al., 2002). The pore distribution and run was characterized by µCT in ceramic (Goebbels et al., 2002) or composite (Despang et al., 2005b) state. Since 2005/6, the anisotropic structures have been subject of research in the area of tissue engineering with human cells for hard tissue (Despang et al., 2005a, Dittrich et al., 2006) and vascularisation (Yamamoto et al., 2010), in *in vitro* and *in vivo* studies in rats for nerve regeneration (Prang et al., 2006) and with murine embryonic stem cells opening opportunities for the formation of many types of tissue (Willenberg et al., 2006). A more detailed and chronological list of scientific contributions to the field with short summaries of their content follows (Table 1).

4.3 Anisotropic hydrogels

The phenomenon of ionotropic gelation was discovered for alginate leading to a hydrogel with parallel aligned, channel-like pores. At the early beginning, the gelation was carried out solely with Cu^{2+} which needs to be replaced in case of medical applications by acidic exchange or ion substitution for a biocompatible one such as Ca^{2+}. Since 2005, hydrogels

Author(s) Year	Content
Thiele, 1947 [in German]	Alignment and gelation of anisometric particles in colloidal solutions (thin layer), resulting in birefringence pattern in polarized light
Thiele & Micke, 1948 [German]	First full article on alignment and gelation of anisometric particles in colloidal solutions, but not yet about capillary formation
Thiele & Kienast, 1952 [German]	Dependence of alignment of anisometric particles on type and concentration of ions of electrolyte including electron microscopy images of sol and thixotropic gel
Thiele & Ander-sen, 1953 [Ger.]	Identical structure and pattern of decalcified femur (collagen) and ionotropic gel (Cu^{2+} gelled pectin) observed in polarised light
Thiele, 1954a [German]	Change in experimental set-up: diffusion of electrolyte from outside into the sol, from thin layer of sol to beads and cylinders, direction of ion diffusion from radial to broad front
Thiele, 1954b	English summary of previous work; differentiation of ionotropic gels from other structures, claim on model for some biological patterns: bone (collagen), see weed (alginate) and ripe fruits (pectin)
Thiele & Ander-sen, 1955a [German]	Transition from inorganic to organic colloids for ionotropic gelation (alginate, pectin); first thoughts on theory of droplet demixing; swelling and birefringence antipodal
Thiele & Ander-sen, 1955b [Ger.]	Effect of chain length of alginate and pectin on ionotropic gelation (viscosity); first images of radial pore channels in multiphasic gels
Schuur, 1955 [Ge.]	Structure formation of ionotropic gels through material flux
Thiele & Kroenke, 1955 [German]	Reversible Pb-based mineralisation of ionotropic gels (cellulose glyconat) within the cavities or pore walls of gel
Thiele & Hallich, 1957 [German]	**Channel-like pores in 3D gels of alginate through ionotr. gelation including images and theory of droplet demixing; influence of type and concentration of cations and sol on pore channel diameter**
Thiele & Hallich, 1959 [German]	Application of capillary structure of ionotropic alginate gels as filters: void volume, permeability (water, gas), pore size distribution
Thiele et al., 1962 [German]	Distinction between 5 zones of ionotropic gels with parallel aligned pores; focus on primary membrane and diffusion induced membrane potential; ion exchange after cross-linking with DIC
Moll, 1963 [German]	Application of Al-alginate gels with channel-like pores as reversible filter for bacteria and viruses, filtering of a 5 nm gold sol
Thiele, 1964 [German]	Diverting overview about ionotropic gelation (theory, helices, mineralisation) as model of biological pattern formation
Thiele et al., 1964 [German]	Ionotropic gelation as principle of biological pattern formation based on similarities to natural tissues in appearance (osteons in bone, layers of pearl) and reversible gelation of eye lens and cornea etc.
Thiele & Cordes, 1967 [German]	Influence of counter ions on gel formation; ligand field theory
Thiele, 1967 [German]	Short summary of principles of structure formation: bone, eye lens, cornea

Author(s) Year	Content
Thiele, 1967b [German book]	Exhaustive summary and overview on ionotropic gelation (book)
Thiele, 1967c [German]	Ionotropic gels as template for oriented intra- or intercapillary mineralisation in native and cross-linked gels by ion waves
Thiele & Awad, 1969	Mineralisation of alginate hydrogels with parallel aligned pores with calcium phosphate phase brushit by ion waves followed by conversion to hydroxyapatite
Purz, 1972	Anisotropic hydrogels based on cellulose-xanthate structured via ionotropic gelation by thallium or zinc ions; SEM investigations
El-Cheik & Awad, 1976	Conductance of ions-free-washed metal alginate inversely proportional to polarisability of gelling cations
Awad et al., 1980	Kinetic of ionotropic gel formation in two steps (quick membrane formation, slow gel growth) evaluated by change in concentration of electrolyte and description as diffusion controlled process
Purz et al., 1985 [German]	Morphology of anisotropic cellulose-derivate gels structured by ions of Tl, Pb, Zn, La and combinations studied by electron microscopy
Hassan et al., 1989	Latest of 3 similar articles on kinetics of sol-gel-transformation of alginate with different ions (nickel, copper and cobalt)
Heinze et al., 1990 [German]	Structure and application of carboxy-containig polysaccharides, especially anisotropic alginate hydrogels for cell immobilisation, drug release; rheological investigations
Hassan et al., 1991	Structure formation of alginate by interaction of cations with two carboxylic and two hydroxy groups
Hassan, 1991	Kinetics of acidic ion exchange of cations (Ni^{2+}, Co^{2+}, Cu^{2+}) in anisotropic alginate hydrogels by conductimetry
Hassan, 1993	Kinetics of anisotropic Ni-alginate gels: idea for application on separation of ion mixtures and capture of isotopes based on selective alginate binding
Kohler & Thumbs, 1995 [German]	New idea on theory of capillary development by ionotropic gelation of alginate as chemically fixed dissipative structure: contraction of alginate during gelling yields a movement of sol next to gelation front which was visualised by adding 0.3 µm glass beads
Thumbs & Kohler, 1996	Mathematical description of ionotropic gelation similar to Rayleigh-Benard convection by Navier-Stokes equation and introduction of critical convection velocity
Weber et al., 1997	**Al_2O_3 membranes with capillaries produced by Cu^{2+}-gelled alginate-Al_2O_3-slurries and change in volume by drying procedures**
Treml & Kohler, 2000	Mathematical description of diffusive mass transport of alginate and gelling ions: correlation of convective transport to bulk concentrations
Dittrich et al., 2002	Synthesis of ceramic membrans (Al_2O_3, TiO_2, HAP) by ionotropic gelation of alginate/ceramic powder-slurries (drying process,

Author(s) Year	Content
	influence of sintering temperature on density, macro-structure)
Goebbels et al., 2002	Non-destructive analysis (μCT) of pore structure of ceramic membranes (Al_2O_3, TiO_2, HAP), synthesised by ionotropic gelation
Khairou et al., 2002	Kinetic study of ionotropic gelation induced by heavy metal ions and interpretation of change of electrolyte concentration: influence of ionic radius and electrolyte density; model of intra- and intermolecular binding of cations to alginate chains
Woelki & Kohler, 2003	Modelling of the integration of alginate chains to the growing gel by conformational changes/degree of contraction (length of chain, velocity of gelation front, velocity of cross-linking reaction)
Treml et al., 2003	**Summary of new theory on capillary formation as chemically fixed dissipative structure depending on bulk concentrations, diffusion constants, properties of alginate chain (number, length of Kuhn segments), rate constant of gelation reaction**
Despang et al., 2005a	Ca-alginate hydrogels and composites of alginate/HAP for bone TE: addition of HAP powder or synchronous mineralisation *in situ*
Despang et al., 2005b	μCT-evaluation of composites of alginate-gelatine, reinforced with HAP (powder and synchronous mineralisation)
Renzo et al., 2005	Pore channels in Cu-alginate microbeads and mineralisation
Dittrich et al., 2006	**Alginate-gelatine-composites reinforced with HAP or ß-TCP mimicking composition of bone (70:30 in- : organic) and biocompatibility test by cultivation of osteogenically induced hMSC**
Willenberg et al., 2006	**Cu-gelled alginate scaffold as polyelectrolyte with chitosan as matrix for TE with murine embryonic stem cells: structure and *in vitro* experiment for 4 days**
Prang et al., 2006	**Oriented axonal regrowth on isocyanate cross-linked, Cu-gelled alginate hydrogels with *in vitro* (entorhinal-hippocampal slice culture) & *in vivo* (spinal cord) experiments in rats**
Mueller et al., 2006	Axonal regrowth on Cu^{2+}-, Ni^{2+}- or Ba^{2+}-alginate hydrogels (after ion exchange) with *in vitro* & *in vivo* experiments in rats
Eljaouhari et al., 2006	Al_2O_3 membrans based on Cu^{2+}- or Ca^{2+}-alginate-slurries including optimized drying procedure, consolidation and permeability data
Dittrich et al., 2007	Influence of processing parameters on pore structure of Ca^{2+}-alginate-HAP-slurries (drying process, pore run (μCT), influence of media on softening, hMSC *in vitro* culture)
Gelinsky et al., 2007	Biphasic but monolithic scaffolds for therapy of osteochondral defect with 2 layers (alginate/hyaluronate and alginate/HAP)
Despang et al., 2008	Scaffolds for bone TE produced by ceramic processing chain; composite, brown-body & ceramic: change of microstructure and biocompatibility of hMSC
Bernhardt et al., 2009	Biocompatibility of alginate-gelatine-HAP-scaffolds evaluated with osteogenically induced human mesenchymal stem cells (hMSC) over 4

Author(s) Year	Content
	weeks (incl. mechanical testing)
Mueller et al., 2009a	Axonal regrowth on Ba- or Ni-gelled alginate with more and longer linear axon ingrowth in dorsal ganglion *in vitro* culture with 10 μm than 120 μm pore diameters
Mueller et al., 2009b	Summary on axonal regrowth guided by anisotropic alginate hydrogels
Khan et al., 2009	Alginate or polyelectrolyte dextran/alginate w/o particle reinforcement of Au, TiO_2 and Fe_3O_4
Yamamoto et al., 2010	Co-culture of HUVEC w/o smooth muscle cells seeded onto Ca-alginate hydrogel for revascularization - static and perfusion cultures

Table 1. Chronology of scientific publications on ionotropic gelation leading to structures with parallel aligned pores (excluding PhD theses and patents); milestones highlighted bold. Abbreviations: DIC - diisocyanate, hMSC - human mesenchymal stem cells, HUVEC - human umbilical vein endothelial cells, HAP – hydroxyapatite.

with channel-like pores created by ionotropic gelation of alginate were in focus for tissue engineering. The idea of creating a tube-like template for capillary tissue structures e. g. for blood vessels (Yamamoto et al., 2010) is fascinating. Depending on the needs, the pore diameter can be adjusted between 30-460 μm by the processing conditions, meanly type and concentration of alginate and electrolyte (Table 2). The swollen hydrogels exhibit a macro-porosity of approx. 30% due to the pore channel diameter but the walls consist of an alginate network with a high nano-porosity. The pore density was found to be 530/mm^2 and the mean pore diameter around 30 μm for Cu^{2+} as cation (Willenberg et al., 2006; Prang et al., 2006). Interestingly, using a different type of alginate gelled with Cu^{2+}, we found a pore density of 124/mm^2 with an mean pore diameter of only 20 μm. Anisotropic hydrogels based on this type of alginate (ISP Manugel DMB) gelled by diffusion of Ca^{2+} ions exhibited a pore density of 77/mm^2 whereas ISP Manucol DM yields 5/mm^2. The mean pore diameter is inversely related to the pore density. Using Ba^{2+} or Ni^{2+} ions instead of Cu^{2+} the pore density was 960/mm^2 and 30/mm^2, respectively, and the mean pore diameter 10 and 120 μm, respectively (Müller et al., 2008).

Target tissue	Dimension (ØH or LWH)	Pore-Ø	Alginate concentr.	Mol. weight	Electrolyte	Reference
	[mm]	[μm]	[Ma.%]	[kDa]	[M]	
Bone	10x5	40-230	2	40-60	1 M $CaCl_2$	Despang et al., 2005a
Embryonic stem cells	7x5x3	30	2	12-80	0.5 M $CuSO_4$	Willenberg et al., 2006
Neuronal tissue	0.5x0.5x3	27	2	100	1 M $Cu(NO_3)_2$	Prang et al., 2006
Vascularisation	5x2	220-460	0.5-4	64-110	0.5-1.5 M $CaCl_2$	Yamamoto et al., 2010

Table 2. Alginate hydrogel scaffolds designed for different tissue engineering applications

The pore diameter is also influenced by the pH value (Fig. 3), mainly, because the alginate conformation (coiled or stretched) can be changed with the pH. Adjusting the pH value, mostly HCl or NaOH is used which also changes the ion strength and therefore the electrostatic conditions within the sol. To achieve a homogenous alginate sol, the aqueous solution should be buffered because at low pH isotropic gelation can occur due to the ability of H^+ ions to interact with the alginate molecules (Thiele & Hallich, 1957).

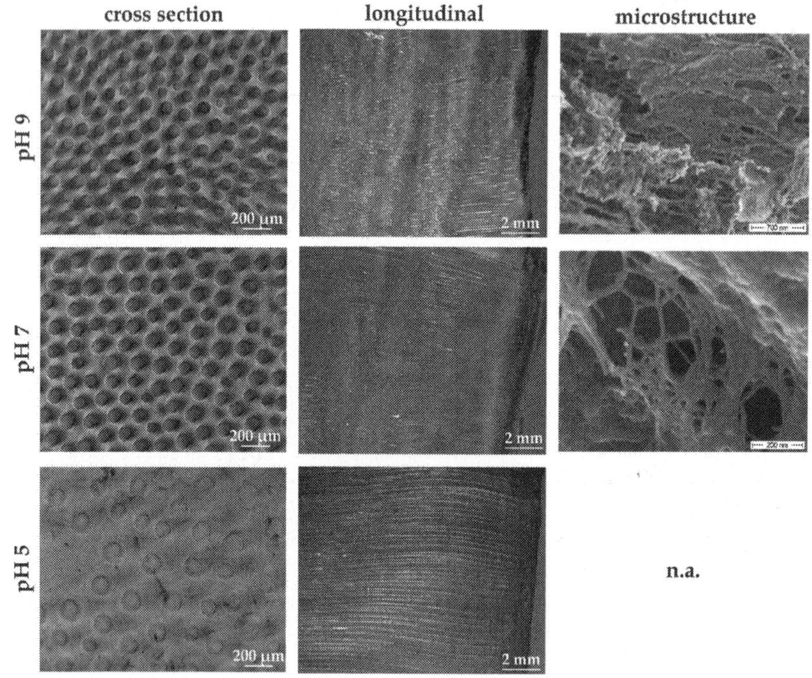

Fig. 3. Variation of pore diameter and pore distribution in the cross section of hydrogels, prepared at different pH values (1% Alginate Manugel, ISP) - microstructure after freeze drying

Up to distinct ranges, other biopolymers can be added to the alginate sol without preventing the process of ionotropic gelation. This also allows to further stabilise the hydrogels by means of covalent cross-linking, e. g. applying carbodiimide chemistry. If a cationic polymer like chitosan is chosen, polyelectrolytic hydrogels which means symplexes of two differently charged polymers are formed (Fig. 4). For a biomimetic approach, we incorporated successfully fibrillar collagen type I as the main component of most mammalian ECMs, but only minor amounts could be used without disturbing the ionotropic gelation process. Also addition of gelatine (thermally denaturised collagen) is possible but the mixture has than to be kept above 30°C to prevent untimely gelation of gelatine.

The most stable (concerning degradation under cell culture conditions) polyelectrolytic hydrogel was found while adding chitosan which additionally facilitated mineralisation by immersion in simulated body fluids (SBF).

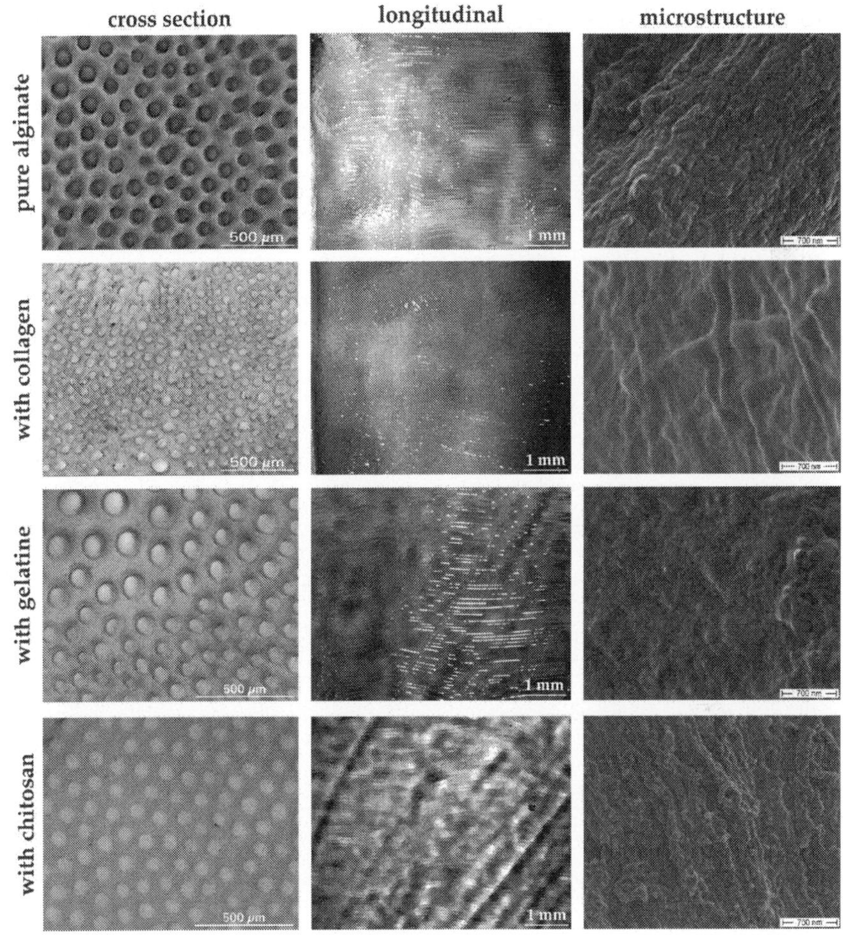

Fig. 4. Polyelectrolytic hydrogels of the negatively charged alginate and positively charged biopolymers (microstructure after air drying)

4.4 Anisotropic composites

Heading for regeneration of hard tissue, the mineral phase of bone, the calcium phosphate hydroxyapatite (HAP), should be incorporated. Alginate-HAP-composites with parallel aligned pores can be achieved following different strategies (Fig. 5), either by mineralisation of the hydrogels after gelation or directly during the sol-gel-process. Possible routes are:

- Immersion of the structured gel in simulated body fluid (SBF) and heterogeneous precipitation of HAP,
- Ion waves, i.e. diffusion of ions (alternating calcium and phosphate ions) in broad front into the hydrogel in some runs creating initially brushit which can be transformed into HAP (Thiele & Awad, 1969),

- Synchronous mineralisation, i.e. precipitation of calcium phosphate during the sol-gel-process (Despang et al., 2005),
- HAP powder, i.e. addition of HAP powder to the alginate sol and structuring of this slurry *via* ionotropic gelation (Despang et al., 2005; Dittrich et al., 2006; Dittrich et al., 2007; Bernhardt et al., 2009),
- Biphasic but monolithic scaffolds for the therapy of osteochondral defects can be produced through deposition of sol layers differing in composition prior to the gelation (Gelinsky et al., 2007).

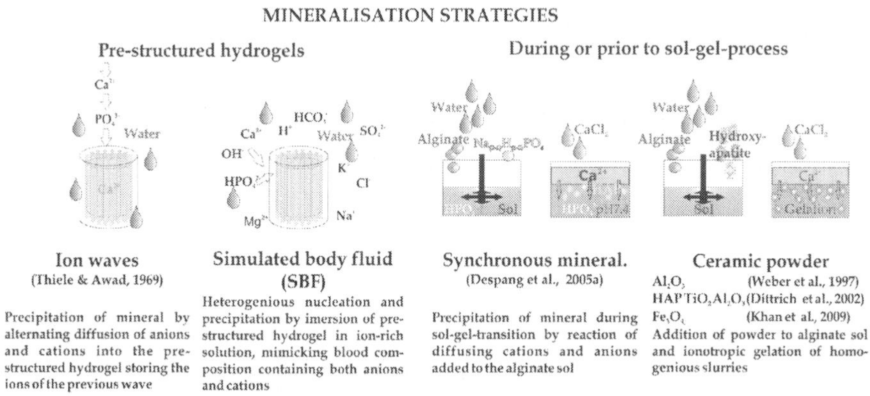

Fig. 5. Strategies of mineralisation – which also can be used in combination

The mineral content of the composites, which was determined by ignition loss, varied between the methods. A dried hydrogel, obtained from a 2% alginate sol without any calcium phosphate phase exhibits approx. 11% of ash due to the gelling ions (Ca^{2+}) and reaction productes ($CaCO_3$ or CaO) during combustion (Despang et al., 2005). 5-9% more mineral content was found for composites which were mineralised simultaneously during the ionotropic gelation. In this case, the Ca^{2+} ions not only orientated the alginate chains but also reacted with the phosphate ions which had been added to the alginate sol before the sol-gel-transition was initiated. Immersion in SBF increased the mineral content up to 11%. Higher contents, mimicking the inorganic-to-organic-ratio of bone (aprox. 70:30), and even more could only be realised by mixing HAP powder to the alginate sol. Thiele reached 50% i.e. a little less than the ratio of bone ECM and each wave led to shrinkage of the structure and therefore the pore diameter decreased (Thiele & Awad, 1969). Interestingly, the place of mineralisation, either intracapillar or in the pore walls, could be adjusted by the processing conditions as well as the shape of the precipitate was changed from round to needle-like by addition of citrate. The different approaches of mineralisation are expressed in varying microstructures (Fig. 6) and change the mechanical properties of the composite materials. The high amount of HAP introduced by addition of ceramic powder results in improved strength compared to the synchronously mineralised composites which was evaluated in wet state (Despang et al., 2005; Bernhardt et al., 2009).

All changes in composition of the sol or slurry prior to ionotropic gelation will influence the pore formation (diameter, length, density) during the sol-gel-process (Dittrich et al., 2007). However, the gel or composite with parallel aligned pores can be influenced after gelation

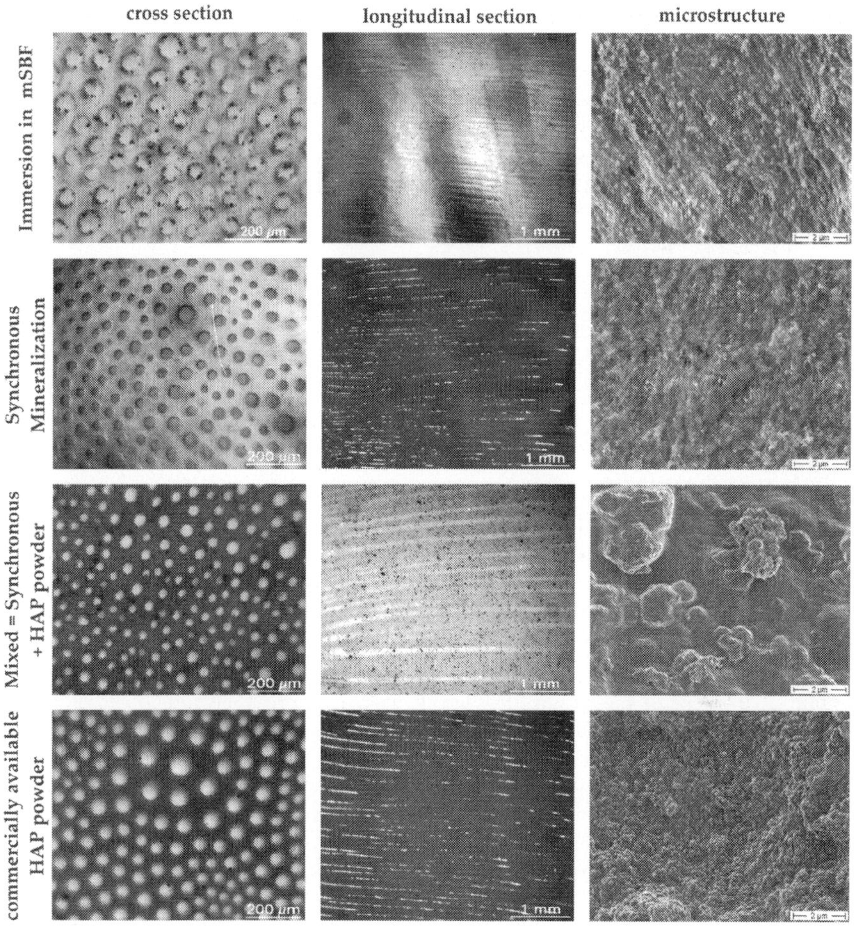

Fig. 6. Composite materials of biopolymer and mineral

by exposure to organic solvents benefiting of the different swelling behaviour. Other strategies are exchange of the gelling ions or different drying procedures. Freeze, air and supercritical drying were studied when the interest on ceramic membranes aroused (Weber et al., 1997) and was further optimised (Dittrich et al., 2002; Eljaouhari et al., 2006). Investigations by micro computer tomography (µCT) revealed that the pore structure was destroyed by ice crystals during freeze drying whereas the structure remained intact when water was exchanged against tert. butanol. Following the run of pore channels, this non destructive method also unveiled that pore channels can merge with distance from the primary membrane (Dittrich et al., 2007).

A mineral gradient in the direction of the long axis of the pore channels can be obtained by carefully covering layers of alginate sol on top of each other which differ in composition (Gelinsky et al., 2007). Bi-phasic but monolithic scaffolds consisting of a hydrogel-part and a mineralised part were under current investigations for regeneration of osteochondral defect. Both parts contain additional components of the respective ECM, i.e. hyaluronic acid for articular cartilage and hydroxyapatite for bone. Furthermore, living chondrocytes were successfully embedded into the cartilage portion and stayed alive within 2 weeks of *in vitro* culture. Incorporating living cells into the process of ionotropic gelation demands of course work under sterile conditions and with sterile components during all process steps.

For medical applications, scaffolds need to be sterile but alginate (like other biopolymers) is affected by all common sterilisation methods (Despang et al., 2008b). Since tissue engineering comprises the degradation of the scaffold after implantation, the sterilisation method enables to adapt this kinetic to the tissue or application of interest. For use in hard tissue regeneration, the type of calcium phosphate powder incorporated in the composites de- or accelerates the degradation because HAP and tricalcium phosphate (TCP) possess different solubility (Dittrich et al., 2006). *In vitro* studies of the degradation kinetics should be carried out under conditions as close as possible to those *in vivo*, i.e. in the incubator at 37°C/5%CO_2 and in cell culture medium (Bernhardt et al., 2009). Also the mechanical stability over time is differently affected by cell culture medium compared to water or PBS (Dittrich et al., 2007).

The biocompatibility of alginate-gelatine-HAP composites with a pore diameter of approx. 90 µm was evaluated by human mesenchymal stem cells (hMSC) which were osteogenically induced. The seeding efficiency was 10-34% and cell number increased by a factor of 4-7 within 4 weeks (Dittrich et al., 2006; Bernhardt et al., 2009). Osteogenic differentiation was confirmed by reverse transcriptase-PCR by gene expression of ALP and BSPII which were not present at day 1 but were found clearly at day 21 (Bernhardt et al., 2009). A clear difference between osteogenically induced and non-induced cells was observed, too. Cells adhere at the face surface but were also found inside the channel-like pores visualised by confocal laser scanning microscopy (Bernhardt et al., 2009).

4.5 Anisotropic ceramics

Two observations paved the road for the synthesis of anisotropic inorganic materials. First of all, the channel-like structure was conserved in the ash after burning the organic part of mineralised alginate which was intended to determine the mineral content (Thiele, 1967c). Additionally, impurities or additives are not segregated like in the case of crystallisation but incorporated into the hydrogel (Thiele, 1964). Only Weber et al. (1997) described the synthesis of ceramic membranes based on structuring via sol-gel-process of ionotropic gelation of alginate/powder-slurries followed by calcination.

Ceramic processing for membrane manufacturing was studied with Al_2O_3 or TiO_2 including development of adapted drying regimes for the wet composites applying method inherent shrinkage, followed by heat treatment to obtain a sintered ceramic without cracks (Weber et al., 1997; Dittrich et al., 2002; Eljaouhari et al., 2006). Dittrich et al. (2002) for the first time synthesised such ceramics consisting of the mineral phase of bone, hydroxyapatite, with parallel aligned pores and investigated their structure by µCT in cooperation with Goebbels et al. (2002). The pore size and wall thickness was adjusted by the ratio of alginate-to-HAP powder (Dittrich et al., 2002).

Anisotropic Al_2O_3 ceramics with a pore diameter of 19 µm (Dittrich et al., 2002), approximately 70 µm (Eljaouhari et al., 2006) or even 250-320 µm (Weber et al. 1997) were manufactured. For TiO_2 ceramics a range of 10-30 µm was reported (Goebbels et al. 2002).

Lower sintering temperatures result in less shrinkage and larger pore diameters (Dittrich et al., 2002). For tissue engineering of bone, pores in the range of 100-300 µm are demanded. Additionally, HAP which was exposed to temperatures of more than ca. 1000°C is no longer resorbable *in vivo* by osteoclasts (the bone degrading cells). Therefore heat treatment at a lower temperature is required to achieve biodegradable implant materials. Sintering is performed for consolidating ceramic materials. A first HAP ceramic without organic components can be derived as intermediate state after bisquit firing, leading to a material called brown body which normally is consolidated in a further sintering step (Fig. 7).

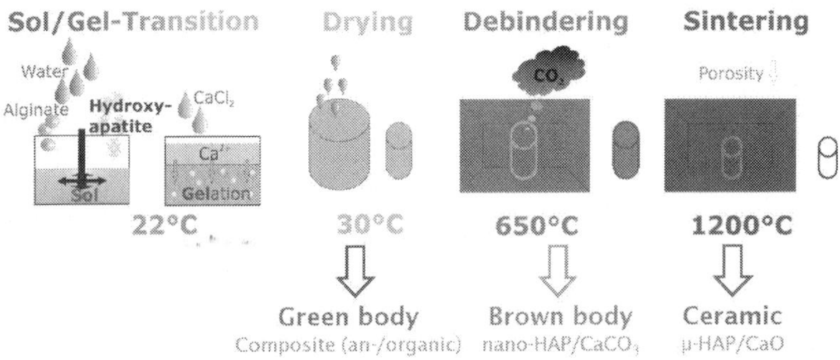

Fig. 7. Sketch of ceramic processing using sol-gel-technique of ionotropic gelation of alginate slurries with ceramic powders

Mechanical tests of HAP brown bodies with parallel aligned pores revealed a compressive strength of 4.5 MPa. This value is quite comparable to that of cancellous bone of human origin (5.9 MPa) tested at the same instrument under similar conditions (Rauh et al., 2009). The brown body exhibited a crystallite size of 41 nm compared to 238 nm of the sintered ceramic after treatment at 1200°C (Despang et al., 2008). Biocompatibility was evaluated by proliferation and differentiation of human mesenchymal stem cells (hMSC). The typical maximum of the specific alkaline phosphatase (ALP) activity was observed at day 14 after seeding. Cell number increase by a factor of 2.5 within 3 weeks for osteogenically induced hMSC cultivated on brown body samples as well as on sintered ceramics (Despang et al., 2008). Osteogenically induced hMSC adhered at the face surface as well as inside the channel-like pores and grew to a confluent layer (Fig. 8).

The pore diameter (40-165 µm) was larger for the brown body than for the sintered ceramics with approximately 30-115 µm (Fig. 9), depending on the type of alginate used for structure formation. The pore density varied between 20-90 pores/mm^2 for the brown bodies and 50-100 pores/mm^2 for the sintered ceramics. Largest samples prepared were 11x8 mm (ØxH).

Since alginate is gelled by many cations, anisotropic ceramics could also be synthesised by different complexing metal ions. Within the non-toxic elements, Zn^{2+} generates hydrogels with pores larger than those derived from Ca^{2+} (Thiele, 1967b). The more the cations orient the alginates molecules, the smaller the pore diameter of the gelled structure which also leads to an increase of the mechanical strength (Thiele & Hallich, 1957). But this does not primarily apply for the ceramics because the fibrous organic part was burnt. Even so using Zn^{2+} for gelling alginate-HAP-slurries led to larger pore channels than Ca^{2+} (Fig. 10), but the biocompatibility was poor i.e. no cell proliferation was observed within 4 weeks on composite material – *in vitro* studies on HAP bioceramics based on Zn-alginate-HAP-slurry still need to be accomplished.

Beside the actual pore size, the specific surface is an important parameter for scaffolds in tissue engineering by regulating protein and growth factor adsorption. The specific surface (BET) was measured for all states of the ceramic processing including the starting HAP powder, green body (composite of alginate and HAP after drying), brown body (thermal removal of organic phase) and consolidated ceramic (Fig. 11). Highest value is reached for the initial powder whereas in the composite material, the alginate is occupying some space and therefore the specific surface decreased. During heat treatment, the organic phase was removed and the consolidation started by sintering. Nano-sized pores of the walls were filled during sintering but the macro-porosity as relevant parameter for cell ingrowth remained unaffected.

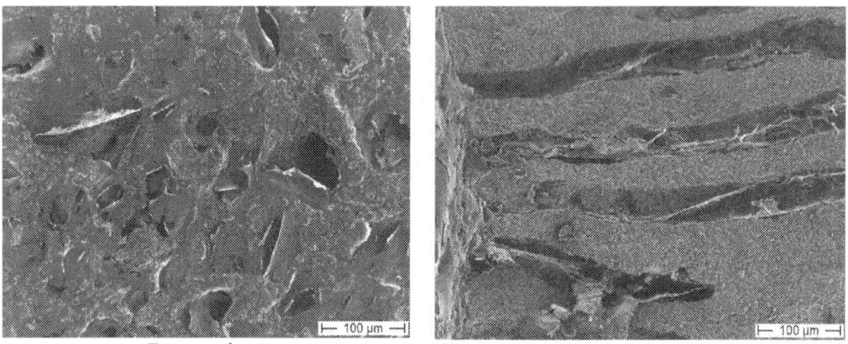

Face surface Longitudinal section

Fig. 8. Osteogenically induced hMSC after 14 days of *in vitro* cultivation on nano-crystalline HAP scaffolds in the state as brown body (Ca^{2+} gelled slurry) - SEM (200x) after supercritical drying

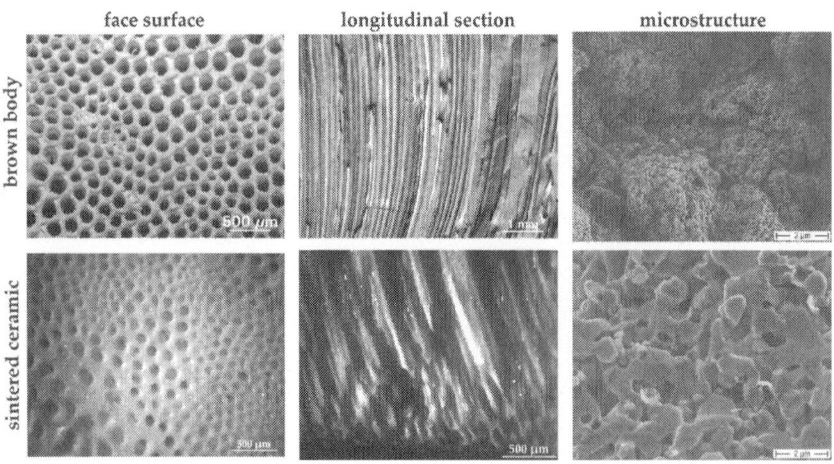

Fig. 9. Hydroxyapatite bioceramic based on Ca-alginate-HAP-slurry (top: state after thermal treatment at 650°C) with channel-like pores (bottom: sintered ceramic)

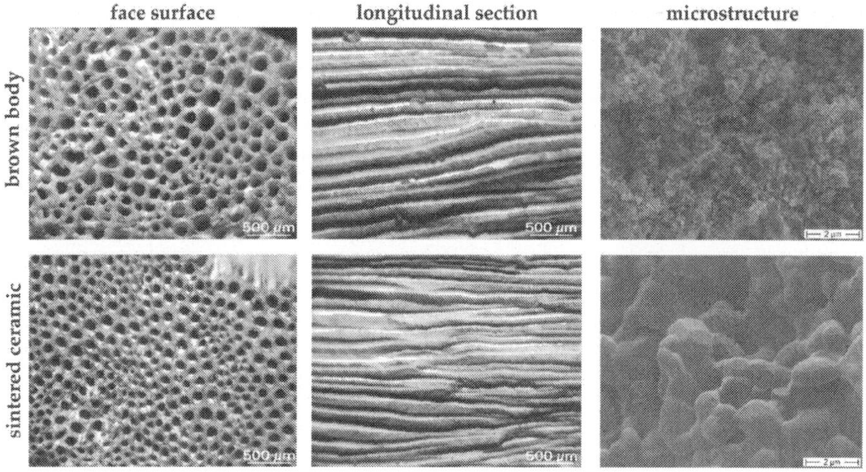

Fig. 10. Ceramics based on Zn-alginate-HAP-slurries (top: brown body, bottom: sintered)

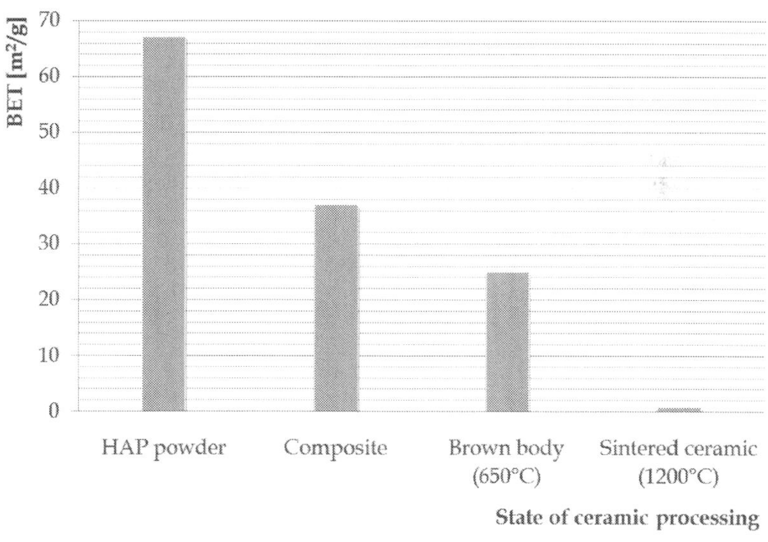

Fig. 11. Change of the specific surface (BET) during ceramic processing through thermal loss of alginate and due to sintering effects

5. Similarities between natural tissues and materials, generated by ionotropic gelation of alginate

In section 3, the highly hierarchical organisation of bone tissue has been described. Many attempts has been undertaken up to now to develop biomimetic materials which resemble the nanocomposite, consisting of collagen type I and nanoscopical HAP crystals and therefore bone ECM at the smallest length scale (Gelinsky & Heinemann, 2010). In contrast, only a few methods are known which opens the possibility to mimic organisation and structure of (compact) bone at the micrometre scale. By applying directed ionotropic gelation of alginate, osteon-like patterns can be achieved. Addition of collagen (or gelatine) and nanoscopical HAP adapts the chemical composition to that of bone ECM and leads also to mechanical strengthening. Finally, also vital cells can be incorporated during the gelation process, leading to a model for living bone tissue which can be utilised for regenerative therapies or research purposes. Figure 12 demonstrates the several levels of hierarchy which can be realised and controlled during ionotropic gelation.

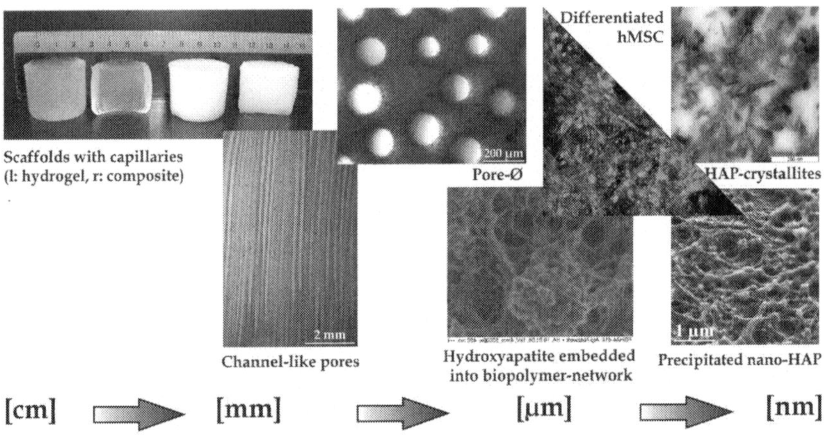

Fig. 12. Example for hierarchically structured composite material synthesised by ionotropic gelation of alginate-gelatine-HAP-slurry; compare with Fig. 2 (hierarchical organisation of cortical bone)

6. Conclusion

With the method of directed ionotropic gelation of alginate-based sols, a variety of materials can be synthesised, mimicking the highly anisotropic properties of natural tissues like bone. By controlling the composition of the starting materials and the reaction conditions, the properties of the product can be adjusted in a wide range. Pure alginate or mixtures of alginate with other biopolymers lead after gelation to elastic hydrogels. By addition of ceramic phases prior to the gelation or mineralisation of the hydrogels afterwards, composites can be achieved with which the composition of bone ECM and the patterns of cortical bone in the micrometre scale nicely can be mimicked.

When applying thermal treatments, the alginate phase is burnt out and pure inorganic materials remain which preserve the fascinating channel-like and aligned pores. Combinations of the calcium phosphate phase HAP and alginate resulted in astonishingly stable brown bodies after alginate burn-out at 650°C. These materials show similar compressive strength than trabecular human bone but are still degradable after implantation due to the small particle size. Further heating to sintering temperatures of 1200°C leads to stable ceramics with higher mechanical strength. But during the sintering step, the HAP grains grow, making the product hardly degradable for osteoclasts (and therefore *in vivo*). Fig. 13 gives an overview about the four main types of materials which can be derived from the process of ionotropic gelation. An increasing number of publications on this topic demonstrates that the phenomenon is still intensively under investigation. Furthermore, more and new fields of application, especially in the biomedical field, have been opened up in the last ten years, including embedding of living human cells during the gelation process. More and astonishing discoveries will follow.

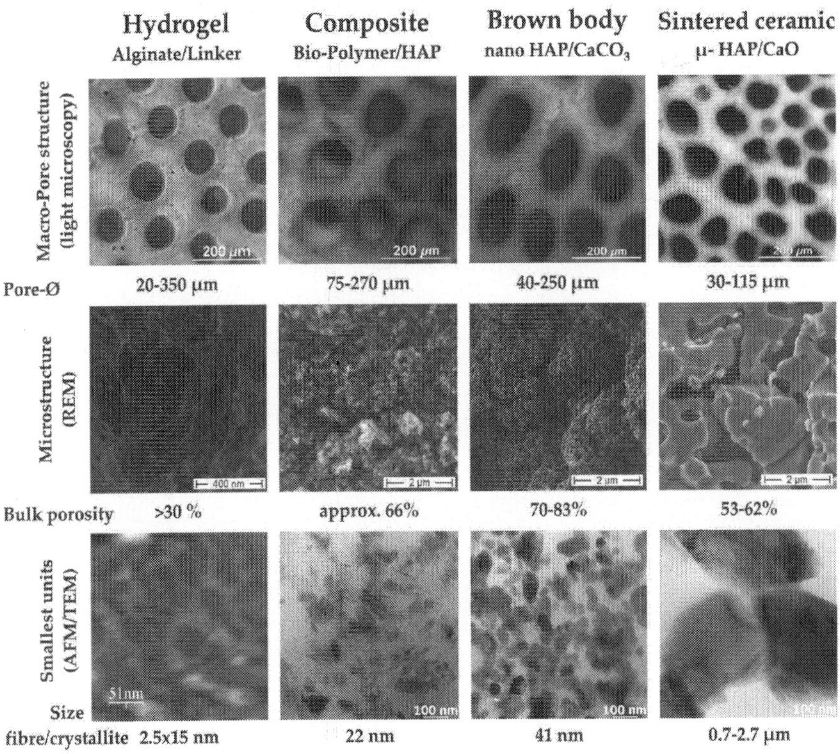

Fig. 13. Overview of anisotropic scaffolds, prepared using the process of ionotropic gelation, consisting of different materials

7. Acknowlegdement

We would like to thank the German Research Foundation (DFG) for financial support of the projects PO392/26-1, TO70/32-1, HE2157/10-2 and GE1133/4-2. We are grateful to Dr. Armin Springer for preparing TEM specimens by ultra microtome. We deeply acknowledge Dr. Anne Bernhardt for evaluation of biocompatibility with human mesenchymal stem cells.

Sincere thanks are given to Dr. Juliane Rauh (Orthopaedic University Hospital, Dresden) for cooperation in mechanical testing of spongy bone of human origin in order to evaluate the effects of sterilisation processes.

8. References

Awad, A.; El-Cheikh, F. & Shaker, A. (1980). Kinetic studies of cobalt alginate gels. *Colloid and Polymer Science*, 258, 1244-1249

Bernhardt, A.; Despang, F.; Lode, A.; Demmler, A.; Hanke, Th. & M. Gelinsky (2009). Proliferation and osteogenic differentiation of human bone marrow stromal cells on alginate-gelatine-hydroxyapatite scaffolds with anisotropic pore structure. *Journal of Tissue Engineering and Regenerative Medicine*, 3, 54-62

Braccini, I.; Grasso, R. P. & Perez, S. (1999). Conformational and configurational features of acidic polysaccharides and their interactions with calcium ions: a molecular modeling investigation. *Carbohydrate Research*, 317, 119-130

Braccini, I. & Perez, S. (2001). Molecular basis of Ca^{2+}-induced gelation in alginates and pectins: the egg-box model revisited. *Biomacromolecules*, 2, 1089-1099.

Despang, F.; Börner, A.; Dittrich, R.; Tomandl, G.; Pompe, W. & Gelinsky, M. (2005a). Alginate/calcium phosphate scaffolds with oriented, tube-like pores. *Materialwissenschaft und Werkstofftechnik*, 36, 761-767

Despang, F.; Bernhardt, R.; Mund, E.; Dittrich, R.; Beckmann, F.; Tomandl, G.; Pompe, W. & Gelinsky, M. (2005b). Investigations of alginate/calcium phosphate scaffolds with oriented tube-like pores by Microcomputed tomography. *Annual Report 2005 of HASYLAB DESY*, 1, 409-410

Despang, F.; Dittrich, R.; Bernhardt, A.; Hanke, Th.; Tomandl, G. & Gelinsky, M. (2008a). Channel-Like Pores in Hap-Containing Scaffolds for Bone Engineering: Hydrogels vs. Ceramics. *Tissue Engineering Part A*, 14, 819

Despang, F; Demmler, A.; Bernhardt, A.; Hanke, Th.; Dittrich, R. & Gelinsky, M. (2008b). Evaluation of sterilisation methods for alginate/hydroxyapatite scaffolds for hard tissue engineering. Proceedings of the 8th World Biomaterials Congress, Amsterdam (The Netherlands), 28.5-1.6.2008

Dittrich, R.; Tomandl, G. & Mangler, M. (2002). Preparation of Al_2O_3, TiO_2 and Hydroxyapatite Ceramics with Pores Similar to a Honeycomb Structure. *Advanced Engineering Materials*, 4, 487-490

Dittrich, R.; Despang, F.; Bernhardt, A.; Mannschatz, A.; Hanke, Th.; Tomandl, G.; Pompe, W. & Gelinsky, M. (2006). Mineralized Scaffolds for hard tissue engineering by ionotropic gelation of alginate, In: Vincenzini, P. *(ed.) Advances in Science and Technology*, Vol. 49, 159-164, trans tech publications inc.

Dittrich, R.; Despang, F.; Bernhardt, A.; Hanke, Th.; Tomandl, G.; Pompe, W. & Gelinsky, M. (2007). Scaffolds for hard tissue engineering by ionotropic gelation of alginate - influence of selected preparation parameters. *Journal of the American Ceramic Society*, 90, 1703-1708

Donati, I.; Holtan, S.; Morch, Y. A.; Borgogna, M.; Dentini, M. & Skjaek-Break, G. (2005). New Hypothesis on the Role of Alternating Sequences in Calcium-Alginate Gels. *Biomacromolecules*, 6, 1031-1040

El-Cheikh, F. & Awad, A. (1976). The electric conductance of some metal alginates. *Colloid and Polymer Science,* 254, 120-120

Eljaouhari, A.; Müller, R.; Kellermeier, M.; Heckmann, K. & Kunz W. (2006). New Anisotropic Ceramic Membranes from Chemically Fixed Dissipative Structures. *Langmuir,* 22, 11353-11359

Gelinsky, M.; Eckert, M. & Despang F. (2007). Biphasic, but monolithic scaffolds for the therapy of osteochondral defects. *International Journal of Materials Research,* 98, 749-755

Gelinsky, M. & Heinemann, S. (2010). Nanocomposites for tissue engineering, In: *Nanocomposites for Life Sciences*, Kumar, Ch. (ed.), 405-434. Wiley-VCH, ISBN 978-3-527-32168-1, Weinheim (Germany)

Goebbels, J.; Weidemann, G.; Dittrich, R.; Mangler, M. & Tomandl, G. (2002). Functionally graded porosity in ceramics - Analysis with high resolution computed tomography, In: *Innovative processing and synthesis of ceramics, glasses and composites V*, Singh, J. & Bansal, N. *(ed.),* Ceramic Transactions Series 129, 113-124, Wiley-VCH

Grant, G. T.; Morris, E. R.; Rees, D.A.; Smith, P. J. C. & Thom, D. (1973). Biological interactions between polysaccharides and divalent cations: The egg-box model. *FEBS Letters,* 32, 195-198

Hassan, R.; Summan, A.; Hassan, M. & El-Shatoury, S. (1989). Kinetics and mechanism of sol-gel transformation on polyelectrolytes of some transition metal ions, especially cobalt alginate ionotropic membranes. *European Polymer Journal,* 25, 25, 1209-1212

Hassan, R. M. (1991). Alginate polyelectrolyte ionotropic gels. Part III: Kinetics of exchange of chelated divalent transition metal ions especially cobalt(II) and copper(II) by hydrogen ions in capillary ionotropic metal alginate polymembrane gels. *Journal of Materials Science,* 26, 5806-5810

Hassan, R. M.; Awad, A. & Hassan, A. (1991). Seperation of metal alginate ionotropic gels to polymembranes with special evidence on the position of chelation in copper alginate complex. *Journal of Polymer Science Part A: Polymer Chemistry,* 29, 1645-1648

Hassan, R. M. (1993). Alginate polyelectrolyte ionotropic gels. *Journal of Materials Science,* 28, 384-388

Heinze, T.; Klemm, D.; Loth, F. & Philipp, B. (1990). Herstellung, Struktur und Anwendung von ionotropen Gelen aus carboxygruppenhaltigen Polysacchariden. Fortschrittsbericht Acta Polymerica, 41, 259-269

Higdon, W. T. (1958). Studies of Ionotropy: A Special Case of Gelation. *Journal of Physical Chemistry,* 62, 10, 1277-1281

Khan, F.; Walsh, D.; Patil, A. J.; Perriman, A. W. & Mann, S. (2009). Self-organized structural hierarchy in mixed polysaccharide sponges. *Soft Matter, 5*, 3081-3085

Khairou, K.; Al-Gethami, W. M. & Hassan, R. M. (2002). Kinetics and mechanism of sol-gel transformation between sodium alginate polyelectrolyte and some heavy divalent metal ions with formation of capillary structure polymembranes ionotropic gels. *Journal of Membrane Science,* 209, 445-456

Kohler, H. H. & Thumbs, J. (1995). Wo kommen die kapillaren im Alginatgel her? *Chemie Ingenieur Technik,* 67, 489-492

Ma, P. X. (2008). Biomimetic materials for tissue engineering. *Advanced Drug Delivery Reviews* 60, 2, 184-198

Moll, G. (1963). Über die löslichen Ultrafilter aus Aluminium- und Lanthan-Alginat und die elektronenmikroskopische Demonstration ihrer Filtrationseigenschaften. *Zeitschrift für Hygiene,* 149, 297-314

Müller, R.; Eljaouhari, A.; Prang, P.; Weidner, N. (2006). Preparation of alginate-based anisotropic capillary hydrogels for the promotion of oriented axonal re-growth in the injured spinal cord. *Cytotherapy,* 8, 55

Müller, R.; Pawar, K.; Weidner, N. (2009a). Alginate-based Anisotropic Capillary Hydrogels as Scaffolds for Guided Axon Regeneration. *Tissue Engineering Part A,* 15, 717-718

Müller, R.; Ferreira, I.; Pawar, K. & Weidner, N. (2009b) Application of Hydrogels to Rewire the Injured Spinal Cord, In *Handbook of Hydrogels: Properties, Preparation & Applications,* Stein, D. B. (Ed.), 397-426, NOVA Publishers, Hauppauge, NY

Prang, P.; Müller, R.; Eljaouhari, A.; Heckmann, K.; Kunz, W.; Weber, T.; Faber, C.; Vroemen, M.; Bogdahn, U. & Weidner, N. (2006). The promotion of oriented axonal regrowth in the injured spinal cord by alginate-based anisotropic capillary hydrogels. *Biomaterials,* 27, 3560-3569

Purz, H. J. (1972). Morphological investigations of ordered gel formation in polyelectrolytes. *Journal of Polymer Science Part C: Polymer Symposia,* 38, 405-417

Purz, H. J.; Tiersch, B. & Philipp, B. (1985). Zur Morphologie ionotroper Gele aus anionischen Cellulosederivaten. *Acta Polymerica,* 36, 569-574

Rauh, J.; Despang, F.; Gelinsky, M.; Pruss, A.; Günther, K.-P. & Stiehler, M. (2009) Einfluss von Peressigsäure-Ethanol Sterilisation auf die biomechanischen Eigenschaften humaner spongiöser Knochentransplantate" Proceedings of the *Deutscher Kongress für Orthopädie und Unfallchirurgie.* Berlin, 21.-24. 10. 2009, *DocPO17-23,* German Medical Science GMS Publishing House

Renzo, F. D.; Valentin, R.; Boissiére, M.; Tourrette, A.; Sparapano, G.; Molvinger, K.; Devoisselle, J.-M.; Gérardin, C. & Quignard, F. (2005). Hierarchical Macroporosity Induced by Constrained Syneresis in Core-Shell Polysaccharide Composites. *Chemistry of Materials,* 17, 4693-4699

Rho, J.Y.; Kuhn-Spearing, L. & Zioupos, P. (1998). Mechanical properties and the hierarchical structure of bone. *Medical Engineering and Physics* 20, 92-102

Schuur, G. (1955). Bemerkungen zu den Untersuchungen Ionotropen Gelen von Polyuronsäuren von H. Thiele und G. Andersen. *Colloid and Polymer Science,* 143, 31-32

Thiele, H. (1947). Richtwirkung von Ionen auf anisotrope Kolloide - Ionotropie. *Naturwissenschaften,* 34, 123

Thiele, H. & Micke, H. (1948). Über Strukturen in ionotropen Gelen. *Colloid and Polymer Science,* 111, 73-79

Thiele, H. & Kienast, G. (1952). Einfluß von Ionen auf die Struktur bei der Gelbildung. *Colloid and Polymer Science,* 127, 134-144

Thiele, H. & Andersen, G. (1953). Modellversuch zum Wachstum der Knochensubstanz. *Naturwissenschaften,* 40, 366-366

Thiele, H. (1954a). Modellversuche zur Synthese mizellarer Strukturen. *Colloid and Polymer Science,* 136, 80-84

Thiele, H. (1954b). Ordered coagulation and gel formation. *Discussions of the Faraday Society,* 18, 294-301

Thiele, H. & Andersen, G. (1955a). Ionotrope Gele von Polyuronsäuren: I. Bildung und Verhalten. *Colloid and Polymer Science,* 140, 76-102

Thiele, H. & Andersen, G. (1955b). Ionotrope Gele von Polyuronsäuren: II Ordnungsgrad. *Colloid and Polymer Science,* 142, 5-24

Thiele, H. & Krönke, H. (1955). Geordnete Kristallisation in ionotropen Gelen. *Naturwissenschaften,* 42, 389-389

Thiele, H. & Hallich, K. (1957). Kapillarstrukturen in ionotropen Gelen. *Colloid and Polymer Science,* 151, 1-12

Thiele, H. & Hallich, K. (1959). Ionotrope Gele mit Kapillarstruktur als Filter. *Colloid and Polymer Science,* 163, 115-122

Thiele, H.; Plohnke, K.; Brandt, E. & Moll, G. (1962). Ordnen von Polyelektrolyten durch Ionendiffusion. *Colloid and Polymer Science,* 182, 24-35

Thiele, H. & Cordes, J. (1967). Zur Theorie der Bildung von Gelen. *Colloid and Polymer Science,* 216/217, 361-370

Thiele, H. (1964). Ordnen von Fadenmolekülen durch Ionendiffusion - ein Prinzip der Strukturbildung. *Protoplasma,* 58, 318-341

Thiele, H.; Joraschky, W.; Plohnke, K.; Wiechen, A.; Wolf, R. & Wollmer, A. (1964). Prinzip einer Strukturbildung Ionen ordnen Fadenmoleküle. *Colloid and Polymer Science,* 197, 26-35

Thiele, H. (1967a). Prinzip einer Strukturbildung. *Naturwissenschaften,* 54, 136-139

Thiele, H. (1967b). *Histolyse und Histogenese: Gewebe und ionotrope Gele - Prinzip einer Strukturbildung.* Akademische Verlagsgesellschaft

Thiele, H. (1967c). Geordnete Kristallisation. Nucleation und Mineralisation. *Journal of Biomedical Materials Research,* 1, 213-238

Thiele, H. & Awad, A. (1969). Nucleation and oriented crystallization apatite in ionotropic gels. *Journal of Biomedical Materials Research,* 3, 431-442

Thumbs, H. & Kohler, H. H. (1996). Capillaries in alginate gels as an example of dissipative structure formation. *Chemical Physics,* 208, 9-24

Treml, H. & Kohler, H. H. (2000). Coupling of diffusion and reaction in the process of capillary formation in alginate gel. *Chemical Physics,* 252, 199-208

Treml, H.; Woelki, S. & Kohler, H. H. (2003). Theory of capillary formation in alginate gels. *Chemical Physics,* 293, 341-353

Weber, K.; Tomandl, G.; Wenger, T. & Heckmann, K. (1997). Preparation of Structured Ceramics for Membrane. *Key Engineering Materials,* 132-136, 1754-1757

Weiner, S. & Wagner, H. D. (1998). The material bone: Structure-mechanical function relations. *Annual Review of Materials Science* 28, 271-298

Wenger, Th. (1998). Herstellung gerichtet-strukturierter Keramiken. Dissertation, University of Regensburg (Germany)

Willenberg, B. J.; Hamazaki, T.; Meng, F. W.; Terada, N. & Batich, C. (2006). Self-assembled copper-capillary alginate gel scaffolds with oligochitosan support embryonic stem cell growth. *Journal of Biomedical Materials Research Part A*, 79A, 440-450

Woelki, S. & Kohler, H. H. (2003). Orientation of chain molecules in ionotropic gels: a Brownian dynamics model. *Chemical Physics*, 293, 323-340

Yamamoto, M.; James, D.; Li, H.; Butler, J.; Rafii, S. & Rabbany, S. Y. (2010). Generation of Stable Co-cultures of Vascular Cells in a Honeycomb Alginate Scaffold. *Tissue Engineering Part A*, 16, 299-308

Zimmermann, H.; Ehrhart, F.; Zimmermann, D.; Müller, K.; Katsen-Globa, A.; Behringer, M.; Feilen, P.; Gessner, P.; Zimmermann, G.; Shirley, S.; Weber, M.; Metze, J. & Zimmermann, U. (2007). Hydrogel-based encapsulation of biological, functional tissue: fundamentals, technologies and applications. *Applied Physics A: Materials Science & Processing*, 89, 909-922

18

Bioinspired and Biomimetic Functional Hybrids as Tools for Regeneration of Orthopedic Interfaces

Gopal Pande, R. Sravanthi and Renu Kapoor
Centre for Cellular and Molecular Biology
Uppal Road Hyderabad 500 007
India

1. Introduction

Multidisciplinary approaches in tissue engineering and nanotechnology have resulted in the availability of new materials whose design and fabrication is inspired by the natural constituents of living organisms. This "bioinspired" approach of designing and manufacturing materials is referred to as biomimetism because materials made by this method exhibit the same structural and functional properties that are seen in naturally occurring biological materials. Thus in general terms, biomimetism or biomimetics as it is also called [Vincent 2003], can be defined as a two way path leading from biology to engineering and back, but in more scientific terms, biomimetic production of materials follows the principles and/or processes of biology to obtain end products that are useful for biological and non biological applications. Some examples of such successfully developed products are: (1) commercially important organic compounds that are made by *in vitro* replication of a specific *in vivo* metabolic pathway e.g. coloring agents - lycopene, β-carotene, and astaxanthin [Dixon 2005, Chemler & Koffas 2008] and anti-cancer drugs - paclitaxel, shikonin, geraniol [Chemler & Koffas 2008; Kolewe et al., 2008] (2) super-hydrophobic and superadhesive glues that are manufactured by imitating processes similar to those seen in the lotus leaf, bee hive, gecko foot and rose petals [Feng & Jiang, 2006; Feng et al., 2003; Nystrom et al., 2006, Nystrom et al., 2010, Lee et al., 2007; Kamino, 2008, Liu et al., 2010] (3) design of anti-fogging and antireflection coatings that are inspired by materials seen in mosquito eyes [Liu et al., 2010]. Along with these successful attempts there are also examples, where the application of biomimetic designing has so far not yielded the desired product. Engineering of Type I collagen is one such case where the natural target molecule exhibits divergent properties in different tissues ranging from the high Young's modulus bearing substance in the matrix of the bone, to being the highly deformable elastomer in tendons, and exhibiting ideal optical properties in the multi-layered corneal tissue but it has not been possible to incorporate all these properties into a biomimetically produced collagen molecule [Weiner & Wagner, 1998, Meek & Fullwood, 2001].

Most strategies in biomimetic material design and manufacturing involve the generation of hierarchical assemblies of multiple components; therefore the bioactive and self healing products that are thus obtained get referred to as "functional hybrids". Although these

products are useful in diverse fields, such as the auto industry, computer logics and the wine industry, their main application is seen in the biomedical field - in particular manufacturing of biomedical devices for orthopedic applications. The design and manufacturing of orthopedic bimimetic implants is meant to replace parts of the hard and weight-bearing bones [Rigo et al., 2004; Chakraborty et al., 2009; Kapoor et al., 2010; Nair et al., 2009; Geary et al., 2008] and replacing soft orthopedic tissue [Balasundaram & Webster, 2007]. Further improvements in the implant's properties, which could include the incorporation of bioactive molecules such as long chain proteins or short peptide sequences [Chakraborty et al., 2009; Kapoor et al., 2010; Balasundaram & Webster, 2007; Keselowsky et al., 2005; Le et al., 2006; Stevens et al., 2008; Sato &Webster, 2004], are necessary to make them more acceptable by the cells at the site and thus ensure their long term success. This is an ongoing process and several new developments have taken in this field in recent years.
In this chapter we have focused on the anatomical organization of the orthopedic interfaces which are mimicked for tissue engineering applications and we have addressed some challenges that need to be met in the design and manufacturing of materials that can be used more effectively to replace damaged, malformed or diseased orthopedic tissue.

2.0 Normal bone anatomy and functions:

In order to efficiently biomimic the structure and function of bone components it is necessary to know the chemical biology and structural organization of the bone and its parts. Since the bone tissue contains uniquely large amounts of inorganic constituents along with the organic material, hence the details of how these two parts are biologically synthesized and combined are very important to be understood before efficient substitutes for them can be designed and manufactured.

2.1 Gross anatomy of the human bones

The simplest classification of the human bone subtypes is shown in Figure 1. It is interesting to note that a significant amount of tissue engineering work on making orthopedic devices has concentrated on the components of the long bones i.e. the 4 limbs of the appendicular skeleton. The internal organization and structure of the axial bones is much more complex than the tubular and cuboidal bones of the appendicular skeleton although the basic constituents of both types of bones are similar. Perhaps it is for this reason that the availability of biomimetically produced tissue engineered orthopedic products is significantly more for the appendicular bone parts than for the axial bone components with the possible exception of products related to teeth and intervertebral discs of the spine.
Each long bone can be divided into three regions, namely the epiphysis, the metaphysis and the diaphysis (Figure 2). The epiphyses make the two rounded ends of the long bone which is supported underneath by the metaphysic layer. In adult bones the two layers encapsulate the growth plate or physis itself which is the main generator of osteogenic cells during the developmental phase. Both the metaphysis and epiphysis are composed of a soft trabecular (spongy) bone that is surrounded by a relatively thin shell of hard cortical bone. The diaphysis which is the hollow cylindrical shaft of the bone is made up of the dense cortical hard bone that surrounds the softer bone marrow area. The main length of the diaphysial hard bone area is lined by two thin connective tissue layers - the periosteum on the outside and endosteum on the inside. Most of the hard region of the bone which makes up the bone

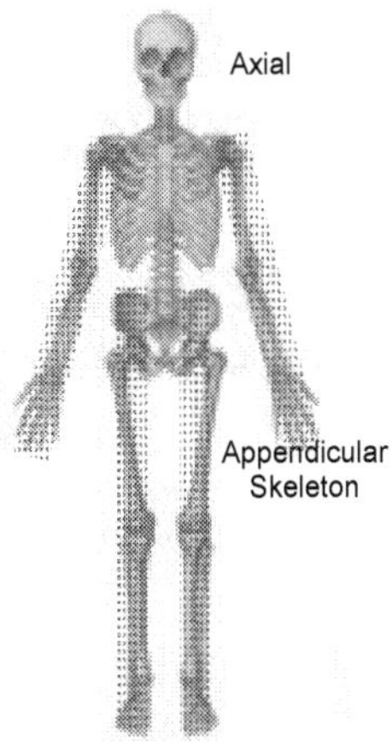

Fig. 1. Classification of bones in the human skeletal system into axial skeleton (yellow color) and appendicular skeleton (green shaded areas). All the long (tubular) bones. e.g. femur, humerus, and short (cuboidal) bones e.g. carpals, tarsals etc. are in the appendicular skeleton whereas the flat and irregular bones e.g. the vertebrae, the maxillofacial bones, bones of the skull etc. constitute the axial skeleton.

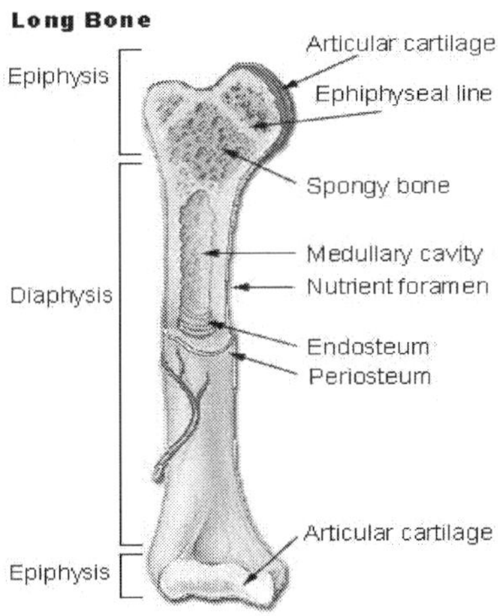

Fig. 2. The gross structure of a long appendicular bone. The epi-physeal regions at the two ends of the bone comprise the softer part of the bone whereas diaphysis constitutes the hard part. The hard of the bone lies in the cortical region and it surrounds a softer part in the medullary region. The medullary region is lined by a membrane supported endosteal layer which acts like a stem cell generating niche. It also acts as the site to produce osteoclast cells which are main cells that take part in bone resorbtion. The periosteum lies as the outer covering the entire bone and is the site of osteoblasts and osteocytes to the cortical bone mass.

mass and is responsible for its rigidity and load bearing capacity lies between these layers; it undergoes the maximum mineralization and therefore it contains the maximum inorganic content in the entire skeletal system. Due to their proximity with the bonemass the periosteum and the endosteum make up the two distinct orthopedic interfaces in long bones. They respectively play key roles in the formation and degeneration of the bone tissue. The cellular and biochemical organization of these two orthopedic interfaces along with the large mass of mineralised bone tissue that lies between them are the main targets of biomimetic designing and manufacturing products for the human skeletal system.

Structurally the periosteum is a vascularised membranous layer that covers the entire outer surface of all bones and functionally it acts as the regenerative orthopedic interface for the entire diaphysial region of the bone,. Externally it combines with the fibers and ligaments of the skeletal muscles and internally it provides attachment to the flattened osteoprogenitor cells which divide by mitosis and differentiate into osteoblasts and then osteocytes. The existence of the periosteum is essential for the regeneration of the bone after trauma injury. The endosteum, which makes the degenerative interface of the bonemass, lines the inner side of the mineralized cortical bone and has two surfaces - one which faces the outer mineralized side of the bone mass and another which faces the inner non mineralized sinusoidal bone marrow. The inner surface of endosteum makes several endosteal niches which harbor multipotent stem cells that generate hematopoietic, muscular, adipose and mesenchymal cell precursors in the marrow region. The outer surface of endosteum acts as the site for producing differentiated osteoclast cells that migrate into the mineralized bone matrix, between the periosteum and endosteum, and participate in its breakdown. Osteoclasts also remove the dead osteocytes that lie embedded in the matrix. The endosteum thus plays a key role in the bone remodeling by actively assisting the bone resorption process through osteoclasts.

2.2 Histological and biochemical organization

In general the bone tissue exhibits a unique histological organization, it exhibits the general properties of vertebrate connective tissues, but its matrix is uniquely dense, semi-rigid, porous and highly calcified because it is made up of an organic matrix and an inorganic mineral component. In a typical appendicular bone the matrix is composed of approximately 30-35% organic and 65-70% inorganic components. The organic component is called the osteoid which is composed of type I collagen and ground substances like glycoproteins, proteoglycans, peptides, carbohydrates and lipids. Mineralization of the osteoid, which can occur by several methods (see Section 3) constitutes the inorganic components of the bone and these constituents include calcium phosphate- hydroxyapatite $Ca_{10}(PO_4)_6(OH)_2$ and calcium carbonate along with similar salts of magnesium, fluoride and sodium in lesser quantity [Clarke 2008; Kalfas 2001].

The cellular component of bone tissue comprises three main cell types: osteoblasts, osteocytes and the osteoclasts. As mentioned above osteoblasts line the periosteal layer and they are cuboidal to flat in shape. They secrete the unmineralized organic matrix which later mineralizes and leads to increase in organic component of bone matrix. Osteoblasts, as they migrate into the matrix or line the canaliculi the thin cylindrical spaces or canals seen in the bone mass, differentiate into osteocytes, which possess long thin cytoplasmic processes called the filopodia. The osteocyte lined canaliculi help in the passage of nutrients and oxygen between the blood vessels and matrix localized osteocytes. Osteocytes also break down the bone matrix by osteocytic osteolysis to release calcium for calcium homeostasis.

They also maintain extracellular phosphorus concentration. The third main category of cells in the bone mass are the osteoclasts. These are bone resorbing cells which are multinucleated and carry out the process of bone resorption. They are generated from the shallow depressions on the inner side of the endosteum called howship lacunae. A schematic representation of the cellular and inorganic organization of the bone mass is seen in Figure 3 below.

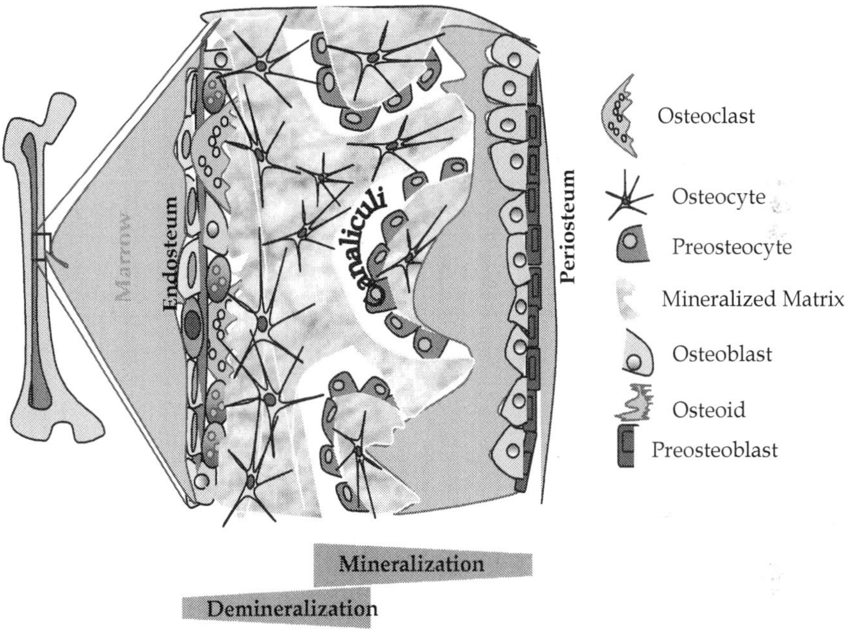

Fig. 3. A figurative description of the cellular organization in two orthopedic interfaces the periosteum and the endosteum that surround the bone matrix in the hard cortical bone.

3. Biomimicry of bone components

The capacity of bone tissue components, both cellular and inorganic, to self-regenerate, particularly after trauma related injuries, has attracted the interest of many scientists [Alves et al., 2010]. During this regeneration process, we observe the recreation of mineral rich tissues of different constitutions and hence this process is also referred to as biomineralization [Palmer, 2008]. Studying the process of biomineralization helps us in understanding the mechanisms by which living organisms deposit mineralized crystals within matrix [Sarikaya, 1999]. Among the approximately 40 different constituents found in the naturally formed biominerals, carbonates, phosphates and silicates of calcium are the most common [Stephen, 1988]. These salts have a significant role to play in determining the physiochemical properties and thermal stability in hard bone tissue [Sarikaya, 1999; Cai & Tang, 2009].

In general terms, biomineralization process can be either biologically induced or biologically controlled. In biologically induced mineralization (BIM) the shape and organization of the crystals is not directly under cellular control and it is determined entirely by inorganic processes. As a result of this the shape and organization of the inorganic compounds made by BIM is of a low order. In contrast to this biologically controlled mineralization (BCM) is cell dependent and it shows a well balanced organization of the mineralizing salts with the organic molecules resulting in well defined crystals of uniform shape, size and orientation [Khaner, 2007; Weiner & Addadi, 1997]. During post trauma osteo-regeneration both types of biomineralization processes are observed however the involvement of BCM is more dominant. Features common to bone mineralization are also seen in the biomineralization of many non skeletal tissues and cells and an examination of those properties helps in understanding the mechanism behind skeletal tissue mineralization.

3.1 Non-skeletal biomineralization

The biomineralization process in non skeletal cells and tissues generates very complex, diverse and interesting mineral forms and this process can be observed in almost in all organisms [Ozawa & Hoshki 2008; Veiss, 2005]. An evolutionary break through about this process was achieved in a report on the formation of magnetites in magnetotactic bacteria which indicated the commonality of biomineralization mechanisms in different biological forms and it also highlighted that this process is regulated by highly complex control systems that are operational even in simple organisms. Several examples of non skeletal biomineralization in multicellular organisms are observed in nature along with the more common unicellular mineral producers. Some of these include silica spicule producing sponges, diatoms and actinopoda; synthesis of amorphous calcium carbonate in ascidians and formation of layered aragonite platelets in the nacreous layer of mollusk shells,few of such examples has been shown in Figure 4 below. [Sarikaya, 1999].

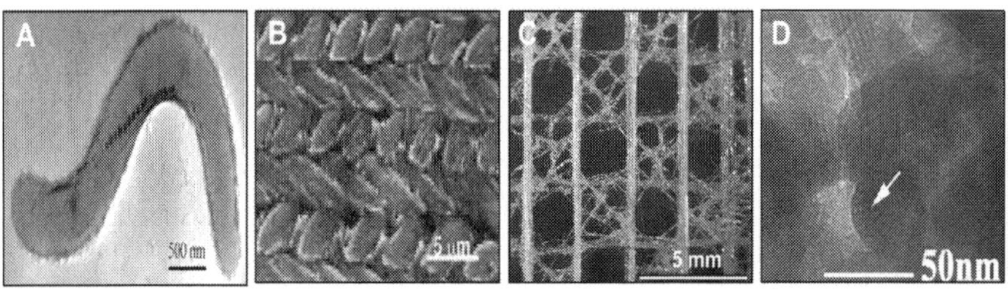

Fig. 4. Biologically controlled mineralization of hierarchical structures observed in A) magnetospirullum magnetium bacteria B) TEM of organic lattice of nacreous shell found in atrina C) finely organized enamel rod structures of mouse tooth D) ordered structures in siliceous skeleton lattice.[Atsushi et al., 2008; Yael et al.,2001;Sarikaya, 1999; James et al., 2007]

3.2 Biomineralization in skeletal tissue

As indicated above, the biomineralization process in the bone tissue is different from what is exhibited by nonskeletal cells and tissues, because in skeletal cells it is primarily cell dependent i.e. it is controlled by BCM mechanisms. At the sub-cellular level biomineralization in bones is mediated by the formation of matrix vesicles (MV) which are membrane encased vesicles of size 20-200nm that are formed by a special exocytic membrane budding process in polarized and differentiatiating osteoblasts/osteocytes of the long bones and also in the hypertrophic chondrocytes of the cartilage and odontoblasts of the growing teeth [Anderson, 2003]. After being secreted out of the cell, the MVs begin to deposit calcium phosphate/apatite crystals within the lumen of the vesicle itself or are specifically transported through the vesicular membrane into the matrix and they mineralize in conjunction with matrix collagen [Ciancaglini, 2006]. This process can thus be divided into 2 phases - in phase I intra-luminal deposition of amorphous calcium phosphate, octa-calcium phosphates and HAp crystals is seen and in phase II seepage of HAp crystals occurs through the MV membrane into extracellular fluid resulting in nucleation of the crystals within collagen fibrils as calcified nodules [Guido & Isabelle, 2004; Kazuhiko et al, 2009]. Type-1 collagen acts as a template for initiating the crystallization of secreted calcium hydroxyapatite crystals [Vincet, 2008] which subsequently gets associated with other ECM components such as proteins, polysaccharides, proteolipids and proteoglycans to support activities such as cell adhesion, transport of ionic molecules, cell signaling etc. Understanding the steps of matrix biomineralization and its degeneration is therefore necessary in order to develop synthetic analogs that would mimic the matrix components that aid in the regeneration of new tissue [Joshua et al., 2009; Alves et al., 2010; Veiss, 2005].

3.3 Steps in bone modeling and remodeling

As mentioned earlier and shown in Figure 3 the process of bone modeling and remodeling is a homeostatic process where the bone formation and resorption processes are observed simultaneously. The two processes are regulated by independent but related controls but since basic steps are very different from one another they need to be understood sperately in order to design materials to replace this integral component of the bone tissue.

3.3.1 Bone modeling

As mentioned above the bone modeling process in long bones is dependent mainly upon the calcification of the collagenous matrix of the bone mass. This process of physiological mineralization of collagen is controlled by the balance of enzymes, such as metalloproteinases, transporters, such as type III Na/Pi co-transporter, and channels, such as the annexin channels, which together aid to efficiently export the mineralizing molecules from the MVs into the matrix. In a recent study, using proteo-liposomal vesicles, it has been shown how to reconstruct a model that would mimic the MV microenvironment and would help us in better understanding the MV microenvironment [Simao et al., 2010]. In addition to the MV associated enzymes, transporters and channels some other molecules in the matrix such as tissue nonspecific alkaline phosphatase (TNAP), the group of docking proteins ankyrins and nucleotide associated inorganic phosphate, that influence the transport of MV pyrophosphate into the matrix and thereby regulate its calcification [Ellis, 2009, Robert, 2001]. These matrix associated molecules exert their effects by directly controlling the amount of free inorganic phosphate in the ECM which in turns determines the transport PPi from the MVs [Ellis, 2009]. The effective role of matrix associated TNAP in controlling vesicle mineralization is highlighted in a disease named hypophosphatasia where TNAP activity is decreased because of a mutation in this gene the mobility of PPi from MVs to the matrix is very high [Robert, 2001]. Mineralization initiation in matrix vesicles is a function of several inhibitors, promoters that needs a proper balance between the elements that maintain them.

In addition to Type I collagen there are some other proteins in the matrix that also associate with the mineralized collagen and then further enhance or inhibit the mineralization process. Some of these proteins observed in bones and teeth are shown in Table 1. Osteopontin[OPN] and Bone Sialoprotein[BSP] are acidic proteins with high affinity for Ca^{2+} ions are localized within the collageneous matrix found adjacent to mineralization front that are involved in determining calcification. BSP are found to be initiator of mineralization whereas OPN affinity for apatite crystal founds to inhibit the crystal maturation process [Hunter et al ., 1996; Bernards et al., 2008].

Bone	Dentin	Enamel
Osteocalcin (OC)	dentin matrix protein 1	Enamelin
Osteopontin (OPN)	dentin sialo-phospho protein	Matrix extracellular phospho-glycoprotein (MEPE)
Osteonectin (ON)	-	-
Bone sialoprotein (BSP)	-	-

Table 1. Major non-collageneous proteins that associate with mineralized ECM in different bone tissues

3.3.2 Bone remodeling

In contrast to the matrix modeling process the remodeling of the mineralized matrix is more complex because it can be controlled by many different mechanisms. In the case of normal bone homeostasis we observe a balance between the calcification and decalcification reactions in the bone matrix where the decalcification of the matrix is facilitated by the removal of the dead osteocytes and discharged MVs from the matrix. This process is primarily carried out by osteoclasts which arise from the endosteum. However, the decalcification process can be disturbed due to several reasons which could be either related to blockages or total stoppage of the calcification process or due to pathological changes in the tissue such as migration of cancer metastatic cells, activation of osteoporotic reactions etc.

The modeling and remodeling of the matrix thus represent the two orthopedic interfaces of the bone which are generated at periosteum and endosteum respectively and their mineralizing and de-mineralizing functions overlap in the matrix as shown in Figure 3.

4. Materials and methods for the mimicry of bone components

Based upon the details of the natural processes that lead to mineralized bone formation and its degradation, as described above, there are several reports in the literature that describe strategies to generate materials *in vitro* that are similar to the *in vivo* physicochemical and/or biological properties of the bone components. In fact bone biomimetism remains as one of the most actively pursued and financially a very rewarding area of human tissue engineering. A brief summary describing the different types of materials and processes that are currently in use to generate bone like materials, for their use as bone implants or substitutes, is provided here.

4.1 Materials useful as substrates or modifiers in bone implants and/or bone substitutes

The choice of materials that can be used to repair or replace a damaged or deformed bone is very wide. An overriding factor in choosing a base material for this purpose is its bioactivity and biocompatibility *in vivo*.

Materials	References
Metals	
Stainless steel AISI 316L, Co-Cr-Mo alloy	Yeung et al.,2007; Aksakal et al., 2008; Seligson et al.,1997; Marti 2000
Ti and its alloys	
Ti6Al4V, TNZT alloys (Ti-Nb-Zr-Ta), Ni Ti, TiNbZr	Aksakal et al., 2008; Chakraborty et al., 2009; Yeung et al.,2007; Banerjee et al., 2004; Banerjee et al., 2006; Niinomi 2003; Ning et al., 2010; Seligson et al.,1997
Ceramics and Bioglass	
α-Al_2O_3, high alumina ceramics, PSZ (partially stabilized zirconia), 45S5 BG, S45P7	Kapoor et al., 2010; Christel et al., 1988; Gorustovich et al., 2010; Yuan et al., 2001
Polymers	
Polyethylene (PE), Polymethacrylic acid (PM MA), polyglycolic acid (PGA), poly lactic acid (PLA), polycarbonate (PC), polypropylene(PP)	Andersson et al., 2004; Reis et al., 2010; Oral et al., 2007; Butler et al., 2001; Athanasiou et al., 1998; Smith et al.,2007; Geary et al., 2008; Shalumon et al., 2009; Jayabalan et al., 2001
Composites	
Mg-Zn-Zr, HA-PEEK poly (aryl-ether-ether-ketone), Polyphospha zenes, BG-COL-HYA-PS (glass-collagen hyaluronic acid-phosphatidylserine)	Ye et al.,2010; Kurtz et al., 2007; Sethuraman et al., 2010; Xu et al., 2010

Table 2. A list of materials in use as base/substrate material in bone implants

Since there is no material available that can per se become a bone substitute, several modifications on the original material are required to make it biocompatible. The aim to do these modifications is that the new material should be nontoxic and biologically inert but yet it should show orthopedic bioactivity and its production should be cost effective. The biocompatibility of the material is also dependent upon certain host factors such as general health, age, tissue perfusion and immunological factors [Wooley et al., 2001] and therefore only certain types of materials have been used so far for this purpose. A list of such materials currently in use is given in Table 2.

Each of the listed materials in the Table has some unique quality that qualifies it to be used as the base material or the substrate of an orthopedic implant. Cationic metals for example can form ionic bonds with non-metals and can be easily converted into alloys which have good ductile properties and heavy load bearing strength. Among the nonmetals, ceramics are interesting because their inter-atomic bonds are either totally ionic or predominantly ionic and they can be covalently bonded to a number of compounds including proteins. Among the polymers for orthopedic use, plastics and elastomers have been the main choice but because of their limited weight bearing capacities their use is restricted. The composites are useful because they can combine the properties of two or more compounds making it a more versatile material to get a functional hierarchy of substances needed to make a bone like substance.

Besides the substances which are used as substrates for making biocompatible materials, there are many other unique elements of bone structure which lend themselves to be mimicked by manmade materials as functionalizing compounds of the substrates. One of the most commonly mimicked biomaterial for this purpose is apatite which is the most abundant phosphate mineral on earth found in mineralizing vertebrates. Among all the calcium phosphate minerals available hydroxyapatite (HAp) is found to be the most thermodynamically stable bioceramic material at physiological environment which helps in faster osteointegration. Hence the most sought after properties that material scientists and bone tissue engineers look for in their apatite are bone bonding ability and osteo-conductivity in addition to their general biocompatibility and bioactivity. The starting compounds used for making HAp is generally calcium phosphate and based on some solution parameters like super saturation, other ionic products and pH we can get many other apatite phases apart from HAp. These non-naturally occurring apatite phases can be more useful than naturally occurring ones.

MINERAL NAME	Ca/P ratio	Abbreviation
Monocalcium phosphate monohydrate	0.5	MCPM
Monocalcium phosphate:dihydrate	0.5	MCPD
Dicalcium phosphate: dehydrate mineral brushite	1.0	(DCPD)
Anhydride mineral monetite	1.0	(DCPA)
Octacalcium phosphate	1.33	(OCP)
α-tricalcium phosphate	1.5	(αTCP)
β-tricalcium phosphate	1.5	(β-TCP)
Whitelock mineral	1.29	
Hydroxyapatite O- HAp	1.67	OHAp
Calcium-deficient hydroxyapatite	1.5-1.67	(CDHA)
Fluorapatite	1.67	(FAp)
Chloroapatite	1.67	(ClAp)
Carbonated apatite TYPE A	1.67	(CO3Ap)
Tetracalcium phosphate, mineral hilgenstokite	2.0	(TTKP or tetcp)

Table 3. Different types of calcium phosphates obtained during preparation of HAp

A list of the various types of apatite phase that can be obtained from different calcium phosphates is given in Table3. Besides using calcium phosphate, a combination of various salts is also used to generate HAp. This process is more close to the natural process because the constituents of starting material are based upon the constituents of the natural body fluid such as blood plasma. The solution that most represents the similarity with blood plasma is referred to as simulated body fluid or SBF and its many constituents have been described elsewhere Tadashi and Hiroaki 2006 and Jalota et al 2006.

		Na^+	K^+	Ca^{2+}	Mg^{2+}	$HCO3^-$	Cl^-	$HPO4^{2-}$	$SO4^{2-}$	Ca/P	Ph
Blood Plasma		142	5	2.5	1.5	27	103	1	0.5	2.5	7.4
SBF Range		127-734	5-10	2.5-12.5	1.5-7.5	4.2-35	111-724	1-5	0.05-1	0-2.5	7.25-7.4
TYPE-1		142	5	2.5	1.5	4.2	148	1.8	----	1.4	7.25
TYPE-2		142	5	2.5	1.5	27	147.8	1	0.5	2.5	7.4
TYPE-3	**c-SBF2 c-SBF3 SBF-JL1 SBF-JL2**	142 142 142 142	5 5 ---	2.5 2.5 2.5 -	1.5 1.5 - -	4.2 35.23 34.9 34.88	147.96 117.62 111 109.9	1 1 1 1.39	0.5 0.5 - -	2.5 2.5 2.5 0	7.4
TYPE-4	**SBF d-SBF**	142 142	5 5	2.5 1.6	1.5 0.7	4. 2 4.2	147.8 144.1	1 1	0.5 0.5	2.5 1.6	7.25 7.25
TYPE-5		142	5	2.5	1.5	4.2	148	1	0.5	2.5	7.4
TYPE-6	**SBF 5XSBF**	142 714.8	5 ----	2.5 12.5	1.5 7.5	4.2 21	147.8 723.8	1 5	0.5 ----	2.5 2.5	7.4 7.6
TYPE-7		127	10	12.5	3	35	123	5	----	2.5	7.4
TYPE-8		142	5	2.5	1.5	4.2	147.8	1	0.05	2.5	7.4
TYPE-9	**SBF-1 5XSBF SBF-2**	142 213 142	5 7.5 5	2.5 3.8 2.5	1.5 2.3 1.5	4.2 6.3 4.2	148 223 148.8	1 1.5 1	0.5 0.75 0.5	2.5 2.53 2.5	7.4
TYPE 10	**SBF-a SBF-b**	714.8 704.2	---- ----	12.5 12.5	7.5 1.5	21 10.5	723.8 711.8	5 5	- -	2.5 2.5	7.4
TYPE-11		142	5	2.5	1.5	4.2	148.8	1	0.5	2.5	7.4
TYPE-12		142	5	2.05	1.5	4.2	148	1		2.05	7.4
TYPE-13		142	5	2.5	1.5	4.2	148.5	1	0.5	2.5	7.4
TYPE-14	**1XSBF 3CaP SBF**	142 109.5	5 6	2.5 7.5	1.5 1.5	4.2 17.5	147.8 110	1 3	0.5 -	2.5 2.5	7.5
TYPE-15	**SBF(N) SBF(O)**	142 142	5 5	2.5 2.5	1.5 -	27 -	123 123	1 1	0.5 0.5	2.5 2.5	7.2
TYPE-16		109.5	6	7.5	1.5	17.5	110	3	0		6.65-6.71 6.55-6.65 6.24-6.42

Table 4. Recipes for making different types of Simulated Body Fluids for biomimetic preparation of Apatite
[Reference for the above Table are a-Liu et al.,1998; b-Kokubo & Kim, 2004; c-Marc & Jacques,2009; d-Chikara et al., 2007; e-Kokubo,1996; f-Bharati et al.,2005; g-Qu & Mei,2008; h-De Medeiros et al., 2008; i-Tsai et al.,2008; j-Habibovic et al.,2002; k-Hyun et al.,1996; l-Silvia et al.,2006; m-Xin et al.,2007; n-Yajing et al.,2009; o-Kapoor et al.,2010; p-Haibo & Mei 2008]

Over the years the constitution of SBF has undergone so many modifications that would be compiled into a list of different SBFs that can used to obtain bone like apatite for bone remodeling purposes. This compilation is shown in Table 4. The original SBF was intended to study mainly the bone-bonding ability of the apatite and it lacked in sulfate ions in relation to original plasma constituents. The SBF constitution was later upgraded with major variations done in chlorine and bicarbonate compositions and to a lesser extent in sulphate ions. SBF with higher Cl^- and lower HCO3- concentrations and variations in buffer systems and pH are found to be in equilibrium with the blood plasma. The physiological pH is maintained in this in vitro system using tris (hydroxymethyl) amino methane (Tris)/HCl.

4.2 Methods for preparing substrates and modifier materials

While the base substrate materials are prepared by conventional metallurgical methods, their bioactivity is induced by functionalizing them with many modifier materials. The modifier materials include proteins, enzymes and most importantly the different types of apatites. There is an endless list of techniques by which apatite deposition can be carried out on orthopedically selected substrates, but the successful methods are those which give high bone bonding ability and good osseointegration. Among the different available techniques, plasma spray, sol-gel synthesis and biomimetic methods are the most successful. Some salient features of the first two and details of the biomimetic approaches are provided here.

4.2.1 Plasma spray

Plasma spray coatings on to metal substrates have gained interest during the past decades due to its high deposition rate and its large scale efficiency. This method is compatible with various platforms including ceramic composites apart from metals. Numerous studies have been carried out on the bone bonding behavior of these coatings with the substrates. The thickness of the coating is of few microns size. The precursor is mainly fed in the form of powder which is released into a plasma gun. A high voltage argon gas generates plasma where the powder gets partly melted and is directed towards the substrate followed by rapid cooling further impelling the substrate thus depositing a coat. This method has been used to deposit different functionalized materials on either metal or non-metal surfaces. [Chen et al., 2008; Chen et al., 2006; Culha et al., 2010]

But the major concerns regarding this process a) is the instability of the coatings therefore poor binding of the coating with the substrate or implant .This necessitates them for further processing to increase the mechanical interlocking of the coating-substrate system. b) High processing temperatures involved lead to changes in CaP phases resulting in the formation of less stable phases thereby reducing the bonding strength between the substrate and the coating. c) These coatings are largely amorphous with less homogeneity over the entire substrate resulting in structures of low crystallinity which signifies that the substrates are not bioactive enough to induce the required bone attachment. Many functionalized scaffolds have been developed by this technique and there biocompatibility was checked *in-vivo* so that these implants can be used for various orthopedic applications [Heimann et al., 2004; Wu et al., 2009]

4.2.2 Sol-gel synthesis

This technique is one of the oldest in developing thin film coating having varied applications like protective coatings, passivation layers, sensors and membranes. The methodology involves the fabrication of materials by using a chemical solution (sol) which acts as the precursor for a specialized integrated network (gel) of either particles or network oligomers/polymers. The unique property of this method is that the kinetics of the reaction can be controlled by monitoring the particle size, porosity and thickness of coating. Hence the fabricated materials can be obtained in the form of films, powders, fibers, processed at a lower temperature which differentiates it form the conventional processing strategies [Podbielska and Ulatowska-arza 2005].

The starting materials used are inorganic or metal-organic precursors (alkoxides). The chemistry of this process involves basically two reactions like hydrolysis and polycondensation. When metal- alkoxides are used the alkoxide is dissolved in alcohol and hydrolyzed by the addition of water, whereas in case of metalloids, acid or base catalyst is added which replaces the alkoxide ligands with hydroxyl groups. In case of inorganic precursors like salts, hydrolysis proceeds by the removal of a proton to form a hydroxo (-OH) or oxo (=O) ligand. Therefore subsequent condensation reactions in case or organic and inorganic produces oligomers or polymers composed of M-O-M or M-μ(OH)-M bonds.

The coating is generally done by depositing the precursor on to the substrate either by dip coating or spin coating, later the samples are dried at high temperature which results in shrinkage and also increases the density of the deposited precursors. The coating thickness is a function of withdrawal speed, concentration and viscosity of the solution hence the porosity of the gel is dependent on the rate at which the solvent is removed. The simplicity of this procedure develops uniform coatings of high homogeneity [Klein, 1988].Many biocompatible, bioactive and stable metals/non-metals and bioglass scaffolds are deveopled by this technique by depositing HAp, various bioactive proteins in the form of thin films and nanoparticles[Weng et al., 2003; Wang etal.,2008; Vijayalakshmi et al.,2008] for hard and soft tissue replacement[Kim et al.,2005; Nguyen et al.,2004; Sepulveda et al.,2002; Zheng et al.,2009].

4.2.3 Biomimetic process

Since the theory of biomimetic process proposed by Kokubo, the study of bioactivity using SBF has been reviewed by many research groups all these years. Why these studies are at a faster pace and what makes this process so challenging from other technologies in predicting bone bioactivity *in vivo*. This process aims at mimicking the blood plasma compositions in acellular conditions using SBF [Tadashi & Hiroaki, 2006]. For natural bone to bond with the implants there must be specific appropriate response which it feels that it can be accepted, is mainly achieved by depositing apatite on to these surfaces termed as bioactivity/bone-bonding ability. Bones ability to deposit calcium phosphate defines its characteristic property as a hard connective tissue. Several results have been obtained using this procedure and they have been summarized in Table 6.

Bio-mimetic Coating Method used to Functionalize Ti-6Al-4V and α-Al_2O_3

Our lab is also developing functionalized scaffolds which can be in long run used for bone engineering applications.

We are working with metal (Ti and its alloys like (Ti-6Al-4V, TiZr, and TiNb), non-metals (Ceramic like α-Al_2O_3) and glass, functionalizing them in order to check the cell behavior *in vitro* and also check there bio-compatibility properties *in vivo*.

There are many methods to functionalize the metal/non-metal surface by using HAp/calcium phosphate which can be done by various methods like plasma spray method, sol-gel coating method, dip coating methods but the most easy and efficient way to mimic the natural component of bone is by Biomimetic coating method, hence we have utilized this process to develop an even, functionalized HAp coating on a titanium alloy (Ti-6Al-4V) and

Cell culture studies and materials used	Objectives	Results	References
Apatite and apatite/ collagen composite coatings on PLLA using Saos-2 osteoblast like cells	Cell attachment, proliferation and differentiation	Biomimetic apatite/collagen coating found to exhibit higher proliferation and differentiation in comparison to apatite coatings	Chen et al., 2008
Biomimetic and electrolyti -cally deposited carbonate apatite on Ti alloy using MC3T3-E1 cells.	Cellular proliferation and differentiation	Higher proliferation and OC and BSP mRNA expression on biomimetically coated substrates than electrolytically deposited method.	Jiawei et al., 2009
Chemically pretreated CP Ti immersed in SBF for 2 and 14 days and tested using human osteoblasts (MG-63) cells.	Cell spreading, proliferation and differentiation	A well spread morphology was observed both functionalized surfaces. TiCT and TiHCA surfaces rendered increased expression of collagen 1 and ALP at 7 and 14 days.	Barbara et al ., 2008
HA deposition on negatively charged SAM coated glass cover slips by culturing human mature OC of bone cell tumor for 24hrs	Osteoclastic activity through F-Actin ring formation, calcium release and formation of resorption pits	Osteoclast were able to attach and resorb on coated glass cover slips	Asiri et al., 2009
Biomimetic apatite deposition on hyaluronic acid (HA)-based polymer scaffold	Osteogenic induction of mesenchymal stromal cells (h-MSCs)	At higher mineralization on HA-based scaffold.	Cristina et al ., 2010
Incorporation of bisphosph -onate sodium clondrate into biomimetically coated apatite on to starch based scaffold using human osteoblast-like cell line (SaOs-2)	Effect of BP on osteoclastic activity and cell morphology, attachment and proliferation	Osteoblastic activity was simulated with bisphopshonates at dose dependent concentration of 0.32mg/ml by enhanced cell viability	Oliveira et al., 2010
BMP-2 into biomimetic apatite coatings using Rat bone marrow stromal cells for 8days on Ti implants	Osteogenic activity	Protein incorporated CaP coatings enhanced the alkaline phophatase activity	Yuelian et al., 2004

Table 6. Cellular responses to biomimetically prepared substrates and coatings

on a bioinert ceramic substrate (α-Al_2O_3). In our method, the metal / ceramic substrates were incubated in simulated body fluid (SBF) at 25°C for different time points with prior treatment with globular protein BSA (bovine serum albumin) [Chakraborty et al., 2009; Kapoor et al., 2010]. This process leads to the formation of HAp coating exhibiting bone like apatite growth on the surface. It may further be noted that bone, a natural composite comprises non stoichiometric calcium hydroxyapatite (HAp) precipitated in a controlled reaction environment of a highly aligned, anisotropic organic template. It differs from stoichiometric hydroxyapatite (HA) in composition, crystallinity and other physical and mechanical properties developed artificially through various methods.

The surface treatment and coating of these materials had shown a better cellular response *in vitro* and also a good biocompatibility property *in vivo* when compared with untreated and uncoated materials. The surface treatment by globular protein i.e., BSA might provide a functionalized template comprising of charged amino-acids which resulted in more nucleation sites [Chakraborty et al., 2009] hence led to the even coverage of HAp (about 280-300μm) by immersion of the materials in SBF at desired temperature of 25°C between the pH range of 5-7, which resulted in the formation 30-40 nm albumin globules, under specified conditions, on both ceramic and Ti-6Al-4V alloy substrates. In comparison with the untreated substrates the coverage of HAp was very much poor(less than 200μm), hence BSA treatment has led to the development of nano-sized globules after HAp coating which have led to the better cellular-activity *in-vitro* which is due to "cooperativity" reaction [Chakraborty et al., 2009] between protein molecules and the charged surface of HAp, depending on the concentration of the protein molecules in the coating [SBF] solutions.

We have done a comparative study of biological properties of the unique coating of HAp developed on both metal and non-metal which is less reported. Based on the methodology of functionalizing these materials we have generated many substrates of Ti and Ceramic which showed a different structural variation and these specific morphological structures of protein and HAp has led to good fibroblast [NIH-3T3] cell response. The Ti-6Al-4V which is BSA treated and coated for 4 days has shown a nano-sized globules (as indicated by arrows) due to globular protein treatment has shown a better *in-vitro* and *in-vivo* activity which can be seen in Figure 1 panel c in comparison with the bare Ti-6Al-4V panel a, BSA treated Ti-6Al-4V panel b and coated Ti-6Al-4V for 4 days without prior treatment with BSA panel d which did not show nano-sized HAp globules.

The unique structural property of HAp coating on Ti-6Al-4V treated with BSA and coated for 4 days is shown in Figure 2 where panel a shows the inter and intra connection of HAp fibers into plates which can be seen in higher magnification in panel b. Panel c shows the femur bone like growth of HAp fibers [Kapoor et al., 2010] which represents the unique methodology in mimicking the bone like components by generating a highly functionalized scaffold for *in-vivo* applications.

On the contrary, micron sized globules of HAp [Figure. 3(c)] were observed on the BSA treated and coated for 2days ceramic substrate surface. This may be attributed to the enhanced hydrophilicity of the BSA treated ceramic substrate (it already has intrinsic hydrophilicity) that accumulates -OH groups throughout the mechanically roughened (grit blasted) surface, on immersion in simulated body fluid (SBF), aqueous medium. These act as nucleation sites and induce Ca^{2+} ions from SBF to be coordinated to the above -OH groups on the substrate, by electrostatic force of attraction. Hence nucleation of a large number of HAp globules takes place and they grow fast into micron sized globules owing to the high surface energy as mentioned, resulting in a dense coverage of substrate surface. Hence due to large deposition of micron-sized HAp globules the NIH-3T3 cellular response was much better on this ceramic substrate in comparison to the bare ceramic (panel a), BSA treated ceramic(panel b) and untreated and coated for 2 days panel d which showed a much bigger HAp deposition.

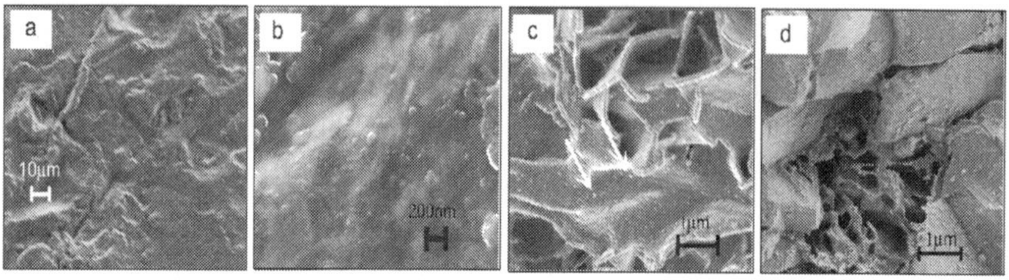

Fig. 4. SEM images of different Ti-6Al-4V where (a)Bare Ti-6Al-4V (b)BSA Treated Ti-6Al-4V (c)BSA Treated and Coated for 4 days Ti-6Al-4V (d) Coated for 4 days Ti-6Al-4V.(Image generated from Kapoor et al., 2010).

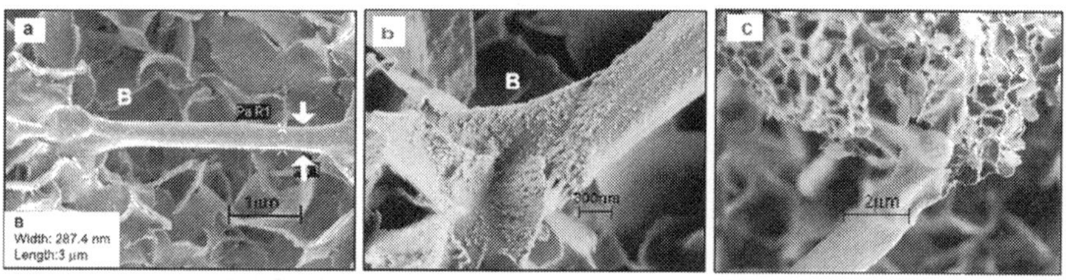

Fig. 5. SEM Images of Ti-6Al-4V substrate which is BSA treated and coated for 4 days where (a) Inter- and intraconnection of the HAp fiber in the crystal plates of 4-day coated substrate. (b) Higher-magnification image of B showing the fiber merges into the crystal plates of the HAp coating. (c) Femur bone-like structure obtained in B4. (Image generated from Chakraborty et al., 2009).

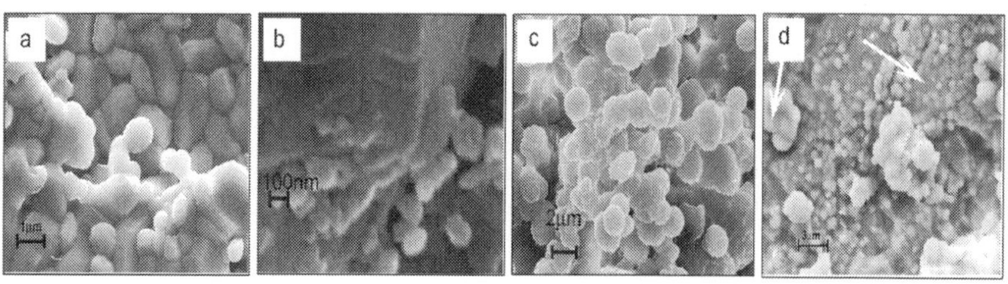

Fig. 6. SEM images of α-Al_2O_3 where (a)Bare α-Al_2O_3 (b)BSA Treated α-Al_2O_3 (c)BSA Treated and Coated for 2 days α-Al_2O_3 (d) Coated for 2 days α-Al_2O_3.(Image generated from Kapoor et al., 2010).

Our *in vivo* experiments also proven that metal/nonmetal implants which are protein treated and coated are more bioactive as they showed no negative response in term of any kind of inflammatory responses.

This comparative assessment of metal/non-metals structural and biological properties showed that metal when treated with protein and biomimtically coated for HAp can be used as a scaffold for many biomedical applications especially for osteoconduction. In modification for the method proposed, many biologically active molecules like osteogenic agents and growth factors can be co-precipitated with apatite crystals onto metal implants for the better osteogenic behavior as this biomimetic coating can be readily absorbed *in-vivo*.

5. Orthopedic challenges

As new methodologies for making functional components of human tissues to rectify a deformity or for developing new treatments of disease and trauma get developed we realize the limitations of the techniques and principles of biomimetic tissue engineering in facing up the real challenges of this approach. While many new methodologies have become available for the management of orthopedic disease and trauma, the computability of the manmade materials in this area is far from ideal. We describe here some of the unmet challenges of this field.

5.1 Biocompatibility and stability of *in-vivo* scaffolds

One of the most important aims of biomimetic design and production of materials for bone implants is to make them stable and compatible to the local bone tissue. Since there is considerable diversity in the details of local anatomies of specific bones the presently available general implant materials are prone to infection, extensive inflammation, and poor osteointegration. Besides their life span is less than 15 years which clearly shows the inability to mimic the longetivity of the molecular components of bone [Harold 2006, Porter 2009]. The implant failure is mainly attributed to acute complications, host responses, prosthesis dislocations and surgery failures seen at initial stages after surgery, and also after several years post surgery when implant loosening, osteolysis, implant wear and tear, instability, infection and fractures are observed.

In order to increase implant life it would be advisable to seed them with young osteoblasts which would sustain the production of bone mass on the implants (Xynos et al., 2001). It would also be useful to use bioactive agents in the coatings that would activate pathways related to cell survival, proliferation and differentiation. Thus it is clear that in order to increase the life of the implanted material it would be advisable to shift the focus of material production from a purely material science outlook to a cell biological and molecular biological approach.

5.2 Materials for osteoporotic applications

Osteoporosis a major health threat to bone degenerations due to decreased bone quality, are characterized by reduction in bone mass and disordered skeletal micro-architecture and are susceptible to fracture risks at sites of hip, spine and wrist [Borges & Bilezikian, 2006]. Much of the concerns regarding this are found in older populations where treatment becomes possible to an extent through regular controlled diet activities. Since the loss in bone mass can be directly attributed to the abnormal remodeling process therefore biomimetic tissue engineering approaches could offer alternate approaches to reduce the hyperactive bone resorption process. One of the targets for this could be the receptor for nuclear factor kappa B which seems to be involved in osteoblast-osteoclast coupling mechanisms.

6. Conclusion

We have shown in this chapter how one can use biomimetic approaches to simulate the osteoregenerative (periosteal surface) and osteo-degenerative (endosteal surface) interfaces of appendicular bones. These processes include novel tissue engineering strategies that combine developments in the field of material science with the cell and molecular biological pathways that are seen in the natural differentiation of osteoblast and osteoclast. We hope that some of these strategies would lead to the better management of trauma and age related degeneration of bone tissues.

7. Acknowlegments

This work is supported by grant Nos. GAP 0311, GAP022 and CMM002 to GP from the Council of Scientific and Industrial Research and Department of Science and Technology Government of India New Delhi. SR is supported with DBT-Indo Australian Biotech Grant (GAP0311) and RK is supported by grant No.GAP220 from the Department of Science and Technology, Government of India.

8. References

Aksakal, B. & Hanyaloglu, C. (2008). Bioceramic dip-coating on Ti-6Al-4V and 316L SS implant Materials. *Mater Sci: Mater Med,* Vol.19, No. , pp. 2097-2104

Anderson, H. (2003). Matrix Vesicles and Calcification. *Curr Opin Rheumatol,* Vol.5, pp.222-226

Andersson, O.H.; Rosenqvist, J. & Karlsson, K.H. (2004).Dissolution, leaching, and Al_2O_3 enrichment at the surface of bioactive glasses studied by solution analysis. *J. Biomed. Mater. Res,* Vol.27, pp. 941-948

Alves,M.; Leonor,B.; Azevedo,H.; Reis,L & Mano,F. (2010).Designing biomaterials based on biomineralization of of bone. *Mater. Chem,* Vol.20, pp. 2911-2921

Asiri, K., Wijenayaka, C., Colby, G. & Atkins, P. (2009).Biomimetic hydroxyapatite coating on glass coverslips for the assay of osteoclast activity in vitro. *J Mater Sci: Mater Med,* Vol.20, pp.1467-1473

Athanasiou, K.A.; Agrawal, C.M.; Barber, F.A. & Burkhart, S.S. (1998). Orthopaedic applications for PLA-PGA biodegradable polymers. *Arthroscopy,* Vol.14, No.7, pp.726-737

Atsushi, A.; Hidekazu, N.; Michiko, N.; Tetsushi ,M. & Tadashi, M.(2008). Formation of magnetite by bacteria and its application. *J. R. Soc. Interface,* Vol.5, pp.977-999

Balasundaram, G. & Webster, T.J. (2007). An Overview of Nano-Polymers for Orthopedic applications. *Macromol Biosci,* Vol.7, pp.635-642

Banerjee, R.;Nag, S.;Samuel, S. & Fraser, H.L. (2004).Strengthening mechanisms in Ti-Nb-Zr-Ta and Ti-Mo-Zr-Fe orthopaedic alloys.*Biomaterials,* Vol. 25, No.17, pp. 3413-3419

Banerjee, R.;Nag, S.;Samuel, S. & Fraser, H.L. (2006).Laser-deposited Ti-Nb-Zr-Ta orthopedic alloys. *J Biomed Mater Res,*Vol. 78A, pp.298-305

Barbara, J.; Lenka, M.; Frank, L.; Andrea, E.; Claudia, B.; Egle, C. & Frank, A. (2008). Osteoblast response to biomimetically altered titanium surfaces. *Acta Biomaterialia,* Vol.4, No.6, pp.1985-1995

Bernards, M.T.;Qin, C. & Jiang, S.(2008). MC3T3-E1 cell adhesion to hydroxyapatite with adsorbed bone sialoprotein, bone osteopontin, and bovine serum albumin. *Colloids Surf B Biointerfaces,* Vol.64, No.2, pp.236-247

Bharati, S.; sinha, m. k & basu,D.(2005).Hydroxyapatite coating by biomimetic method on titanium alloy using concentrated sbf. Bull. Mater. Sci, Vol. 28, pp. 617–621

Butler, K.; Benghuzzi, H. & Tucci, S. (2001).Tissue-implant response following soft tissue implantation of poly-L-lysine coated UHMW-polyethylene into adult male rats. *Biomed Sci Instrum,* Vol.37, pp.19-24

Cai,Y. &Tang,R.(2009). Towards understanding biomineralization: calcium phosphate in a biomimetic mineralization process. *Front. Mater. Sci. China,*Vol.3,No.2,pp.124-131

Ciancaglini,P.; Simão, S.; Camolezi,L.; Millán,J. & Pizauro,M. (2006). Contribution of matrix vesicles and alkaline phosphatase to ectopic bone formation. *Braz J Med Biol Res,* Vol.39, No.5, pp.603-610

Chakraborty, J.; Mazaj, M.; Kapoor, R.; Gouri, S.P.; Daneu, N.; Sinha, M.K.; Pande, G . & Basu, D. (2009).Bone-like growth of hydroxyapatite in the biomimetic coating of Ti-6Al-4V alloy pretreated with protein at 25°C. *J Mat Res,*Vol.24,pp.2145-2153

Chen, C.C.; Huang, T.H.; Kao, C.T. & Ding, S.J. (2006).Characterization of Functionally Graded Hydroxyapatite/Titanium Composite Coatings Plasma-Sprayed on Ti Alloys. *J Biomed Mater Res Part B: Appl Biomater,* Vol.78B, pp. 146–152

Chen, D.; Jordan, E.H. & We, M.G.M. (2008).Apatite formation on alkaline-treated dense TiO2 coatings deposited using the solution precursor plasma spray process. *Acta Biomaterialia,*Vol. 4,pp.553-559

Chen, Y., Mak,A., Wang, M., Li, J. & Wong, J. (2008). In vitro behavior of osteoblast-like cells on PLLA films with a biomimetic apatite or apatite/collagen composite coating. *J Mater Sci: Mater Med,* Vol.19, pp.2261–2268

Chikara, O.; Masanobu, K & Toshiki, M. (2007).Coating bone-like apatite onto organic substrates using solutions mimicking body fluid. *J Tissue Eng Regen Med,* Vol.1, pp. 33–38

Christel, P.; Meunier, A.; Dorlot, J.M.; Crolet, J.M.; Witvoet, J.; Sedel, L. & Boutin, P.(1988).Biomechanical Compatibility and Design of Ceramic Implants for Orthopedic Surgery. *Ann. N. Y. Acad. Sci,* Vol. 523, pp. 234–256

Clarke, B. (2008).Normal Bone Anatomy and Physiology. *Clin J Am Soc Nephrol,*Vol. 3, pp.S131–S139

Cristina, M., Vincenzo, G., Nicoletta, Z., Maria, G., Andrea, F., Francesco, G., Elena, G., Stefano, S., Andrea, F., Luigi, A. & Gina, L. (2010). Mineralization behavior with mesenchymal stromal cells in a biomimetic hyaluronic acid-based scaffold. *Biomaterials,* Vol.31, No.14, pp.3986-3996

Culha, O.; Tekmen, C.; Toparli, M. & Tsunekawa, Y. (2010).Mechanical properties of in situ Al2O3 formed Al–Si composite coating via atmospheric plasma spraying. *Materials & Design,* Vol.31, pp.533-544

De Medeiros, W.S.; De Oliveira, M. V.; Pereira, L. C & De Andrade, M. C.(2008).Bioactive Porous Titanium: An Alternative to Surgical Implants . *Artif Organs,* Vol. 32, pp. 277–282

Dreinhofer,K.; Feron, J.; Herrera, A.; Hube, R.; Johnell, O.; Lidgren, L.; Miles,K.; Panarella, L.; Simpson, H. & Wallace, A. (2004).Orthopaedic surgeons and fragility fractures. *J Bone Joint Surg [Br],* Vol.86-B, pp.958-961

Dixon, R.A. (2005).Engineering of plant natural product pathways. Curr Opin Plant,Vol. 8, pp.329–336

Elliott, J.C.; Wilson, R.M. & Dowker, S.E.P. (2002).Apatite structures. Adv X Ray Anal,Vol.45, pp.172-181

Ellis, E. (2009). Role of matrix vesicles in biomineralization. *Biochimica et Biophysica Acta 1790*, pp.1592–1598

Feng, L.; Song, Y.; Zhai, J.; Liu, B.; Xu, J.; Jiang, L. & Zhu, D. (2003).Creation of a Superhydrophobic Surface from an Amphiphilic Polymer. *Angew. Chem. Int. Ed*, Vol.42, No. 7, pp.800-802

Feng, X. & Jiang, L. (2006).Design and Creation of Superwetting/Antiwetting Surfaces. *Adv.Mater*,Vol. 18, pp.3063-3078

Geary, C.; Birkinshaw, C. & Jones, E. (2008). Characterisation of Bionate polycarbonate polyurethanes for orthopaedic applications. *J Mater Sci: Mater Med*,Vol. 19, pp.3355–3363

Gorustovich, A.A.; Steimetz, T.; Cabrini, R.L. & Lopez, J.M.P. (2010).Osteoconductivity of strontium-doped bioactive glass particles: A histomorphometric study in rats. *J Biomed Mater Res*,Vol. 92A, pp. 232–237

Guido, M. & Isabelle, J. (2004). *Cells, tissues, and disease: principles of general pathology*, Oxford University Press, 0-19-514090-7, New York

Habibovic, P.; Florence, B.; Clemens, A.B.; De Groot, K & Layrolle, P. (2002). Biomimetic Hydroxyapatite Coating on Metal Implants. *J. Am. Ceram. Soc*, Vol. 85, pp. 517–522

Haibo, Qu & Mei, W. (2008). Effect of temperature and intital ph on biomimetic apatite coating. *J Biomed Mater Res Part B: Appl Biomater 87B*, pp. 204–212

Harold, C.;Slavkin,P. & Bartold, M. (2006).Challenges and potential in tissue engineering. *Periodontol 2000*, Vol. 41, pp.9–15

Heimann, B.R.;Suhurmann, N. & Muller, T.R. (2004).*In vitro* and *in vivo* performance of Ti6Al4V implants with plasma sprayed osteoconductive hydroxyapaptite-bioinert titania bond coat "duplex" systems: an experimental study in sheep.*J Mater Sci:Mater Med*,Vol.15, pp.1045-1052.

Hunter, K.; Hauschka,V.; Poole, A.; Rosenberg,C. & Harvey, A. (1996). Nucleation and inhibition of hydroxyapatite formation by mineralized tissue proteins. *International Review of Cytology*, Vol.242, pp.121-156.

Hyun,M.K.; Fumiaki, M.; Tadashi, K & Takashi, N.(1996).Preparation of bioactive Ti and its alloys via simple chemical surface treatment. *Journal of Biomedical Materials Research*, Vol. 32, pp. 409-417

James, C.; Joanna, A.; Georg, E.; David, K.; Alexander, W.; Peter, A.; Kirk, F.; Michael, J.; Frank, W.; Paul, K.; Peter, F. & Daniel, E. (2007)Hierarchical assembly of the siliceous skeletal lattice of the hexactinellid sponge Euplectella aspergillum. *Journal of Structural Biology*, Vol.158, pp.93–106

Jayabalan, M.; Thomas, V. & Rajesh, P.N. (2001).Polypropylene fumarate/phloroglucinol triglycidyl methacrylate blend for use as partially biodegradable orthopaedic cement. *Biomaterials*, Vol.22, No.20, pp.2749-57

Jiawei, W., Jan de, B. & Klaas de, G. (2009). Proliferation and differentiation of osteoblast-like MC3T3-E1 cells on biomimetically and electrolytically deposited calcium phosphate coatings. *J Biomed Mater Res*,Vol. 90A, pp.664–670

Joshua, R.; Timothy, T.; Popat, R.K.(2009). Bone Tissue Engineering: A Review in Bone Biomimetics and Drug Delivery Strategies. *Biotechnol. Prog*, Vol.25, No.6, pp.1539–1560

Kalfas, I.H. (2001).Principles of bone healing. *Neurosurg Focus*, Vol.10, No. 4, pp.7-10

Kamino, K. (2008). Underwater Adhesive of Marine Organisms as the Vital Link between Biological Science and Material Science. *Mar Biotechnol*, Vol.10, pp.111-121

Kapoor, R.; Gouri, S.P.; Kumar, J.M.; Raj, A. T.; Srinivas, G.; Chakraborty, J.;Sinha, M. K,.;Basu, D. & Pande, G. (2010).Comparative assessment of structural and biological properties of biomimetically coated hydroxyapatite on alumina (α-Al2O3) and titanium (Ti-6Al-4V) alloy substrates. *J Biomed Mat Res Part A*, Vol.94A, pp.913-926

Kazuhiko, K.;Buchanan,V.& Weiss,M.(2009). Biomineralization in Humans: Making the Hard Choices in Life. *Annu. Rev. Genet*, Vol.43,pp.119-142

Keselowsky, B. G.; Collard, D. M. & Garcia, A. J. (2005).Integrin binding specificity regulates biomaterial surface chemistry effects on cell differentiation. *PNAS*, Vol. 102, pp.5953-5957

Khaner, O. (2007). Evolutionary innovations of the vertebrates. *Integrative Zoology*, Vol.2, pp.60-67

Kim, H.W.; Kim, H.E.; Salih, V. & Knowles, J.C. (2005).Hydroxyapatite and Titania Sol-Gel Composite Coatings on Titanium for Hard Tissue Implants; Mechanical and *In Vitro* Biological Performance. *J Biomed Mater Res Part B: Appl Biomater*, Vol.72B: pp.1- 8

Klein, L.C. (1988) Sol-Gel Technology for Thin Films, Fibers, Preforms, Electronics and Specialty Shapes, Noyes Publications, 0-8155-1154,USA

Kokubo,T.(1996). Formation of biologically active bone like apatite on metals and polymers by a biomimetic process. *Thermochemica acta*, Vol. 280/281, pp.479-490

Kokubo, T.; Kim, H.M.; Kawashita,M.; Nakamura,T.(2004).Bioactive Metals: Preparation and Properties. *J Mater Sci Mater Med*, Vol.15, pp.99-107

Kurtz, S.M. & Devine, J.N. PEEK. (2007).Biomaterials in Trauma, Orthopedic, and Spinal Implants. *Biomaterials*, Vol.28,No.32, pp. 4845-4869

Lawrence, G. (2005).Pathogenesis of osteoporosis: concepts, conflicts, and prospects. *J. Clin. Invest*, Vol.115, pp. 3318-3325

Le, M.H.; Ducheyne, P.; Lynch, L.; Boettiger, D. & Composto, R. J. (2006). Effect of biomaterial surface properties on fibronectin-$a5\beta1$ integrin interaction and cellular attachment. *Biomaterials*, Vol.27, pp.1907-1916

Lee, H.; Lee, B.P. & Messersmith P.B. (2007).A reversible wet/dry adhesive inspired by mussels and geckos. *Nature*, Vol.448, pp.338-341

Liu, Y.; Huang, B.; Ruan, J. & He, Y. (1998). Behaviour of Composite Ca/P Bioceramics in Stimulated Body Fluid. *J. Mater.Sci.Technol*, Vol.14, pp. 533-537

Liu, K.; Yao, X. & Jiang, L. (2010).Recent developments in bio-inspired special wettability. *Chem. Soc. Rev*, (In press)

Marc, B & Jacques, L. (2009).Can bioactivity be tested in vitro with SBF solution? *Biomaterials*, Vol. 30, pp. 2175-2179

Marti, A. (2000).Cobalt-base alloys used in bone surgery. *Injury*, Vol. 31, No. 4, pp.18-21

Meek, K.M. & Fullwood, N.J. (2001).Corneal and scleral collagens - a microscopist's perspective. *Micron*, Vol.32, pp.261-272

Mueller, G. & Russell, R. (2003). Osteoporosis: pathogenesis and clinical intervention. Biochem. Syst. Ecol, Vol. 31, No. 2, pp.462-464

Nair, M.B.; Varma, H.K.; Menon, K.V.; Shenoy, S.J. & John, A. (2009).Tissue regeneration and repair of goat segmental femur defect with bioactive triphasic ceramic-coated hydroxyapatite scaffold. *J Biomed Mater Res*, Vol. 91A, pp.855-865

Nguyen, H.Q.; Deporter, D.A.; Pilliar, R.M.;Valiquette, N. & Yakubovich, R. (2004).The effect of sol-gel-formed calcium phosphate coatings on bone ingrowth and osteoconductivity of porous-surfaced Ti alloy implants. *Biomaterials*,Vol.25, pp.865-876

Niinomi, M. (2003).Fatigue performance and cyto-toxicity of low rigidity titanium alloy, Ti-29Nb-13Ta-4.6Zr.*Biomaterials*, Vol.24, No.16, pp.2673-2683

Ning, C.; Ding, D.;Dai, K.; Zhai, W. & Chen, L. (2010).The effect of Zr content on the microstructure, mechanical properties and cell attachment of Ti-35Nb-xZr alloys. *Biomed Mater*, (In press)

Nystrom, D.; Lindqvist, J.;Ostmark, E.; Hult, A. & Malmstrom, E. (2006).Superhydrophobic bio-fibre surfaces via tailored grafting architecture. *Chem. Commun*, pp.3594-3596

Nystrom, D.; Malmstrom, E.; Hult, A.; Blakey, I.; Boyer, C.;Davis, T.P. & Whittaker, M.R. (2010).Biomimetic Surface Modification of Honeycomb Films via a "Grafting From" Approach. *Langmuir*, (In press)

Oliveira,A.; Pedro,A.; Saiz,C.; Mano,J.; Rodriguez,G.; San, J. & Reis,R. (2010). Biomimetic Ca-P Coatings Incorporating Bisphosphonates Produced on Starch-Based Degradable Biomaterials. *J Biomed Mater Res Part B: Appl Biomater*, Vol.92B, pp.55-67

Oral, E. & Muratoglu, O.K. (2007).Radiation cross-linking in ultra-high molecular weight polyethylene for orthopaedic applications. *Nucl Instrum Methods Phys Res B*, Vol.265, No.1, pp. 18-22

Ozawa,H.;Hoshi,K. & Amizuka,N.(2008).Current concepts of bone mineralization. . *J.Oral Biosci*, Vol.50, No.1, pp.1-14

Palmer,C.;Christina,J.;Kaltz,R. & Spoerke,D.(2008). Biomimetic Systems for Hydroxyapatite Mineralization Inspired By Bone and Enamel. *Chem. Rev*, Vol.108.pp. 4754-4783

Podbielska, H. & Ulatowska-jarza,A. (2005). Sol-gel technology for biomedical engineering. *Bull. Pol. Ac.: Tech.* Vol.53, No.3, pp.261-271

Porter, J.R.; Ruckh, T.T. & Popat, K.C. (2009).Bone Tissue Engineering: A Review in Bone Biomimetics and Drug Delivery Strategies. *Biotechnol. Prog*, Vol.25, pp.1539-1560

Puleo, D.A. & Nanci, A. (1999).Understanding and controlling the bone-implant interface. *Biomaterials*, Vol. 20, pp. 2311- 2321

Qu, H & Mei, W. (2008). Improvement of Bonding Strength between Biomimetic Apatite Coating and Substrate. *J Biomed Mater Res Part B: Appl Biomater*, Vol.84B, pp. 436-443

Reis, J.; Kanagaraj S.; Fonseca, A.; Mathew, M.T.; Capela-Silva, F, Potes J, Pereira A, Oliveira, M.S, Simoes, J.A. (2010).In vitro studies of multiwalled carbon nanotube/ultrahigh molecular weight polyethylene nanocomposites with osteoblast-like MG63 cells. *Braz J Med Biol Res*. Vol.43,No.5, pp.476-82

Rigo, E.C.S.; Boschi, A.O.; Yoshimoto, M.; Allegrini, S.;Konig, B. & Carbonari, M.J. (2004).Evaluation in vitro and in vivo of biomimetic hydroxyapatite coated on titanium dental implants. *Mater Sci and Eng:C*, Vol. 24, pp.647-651

Robert, M.; David, F.; Dorothy, A. & Clifford, J. (2001). *Osteoporosis*. Third edition-Volume 1, Eli Lilly & Company, 978-0-12-370545-7,London,UK

Sarikaya, M. (1999).Biomimetic fabrication of apatite related biomaterials.*PNAS*, Vol.96, No.25, pp.14183-14185

Sato, M. & Webster, T.J. (2004).Nanobiotechnology: implications for the future of nanotechnology in orthopedic applications. *Expert Rev. Medical devices*, Vol.1, pp.105-114

Seligson, D.; Mehta, S.; Mishra, A.K.; FitzGerald, T.J.; Castleman, D.W.; James, A.H.; Voor, M.J.; Been, J. & Nawab, A. (1997). In vivo study of stainless steel and Ti-13Nb-13Zr bone plates in a sheep model. *Clin Orthop Relat Res*, Vol.343, pp.213-23

Sepulveda, P.; Jones, J.R. & Hench, L.L. (2002).Bioactive sol-gel foams for tissue repair. *J Biomed Mater Res*, Vol.59, pp. 340–348

Sethuraman, S.; Nair, L.S.; El-Amin, S.; Nguyen, M.T.; Singh, A.; Greish, Y.E.; Allcock, H.R.; Brown, P.W. & Laurencin C.T.(2010).Development and Characterization of Biodegradable Nanocomposite Injectables for Orthopaedic Applications Based on Polyphosphazenes.*J Biomater Sci Polym Ed*, (In press)

Shalumon, K.T. & Jayabalan, M. (2009). Studies on biodegradation of crosslinked hydroxyl terminated-poly (proplyene fumarate) and formation of scaffold for orthopedic applications. *J Mater Sci: Mater Med*, Vol. 20, pp.S161–S171

Silvia, F.; Sally, J. M.; Eduardo, S.; Antoni, P. T. & Grayson, W. M. (2006). Functionally graded bioactive coatings: Reproducibility and stability of the coating under cell culture conditions. *Acta Biomaterialia,*Vol. 2, pp. 133–142

Simao, S.; Yadav,C.; Ciancaglini, P. & Millan, L.(2010). Proteoliposomes as matrix vesicles biomimetics to study the initiation of skeletal mineralization. *Braz J Med Biol Res,* Vol.43, No.3, pp.234-241

Smith, L.J.; Swaim, J.S.; Yao, C.; Haberstroh, K.M.; Nauman, E.A. & Webster, T.J.(2007).Increased osteoblast cell density on nanostructured PLGA-coated nanostructured titanium for orthopedic applications. *Int J Nanomedicine*, Vol.2, No.3, pp.493–499

Stephen,M.(1988). Molecular recongnistion in biomimeralization. *Nature,* Vol.332, pp.119 - 124.

Stevens, B.; Yang, Y.; Mohandas, A.; Stucker, B. & Nguyen, K.T. (2008). A Review of Materials, Fabrication Methods, and Strategies Used to Enhance Bone Regeneration in Engineered Bone Tissues. *J Biomed Mater Res Part B: Appl Biomater,* Vol. 85B, pp.573–582

Tadashi, K. & Hiroaki, T. (2006). How useful is SBF in predicting in vivo bone bioactivity. *Biomaterials*, Vol.27, pp.2907–2915.

Tsai, S.W.; Hsu, F.Y & Chen, P.L. (2008). Beads of collagen–nanohydroxyapatite composites prepared by a biomimetic process and the effects of their surface texture on cellular behavior in MG63 osteoblast like cells. *Acta Biomater*, Vol. 4, pp. 1332-41

Veiss,A.(2005). A Window on Biomineralization. *Science*, Vol.4, No.307 (5714), pp.1419-1420.

Vijayalakshmi, U.; Prabakaran, K. & Rajeswari, S. (2008).Preparation and characterization of sol–gel hydroxyapatite and its electrochemical evaluation for biomedical applications. *J Biomed Mater Res*. Vol. 87A, pp.739–749

Vincent, J.F.V. (2003). Biomimetic modeling. *Phil. Trans. R. Soc. Lond. B*, Vol.358, pp.1597–1603.

Wang, D.; Chen, C.; He, T. & Lei, T. (2008). Hydroxyapatite coating on Ti6Al4V alloy by a sol–gel method. *J Mater Sci: Mater Med,* Vol.19, pp.2281–2286

Weiner,S .& Addadi,L. (1997). Design strategies in mineralized biological materials. *J. Mater. Chem*, Vol.7, No.5, pp. 689–702

Weiner, S. & Wagner, H.D. (1998).The material bone: structure-mechanical function relations. *Annu. Rev. Mater. Sci*, Vol.28, pp.271–298

Weng W.; Zhang, S.; Cheng, K.; Qu, H.; Du, P.; Shen,G.; Yuan, J. & Han, G. (2003). Sol–gel preparation of bioactive apatite films *Surface and Coatings Technology,* Vol.167, pp.292–296

Wooley, P.H.; Morren, R.; Andary, J.; Sud, S.; Yang, S.Y.; Mayton, L.; Markel, D.; Sieving, A. & Nasser, S. (2002).Inflammatory responses to orthopaedic biomaterials in the murine air pouch. *Biomaterials*, Vol.23, No.2, pp.517-526

Wu, C.; Ramaswamy, Y.; Liu, X.; Wang, G. & Zreiqat, H. (2009).Plasma-sprayed CaTiSiO5 ceramic coating on Ti-6Al-4V with excellent bonding strength, stability and cellular bioactivity. *J. R. Soc. Interface*, Vol. 6, pp.159–168

Xin,Y.; Liu,C.; Zhang,X.; Tang, G.; Tian,X. & Chu, P. K.(2007) Corrosion behavior of biomedical AZ91 magnesium alloy in simulated body fluid. *J. Mater. Res*, Vol. 22, No. 7, pp.2004-2011

Xu, C.; Su, P.; Wang, Y.; Chen, X.; Meng, Y.; Liu, C.; Yu, X.; Yang, X.; Yu, W.; Zhang, X. & Xiang, A.P. (2010).A novel biomimetic composite scaffold hybridized with mesenchymal stem cells in repair of rat bone defects models. J Biomed Mater Res Part A, (In Press)

Xynos, I.D.; Edgar, A.J.; Buttery, L.D.K.; Hench, L.L. & Polak, J.M. (2001). Gene-expression profiling of human osteoblasts following treatment with the ionic products of Bioglass 45S5 dissolution. *J. Biomed. Mater.Res*, Vol. 55A, pp. 151–157

Yael, K.; Giuseppe, F.; Lia, A. & Steve, W. (2001). Structure of the Nacreous Organic Matrix of a Bivalve Mollusk Shell Examined in the Hydrated State Using Cryo-TEM. *Journal of Structural Biology*, Vol.135, pp.8–17

Yajing, Z.; Guozhi, Z. & Mei, Wei. (2009)Controlling the Biodegradation Rate of Magnesium Using biomimetic apatite coating. *J Biomed Mater Res Part B: Appl Biomater 89B*, pp. 408–414

Ye, X.; Chen, M.; Yang, M.; Wei, J. & Liu, D. (2010).In vitro corrosion resistance and cytocompatibility of nano-hydroxyapatite reinforced Mg–Zn–Zr composites. *J Mater Sci: Mater Med*, Vol.2, pp.1321–1328

Yeung, K.W.K.; Poon, R.W.Y.; Chu, P.K.; Chung, C.Y.; Liu, X.Y.; Lu, W.W.; Chan, D.; Chan, S.C.W.; Luk, K.D.K. & Cheung, K.M.C. (2007).Surface mechanical properties, corrosion resistance, and cytocompatibility of nitrogen plasma-implanted nickel-titanium alloys: A comparative study with commonly used medical grade materials. *J Biomed Mater Res*, Vol.82A, pp.403–414

Yuan, H.; De Bruijn, J.D.; Zhang, X.; van Blitterswijk, C.A. & de Groot K. (2001).Bone Induction by Porous Glass Ceramic Made from BioglassT (45S5). *J Biomed Mater Res (Appl Biomater)*, Vol.58, No.3, pp.270–276

Yuelian, L., Ernst, B., Pierre L., Joost, D., De, B. & Klaas, D.(2004). Tissue Engineering Bone Morphogenetic Protein 2 Incorporated into Biomimetic Coatings Retains Its Biological Activity. *Tissue Engineering*, Vol.10, No.1-2, pp.101-108

Zheng, Y.; Lv, H.; Wang, Y.; Lu, H.; Qing, L. & Xi, T. (2009).Performance of novel bioactive hybrid hydrogels in vitro and in vivo used for artificial cartilage. *Biomed Mater*, Vol.4, No.1, pp.015015

19

Advances in Biomimetic Apatite Coating on Metal Implants

C.Y. Zhao, H.S. Fan and X.D. Zhang
National Engineering Research Center for Biomaterials,
Sichuan University, Sichuan, Chengdu 610064
China

1. Introduction

Artificial implants are generally encapsulated by a fibrous tissue when implanted into bone defects. However, Hench et al. showed that bioglass directly bonded to living bone via a biologically active bone-like apatite layer instead of the formation of surrounding fibrous tissue(Hench et al., 1971). Meanwhile, with the mineral compositional resemblance with the inorganic phase of human bone, calcium phosphate ceramics possessed excellent biocompatibility and osteoconductivity, and it also showed bone-bonding ability via a biologically active bone-like apatite layer(W.P. Cao & Hench, 1996; Hench, 1998). Nowadays, they are both extensively used as hard tissue repair or substitution materials in clinic. However, these materials cannot be used under load-bearing conditions such as femur, tibia and spinal interbody, because they are usually very stiff and brittle, and have low impact resistance and relatively low tensile strength(Rezwan et al., 2006).

Titanium and its alloys are widely used as orthopaedic implants due to their superior mechanical properties and excellent biocompatibility(X.Y. Liu et al., 2004; Ratner, 2001). However, their bioactivity are not as good as that of calcium phosphate ceramics and during implantation they can only form osteointegration at the interface of titanium and bone tissue, instead of bone-bonding(Feng et al., 2002). To overcome these disadvantages, various methods of coating the titanium surface have been developed to combine the mechanical properties of metals with bone-bonding ability of bioactive ceramics, such as ion-beam(Ong et al., 1992) or radiofrequency magnetron sputter deposition(Wolke et al., 1998), sol-gel method (Brendel et al., 1992; Weng & Baptista, 1999) et al, with plasma spraying being the most popular(Y. Cao et al., 1996; J. Chen et al., 1994). However, each of them has its own technical limitations, for example, the inability to coat those complex-shaped implants with internal cavities or porous implants and incorporate biologically active agents. Therefore, an optimal technique for apatite coatings on complex-shaped or porous implants still has to be developed.

One alternative method is the so-called biomimetic apatite coating, which consists of mimicking the bone mineralization process by immersing implants in simulated body fluid (SBF) that mimics the inorganic composition, pH, and temperature of human blood plasma(Abe et al., 1990). As a result of the low temperature conditions of this technique, diverse Ca-P phases such as amorphous calcium phosphate (ACP), octacalcium phosphate (OCP) or carbonated apatite (CA), some of which are stable only at low temperatures, can be deposited on the metal implants(Barrère et al., 1999, 2001, 2002a, b; Habibovic et al., 2002). Compared with the above mentioned techniques, biomimetic technique might have the following advantages: (1) it is expected to endow the materials with high bioactivity, and the properties of the coating such as phase composition, crystallinity and dissolution can be adjusted by controlling the process parameters to meet specific clinic needs, (2) it is a low-temperature process, free of adverse heat effect on substrates, and even heat-sensitive substrates including polymers can be coated, (3) it can be used to produce biomimetic apatite coating on/or even into porous or complex-shaped implants, (4) it can incorporate biologically active agents or drugs into biomimetic apatite coating through coprecipitation rather than merely absorb on the surface. The degradation of these coatings would result in a gradual release of biologically active agents or drugs rather than in a single rapid burst, (5) it is a simple and cost-effective way(Habibovic et al., 2004a; Wen et al., 1998). Two conditions, however, must be met in order to insure an effective biomimetic apatite deposition: (1) pretreatments of the metal surface, and (2) supersaturation of calcium and phosphate in the solution(Narayanan et al., 2008; Q.Y. Zhang & Leng, 2005). Regarding the pretreatments, surface morphology of metal implants such as surface roughness can affect the nucleation and growth of apatite coating from the simulated body fluid, and the surface chemistry such as hydroxyl groups on the titanium surface is beneficial for the chemical bonding with calcium and phosphate ions (Barrère et al., 2004; Leitão et al., 1997). Regarding the degree of supersaturation in the solution, it influences the calcification ability of metal implants(Barrère et al., 2004). Both factors determine its in vitro and in vivo biological effects. In this chapter, the effects of both factors including pretreatments of the metal surface and the simulated body fluid on biomimetic coating as well as the possibility to incorporate biologically active agents and drugs into the biomimetic apatite coatings are introduced. The in vitro and in vivo biological performances of these biomimetic apatite coatings are also described.

2. Effect of pretreatments on biomimetic apatite coating

During the biomimetic deposition process, the heterogeneous nucleation ability of Ca^{2+} and PO_4^{3-} ions are directly dependent on the activation of metal surface in the pretreatment process. The purpose of the pretreatments is mainly to modify the surface topography, and/or modify the chemical composition or structure of the oxide layer or form a new surface layer. The solvent cleaning to remove the surface contaminants such as oils, greases is not included in this chapter as a pretreatment(Lausmaa, 2001). The main pretreatments are summarized as follows:

2.1 Physical methods to modify the surface topography

The metal surface becomes coarse and porous through special treatments, such as grit blasting or other methods to form porous structure(Barrère et al., 2003a; Habibovic et al., 2002; Ryan et al., 2006). After immersion in supersaturated calcium phosphate solution, the Ca^{2+} and PO_4^{3-} ions adhere to these coarse and/or porous surfaces through mechanical interlocking. Regarding the effects of surface topography on biomimetic apatite coating, previous study showed that the nucleation and morphology of apatite coating could be affected by the surface roughness of the substrate after immersion in Hank's balanced salt solution (HBSS)(Leitão et al., 1997). Furthermore, the adhesion strength of the biomimetic apatite coating was dependent on the mechanical interlock between biomimetic coating and implant surface(Leitão et al., 1997). There were many types of methods for the fabrication of coarse surface or porous structure. For example, the rough surface on Ti6Al4V plates was obtained via grit blasting by using alumina particles and an average surface roughness of 3.5 μm was required for an optimal apatite coating(Habibovic et al., 2002). The porous implants, such as porous tantalum implants manufactured by chemical vapor infiltration to deposit pure tantalum onto vitreous carbon foams, porous Ti6Al4V implants produced by a positive replica technique, were in favor of apatite deposition(Barrère et al., 2003a; Habibovic et al., 2005). OCP or CA coating was successfully deposited on or into the porous tantalum or porous Ti6Al4V implants by immersion into a highly concentrated simulated body fluid(Barrère et al., 2003a; Habibovic et al., 2005).

2.2 Chemical and electrochemical methods

Chemical and electrochemical treatments of titanium and its alloys, such as acid treatment, alkali or alkali-heat treatment, acid-alkali treatment, hydrogen peroxide (H_2O_2) treatment, anodic (microarc) oxidation, are mainly based on chemical or electrochemical reactions occurring at the interface between titanium and a solution, and a porous sodium titanate gel or titania-based film forms on the substrate(Lausmaa, 2001). After immersion in SBF, a bone-like apatite coating spontaneously deposits on its surface. The mechanism of apatite formation can be interpreted as the electrostatic interaction between Ti-OH functional groups on the film and Ca^{2+}, PO_4^{3-} ions in the simulated body fluid and/ or the matching of crystal structure between the titania and apatite(Kim H.M. et al., 1996; Wang et al., 2000). Chemical methods are substantially biomimetic in nature.

2.2.1 Acid treatment

Acid treatment is often used to remove surface oxide and contamination in order to obtain clean, uniform and rough surface finishes. The mixed acid of 10–30 vol% of HNO_3 and 1–3 vol%of HF in distilled water is the most commonly used and is recommended to be a standard solution as a pre-treatment. The ratio of nitric acid to hydrofluoric acid at 10:1 is preferred to minimize the formation of free hydrogen. The free hydrogen results from the reaction between titanium and hydrofluoric acid and can adsorb on the titanium surface to cause embrittlement of the surface layer(ASTM standard B600, 1997; Lausmaa, 2001). The acid etching of titanium in HCl under inert atmosphere as a pretreatment was used to obtain a uniform initial micro-roughened surface before alkali treatment, which provided an improved condition for a homogenous hydroxycarbonated apatite precipitation after exposition in SBF(Jonášová et al., 2004). Nitric acid passivation was also used as a pretreatment before alkaline treatment to form a microporous surface on NiTi alloy(M.F. Chen et al., 2003). Wen et al. employed a mixture of 100ml HCl(18mass%) and 100ml H_2SO_4 (48 mass%) before alkaline treatment to obtain a microporous surface(Wen et al., 1997, 1998). However, titanium with only acid treatment could not spontaneously induce apatite deposition in SBF. Lately, Lu et al firstly revealed that titanium with nitric acid treatment could induce biomimetic apatite coatings formation in SBF. They confirmed that nitric acid treatment did not increase the oxide thickness on the Ti substrates, but the increase of the nitric acid treatment temperature and duration helped to improve its apatite-forming ability(Lu et al., 2007).

2.2.2 Alkaline treatment

Kim et al established a simple chemical treatment, i.e. an alkali and heat(AH) treatment process, for spontaneously inducing a uniform bonelike apatite layer on titanium surface in

SBF (H.M. Kim et al., 1996). Treatment of titanium in 5-10M NaOH or KOH solution at 60°C for 24h produced a microporous and graded alkali titanate hydrogel layer(H.M. Kim et al., 1996, 1998,1999; Kokubo et al., 1996). The as-formed gel layer, however, was mechanically unstable. Subsequent heat treatment of the alkali-treated Ti at 600°C for 1h made the hydrogel layer dehydrated and densified to form a cystalline alkali titanate layer. The heat treatment considerably increased the mechanical strength of the surface gel layer to its substrates, but it slightly lowered the bioactivity of the alkali titanate gel layer on NaOH-treated Ti surfaces. That's to say, it would take a little longer time to induce the apatite formation on the titanium surface in SBF(H.M. Kim et al., 1997). The mechanism of apatite formation on AH treated titanium in SBF is as follows: When AH-treated titanium is exposed to SBF, the alkali ions are released from the alkali titanate layer and hydronium ions enter into the surface layer via ions exchange, which result in the formation of negatively charged Ti-OH groups in the surface. At the same time, the released Na^+ ions increase the degree of supersaturation with respect to apatite by increasing pH. Because of the electrostatic interaction, the negatively charged Ti-OH groups combine selectively with the positively charged Ca^{2+} in the fluid to form calcium titanate. Calcium titanate takes the phosphate ions as well as the calcium ions in the fluid to form the apatite nuclei. Once the apatite nuclei are formed, they spontaneously grow by consuming the calcium and phosphate ions from SBF(H.M. Kim et al., 1996; Takadama et al., 2001a, b). The order of calcium and phosphate ion deposition on AH-treated titanium surface is that the precipitation of Ca ions is prior to that of phosphate ions(B.C.Yang et al., 1999).

AH treatment is a simple and economical method. It affects only the top 1 μm of the surface and its effects can extend all over the irregular surface of the implant, which is especially important for porous and porous-coated implants. The AH treatment can provide porous and porous-coated implants with bioactive surface while does not reduce the pore space available for bone ingrowth(Nishiguchi et al., 2001; Takemoto et al., 2005a).

Based on the AH treatment to improve the bioactivity of titanium and its alloys, many researchers have further optimized the treatment process for better bioactivity. Wei et al optimised the bioactivity of alkaline-treated titanium alloy by changing a variety of conditions for the AH treatments of Ti6Al4V alloy, and found that the rate of apatite formation on AH-treated titanium alloy could be significantly accelerated(M. Wei et al., 2002). Uchida et al conjoined the hot water and heat treatments after alkali treatment (Water-AH) to convert the sodium titanate gel into anatase, which significantly improved the apatite-forming ability of the metal in SBF(Uchida et al., 2002). Some researchers have successfully applied these techniques to porous or porous-coated metal implants, and these treated implants all showed apatite-forming ability in SBF(Fujibayashi et al., 2004; Nishiguchi et al., 2001; Takemoto et al., 2005a, 2006). Takemoto et al developed a dilute hydrochloric acid (HCl) treatment between alkali treatment and heat treatment (HCl-AH) for porous titanium implants, which could remove sodium from the alkali-treated porous titanium more effectively than conventional hot water treatment, and the subsequent heat treatment converted titania into anatase. The surface of HCl-AH implants possessed a more complex porous structure than the others, which showed a combination of large and small microporous structures. Both water-AH treated and HCl-AH treated porous titanium showed high apatite-forming ability after immersion in SBF. Island-like apatite deposits could be recognized on the surface of both implants within 1 day. There was larger size of the apatite deposits in the HCl-AH treated implants and higher number of spherulites in the Water-AH group(Fujibayashi et al., 2004; Takemoto et al., 2006).

In addition to titanium and its alloy, the AH treatment was also applied to other metals. Miyazaki et al treated tantalum in a 0.2 or 0.5M NaOH aqueous solution at 60°C for 24 h and the treated tantalum metal induced apatite deposition within 1 week in SBF(Miyazaki et al., 2000, 2001, 2002). High temperature and high pressure were also applied to the alkaline treatment in order to promote the deposition of apatite on the substrate from SBF(De Andrade et al., 2000).

2.2.3 Acid-alkali treatment

The main idea of acid-alkali (AA) treatment is to etch the metal surface with acid solution to acquire a uniform and rough surface, and the subsequent alkali treatment might have two concurrent effects: that is the formation of a microporous surface layer on the acid-etched surface and the formation of more titanium oxide layer on this microporous layer. Both steps are helpful to improve the bioactivity of titanium implants(Wen et al., 1997, 1998).

Wen et al used a mixture of 100 ml 18 wt% HCl and 100 ml 48 wt% H_2SO_4 solutions to etch titanium for 30 min and then treated them in boiling 0.2 M NaOH solution at 140°C for 5 h. Many micrometre-sized acid etched pits or grooves formed on the titanium surface by acid treatment, and large amounts of nanosized fine pits with more titanium oxide layer were produced on the surface by the alkali treatment. Combined acid treatment with alkali treatment, a completely microporous titanium oxide surface on a submicrometre scale was formed. Conformal and adherent apatite coating were rapidly precipitated on the AA-treated surfaces after soaking in supersaturated calcification solution (SCS)(Wen et al., 1997, 1998). When AA treatment was applied to porous titanium, it could induce apatite deposition on its inner pores(Zhao et al., 2010). HNO_3 and NaOH solution were also employed to prepare a bioactive layer on the surface of NiTi alloy, and an apatite layer was spontaneously deposited on the treated titanium surface after soaked in SBF(M.F.Chen et al., 2003).

In order to solve the inhomogeneous and non-uniform apatite deposition of NaOH-treated titanium after exposition in SBF, acid etching of titanium in HCl under inert atmosphere was used as a pretreatment to obtain a uniform micro-roughened surface before alkali treatment, and the acid etching provided an improved condition for homogenous apatite deposition(Jonášová et al., 2004).

Though NaOH-treated titanium could form a bone-like apatite layer on its surface in SBF via the release of Na^+, the inflammation response and cell death would occur if the released Na^+ increased external alkalinity (Silver et al., 2001). Therefore, it would be beneficial to decrease the release of Na^+ into the surrounding tissue. Jonášová et al washed NaOH-treated titanium with distilled water to lower the amount of Na^+ in the surface layer, and they found that the rate of apatite formation was not significantly influenced by a lower amount of Na^+ in the surface layer(Jonášová et al., 2002). Hot water or dilute HCl immersion were also used to partially or almost completely remove Na^+, and this had already been described above(Fujibayashi et al., 2004; Takemoto et al., 2006; Uchida et al., 2002).

2.2.4 Precalcification

The calcium ion implantation process developed by Hanawa et al was reported to form a continuous interface between the surface-modified layer and substrate, which was expected to prevent the interface fracture. Furthermore, the implanted calcium ions formed calcium titanate in the surface oxide layer, which could possibly accelerate apatite precipitation (Hanawa et al., 1994). However, the calcium ion implantation process required a special apparatus. Therefore, some simple processes for forming a calcium-ion-containing surface layer on titanium were explored. Hanawa et al reported that titanium plates were immersed in the calcium-ion-containing solutions, including calcium nitrate, calcium chloride and calcium oxide solution, at ambient temperature for 7 days, and a surface-modified layer consisting of calcium hydroxide and/or calcium titanate was formed on its surface. The surface-modified layer in which titanium was modified by calcium oxide was thickest. Apatite was deposited on the surface-modified titanium after immersion in HBSS(Hanawa et al., 1997).

Surface modification of titanium in CaO solution with hydrothermal treatment in an autoclave was also performed. This process enhanced apatite precipitation on the modified surface in HBSS, which resulted from the effects of high pH, high pressure and high temperature of the CaO solution on titanium surface(Hamada et al., 2002). Heat treatment above 600°C of hydrothermal-modified titanium in CaO solution could enhanced the apatite formation in SBF (Sultana et al., 2009). Hydrothermally deposit Ca ions on porous titanium in calcium hydroxide ($Ca(OH)_2$) solutions as a pre-treatment also endowed porous titanium with apatite-inducing ability(X.B.Chen et al., 2009). In addition, precalcification with boiling saturated $Ca(OH)_2$ solution was used to bioactivate titanium. After precalcification, a uniform calcium phosphate rapidly precipitated onto the surfaces of titanium in SCS(Feng et al., 2002a). Later, heat-treatment in water vapor was carried out prior to precalcification to improve the bond strength of the apatite coating to substrate(Feng et al., 2002b). Precalcification was also applied to AA- or AH-treated titanium by soaking them in Na_2HPO_4 and then saturated $Ca(OH)_2$ solution before immersion in SCS or SBF to speed up the formation of apatite(Liang et al., 2003; Wen et al., 1997).

2.2.5 H_2O_2 treatment

Titania gels were able to induce the precipitation of apatite when soaked in SBF(P. Li et al., 1994). The formation of titania gels on the surface of implant was therefore considered to be one of the potential approaches to improve the bioactivity of implant(P. Li & de Groot K., 1993; P. Li et al., 1994). It was known that biomaterials implanted into the body would cause inflammatory responses, which then resulted in generation of H_2O_2 around the implant(Tengvall et al., 1989a). The interaction between H_2O_2 and titanium implants were thought to be beneficial for the biocompatibility of the titanium(Baker et al., 2009; Tengvall et al., 1989b). Some reports showed that titanium could react with a H_2O_2 solution and formed titania gel(Tengvall & Lundström, 1992; Tengvall et al., 1989b, 1989c). Obviously, it could be an effective and convenient technique as a pretreatment of titanium. Depending on the H_2O_2 concentration and the treatment time, exposure titanium to H_2O_2 solution led to roughening and thickening of its surface oxide(MacDonald et al., 2004; Pan et al., 1996, 1998; Wälivaara et al., 1993). Pan et al. reported that the oxide was composed of a double layer structure with a thin and dense inner oxide and an porous outer layer(Pan et al., 1996, 1998). When titanium was treated in a H_2O_2/0.1M HCl solution at 80°C, an amorphous titania gel layer was formed on its surface. The thickness of the titania gel layers depended almost linearly on the period of time of the chemical treatment. The subsequent heat treatment above 300°C transformed the amorphous gel to crystalline anatase. The presence of rutile and the densification of the gel occurred concurrently when the temperature was raised

above 600°C. The minimum thickness of the titania gel layer reached about 0.2μm and the temperature of heat treatment between 400-500 exhibited excellent apatite-forming ability(Wang et al., 2002).
Titanium treated with a H_2O_2/3mM $TaCl_5$ solution at 80°C also yielded an amorphous titania gel on its surface. The subsequent heat treatment between 300-600°C transformed the amorphous gel to crystalline anatase. The anatase titania layer could induce apatite deposition within 1 day of immersion in SBF, and the thicker titania gels deposited more apatite than that of the thinner one. The nucleation of apatite preferentially took place inside the cracks in the thicker gel layers(Wang et al., 2000).
Although heat treatment after immersion in H_2O_2/0.1M HCl or H_2O_2/3mM $TaCl_5$ solution could induce crystallization of the amorphous titania, it was supposed to cause the loss of the Ti-OH groups that played an important role in initiating the deposition of apatite(H.M. Kim et al., 1997; Wang et al., 2000, 2002). Therefore, a low-temperature mild condition approach to prepare bioactive surface through interactions between titanium and H_2O_2 solutions was of great interest. Ohtsuki et al. reported that titanium treated with H_2O_2/$TaCl_5$ or H_2O_2/$SnCl_2$ solution at 60°C for 24h gave it apatite-forming ability after immersion in SBF. They thought that basic Ti-OH groups in titania hydrogel layers on their surfaces were responsible for apatite nucleation and growth(Ohtsuki et al., 1997). Wu et al soaked titanium in H_2O_2/3mM $TaCl_5$ solution at 80°C for 3 days, on which crystalline titania layers consisting of anatase and rutile were deposited. Those titania layers, regardless of the fraction of anatase and rutile, showed excellent ability to induce deposition of apatite(J.M.Wu et al., 2004).

2.2.6 Electrochemical methods

Electrochemical methods, including electrocrystallization(J.S. Chen et al., 1998; Shirkhanzadeh, 1995), electrophoretic deposition (Zhitomirsky & Gal-Or, 1997)and anodic oxidation(micro-arc oxidation)(Lausmaa, 2001; X.Y. Liu et al., 2004), are based on different chemical reactions occurring at an electrically energized surface (electrode) placed in an electrolyte. In this section, only the anodic oxidation (micro-arc oxidation) is introduced.
Micro-arc oxidation (MAO) is also called anodic spark oxidation or plasma electrolytic oxidation. It is a relatively convenient technique to form ceramic coatings on the surface of metals, such as Ti, Al, Mg and their alloys. The in situ formed ceramic coatings are porous and firmly bond to metal substrate. Furthermore, it is very suitable for modifying metal surfaces with complex geometries, even porous structure(Sun et al., 2008). Since Ishizawa and Ogino first developed anodic titanium oxide coatings containing Ca and P on titanium by using this technique(Ishizawa & Ogino, 1995a, b), the titania-based coatings formed by MAO can be divided into two categories. One is titania-based composite coatings consisting of TiO_2, $CaTiO_3$, $Ca_2P_2O_7$ and $Ca_3(PO_4)_2$ (Han et al., 2003; Huang et al., 2005; Song et al., 2004) or TiO_2 and hydroxyapatite (HA)(M. Kim et al., 2007; Sun et al., 2007), which was produced in electrolytes containing Ca and P at high applied voltage and could induce the formation of apatite on its surface. The other is monophasic TiO_2 coatings, which was produced in electrolytes containing Ca and P at applied voltages lower than 400 V(Ishizawa & Ogino, 1995a, b; D.Q. Wei et al., 2007; Zhu et al., 2001) or in electrolytes containing H_2SO_4, H_3PO_4 or HCl(Das et al., 2007; B.C. Yang et al., 2004). Although most monophasic TiO_2 coatings formed by MAO had no apatite-forming ability, the titanium anodically oxidized in H_2SO_4 solution under the conditions with spark-discharge could induce apatite formation on its surface after immersion in SBF. The increase of the amount of either anatase or rutile by conditioning the

anodic oxidation was helpful to shorten the induction period of apatite formation. However, the titanium anodically oxidized under the condition without spark discharge could not induce apatite formation, even though the anatase was also formed on its surface(B.C. Yang et al., 2004). In view of this, subsequent activation methods such as heat treatment(Das et al., 2007; B.C. Yang et al., 2004), hydrothermal treatment(Huang et al., 2004; Ishizawa & Ogino, 1995a), chemical treatment (D.Q. Wei et al., 2007)and ultraviolet (UV) irradiation(Han et al., 2008) were carried out to improve the bioactivity of the MAO-formed monophasic TiO_2 coatings. Micro-arc oxidation in the aqueous electrolytes containing NaOH was also used to treat porous titanium, and the bioactive thin films were formed on the porous titanium inner-pore walls. The thus-treated porous titanium showed apatite-forming ability in SBF(Sun et al., 2008).

2.3 Surface-induced mineralization (SIM)

Surface-induced mineralization (SIM) is based on the observation that in nature organisms use biopolymers to produce ceramic composites, such as teeth, bones, and shells. The SIM process includes modification of a surface to introduce surface functionalization followed by immersion in aqueous supersaturated calcium phosphate solutions. In short, this technique is based on crystal nucleation and growth onto functionalized interfaces(Bunker et al., 1994; Campbell et al., 1996).

Various functional groups have been introduced onto the surface of Ti and its alloys to functionalize the surface capable of nucleating apatite. Campbell et al. introduced the functionalized end groups including -COOH, $-SO_3H$, $-PO_4H_2$, $-CH_3$, and $-NH_2$ to the surface of Ti to initiate calcium phosphate deposition(Campbell et al., 1996). Mao et al. introduced highly organized arrangement of carboxyl and hydroxyl groups on the surface of hydroxylated titanium with strong (0001) texture through self-assembly of vinyltriethoxysilane. The functionalized substrate showed the ability to induce oriented nucleation and growth of HA (Mao et al., 1998). Majewski et al coated titanium with self-assembled monolayers (SAMs), NH_2-, SH-, and SO_3H-SAMs, respectively. The results showed apatite deposition from SBF and SH-SAM appeared to favor the formation of apatite(Majewski & Allidi, 2006). In another study, various functional groups were introduced onto the surface of commercially pure titanium foils using a SAM technique, and the results suggested that the pre-deposition of HA onto these functionalized SAM surfaces might be an effective and fast way to prepare biomimetic apatite coatings on surgical implants. These results suggested that surface functional groups could play a critical role in inducing Ca/P nucleation(Q. Liu et al., 2002).

3. Effect of simulated body fluid on biomimetic apatite coating

The simulated body fluid plays a significant role in determining the phase composition, crystallization, growth rate of biomimetic apatite coating, which actually are affected by the composition, concentration, pH, flowing state of simulated body fluid and its additives, such as trace elements, proteins and drugs.

3.1 History of the simulated body fluid

Human blood plasma has a Ca/P molar ratio of 2.50(Gamble, 1967). Many researchers try to develop the acellular simulated body fluid (SBF) by mimicking the inorganic ion concentrations of human blood plasma(Kokubo & Takadama, 2006; Kokubo, 1990a). The historical development of SBF which claims to imitate the human plasma or the extracellular fluid is given in Table 1. In the earlier solutions, Ringer's(Ringer, 1883), Earle's (EBSS, Earle's Balanced Salt Solution)(Earle, 1943) and Hank's (HBSS)(Hanks, 1975; Hanks & Wallace, 1949) solutions were very popular. Later, the pH values of SBF solutions were fixed at 7.4 by using TRIS (tris-hydroxymethyl-aminomethane)-HCl (hydrochloric acid) buffer solution, and the Ca/P molar ratio was raised to 2.50 (Kokubo et al., 1990b). However, the original SBF used by Kokubo et al. (Kokubo et al., 1990b) and Hench et al. (Filgueiras et al., 1993)

	Na^+	K^+	Mg^{2+}	Ca^{2+}	Cl^-	HCO_3^-	HPO_4^-	SO_4^{2-}	Buffer
Human blood plasma (Gamble, 1967)	142.0	5.0	1.5	2.5	103.0	27.0	1.0	0.5	
Ringer(Ringer,1883)	130	4.0		1.4	109.0				
EBSS(Earle, 1943)	143.5	5.37	0.8	1.8	123.5	26.2	1.0	0.8	
HBSS(Hanks,1975; Hanks.&Wallace, 1949)	142.1	5.33	0.9	1.26	146.8	4.2	0.78	0.41	
Original SBF (Kokubo et al., 1990b)	142.0	5.0	1.5	2.5	148.8	4.2	1.0	0	TRIS
c-SBF(Cho et al., 1995; Kokubo, 1991; Ohtsuki et al., 1991)	142.0	5.0	1.5	2.5	147.8	4.2	1.0	0.5	TRIS
Tas-SBF(Tas, 2000)	142.0	5.0	1.5	2.5	125.0	27.0	1.0	0.5	TRIS
Bigi-SBF(Bigi et al., 2000)	141.5	5.0	1.5	2.5	124.5	27.0	1.0	0.5	HEPES
r-SBF(Oyane et al., 2003)	142.0	5.0	1.5	2.5	103.0	27.0	1.0	0.5	HEPES
m-SBF(Oyane et al., 2003)	142.0	5.0	1.5	2.5	103.0	10.0	1.0	0.5	HEPES
i-SBF(Oyane et al., 2003)	142.0	5.0	1.0	1.6	103.0	27.0	1.0	0.5	HEPES
n-SBF(Takadama et al., 2004)	142.0	5.0	1.5	2.5	103.0	4.2	1.0	0.5	TRIS
SBF×5(Barrère et al.,2000a; Habibovic et al., 2002)	714.8		7.5	12.5	723.8	21.0	5.0		
SBFB×5(Habibovic et al., 2002)	704.2		1.5	12.5	711.8	10.5	5.0		
SCS1(Habibovic et al., 2005)	140.4			3.1	142.9		1.86		TRIS
SCS(Wen et al., 1997)	136.8	3.71		3.1	144.5		1.86		TRIS

Table 1. Ion concentrations of SBFs and human blood plasma

lacked the SO_4^{2-} ions which were contained in human blood plasma. In 1991, the corrected SBF papers were published by Kokubo et al(Kokubo, 1991; Ohtsuki C. et al., 1991), and the detailed recipe for preparation of SBF was reported in 1995 by Cho et al due to the difficulty to prepare clear SBF with no precipitation(Cho et al., 1995).
Since the corrected SBF was proposed by Kokubo et al, it still had higher Cl^- ion and lower HCO_3^- ion concentrations than human blood plasma, as could be seen from Table 1. Therefore, a number of slightly different compositions were proposed. Tas et al. used di-sodium hydrogen phosphate in place of di-potassium hydrogen phosphate to raise the HCO_3^- concentration to 27 mM in a TRIS-HCl buffered SBF solution (i.e., Tas-SBF)(Tas, 2000). Bigi et al. increased the content of carbonate ions to 27mM HCO_3^- in a HEPES-NaOH-buffered SBF solution (i.e., Bigi-SBF)(Bigi et al., 2000). Oyane et al. tried to correct this difference. They prepared r-SBF and i-SBF, which had ion concentrations equal to those of blood plasma, and m-SBF, which had ion concentrations equal to those of blood plasma except for the HCO_3^- concentration. However, r-SBF and i-SBF lacked long-term stability due to a strong tendency to precipitate both apatite and calcite from these SBF(Oyane et al., 2003). It was reported that the buffering agent TRIS present in conventional SBF (c- and Tas-SBF) formulations could form soluble complexes with several cations, including Ca^{2+}, which further reduced the concentration of free Ca^{2+} ions available for apatite formation, while HEPES did not show this behavior(Jalota et al., 2007; Serro & Saramago, 2003). Takadama et al. reported a newly improved SBF (n-SBF). They decreased the Cl^- ion concentration equal to those of blood plasma, but maintained the HCO_3^- ion concentration equal to that of the corrected SBF (c-SBF)(Takadama et al., 2004). After comparison with c-SBF, the n-SBF did not differ from c-SBF in stability and reproducibility. In 2003, conventional SBF with the refined recipe was proposed to a standard solution for in vitro measurement of apatite-forming ability of implant materials (Kokubo & Takadama, 2006).
Although SBF mimicked the inorganic composition and the pH of human blood plasma and it was employed by many investigators to produce biomimetic apatite coating on implant surfaces, it would take several days with daily refreshments of SBF solution due to the slow apatite nucleation process(P. Li et al., 1994; P. Li & Ducheyne, 1998; Peltola et al., 1998). In order to shorten the apatite nucleation time, more concentrated SBFs, such as 1.5 SBF(Abe et al., 1990), SBF×5(Barrère et al., 2000a, 2001; Habibovic et al., 2002) or SBF×10(Tas & Bhaduri, 2004), were used. It should be note that SBF×5 was five times more concentrated than c-SBF recipe, but TRIS- or HEPES-free. Instead of activating the metal surface by the above methods, non-bioactive materials could also be coated by SBF×5 immersion, and the induction time of apatite was shortened when compared to incubation in 1.0 SBF(Barrère et al., 2000a, 2001; Habibovic et al., 2002).

3.2 Effects of ion concentration and type in simulated body fluid on biomimetic apatite coatings

Biomimetic apatite coatings based on heterogeneous nucleation of apatite have been successfully obtained after immersion the pretreated metal implants in SBF. However, it would take several days with daily refreshing of SBF solution due to the metastability of SBF at physiological conditions (P. Li et al., 1994; P. Li & Ducheyne, 1998; Peltola et al., 1998). In order to accelerate the coating process, one approach was to pretreat metal implants with more effective methods to enhance the deposition of apatite as described above. Another possibility for shortening the coating process was by concentrating the SBF solution. A 5 times more concentrated SBF (so-called SBF×5) was developed by decreasing pH with carbon dioxide gas. The subsequent release of carbon dioxide resulting in a pH increase and thus increasing supersaturation of SBF×5 solution. This process allowed the deposition of a uniform apatite coating within 24 h without refreshing the metastable solution. The coating was dense and composed of globules with amorphous carbonated apatite(Barrère et al., 2000a).

The formation and properties of biomimetic apatite coatings on titanium were strongly related to the ionic strength, carbonate and magnesium contents in the SBF×5 solution.

NaCl controlled the ionic strength of the solution, and thereby controlled CO_2 release, i.e. pH profile. Low ionic strength in SBF×5 solution led to the earlier precipitation in the solution resulting in later and thinner formation of apatite coating on Ti6Al4V, while high ionic strength delayed precipitation in the solution and favored apatite heterogeneous nucleation on Ti6Al4V(Barrère et al., 2002a).

HCO_3^- content increased the pH of the solution due to its buffering capacity and influenced the release rate of dissolved CO_2. Thus, HCO_3^- content strongly affected the supersaturation and apatite structure. Furthermore, HCO_3^- favored the attachment of apatite on Ti6Al4V by decreasing apatite crystal size resulting in a better physical attachment of apatite coating on Ti6Al4V substrate(Barrère et al., 2002a).

The formation and attachment of apatite coating was strongly related to Mg^{2+} content. Mg^{2+} inhibited precipitation in the solution and favored the formation of apatite coating due to its relatively high concentration at the coating/substrate interface. It had a stronger inhibitory effect on apatite crystal growth than HCO_3^-. Mg^{2+} content in SBF×5 solution also changed the phase composition and crystallinity of the coating(Barrère et al., 2002b).

A two-step method was developed to deposit CA or OCP coating on titanium implants. The implants were first soaked in a SBF×5 solution for 24 h to seed the metal surface with calcium phosphate nuclei. Then, the implants were soaked for another 24 h in a SBFB×5 solution to induce the fast growth of CA coating. The CA coating consisted of well-formed crystals 1-3μm in size uniformly precipitated on the surface of implant. The thickness of coating was approximately 30μm, the crystallinity was around 75% and Ca/P ratio was 1.67. A homogeneous CA coatings in thickness was deposited on the entire surface of porous implants(Barrère et al., 2003c; Habibovic et al., 2002).

By changing the SBFB×5 into SCS 1 and prolonging the immersion time to 48h, OCP coating with a 55 μm in thickness homogeneously was deposited on the surface of the metal. Large crystals 30-60 μm in size perpendicularly grew onto the metal surface. The crystallinity of the coating was around 100% and its Ca/P ratio 1.33(Barrère et al., 2001). However, the thickness of the OCP coating was not the same throughout the porous implant. It was thicker at the exterior of the porous implant than that of the interior(Barrère et al., 2003a; Habibovic et al., 2005).

3.3 Effects of pH of simulated body fluid on biomimetic apatite coatings

Barrère et al. systematically investigated the interdependence of ionic strength, pH, carbonate concentration in SBF×5 solution, and their influences on the formation of the resultant apatite(Barrère et al., 2002a). Later, the influence of Mg^{2+} on pH was investigated(Barrère et al., 2002b). However, the pH in these studies was indirectly controlled by ionic strength, carbonate concentration or Mg^{2+} of SBF×5 solution. Li et al reported that Ca/P molar ratios and chemical compositions of the calcium phosphate precipitates were affected by the pH of the SBF, and an apatite with Ca/P molar ratio close to the HA was obtained if the pH of the solution was continuously adjusted to 7.26 during calcium phosphate precipitated from SBF(J.G. Li, et al., 1997). Chou et al used two-step immersion process to investigate the influence of solution pH of initial SBF×5 solution on micro-structural evolution and final apatite structure. They first immersed the argon plasma etched polystyrene culture dishes into SBF×5 solution with different pH (5.8 or 6.5), then immersed into the identical Mg^{2+} and HCO_3^--free SBF×5 (pH=6.0). The results showed that the pH of the initial SBF×5 solution influenced the final structure of the crystalline apatite. Precursor spheres formed with high initial pH of SBF×5 (pH 6.5) transformed into larger, single crystals plates, while precursor spheres formed with low initial pH of SBF×5 (pH 5.8) developed minute, polycrystalline plate-like structures over predominantly spherical precursor substrate(Chou et al., 2004).

3.4 Effects of flowing state of simulated body fluid on biomimetic apatite coatings

The immersion process in simulated body fluid required daily refreshment of SBF to maintain ions concentration and a constant pH for apatite growth. However, most of soaking processes were maintained under static conditions without fluid flow, which might lead to local precipitation or uneven coatings (Habibovic et al, 2004a). Body fluid of human was a dynamic circulating system, so the flowing SBF was better in mimicking the living body fluid than static one. Habibovic et al soaked the implants into more concentrated body fluids with stirring at a speed of 250 rounds per minute to make the SBF homogeneous(Habibovic et al., 2002). Siriphannon et al investigated the formation of HA in simulated body fluid under static and flowing systems, and found that compared with static systems, the formation of HA layer under flowing SBF differed in the formation rates, formation behavior, and microstructure(Siriphannon et al., 2002). Papadopoulou et al investigated the surface changes of dental ceramics coated with bioactive glass after exposure in a simulated body fluid under static and dynamic conditions. The CA layer formed on the surface of material in static environment was more dense and compact than that formed under dynamic conditions(Papadopoulou et al., 2003). Deng et al investigated the influence of dynamic flow rate on bone-like apatite formation in porous calcium phosphate ceramic in revised simulated body fluid (r-SBF). They reported that the crystal shape of bone-like apatite changed with the flow rate(Deng et al., 2005).

3.5 Effects of trace elements in simulated body fluid on biomimetic apatite coatings

Bone mineral contains calcium, phosphate,carbonate and other inorganic compounds such as sodium, fluoride, chloride, magnesium, strontium, zinc, copper and iron in varying quantities. These elements can affect bone mineral characteristics, such as crystallinity, degradation behavior and mechanical properties(Becker et al., 1968; L.Yang et al., 2010). Many researchers studied the possibility to incorporate different ions into the apatite by a biomimetic method.

Oliveira et al incorporated different amounts of Sr into nano-apatite coatings by adding $SrCl_2$ in SBF solution with higher concentrations of Ca^{2+} and HPO_4^{2-} than that of human blood plasma. The presence of Sr ions in solution inhibited the apatite formation and resulted in the decrease of coating thickness, and it incorporated in the apatite layer by replacing Ca in the apatite lattice(Oliveira et al., 2007). Bracci et al employed a modified calcium phosphate calcifying solution by replacing part of Ca^{2+} ions with Sr^{2+} and Mn^{2+} ions to investigate the influences of Sr^{2+} and Mn^{2+} ions on the chemical, structural and morphology of coatings deposited on metallic substrates. A Sr-containing hydroxyapatite was deposited on metallic substrates in a few hours, but the presence of Sr^{2+} inhibited apatite precipitation, reduced the dimensions of the spherical aggregates and decreased the degree of crystallinity of apatite. Mn^{2+} ions completely hindered the precipitation of apatite and yielded an amorphous phosphate relatively rich in Mn(Bracci et al., 2009). In addition, cobalt, copper, zinc, strontium and fluoride with varying concentrations were incorporated in the calcium phosphate films by using a biomimetic approach consisting of precalcification and calcification steps. The additives affected morphology and composition of calcium phosphate films to different extent by a dose dependent manner(Patntirapong et al., 2009; L.Yang et al., 2010).

3.6 Effects of protein addition in simulated body fluid on biomimetic apatite coatings

With the plasma-spraying technique, it is impossible for biologically active molecules such as osteogenetic agents and growth factors to incorporate the HA coating during spray process due to the extremely high temperatures(>10,000°C). However, the development of biomimetic coating techniques make it possible, which involves soaking the implants in supersaturated calcium phosphate solutions at physiological temperatures(Abe et al., 1990). By this technique, biologically active molecules can be coprecipitated with apatite crystals onto metal implants rather than being merely adsorbed on its surface(Y. Liu et al., 2001, 2003, 2006; Wen et al., 1999). Therefore, the biomimetic apatite coating can be used as the carriers for biologically active molecules. After implantation in vivo, the degradation of these biomimetic coatings would lead to the gradual exposure and release of incorporated molecules from these coatings rather than in a single rapid burst, which also renders the biomimetic coatings of great potential value as a drug-carrier system in orthopedics(Y. Liu et al., 2006).

Liu et al first biomimetically precoated titanium alloy implants with a thin and dense layer of calcium phosphate, and then incubated in a supersaturated solution of calcium phosphate with bovine serum albumin (BSA) at various concentrations under physiological conditions for 48 h. BSA successfully coprecipitated with the Ca^{2+} and PO_4^{3-} ions on the surface of Ti alloy implants, and the release of this protein from the biomimetic coatings took place gradually over the span of several days. BSA influenced the properties of biomimetic coating in a concentration-dependent manner. With the increase of BSA concentration, the coatings became denser and thinner, and showed smaller crystal size and lower crystallinity. Crystal geometry changed more curve, and crystal structure of the coating transformed from an OCP to a CA(Y. Liu et al., 2001). Wen et al pretreated titanium by acid etching, boiling diluted alkali incubation, precalcification, and immersed it in SCS with or without containing BSA. Their results also showed that the incorporation of BSA significantly modified the morphology, composition, and crystallinity of the apatite coating(Wen et al., 1999). The release rate of Ca^{2+} ions from these BSA-containing apatite layers was slower than from non-protein-containing ones within the bathing medium, which indicated that BSA bonded strongly to Ca^{2+} ions within the crystal lattice. BSA incorporated into the crystal lattice enhanced the mechanical strength of coating in a concentration-dependent manner within the bathing medium (Y. Liu et al., 2003).

Fibronectin is known to promote cell adhesion, which plays a special role in the process of osteointegration due to its ability to attach osteoblasts to the extracellular matrix components, in spite of its low concentration (~0.2 mg/ml) in biological fluids(Tamada &

Ikada, 1993). Furthermore, it contains calcium-sensitive heparin binding sites, which should interfere with the apatite deposition. When fibronectin was dissolved in HBSS, the influence of fibronectin on apatite deposition was found to be concentration-dependent. Low concentration of fibronectin (0.01 mg/ml) did not significantly affect apatite precipitation, but when increased to 0.05 mg/ml, it strongly inhibited the apatite nucleation(do Serro et al., 2000).
In a study by Liu et al. Recombinant Human Bone Morphogenetic Protein -2(rh-BMP-2) was incorporated in a dose-dependent manner into biomimetic apatite coatings on titanium implants. The incorporated BMP-2 underwent gradual release (over a period of weeks) into the surrounding tissue wherein it retained its biological activity. Its biological performance will be described later(Y. Liu et al., 2006). Uchida et al immobilized laminin on titanium by immersion the AH -treated titanium in a calcium phosphate solution containing laminin at 25°C for 1 day(Uchida et al., 2004).

3.7 Effects of drugs in simulated body fluid on biomimetic apatite coatings

Bone infections still represent a challenging problem for orthopaedic implant surgery, which result from the poor access to the bone-infected site by systemically administered antibiotics. Local therapy is therefore desired and can be achieved by using a suitable carrier for a controlled drug delivery(Radin et al., 1997). Polymethylmethacrylate (PMMA) cement is a standard antibiotic carrier used in clinic, and PMMA beads loaded with antibiotics is frequently used for the treatment of infections(Buchholz et al., 1984; Garvin et al., 1988; Henry et al., 1991; Josefsson et al., 1990). However, the need for a second operation to remove the non-absorbable PMMA beads and the possibility of thermal damage to the antibiotics caused by the exothermic polymerization reaction of the cement is still a problem(Radin et al., 1997). Furthermore, the non-absorbable drug carrier like PMMA, and the biodegradable drug carriers, such as poly(lactide/glycolide) copolymer and poly(propylene glycol-fumerate)/methyl methacrylate composite are non-bioactive(Gerhart et al., 1993; Garvin & Feschuk, 2005; Henry et al., 1991). Therefore, combining osteoconductive properties of bioactive materials with a local and sustained release of antibiotic can be used to not only enhance early osteointegration of implants, but also prevent post-surgical infections. However, like proteins and biologically active agents, the antibiotic can not be incorporated during the preparation of plasma-sprayed HA coating or ceramics due to the extremely high processing temperature. The adsorption of these antibiotic drugs on the surface of these bioactive materials limits their loading and release characteristics.
Loading antibiotic by using a biomimetic method attracted much attention. Campbell and coworkers incorporated an antibiotic chlorhexidine into apatite coatings by using a surface induced mineralization approach. After treating with silane-coupling molecules and sulfonation, the substrates were immersed into various chlorhexidine solutions between mineralization cycles. The release test showed an initial rapid antibiotic release followed by a period of slower sustained release. The apatite containing chlorhexidine showed good anti-microbial efficacy(Campbell et al., 2000).
In a study by Stigter et al., the metal implants were first immersed into a SBF×5 at 37°C for 24 h to obtain a thin ACP coating for inducing the subsequent precipitation. The ACP-coated implants were then immersed in a supersaturated calcium phosphate (SCP) solution containing various concentrations of tobramycin at 37°C for 48 h, and different quantities of tobramycin was co-precipitated with a CA coating on the surface of

implants. With the increase of the amount of incorporated tobramycin, the thickness of coating decreased, but it did not change the morphology of the coating. The dissolution of coating showed a fast initial dissolution of the coating followed by a plateau at both pH 7.3 and at pH 5, initial dissolution rate and at total release of calcium at pH 7.3 were slower and lower than that at pH 5. The release rate of tobramycin was gradual and faster at pH 7.3 than at pH 5. Tobramycin released from the biomimetic apatite coating could inhibit growth of Staphylococcus aureus bacteria in vitro(Stigter et al., 2002). Later, different antibiotics including acidic antibiotics with almost similar chemical structure such as cephalothin, cefamandol, amoxicillin and carbenicillin and basic antibiotics such as vancomycin, gentamicin and tobramycin were incorporated into the CA coatings, and their release and efficacy against bacteria growth were investigated in vitro. With the increase of concentrations of antibiotics in SCP solution, more antibiotic incorporated into the CA coating. The incorporation efficiency of antibiotic was strongly related to their chemical structure. Antibiotics containing carboxylic groups were better incorporated than that lacking these groups, but slower released from the CA coating, which probably resulted from the binding or chelating between carboxylic groups in their chemical structure and calcium. All antibiotics that were released from the CA coating showed inhibition of growth of Staphylococcus aureus bacteria(Stigter et al., 2004). In another study, antibiotics cephradine containing carboxylic groups in simulated body fluid was also found to be beneficial for the apatite coprecipitation. However, the coprecipitation did not take place between apatite and a traditional Chinese medicine salviae miltlorrhizae (SM). The authors speculated that Chinese medicine SM was probably more absorbed on the surface of the Ti, when calcium and phosphate ions precipitated(Z. Wu et al., 2008).

4. Biological performance of biomimetic apatie coatings

The purpose of pretreatments and the biomimetic apatite coating process was to obtain satisfactory biological performance. The biomimetic apatite coating formed in vitro and in vivo determined its biological performance.

4.1 Effects of biomimetic apatite coatings on in vitro behavior of osteoblasts and osteoclasts

Leeuwenburgh et al investigated the resorption behavior of three different biomimetic calcium phosphate coatings (ACP, CA and OCP) by using osteoclast-enriched mouse bone-marrow cell cultures for 7 days. No release of particles and morphologic changes could be observed for all biomimetic coatings after preincubation for 7 days in α-minimal essential medium(α-MEM). However, both CA and OCP coatings degraded in the presence of cells. Osteoclasts degraded the CA coatings by normal osteoclastic resorption, but the resorption pattern of the OCP coatings differed from that of CA coatings. It seemed that ACP coating was too thin to detect resorption lacunae, if there were any. The nature of the apatite coatings such as crystal size and chemical composition influenced the cell-mediated degradation(Leeuwenburgh et al., 2001).

The biomimetic apatite on the surface of AH-treated titanium through immersion in SBF could promote differentiation of bone marrow stromal cells along osteogenic lineage(Nishio et al., 2000). Jalota et al showed that, compared with the neat and NaOH-treated titanium foams, biomimetically apatite coating on the surface of titanium foams formed in 1.5×Tas-

SBF exhibited the highest protein production and rat osteoblasts attachment (Jalota et al., 2007).

Trace elements in the biomimetic coating also influenced the cell behavior. Mg-containing apatite, Sr-containing apatite and an amorphous phosphate relatively rich in Mn coating promoted human osteoblast-like MG-63 cells differentiation and mineralization due to the presence of the ions, and the differentiation and mineralization followed the order: $Mg^{2+} < Sr^{2+} < Mn^{2+}$. Mg^{2+} and Sr^{2+} apatite coatings promoted proliferation and expression of collagen type I while the relatively high content of Mn^{2+} in the phosphate had a significant beneficial effect on osteocalcin production(Bracci et al., 2009).

Yang et al investigated the effects of inorganic additives (copper, zinc, strontium, fluoride and carbonate) to calcium phosphate coating on in vitro behavior of osteoblasts and osteoclasts by a medium-throughput system based on deposition of calcium phosphate films in multi-well tissue culture plates. The proliferation and differentiation of MC3T3-E1 osteoblasts on these films depended on the inorganic additives and concentration tested. In general, copper and zinc ions inhibited osteoblast proliferation, but had no effect or mild inhibitory on osteoblast differentiation. The effect of strontium on osteoblast proliferation was concentration-dependent, whereas both films containing fluoride and carbonate augmented osteoblast proliferation. Compared with the control films without additives, strontium, fluoride and carbonate ions clearly decreased osteoblast differentiation. The resorptive activity of primary rabbit osteoclasts cultured on calcium phosphate films containing additives significantly decreased and it was concentration-dependent as compared to the control, independent of the element incorporated. The elements in the tested concentrations showed no cytotoxic effect(L.Yang et al., 2010). In another study by Patntirapong et al, calcium phosphate film with Co^{2+} incorporation increased both osteoclast differentiation and resorptive function(Patntirapong et al., 2009).

4.2 Bone tissue engineering on apatite-coated titanium discs

Bone tissue engineering has already been proven to be feasible in porous scaffold by many research groups, and the in vitro bone tissue engineering constructs can provide implants with better fixation(Burg et al., 2000; Hutmacher, 2000; Rezwan et al., 2006; Rose & Oreffo, 2002). Dekker et al first showed that tissue engineering technology was effective on flat surfaces. They seeded both primary and subcultured rat bone marrow cells on biomimetic amorphous calcium phosphate-coated titanium plates and cultured in the presence or absence of dexamethasone for 7 days, then subcutaneously implanted in nude mice for 4 weeks. De novo bone formation was detected on the calcium phosphate-coated plates with primary or subcultured cells, which had been continuously cultured in medium with dexamethasone(Dekker et al., 1998).

In another study by Dekker et al, subcultured rat bone marrow cells were seeded on the amorphous CA and crystalline OCP-coated discs for their use in bone tissue engineering. After 1 week of culture, the cells covered the entire surface of all substrates with a continuous multi-layer. The crystalline OCP-coated discs were higher in the amount of cells while the amorphous CA-coated discs exhibited a visually higher in the amount of mineralized extracellular matrix. After subcutaneously implanted in nude mice for 4 week, clear de novo bone formation was observed on all discs with cultured cells. Compared to the amorphous CA-coated discs, the newly formed bone on the crystalline OCP-coated discs was more organized and showed a significantly higher volume and the percentage of bone contact(Dekker et al., 2005).

4.3 Effects of biomimetic apatite coatings on osteoinduction of implants

Yuan et al. reported that OCP-coated porous tantalum implants induced bone formation after implantation in the dorsal muscles of adult dogs for 3 months, while the uncoated one did not(Yuan, 2001).

In the goat study by Barrère et al. porous Ta and dense Ti alloy (The alloy had a dense surface, but it had a center hole with a diameter of 2.5 mm, with one side open and the other side closed) with OCP coating were implanted in the dorsal muscles of goats at 12 and 24 weeks. Both OCP-coated implants induced ectopic bone formation, and the newly formed bone was observed either in the inner pores of porous Ta or in the inner cavity of the dense Ti alloy, but not on flat surface of dense Ti alloy. The formed bone was in direct contact with the implants without the intervention of fibrous tissue. On the other hand, uncoated implants did not show any ectopic bone formation. This study indicated that both the presence of a Ca-P coating and the architecture of the implant were important factors for inducing ectopic bone formation(Barrère et al., 2003a). A similar study by Habibovic et al. showed that OCP-coated porous Ti alloy implants could also induce ectopic bone formation after implanted intramuscularly for 6 and 12 weeks in goats(Habibovic et al., 2005).

Another goat study by Habibovic et al. investigated the influence of OCP coating on osteoinductive performance of different porous materials. Their results showed that the OCP coating could improve the osteoinductive potential of different kinds of orthopedic implants(Habibovic et al., 2004b).

In a study by Liu et al. rh-BMP-2 was incorporated into OCP coating on Ti alloy implants, and subsequently implanted in a rat model to investigate protein release and osteoinduction. The incorporated BMP-2 which retained its biological activity was gradually released from the coating and induced the formation of bone tissue not only upon the implant surface but also within its immediate surroundings(Y. Liu et al., 2006).

Apart from coating implants with apatite in vitro, the bioactive implants which could induce bone-like apatite in vivo also had the ability to induce ectopic bone formation. Fujibayashi et al first reported that the non-soluble plasma-sprayed porous titanium metal that contained no calcium or phosphorus could induce ectopic bone formation when treated by water-AH treatments to form an appropriate microstructure(Fujibayashi et al., 2004). The water-AH treated porous titanium showed an in vitro apatite-forming ability after soaked in the SBF within a 7-day period(Fujibayashi et al., 2004). Though the in vitro apatite-forming ability of the samples could not reflect completely its in vivo behavior, it was widely believed that bone-like apatite layer formation on the pore surface in the early stages was a key factor for bone induction by non-CaP biomaterials and CaP-based porous ceramics(Habibovic & de Groot, 2007; X.D. Zhang et al., 2000). Takemoto et al. had partially confirmed the existence of bone-like apatite on the porous bioactive titanium by SEM-EDX, which were implanted in the dorsal muscles of beagle dogs(Takemoto et al., 2006). Later, our group found that porous titanium with a series of surface treatments, such as AA treatment(Zhao et al. 2010b), H_2O_2 treatment and $H_2O_2/TaCl_5$ treatment(unpublished data), could induce ectopic formation after implantation in the dorsal muscles of dogs for 3 or 5 months. Porous titanium with those treatments all showed in vitro apatite-forming ability after immersion in SBF for only one day(Zhao et al. 2010b).

Although the exact mechanism of osteoinduction by biomaterials was still not well understood, some previous studies reported that osteoinductive biomaterials showed better performance than non-osteoinductive one at orthotopic sites(Habibovic & de Groot, 2007; Habibovic et al., 2005, 2006). Therefore, the osteoinductive porous metals with good biomechanical compatibility were attractive in clinical application under load-bearing conditions.

4.4 Effects of biomimetic apatite coatings on osteointegration or osteogenecity of implants

In a study by Barrère et al, uncoated and bone-like carbonated apatite (BCA)-coated dense titanium alloy (Ti6Al4V) and porous Ta cylinders were implanted in the femoral diaphysis of adult female goats in a press-fit manner for 6, 12, and 24 weeks. Bone contact was always found significantly higher for BCA-coated dense Ti6Al4V and porous Ta cylinders than the corresponding uncoated one, which indicated that BCA coating enhanced the bone integration as compared to the uncoated implants and was highly beneficial for the long-term fixation of metal prostheses in load-bearing applications(Barrère et al., 2003c).

In another study, Barrère et al compared the osteogenic potentials of BCA-coated, OCP-coated, and bare porous tantalum cylinders in a gap of 1 mm created in the femoral condyle of a goat at 12 weeks. After 12 weeks, bone did not fill the gap in any of the porous implants, but OCP-coated porous cylinders exhibited bone formation in the center of the implant compared to the two other groups. This study suggested that the nature of the Ca-P coating, via its microstructure, dissolution rate, and specific interactions with body fluid, might influence the osteogenecity of the Ca-P biomaterial(Barrère et al., 2003a). Similar to the previously described study, Habibovic et al. found that the application of OCP coating on porous Ti6Al4V implants could improve its performance in bone healing process in femoral defects of goats(Habibovic et al., 2005). In a study, AA- or AH-pretreated porous titanium with biomimetic apatite coatings were hemi-transcortically implanted into the femurs of dogs for 2 months, and they showed excellent osteointegration with host bone(Zhao et al., 2010a).

Yan et al investigated the effects of AH treatment, and bone-like apatite-formed on titanium after such treatment on the bone-bonding ability of Ti implants by implanted into the tibial metaphyses of mature rabbits. Both treated implants exhibited significantly higher failure loads compared with untreated Ti implants at all time periods and directly bonded to bone tissue during the early post-implantation period. Scanning electron microscopy-energy dispersive X-ray microanalysis (SEM-EMPA) showed a uniform calcium- and phosphorus-rich layer was detected at the interface between the treated implants and bone, which indicated that Ti implants with AH treatment could induce bone-like apatite deposition in vivo, and therefore accelerated the bone-bonding behavior of implants and enhanced the strength of bone-implant bonding(Yan et al., 1997a, 1997b). Titanium alloys with AH treatment showed a similar enhancement of the bonding strength(Nishiguchi et al., 1999a). However, heat treatment after alkali treatment was an essential step for good bone-bonding ability. The unstable reactive surface layer of alkali-treated titanium would result in no bone-bonding ability(Nishiguchi et al., 1999b). AH-treated titanium cylindrical mesh cage was successfully used to repair a segmental rabbit femur defect, and it enhanced the bone repairing process and achieved faster repair of long bone segmental defects(Fujibayashi et al., 2003). It could also provide porous titanium coating implants with earlier stable fixation(Nishiguchi et al., 2001).

Water-AH-treated Ti could achieve earlier fixation than AH-treated one because of the formation of anatase, but sodium removal decreased the bonding strength between the implants and bones due to the loss of the surface graded structure of the bioactive layer(Fujibayashi et al., 2001). On the other hand, Water-AH-treated porous titanium enhanced bone ingrowth and apposition(Takemoto et al., 2005b). In addition, AH-treated tantalum implants also could bond to bone(Kato et al., 2000).

Hydrogen peroxide solution containing tantalum chloride ($H_2O_2/TaCl_5$) treatment was also used to provide titanium with the apatite-forming ability in SBF(Ohtsuki et al., 1997). $H_2O_2/TaCl_5$ -treated titanium implants showed higher bonding strength with living bone than untreated one after implantation in rabbit tibia, which was attributed to high potential of osteoconductive properties and/or direct bonding to living bone(Kaneko et al., 2001). It was reported that bonding phenomena between implants and living bone was initiated by the formation of a bone-like apatite layer on the surface of implants(Neo et al., 1993). Titanium fiber mesh treated by the same method enhanced bone growth and achieved faster tight bonding with bone than untreated titanium fiber mesh(T. Kim et al., 2003).

4.5 In vitro and in vivo degradation of biomimetic apatite coating

When biomimetic apatite-coated metal was implanted in vivo, they reacted dynamically towards the surrounding body fluids and showed a series of different biological behavior such as enhancing bone integration, inducing ectopic bone formation and combining with cultured bone marrow cells to inducing bone formation, which was closely related to the degradation behavior of the coating (Barrère et al., 2003a, 2003c; Dekker et al., 1998, 2005; Habibovic et al., 2005).

In a simulated physiological solution CA and OCP coatings showed different dissolution rates. CA dissolved faster than OCP at pH = 7.3 while CA dissolved slower than OCP at pH = 5.0(Barrère et al., 2000b). When the coated plates were soaked in α-MEM for 1, 2, and 4 weeks and were implanted subcutaneously in Wistar rats for similar periods. A carbonate apatite formed onto CA and OCP coatings via a dissolution-precipitation process both in vitro and in vivo, and organic compounds incorporated the carbonate apatite coating in vivo. However, both coatings dissolved overtime in vitro, whereas in vivo CA calcified and OCP partially dissolved after 1 week. Specific incorporations of organic compounds, different surface microstructure, different thermodynamic stability, or a combination of all these factors could contribute to the different degradation behavior of OCP and CA coatings(Barrère et al., 2003b).

In the study of femoral diaphysis of goats by Barrère et al, CA coating completely dissolved in the medullar cavity after 6 weeks of implantation. On the other hand, the coating thickness decreased with time and it was still present even after 24 weeks of implantation in the cortical region. The coating only remained on the implants when it was integrated in the newly formed bone. The in vivo degradation of CA coating was related to mechanical forces, dissolution, cellular activity, or combinations of those effects(Barrère et al., 2003c).

Intramuscular implantation of OCP-coated Ti6Al4V cylinders and porous tantalum cylinders in the goat showed that, after 12 and 24 weeks, the OCP coating had dissolved extensively and remained in only some places after 12 weeks of implantation. The remaining OCP coating on porous tantalum cylinders was detected as an integrated layer in the newly formed bone. After 12 weeks of gap-healing implantation in the femoral condyle of goat, the CA coating on porous tantalum cylinders had almost completely disappeared while the OCP coating partially remained after 12 weeks of implantation. In a bony environment, physic-chemistry of the Ca-P coating determined the osteoclastic activity. The osteoclastic activity of CA coating was supposed to by higher in vivo than that of OCP coatings(Barrère et al., 2003a). In a in vitro study by Leeuwenburgh et al. CA coatings were

resorbed by osteoclasts in a normal osteoclastic resorption manner while OCP coatings were degraded not by classical pit formation(Leeuwenburgh et al., 2001).
In another study by Habibovic et al, OCP-coated porous Ti6Al4V implants was implanted in the back muscle and femur of goats for 6 and 12 weeks. The in vivo dissolution behavior of the OCP coating was similar to that on porous tantalum cylinders. After 6 weeks of intramuscular implantation, the OCP coating had extensively dissolved. In the remaining OCP coating areas, signs of its resorption by multinucleated cells could be observed. After 12 weeks of implantation, the coating was further degraded and could only occasionally be detected. The remaining OCP coating was often observed to incorporate into the newly formed bone(Habibovic et al., 2005).

5. Conclusions

Biomimetic coating process allows the deposition of an apatite layer on the complex-shaped implant or within the porous implant at low temperature. The thus-treated implants show excellent bioactivity and can bond to living bone directly. The properties of the biomimetic coatings can be adjusted by controlling the process parameters to meet specific clinic needs. The biomimetic apatite coating also can be used as a carrier of biologically active molecules, such as osteogenetic agents and growth factors, or drugs. Furthermore, it is simple and cost-effective. It offers the most promising alternative to plasma spraying and other coating methods. However, the biomimetic apatite coatings are still unsatisfactory and remain under investigation. The lower bond strengths between biomimetic-deposited apatite coating and its underlying substrate have limited their applications for clinical use. The in vivo cirumstances are far more complex than that of in vitro biomimetic process. Therefore, the mechanism of biomineralization is needed to be further investigated and combine the biomimetic process to develop implants with better performance. On the other hand, the pretreatments on metals that can induce bone-like apatite deposition in vivo provide another promising process for better biological performance. The pretreatments that can induce faster bone-like apatite deposition in vivo and earlier fixation with bone tissue are needed to be developed.

6. References

Abe, Y., Kokubo T., & Yamamuro T. (1990). Apatite coating on ceramics, metals and polymers utilizing a biological process. *Journal of Materials Science: Materials in Medicine*, Vol. 1, No.4, pp. 233-238.

ASTM standard B600. (1997). Standard guide for descaling and cleaning titanium and titanium alloy surfaces, In: *Annual Book of ASTM Standard*, Vol. 2.04, pp. 6-8, American Society for Testing and Materials, Philadelphia, PA.

Baker, M.A., Assis, S.L., Higa, O.Z., & Costa, I. (2009). Nanocomposite hydroxyapatite formation on a Ti-13Nb-13Zr alloy exposed in α-MEM cell culture medium and the effect of H_2O_2 addition. *Acta Biomaterialia*, Vol. 5, No.1, pp. 63-75.

Barrère, F., Layrolle, P., Van Blitterswijk, C.A., & De Groot, K. (1999). Biomimetic calcium phosphate coatings on Ti6Al4V: A crystal growth study of octacalcium phosphate and inhibition by Mg^{2+} and HCO_3^-. *Bone*, Vol. 25, No. 2 suppl, pp. 107S-111S.

Barrère F., Layrolle P., van Blitterswijk., & de Groot K. (2000a). Fast formation of biomimetic Ca-P coating on Ti6Al4V, *Symposium on Mineralization in Natural and Synthetic Biomaterials*, Vol. 599, pp. 135-140, Boston, MA, November 29-December 01, 1999

Barrère, F., Stigter, M., Layrolle, P., van Blitterswijk, C.A. & de Groot, K. (2000b). In vitro dissolution of various calcium-phosphate coatings on Ti6Al4V, *13th International Symposium on Ceramic in Medicine/Symposium on Ceramic Materials in Orthopaedic Surgery: Clinical Results*, Vol. 192-195, pp. 67-70, Bologna, Italy, November 22-26, 2000.

Barrère, F., Layrolle, P., van Blitterswijk, C.A., & de Groot, K. (2001). Biomimetic coatings on titanium: a crystal growth study of octacalcium phosphate. *Journal Of Materials Science-Materials In Medicine*, Vol. 12, No.6, pp. 529-534.

Barrère, F., van Blitterswijk, C.A., de Groot, K. & Layrolle, P. (2002a). Influence of ionic strength and carbonate on the Ca-P coating formation from SBFx5 solution. *Biomaterials*, Vol. 23, No.9, pp. 1921-1930.

Barrère, F., van Blitterswijk, C.A., de Groot, K. & Layrolle, P. (2002b). Nucleation of biomimetic Ca-P coatings on Ti6Al4V from a SBFx5 solution: influence of magnesium. *Biomaterials*, Vol. 23, No.10, pp. 2211-2220.

Barrère, F., van der Valk, C., Dalmeijer, R., Meijer, G., van Blitterswijk, C., de Groot, K., & Layrolle, P. (2003a). Osteogenecity of octacalcium phosphate coatings applied on porous metal implants. *Journal of Biomedical Materials Research Part A*, Vol. 66, No.4, pp. 779-788.

Barrère, F., Van Der Valk, C., Dalmeijer, R., Van Blitterswijk, C., de Groot, K., & Layrolle, P. (2003b). In vitro and in vivo degradation of biomimetic octacalcium phosphate and carbonate apatite coatings on titanium implants. *Journal of Biomedical Materials Research Part A*, Vol. 64, No.2, pp. 378-387.

Barrère, F., Van der Valk, C., Meijer, G., Dalmeijer, R., De Groot, K., & Layrolle, P. (2003c). Osteointegration of biomimetic apatite coating applied onto dense and porous metal implants in femurs of goats. *Journal of Biomedical Materials Research Part B: Applied Biomaterials*, Vol. 67, No.1, pp. 655-665.

Barrère, F., Snel, M.M.E., van Blitterswijk, C.A., de Groot, K., & Layrolle, P. (2004). Nano-scale study of the nucleation and growth of calcium phosphate coating on titanium implants. *Biomaterials*, Vol. 25, No.14, pp. 2901-2910.

Becker, R., Spadaro, J., & Berg, E. (1968). The trace elements of human bone. *The Journal of Bone and Joint Surgery*, Vol. 50, No.2, pp. 326-334.

Bigi, A., Boanini, E., Panzavolta, S., & Roveri, N. (2000). Biomimetic growth of hydroxyapatite on gelatin films doped with sodium polyacrylate. *Biomacromolecules*, Vol. 1, No.4, pp. 752-756.

Bracci, B., Torricelli, P., Panzavolta, S., Boanini, E., Giardino, R., & Bigi, A. (2009). Effect of Mg^{2+}, Sr^{2+}, and Mn^{2+} on the chemico-physical and in vitro biological properties of calcium phosphate biomimetic coatings. *Journal of Inorganic Biochemistry*, Vol. 103, No.12, pp. 1666-1674.

Brendel, T., & Engel A, Rüssel C. (1992). Hydroxyapatite coatings by a polymeric route. *Journal of Materials Science: Materials in Medicine*, Vol. 3, No.3, pp. 175-179.

Buchholz, H., Elson, R., & Heinert, K. (1984). Antibiotic-loaded acrylic cement: current concepts. *Clinical Orthopaedics and Related Research*, Vol. 190, No.3, pp. 96-108.

Bunker B.C., Rieke P.C., Tarasevich B.J., Campbell A.A., Fryxell G.E., Graff G.L., Song L., Liu J., Virden J.W., & McVay G.L. (1994). Ceramic Thin-Film Formation on Functionalized Interfaces Through Biomimetic Processing. *Science,* Vol. 264, No.5155, pp. 48-55.

Burg, K.J.L., Porter, S., & Kellam, J.F. (2000). Biomaterial developments for bone tissue engineering. *Biomaterials,* Vol. 21, No.23, pp. 2347-2359.

Campbell, A.A., Fryxell, G.E., Linehan, J.C., & Graff, G.L. (1996). Surface-induced mineralization: A new method for producing calcium phosphate coatings. *Journal of Biomedical Materials Research,* Vol. 32, No.1, pp. 111-118.

Campbell, A.A., Song, L., Li, X.S., Nelson, B.J., Bottoni, C., Brooks, D.E., & DeJong, E.S. (2000). Development, characterization, and anti-microbial efficacy of hydroxyapatite-chlorhexidine coatings produced by surface-induced mineralization. *Journal Of Biomedical Materials Research Part B-Applied Biomaterials,* Vol. 53, No.4, pp. 400-407.

Cao, W.P., & Hench, L.L. (1996). Bioactive Materials. *Ceramics International,* Vol. 22, No.6, pp. 493-507.

Cao, Y., Weng, J., Chen, J.Y., Feng, J.M., Yang, Z.J., & Zhang, X.D. (1996). Water vapour-treated hydroxyapatite coatings after plasma spraying and their characteristics. *Biomaterials,* Vol. 17, No. 4, pp. 419-424.

Chen, J., Wolke, J.G.C., & de Groot, K. (1994). Microstructure and crystalilinity in hydroxyapatite coatings. *Biomaterials,* Vol. 15, No. 5, pp. 396-399.

Chen, J.S., Juang, H.Y., & Hon, M.H. (1998). Calcium phosphate coating on titanium substrate by a modified electrocrystallization process. *Journal of Materials Science-Materials in Medicine,* Vol. 9, No. 5, pp. 297-300.

Chen, M.F., Yang, X.J., Liu, Y., Zhu, S.L., Cui, Z.D., & Man, H.C. (2003). Study on the formation of an apatite layer on NiTi shape memory alloy using a chemical treatment method. *Surface and Coatings Technology,* Vol. 173, No.2-3, pp. 229-234.

Chen, X.B., Li, Y.C., Du Plessis, J., Hodgson, P.D., & Wen, C. (2009). Influence of calcium ion deposition on apatite-inducing ability of porous titanium for biomedical applications. *Acta Biomaterialia,* Vol. 5, No.5, pp. 1808-1820.

Cho, S.B., Nakanishi, K., Kokubo, T., Soga, N., Ohtsuki, C., Nakamura, T., Kitsugi, T., & Yamamuro, T. (1995). Dependence of Apatite Formation on Silica Gel on Its Structure: Effect of Heat Treatment. *Journal of the American Ceramic Society,* Vol. 78, No.7, pp. 1769-1774.

Chou, Y., Chiou, W., Xu, Y., Dunn, J., & Wu, B. (2004). The effect of pH on the structural evolution of accelerated biomimetic apatite. *Biomaterials,* Vol. 25, No.22, pp. 5323-5331.

Das, K., Bose, S., & Bandyopadhyay, A. (2007). Surface modifications and cell-materials interactions with anodized Ti. *Acta Biomaterialia,* Vol. 3, No. 4, pp. 573-585.

De Andrade, M.C., Sader, M.S., Filgueiras, M.R.T., & Ogasawara, T. (2000). Microstructure of ceramic coating on titanium surface as a result of hydrothermal treatment. *Journal of Materials Science-Materials in Medicine,* Vol. 11, No. 11, pp. 751-755.

Dekker, R., De Bruijn, J., Van Den Brink, I., Bovell, Y., Layrolle, P., & Van Blitterswijk, C. (1998). Bone tissue engineering on calcium phosphate-coated titanium plates utilizing cultured rat bone marrow cells: a preliminary study. *Journal of Materials Science: Materials in Medicine,* Vol. 9, No. 12, pp. 859-863.

Dekker, R., de Bruijn, J., Stigter, M., Barrère, F., Layrolle, P., & van Blitterswijk, C. (2005). Bone tissue engineering on amorphous carbonated apatite and crystalline octacalcium phosphate-coated titanium discs. *Biomaterials*, Vol. 26, No. 25, pp. 5231-5239.

Deng, C.L., Chen, J.Y., Fan, H.S., & Zhang, X.D. (2005). Influence of dynamic flow speed on bonelike apatite formation in porous calcium phosphate ceramic in RSBF, *6th Asian Symposium on Biomedical Materials*, Vol. 288-289, pp. 273-276, Emei, China, July 19-22, 2004.

do Serro, A.P.V.A., Fernandes, A.C., & Saramago, B.de J.V. (2000). Calcium phosphate deposition on titanium surfaces in the presence of fibronectin. *Journal of Biomedical Materials Research*, Vol. 49, No. 3, pp. 345-352.

Earle, W. (1943). Production of malignancy in vitro. IV. The mouse fibroblast cultures and changes seen in the living cells. *Journal of the National Cancer Institute*, Vol. 4, pp. 165-212.

Feng, B., Chen, J.Y., Qi, S.K., He, L., Zhao, J.Z., & Zhang, X.D. (2002a). Carbonate apatite coating on titanium induced rapidly by precalcification. *Biomaterials*, Vol. 23, No. 1, pp. 173-179.

Feng, B., Chen, Y., & Zhang, X.D. (2002b). Effect of water vapor treatment on apatite formation on precalcified titanium and bond strength of coatings to substrates. *Journal of Biomedical Materials Research*, Vol. 59, No. 1, pp. 12-17.

Filgueiras, M.R., La Torre, G., & Hench, L.L. (1993). Solution effects on the surface reactions of three bioactive glass compositions. *Journal of Biomedical Materials Research*, Vol. 27, No. 12, pp. 1485-1493.

Fujibayashi, S., Nakamura, T., Nishiguchi, S., Tamura, J., Uchida, M., Kim, H.M., & Kokubo, T. (2001). Bioactive titanium: Effect of sodium removal on the bone-bonding ability of bioactive titanium prepared by alkali and heat treatment. *Journal Of Biomedical Materials Research*, Vol. 56, No. 4, pp. 562-570.

Fujibayashi, S., Kim, H.M., Neo, M., Uchida, M., Kokubo, T., & Nakamura, T. (2003). Repair of segmental long bone defect in rabbit femur using bioactive titanium cylindrical mesh cage. *Biomaterials*, Vol. 24, No. 20, pp. 3445-3451.

Fujibayashi, S., Neo, M., Kim, H.M., Kokubo, T., & Nakamura, T. (2004). Osteoinduction of porous bioactive titanium metal. *Biomaterials*, Vol. 25, No. 3, pp. 443-450.

Gamble, J.E. (1967). *Chemical anatomy, physiology and pathology of extracellular fluid*. Harvard University Press, Cambridge, MA.

Garvin, K., Salvati, E., & Brause, B. (1988). Role of gentamicin-impregnated cement in total joint arthroplasty. *The Orthopedic clinics of North America*, Vol. 19, No. 3, pp. 605-610.

Garvin, K., & Feschuk, C. (2005). Polylactide-polyglycolide antibiotic implants. *Clinical Orthopaedics and Related Research*, No. 437, pp. 105-110.

Gerhart, T., Roux, R., Hanff, P., Horowitz, G., Renshaw, A., & Hayes, W. (1993). Antibiotic-loaded biodegradable bone cement for prophylaxis and treatment of experimental osteomyelitis in rats. *Journal of Orthopaedic Research*, Vol. 11, No. 2, pp. 250-255.

Habibovic, P., Barrère, F., van Blitterswijk, C.A., de Groot, K., & Layrolle, P. (2002). Biomimetic hydroxyapatite coating on metal implants. *Journal Of The American Ceramic Society*, Vol. 85, No. 3, pp. 517-522.

Habibovic, P., Barrère, F., & De Groot, K. (2004a). New biomimetic coating technologies and incorporation of bioactive agents and proteins, In: *Learning from nature how to design new implantable biomaterials*, Reis R.L., & Weiner S. (Eds.). pp. 105-121, Kluwer Academic Publishers, the Netherlands.

Habibovic, P., Van der Valk, C.M., Van Blitterswijk, C.A., De Groot, K., & Meijer, G. (2004b). Influence of octacalcium phosphate coating on osteoinductive properties of biomaterials. *Journal of Materials Science-Materials in Medicine*, Vol. 15, No. 4, pp. 373-380.

Habibovic, P., Li, J.P., van der Valk, C.M., Meijer, G., Layrolle, P., van Blitterswijk, C.A., & de Groot, K. (2005). Biological performance of uncoated and octacalcium phosphate-coated Ti6A14V. *Biomaterials*, Vol. 26, No. 1, pp. 23-36.

Habibovic, P., Yuan, H.P., Van den Doel, M., Sees, T.M., Van Blitterswiik, C.A., & De Groot, K. (2006). Relevance of osteoinductive biomaterials in critical-sized orthotopic defect. *Journal Of Orthopaedic Research*, Vol. 24, No. 5, pp. 867-876.

Habibovic, P., & de Groot, K. (2007). Osteoinductive biomaterials - properties and relevance in bone repair. *Journal Of Tissue Engineering And Regenerative Medicine*, Vol. 1, No. 1, pp. 25-32.

Hamada, K., Kon, M., Hanawa, T., Yokoyama, K., Miyamoto, Y., & Asaoka, K. (2002). Hydrothermal modification of titanium surface in calcium solutions. *Biomaterials*, Vol. 23, No. 10, pp. 2265-2272.

Han, Y., Hong, S., & Xu, K. (2003). Structure and in vitro bioactivity of titania-based films by micro-arc oxidation. *Surface and coatings technology*, Vol. 168, No. 2-3, pp. 249-258.

Han, Y., Chen, D.H., Sun, J.F., Zhang, Y.M., & Xu, K.W. (2008). UV-enhanced bioactivity and cell response of micro-arc oxidized titania coatings. *Acta Biomaterialia*, Vol. 4, No. 5, pp. 1518-1529.

Hanawa, T., Murakami, K., & Kihara, S. (1994). Calcium phosphate precipitation on calcium-ion-implanted titanium in electrolyte, In: *Characterization and performance of calcium phosphate coatings for implants*, Horowitz, E., & Parr, J.E. (Eds.), pp. 170-184, American Society for Testing and Materials, Philadelphia.

Hanawa, T., Kon, M., Ukai, H., Murakami, K., Miyamoto, Y., & Asaoka, K. (1997). Surface modification of titanium in calcium-ion-containing solutions. *Journal of Biomedical Materials Research*, Vol. 34, No. 3, pp. 273-278.

Hanks, J. H., & Wallace, R. E. (1949). Relation of oxygen and temperature in the preservation of tissues by refrigeration. *Proceedings of the Society for Experimental Biology and Medicine*, Vol. 71, No. 2, pp. 196-200.

Hanks, J.H. (1975). Hanks' balanced salt solution and pH control. *Methods in Cell Science*, Vol. 1, No. 1, pp. 3-4.

Hench, L.L., Splinter, R.J., Allen, W.C., Greenlee, K. (1971). Bonding mechanisms at the interface of ceramic prosthetic materials. *Journal of Biomedical Materials Research*, Vol. 5, No. 3, pp. 117-141.

Hench, L.L. (1998). Bioactive materials: The potential for tissue regeneration. *Journal of Biomedical Materials Research*, Vol. 41, No. 4, pp. 511-518.

Henry, S., Seligson, D., Mangino, P., & Popham, G. (1991). Antibiotic-impregnated beads. Part I: Bead implantation versus systemic therapy. *Orthopaedic review*, Vol. 20, No. 3, pp. 242-247.

Huang, P., Zhang, Y., Xu, K., & Han, Y. (2004). Surface modification of titanium implant by microarc oxidation and hydrothermal treatment. *Journal of Biomedical Materials Research Part B: Applied Biomaterials*, Vol. 70, No. 2, pp. 187-190.

Huang, P., Xu, K., & Han, Y. (2005). Preparation and apatite layer formation of plasma electrolytic oxidation film on titanium for biomedical application. *Materials Letters*, Vol. 59, No. 2-3, pp. 185-189.

Hutmacher, D. (2000). Scaffolds in tissue engineering bone and cartilage. *Biomaterials*, Vol. 21, No. 24, pp. 2529-2543.

Ishizawa, H., & Ogino, M. (1995a). Characterization of thin hydroxyapatite layers formed on anodic titanium oxide films containing Ca and P by hydrothermal treatment. *Journal of Biomedical Materials Research*, Vol. 29, No. 9, pp. 1071-1079.

Ishizawa, H., & Ogino, M. (1995b). Formation and characterization of anodic titanium oxide films containing Ca and P. *Journal of Biomedical Materials Research*, Vol. 29, No. 1, pp. 65-72.

Jalota, S., Bhaduri, S.B., & Tas, A.C. (2007). Osteoblast proliferation on neat and apatite-like calcium phosphate-coated titanium foam scaffolds. *Materials Science and Engineering C-Biomimetic and Supramolecular Systems*, Vol. 27, No. 3, pp. 432-440.

Jonášová, L., Muller, F.A., Helebrant, A., Strnad, J., & Greil, P. (2002). Hydroxyapatite formation on alkali-treated titanium with different content of Na^+ in the surface layer. *Biomaterials*, Vol. 23, No. 15, pp. 3095-3101.

Jonášová, L., Müller, F.A., Helebrant, A., Strnad, J., & Greil, P. (2004). Biomimetic apatite formation on chemically treated titanium. *Biomaterials*, Vol. 25, No. 7-8, pp. 1187-1194.

Josefsson, G., Gudmundsson, G., Kolmert, L., & Wijkström, S. (1990). Prophylaxis with systemic antibiotics versus gentamicin bone cement in total hip arthroplasty: a five-year survey of 1688 hips. *Clinical Orthopaedics and Related Research*, No. 253, (April 1990), pp. 173-178.

Kaneko, S., Tsuru, K., Hayakawa, S., Takemoto, S., Ohtsuki, C., Ozaki, T., Inoue, H., & Osaka, A. (2001). In vivo evaluation of bone-bonding of titanium metal chemically treated with a hydrogen peroxide solution containing tantalum chloride. *Biomaterials*, Vol. 22, No. 9, pp. 875-881.

Kato, H., Nakamura, T., Nishiguchi, S., Matsusue, Y., Kobayashi, M., Miyazaki, T., Kim, H.M., & Kokubo, T. (2000). Bonding of alkali- and heat-treated tantalum implants to bone. *Journal Of Biomedical Materials Research*, Vol. 53, No. 1, pp. 28-35.

Kim, H.M., Miyaji, F., Kokubo, T., & Nakamura, T. (1996). Preparation of bioactive Ti and its alloys via simple chemical surface treatment. *Journal Of Biomedical Materials Research*, Vol. 32, No. 3, pp. 409-417.

Kim, H.M., Miyaji, F., Kokubo, T., & Nakamura, T. (1997). Effect of heat treatment on apatite-forming ability of Ti metal induced by alkali treatment. *Journal Of Materials Science-Materials In Medicine*, Vol. 8, No. 6, pp. 341-347.

Kim, H.M., Miyaji, F., & Kokubo, T. (1998). Preparation of functionally graded bioactive titanium and its alloys by chemical treatment. *Journal Of The Japan Institute Of Metals*, Vol. 62, No. 11, pp. 1102-1107.

Kim, H.M., Miyaji, F., Kokubo, T., Nishiguchi, S., & Nakamura, T. (1999). Graded surface structure of bioactive titanium prepared by chemical treatment. *Journal Of Biomedical Materials Research*, Vol. 45, No. 2, pp. 100-107.

Kim, M., Ryu, J., & Sung, Y. (2007). One-step approach for nano-crystalline hydroxyapatite coating on titanium via micro-arc oxidation. *Electrochemistry communications*, Vol. 45, No. 8, pp. 1886-1891.

Kim, T., Suzuki, M., Ohtsuki, C., Masuda, K., Tamai, H., Watanabe, E., Osaka, A., & Moriya, H. (2003). Enhancement of bone growth in titanium fiber mesh by surface modification with hydrogen peroxide solution containing tantalum chloride. *Journal of Biomedical Materials Research Part B-Applied Biomaterials*, Vol. 64, No. 1, pp. 19-26.

Kokubo, T. (1990a). Surface chemistry of bioactive glass-ceramics. *Journal of Non-Crystalline Solids*, Vol. 120, No. 1-3, pp. 138-151.

Kokubo, T., Kushitani, H., Sakka, S., Kitsugi, T., & Yamamuro, T. (1990b). Solutions able to reproduce in vivo surface-structure changes in bioactive glass-ceramic A-W. *Journal of Biomedical Materials Research*, Vol. 24, No. 6, pp. 721-734.

Kokubo, T. (1991). Bioactive glass ceramics: properties and applications. *Biomaterials*, Vol. 12, No. 2, pp. 155-163.

Kokubo, T., Miyaji, F., Kim, H.M., & Nakamura, T. (1996). Spontaneous formation of bonelike apatite layer on chemically treated titanium metals. *Journal Of The American Ceramic Society*, Vol. 4, No. 1, pp. 1127-1129.

Kokubo, T., & Takadama, H. (2006). How useful is SBF in predicting in vivo bone bioactivity? *Biomaterials*, Vol. 27, No. 15, pp. 2907-2915.

Lausmaa, J. (2001). Mechanical, thermal, chemical and electrochemical surface treatment of titanium, In: *Titanium in medicine*, Brunette, D.M., Tengvall, P., Textor, M., & Thomsen, P. (Ed.), pp. 231-266, Springer-verlag, Berlin, Heidelberg, New York.

Leeuwenburgh, S., Layrolle, P., Barrère, F., De Bruijn, J., Schoonman, J., Van Blitterswijk, C., & De Groot, K. (2001). Osteoclastic resorption of biomimetic calcium phosphate coatings in vitro. *Journal of Biomedical Materials Research Part A*, Vol. 56, No. 2, pp. 208-215.

Leitão, E., Barbosa, M.A., & de Groot, K. (1997). Influence of substrate material and surface finishing on the morphology of the calcium-phosphate coating. *Journal of Biomedical Materials Research*, Vol. 36, No. 1, pp. 85-90.

Li, J.G., Liao, H.H., & Sjöström, M. (1997). Characterization of calcium phosphates precipitated from simulated body fluid of different buffering capacities. *Biomaterials*, Vol. 18, No. 10, pp. 743-747.

Li, P., & Ducheyne, P. (1998). Quasi-biological apatite film induced by titanium in a simulated body fluid. *Journal of Biomedical Materials Research Part A*, Vol. 41, No. 3, pp. 341-348.

Li, P., & de Groot, K. (1993). Calcium phosphate formation within sol-gel prepared titania in vitro and in vivo. *Journal of Biomedical Materials Research*, Vol. 27, No. 12, pp. 1495-1500.

Li, P., Kangasniemi, I., de Groot, K., & Kokubo, T. (1994). Bonelike hydroxyapatite induction by a gel-derived titania on a titanium substrate. *Journal of the American Ceramic Society*, Vol. 77, No. 5, pp. 1307-1312.

Liang, F.H., Zhou, L., & Wang, K.G. (2003). Enhancement of the bioactivity of alkali-heat treated titanium by pre-calcification. *Journal of Materials Science Letters*, Vol. 22, No. 23, pp. 1665-1667.

Liu, Q., Ding, J., Mante, F.K., Wunder, S.L., & Baran, G.R. (2002). The role of surface functional groups in calcium phosphate nucleation on titanium foil: a self-assembled monolayer technique. *Biomaterials*, Vol. 23, No. 15, pp. 3103-3111.

Liu, X.Y., Chu, P.K., & Ding, C.X. (2004). Surface modification of titanium, titanium alloys, and related materials for biomedical applications. *Materials Science and Engineering R-Reports*, Vol. 47, No. 3-4, pp. 49-121.

Liu, Y., Layrolle, P., de Bruijn, J., van Blitterswijk, C., & de Groot, K. (2001). Biomimetic coprecipitation of calcium phosphate and bovine serum albumin on titanium alloy. *Journal of Biomedical Materials Research Part A*, Vol. 57, No. 3, pp. 327-335.

Liu, Y., Hunziker, E., Randall, N., De Groot, K., & Layrolle, P. (2003). Proteins incorporated into biomimetically prepared calcium phosphate coatings modulate their mechanical strength and dissolution rate. *Biomaterials*, Vol. 24, No. 1, pp. 65-70.

Liu, Y., Li, J., Hunziker, E., & De Groot, K. (2006). Incorporation of growth factors into medical devices via biomimetic coatings. *Philosophical Transactions of the Royal Society A: Mathematical, Physical and Engineering Sciences*, Vol. 364, No. 1838, pp. 233-248.

Lu, X., Zhao, Z.F., & Leng, Y. (2007). Biomimetic calcium phosphate coatings on nitric-acid-treated titanium surfaces. *Materials Science and Engineering C-Biomimetic and Supramolecular Systems*, Vol. 27, No. 4, pp. 700-708.

MacDonald, D.E., Rapuano, B.E., Deo, N., Stranick, M., Somasundaran, P., & Boskey, A.L. (2004). Thermal and chemical modification of titanium-aluminum-vanadium implant materials: effects on surface properties, glycoprotein adsorption, and MG63 cell attachment. *Biomaterials*, Vol. 25, No. 16, pp. 3135-3146.

Majewski, P.J., & Allidi, G. (2006). Synthesis of hydroxyapatite on titanium coated with organic self-assembled monolayers. *Materials Science and Engineering A-Structural Materials Properties Microstructure and Processing*, Vol. 420, No. 1-2, pp. 13-20.

Mao, C., Li, H., Cui, F., Feng, Q., Wang, H., & Ma, C. (1998). Oriented growth of hydroxyapatite on (0001) textured titanium with functionalized self-assembled silane monolayer as template. *Journal of Materials Chemistry*, Vol. 8, No. 12, pp. 2795-2801.

Miyazaki, T., Kim, H.M., Miyaji, F., Kokubo, T., Kato, H., & Nakamura, T. (2000). Bioactive tantalum metal prepared by NaOH treatment. *Journal Of Biomedical Materials Research*, Vol. 50, No. 1, pp. 35-42.

Miyazaki, T., Kim, H.M., Kokubo, T., Miyaji, F., Kato, H., & Nakamura, T. (2001). Effect of thermal treatment on apatite-forming ability of NaOH-treated tantalum metal. *Journal of Materials Science-Materials in Medicine*, Vol. 12, No. 8, pp. 683-687.

Miyazaki, T., Kim, H.M., Kokubo, T., Ohtsuki, C., Kato, H., & Nakamura, T. (2002). Mechanism of bonelike apatite formation on bioactive tantalum metal in a simulated body fluid. *Biomaterials*, Vol. 23, No. 3, pp. 827-832.

Narayanan, R., Seshadri, S.K., Kwon, T.Y., & Kim, K.H. (2008). Calcium phosphate-based coatings on titanium and its alloys. *Journal of Biomedical Materials Research Part B-Applied Biomaterials*, Vol. 85, No. 1, pp. 279-299.

Neo, M., Nakamura, T., Ohtsuki, C., Kokubo, T., & Yamamuro, T. (1993). Apatite formation on three kinds of bioactive material at an early stage in vivo: a comparative study by transmission electron microscopy. *Journal of Biomedical Materials Research*, Vol. 27, No. 8, pp. 999-1006.

Nishiguchi, S., Kato, H., Fujita, H., Kim, H.M., Miyaji, F., Kokubo, T., & Nakamura, T. (1999a). Enhancement of bone-bonding strengths of titanium alloy implants by alkali and heat treatments. *Journal Of Biomedical Materials Research*, Vol. 48, No. 5, pp. 689-696.

Nishiguchi, S., Nakamura, T., Kobayashi, M., Kim, H.M., Miyaji, F., & Kokubo, T. (1999b). The effect of heat treatment on bone-bonding ability of alkali-treated titanium. *Biomaterials*, Vol. 20, No. 5, pp. 491-500.

Nishiguchi, S., Kato, H., Neo, M., Oka, M., Kim, H.M., Kokubo, T., & Nakamura, T. (2001). Alkali- and heat-treated porous titanium for orthopedic implants. *Journal Of Biomedical Materials Research*, Vol. 54, No. 2, pp. 198-208.

Nishio, K., Neo, M., Akiyama, H., Nishiguchi, S., Kim, H., Kokubo, T., & Nakamura, T. (2000). The effect of alkali-and heat-treated titanium and apatite-formed titanium on osteoblastic differentiation of bone marrow cells. *Journal of Biomedical Materials Research Part A*, Vol. 52, No. 4, pp. 652-661.

Ohtsuki C., Kushitani H., Kokubo T., Kotani S., & Yamamuro T. (1991). Apatite formation on the surface of ceravital-type glass-ceramic in the body. *Journal of Biomedical Materials Research*, Vol. 25, No. 11, pp. 1363-1370.

Ohtsuki, C., Iida, H., Hayakawa, S., & Osaka, A. (1997). Bioactivity of titanium treated with hydrogen peroxide solutions containing metal chlorides. *Journal of Biomedical Materials Research*, Vol. 35, No. 1, pp. 39-47.

Oliveira, A., Reis, R., & Li, P. (2007). Strontium-substituted apatite coating grown on Ti6Al4V substrate through biomimetic synthesis. *Journal of Biomedical Materials Research Part B: Applied Biomaterials*, Vol. 83, No. 1, pp. 258-265.

Ong J.L., Lucas L.C., Lacefield W.R., & Rigney E.D. (1992). Structure, solubility and bond strength of thin calcium phosphate coatings produced by ion beam sputter deposition. *Biomaterials*, Vol. 13, No. 4, pp. 249-254.

Oyane, A., Onuma, K., Ito, A., Kim, H.M., Kokubo, T., & Nakamura, T. (2003). Formation and growth of clusters in conventional and new kinds of simulated body fluids. *Journal of Biomedical Materials Research Part A*, Vol. 64, No. 2, pp. 339-348.

Pan, J., Thierry, D., & Leygraf, C. (1996). Hydrogen peroxide toward enhanced oxide growth on titanium in PBS solution: Blue coloration and clinical relevance. *Journal of Biomedical Materials Research*, Vol. 30, No. 3, pp. 393-402.

Pan, J., Liao, H., Leygraf, C., Thierry, D., & Li, J. (1998). Variation of oxide films on titanium induced by osteoblast-like cell culture and the influence of an H_2O_2 pretreatment. *Journal of Biomedical Materials Research*, Vol. 40, No. 2, pp. 244-256.

Papadopoulou, L., Kontonasaki, E., Zorba, T., Chatzistavrou, X., Pavlidou, E., Paraskevopoulos, K., Sklavounos, S., & Koidis, P. (2003). Dental ceramics coated with bioactive glass: Surface changes after exposure in a simulated body fluid under static and dynamic conditions. *Physica Status Solidi (a)-Applied Research*, Vol. 198, No. 1, pp. 65-75.

Patntirapong, S., Habibovic, P., & Hauschka, P. (2009). Effects of soluble cobalt and cobalt incorporated into calcium phosphate layers on osteoclast differentiation and activation. *Biomaterials*, Vol. 30, No. 4, pp. 548-555.

Peltola, T., P tsi, M., Rahiala, H., Kangasniemi, I., & Yli-Urpo, A. (1998). Calcium phosphate induction by sol-gel-derived titania coatings on titanium substrates in vitro. *Journal of Biomedical Materials Research Part A*, Vol. 41, No. 3, pp. 504-510.

Radin, S., Campbell, J.T., Ducheyne, P., & Cuckler, J.M. (1997). Calcium phosphate ceramic coatings as carriers of vancomycin. *Biomaterials*, Vol. 18, No. 11, pp. 777-782.

Ratner, B.D. (2001). A perspective on titanium biocompatibility, In: *Titanium in medicine*, Brunette, D.M., Tengvall, P., Textor, M., & Thomsen, P. (Ed.), pp.1-12, Springer-verlag, Berlin, Heidelberg, New York.

Rezwan, K., Chen, Q., Blaker, J., & Boccaccini, A. (2006). Biodegradable and bioactive porous polymer/inorganic composite scaffolds for bone tissue engineering. *Biomaterials*, Vol. 27, No. 18, pp. 3413-3431.

Ringer, S. (1883). A further contribution regarding the influence of the different constituents of the blood on the contraction of the heart. *Journal of Physiology*, Vol. 4, No. 1, pp. 29-42.

Rose, F., & Oreffo, R. (2002). Bone tissue engineering: hope vs hype. *Biochemical and biophysical research communications*, Vol. 292, No. 1, pp. 1-7.

Ryan, G., Pandit, A., & Apatsidis, D. (2006). Fabrication methods of porous metals for use in orthopaedic applications. *Biomaterials*, Vol. 27, No. 13, pp. 2651-2670.

Serro, A.P., & Saramago, B. (2003). Influence of sterilization on the mineralization of titanium implants induced by incubation in various biological model fluids. *Biomaterials*, Vol. 24, No. 13, pp. 4749-4760.

Shirkhanzadeh, M. (1995). Calcium phosphate coatings prepared by electrocrystallization from aqueous electrolytes. *Journal of Materials Science-Materials in Medicine*, Vol. 6, No. 2, pp. 90-93.

Silver, I.A., Deas, J., & Erecinska, M. (2001). Interactions of bioactive glasses with osteoblasts in vitro: effects of 45S5 Bioglass (R), and 58S and 77S bioactive glasses on metabolism, intracellular ion concentrations and cell viability. *Biomaterials*, Vol. 22, No. 2, pp. 175-185.

Siriphannon, P., Kameshima, Y., Yasumori, A., Okada, K., & Hayashi, S. (2002). Comparative study of the formation of hydroxyapatite in simulated body fluid under static and flowing systems. *Journal of Biomedical Materials Research*, Vol. 60, No. 1, pp. 175-185.

Song, W., Jun, Y., Han, Y., & Hong, S. (2004). Biomimetic apatite coatings on micro-arc oxidized titania. *Biomaterials*, Vol. 25, No. 17, pp. 3341-3349.

Stigter, M., De Groot, K., & Layrolle, P. (2002). Incorporation of tobramycin into biomimetic hydroxyapatite coating on titanium. *Biomaterials*, Vol. 23, No. 20, pp. 4143-4153.

Stigter, M., Bezemer, J., de Groot, K., & Layrolle, P. (2004). Incorporation of different antibiotics into carbonated hydroxyapatite coatings on titanium implants, release and antibiotic efficacy. *Journal of Controlled Release*, Vol. 99, No. 1, pp. 127-137.

Sultana, R., Hamada, K., Ichikawa, T., & Asaoka, K. (2009). Effects of heat treatment on the bioactivity of surface-modified titanium in calcium solution. *Bio-Medical Materials and Engineering*, Vol. 19, No. 2-3, pp. 193-204.

Sun, J.F., Han, Y., & Huang, X. (2007). Hydroxyapatite coatings prepared by micro-arc oxidation in Ca-and P-containing electrolyte. *Surface and coatings technology*, Vol. 201, No. 9-11, pp. 5655-5658.

Sun, J.F., Han, Y., & Cui, K. (2008). Microstructure and apatite-forming ability of the MAO-treated porous titanium. *Surface and Coatings Technology*, Vol. 202, No. 17, pp. 4248-4256.

Takadama, H., Kim, H.M., Kokubo, T., & Nakamura, T. (2001a). TEM-EDX study of mechanism of bonelike apatite formation on bioactive titanium metal in simulated body fluid. *Journal Of Biomedical Materials Research*, Vol. 57, No. 3, pp. 441-448.

Takadama, H., Kim, H.M., Kokubo, T., & Nakamura, T. (2001b). An X-ray photoelectron spectroscopy study of the process of apatite formation on bioactive titanium metal. *Journal Of Biomedical Materials Research*, Vol. 55, No. 2, pp. 185-193.

Takadama, H., Hashimoto, M., Mizuno, M., & Kokubo, T. (2004). Round-robin test of SBF for in vitro measurement of apatite-forming ability of synthetic materials. *Phosphorus Research Bulletin*, Vol. 17, pp. 119-125.

Takemoto, M., Fujibayashi, S., Matsushita, T., Suzuki, J., Kokubo, T., & Nakamura, T. (2005a). Mechanical properties and osteoconductivity of porous bioactive titanium metal, *17th International Symposium on Ceramics in Medicine*, Vol. 284-286, pp. 263-266, New Orleans, LA, December 08-12, 2004.

Takemoto, M., Fujibayashi, S., Neo, M., Suzuki, J., Kokubo, T., & Nakamura, T. (2005b). Mechanical properties and osteoconductivity of porous bioactive titanium. *Biomaterials*, Vol. 26, No. 30, pp. 6014-6023.

Takemoto, M., Fujibayashi, S., Neo, M., Suzuki, J., Matsushita, T., Kokubo, T., & Nakamura, T. (2006). Osteoinductive porous titanium implants: Effect of sodium removal by dilute HCl treatment. *Biomaterials*, Vol. 27, No. 13, pp. 2682-2691.

Tamada, Y., & Ikada, Y. (1993). Effect of preadsorbed proteins on cell adhesion to polymer surfaces. *Journal of colloid and interface science*, Vol. 155, No. 2, pp. 334-339.

Tas, A.C. (2000). Synthesis of biomimetic Ca-hydroxyapatite powders at 37°C in synthetic body fluids. *Biomaterials*, Vol. 21, No. 14, pp. 1429-1438.

Tas, A.C., & Bhaduri, S.B. (2004). Rapid coating of Ti6Al4V at room temperature with a calcium phosphate solution similar to 10× simulated body fluid. *Journal of Materials Research*, Vol. 19, No. 9, pp. 2742-2749.

Tengvall, P., Lundström, I., Sjöqvist, L., Elwing, H., Bjursten, L.M. (1989a). Titanium-hydrogen peroxide interaction: Model studies of the influence of the inflammatory response on titanium implants. *Biomaterials*, Vol. 10, No. 3, pp. 166-175.

Tengvall, P., Elwing, H., Sjöqvist, L., Lundström, I., & Bjursten, L.M. (1989b). Interaction between hydrogen peroxide and titanium: a possible role in the biocompatibility of titanium. *Biomaterials*, Vol. 10, No. 2, pp. 118-120.

Tengvell, P., Elwing, H., & Lundström, I. (1989c). Titanium gel made from metallic titanium and hydrogen peroxide. *Journal of colloid and interface science*, Vol. 130, No. 3, pp. 405-413.

Tengvall, P., & Lundström, I. (1992). Physico-chemical considerations of titanium as a biomaterial. *Clinical Materials*, Vol. 9, No. 2, pp. 115-134.

Uchida, M., Kim, H.M., Kokubo, T., Fujibayashi, S., & Nakamura, T. (2002). Effect of water treatment on the apatite-forming ability of NaOH-treated titanium metal. *Journal Of Biomedical Materials Research*, Vol. 63, No. 5, pp. 522-530.

Uchida, M., Oyane, A., Kim, H., Kokubo, T., & Ito, A. (2004). Biomimetic coating of laminin-apatite composite on titanium metal and its excellent cell-adhesive properties. *Advanced Materials*, Vol. 16, No. 13, pp. 1071-1074.

Wälivaara, B., Lundström, I., Tengvall, P. (1993). An in-vitro study of H_2O_2-treated titanium surfaces in contact with blood plasma and a simulated body fluid. *Clinical Materials*, Vol. 12, No. 2, pp. 141-148.

Wang, X.X., Hayakawa, S., Tsuru, K., & Osaka, A. (2000). Improvement of bioactivity of $H_2O_2/TaCl_5$-treated titanium after subsequent heat treatments. *Journal of Biomedical Materials Research*, Vol. 52, No. 1, pp. 171-176.

Wang, X.X., Hayakawa, S., Tsuru, K., & Osaka, A. (2002). Bioactive titania gel layers formed by chemical treatment of Ti substrate with a H_2O_2/HCl solution. *Biomaterials*, Vol. 23, No. 5, pp. 1353-1357.

Wei, D.Q., Zhou, Y., Jia, D.C., & Wang, Y.M. (2007). Characteristic and in vitro bioactivity of a microarc-oxidized TiO_2-based coating after chemical treatment. *Acta Biomaterialia*, Vol. 3, No. 5, pp. 817-827.

Wei, M., Kim, H.M., Kokubo, T., & Evans, J.H. (2002). Optimising the bioactivity of alkaline-treated titanium alloy. *Materials Science and Engineering C-Biomimetic And Supramolecular Systems*, Vol. 20, No. 1-2, pp. 125-134.

Wen, H.B., Wolke, J.G.C., deWijn, J.R., Liu, Q., Cui, F.Z., & de Groot, K. (1997). Fast precipitation of calcium phosphate layers on titanium induced by simple chemical treatments. *Biomaterials*, Vol. 18, No. 22, pp. 1471-1478.

Wen, H.B., Liu, Q., De Wijn, J.R., De Groot, K., & Cui, F.Z. (1998). Preparation of bioactive microporous titanium surface by a new two-step chemical treatment. *Journal Of Materials Science-Materials In Medicine*, Vol. 9, No. 3, pp. 121-128.

Wen, H.B., De Wijn, J., Van Blitterswijk, C., & De Groot, K. (1999). Incorporation of bovine serum albumin in calcium phosphate coating on titanium. *Journal of Biomedical Materials Research Part A*, Vol. 46, No. 2, pp. 245-252.

Weng, W.J., & Baptista, J.L. (1999). Preparation and characterization of hydroxyapatite coatings on Ti6Al4V alloy by a sol-gel method. *Journal of the American Ceramic Society*, Vol. 82, No. 1, pp. 27-32.

Wolke, J.G.C., de Groot, K., & Jansen, J.A. (1998). In vivo dissolution behavior of various RF magnetron sputtered Ca-P coatings. *Journal of Biomedical Materials Research*, Vol. 39, No. 15, pp. 524-530.

Wu, J.M., Hayakawa, S., Tsuru, K., & Osaka, A. (2004). Low-temperature preparation of anatase and rutile layers on titanium substrates and their ability to induce in vitro apatite deposition. *Journal of the American Ceramic Society*, Vol. 87, No. 9, pp. 1635-1642.

Wu, Z., Feng, B., Weng, J., Qu, S., Wang, J., & Lu, X. (2008). Biomimetic apatite coatings on titanium coprecipitated with cephradine and salviae miltlorrhizae. *Journal of Biomedical Materials Research Part B: Applied Biomaterials*, Vol. 84, No. 2, pp. 486-492.

Yan, W.Q., Nakamura, T., Kawanabe, K., Nishigochi, S., Oka, M., & Kokubo, T. (1997a). Apatite layer-coated titanium for use as bone bonding implants. *Biomaterials*, Vol. 18, No. 17, pp. 1185-1190.

Yan, W.Q., Nakamura, T., Kobayashi, M., Kim, H.M., Miyaji, F., & Kokubo, T. (1997b). Bonding of chemically treated titanium implants to bone. *Journal Of Biomedical Materials Research*, Vol. 37, No. 2, pp. 267-275.

Yang, B.C., Weng, J., Li, X.D., & Zhang, X.D. (1999). The order of calcium and phosphate ion deposition on chemically treated titanium surfaces soaked in aqueous solution. *Journal of Biomedical Materials Research*, Vol. 47, No. 2, pp. 213-219.

Yang, B.C., Uchida, M., Kim, H.M., Zhang, X..D., & Kokubo, T. (2004). Preparation of bioactive titanium metal via anodic oxidation treatment. *Biomaterials*, Vol. 25, No. 6, pp. 1003-1010.

Yang, L., Perez-Amodio, S., Barrère-de Groot, F., Everts, V., van Blitterswijk, C., & Habibovic, P. (2010). The effects of inorganic additives to calcium phosphate on in vitro behavior of osteoblasts and osteoclasts. *Biomaterials*, Vol.31, No. 11, pp. 2976-2989.

Yuan, H. (2001). *Osteoinduction by calcium phosphates* [PhD thesis]. Leiden University, The Netherlands.

Zhang, Q.Y., & Leng, Y. (2005). Electrochemical activation of titanium for biomimetic coating of calcium phosphate. *Biomaterials*, Vol. 26, No. 18, pp. 3853-3859.

Zhang, X.D., Yuan, H.P., & de Groot., K. (2000). Calcium phosphate biomaterials with intrinsic osteoinductivity, Notebook: Workshop 1#, Biomaterials with Intrinsic Osteoinductivity, *The 6th world biomaterials conference*. Hawaii, USA, May 15-20, 2000.

Zhao, C.Y., Zhu, X.D., Yuan, T., Fan, H.S., & Zhang, X.D. (2010a). Fabrication of biomimetic apatite coating on porous titanium and their osteointegration in femurs of dogs. *Materials Science and Engineering C-Materials for Biological Applications*, Vol. 30, No. 1, pp. 98-104.

Zhao, C.Y., Zhu, X.D., Liang, K.L., Ding, J.T., Xiang, Z., Fan, H.S., & Zhang, X.D., Osteoinduction of Porous Titanium: A Comparative Study Between Acid-Alkali and Chemical-Thermal Treatments. *Journal of Biomedical Materials Research: Part B - Applied Biomaterials*, Vol. 95, No. 2, pp. 387-396.

Zhitomirsky, I., & Gal-Or, L. (1997). Electrophoretic deposition of hydroxyapatite. *Journal of Materials Science-Materials in Medicine*, Vol. 8, No. 4, pp. 213-219.

Zhu, X., Kim, K., & Jeong, Y. (2001). Anodic oxide films containing Ca and P of titanium biomaterial. *Biomaterials*, Vol. 22, No. 16, pp. 2199-2206.

20

Biomimetic Hydroxyapatite Deposition on Titanium Oxide Surfaces for Biomedical Application

Wei Xia[1,2], Carl Lindahl[1,2], Jukka Lausmaa[2,3] and Håkan Engqvist[1,2]
[1]Angstrom Laboratory, Department of Engineering Sciences, Uppsala University, Uppsala
[2]BIOMATCELL, VINN Excellence Center of Biomaterials and Cell Therapy, Gothenburg
[3]Department of Chemistry and Materials Technology, SP Technical Research Institute of Sweden
Sweden

1. Introduction

Titanium is widely used as material for permanent implants in orthopedic and dental applications. It is well known that Ti shows a mechanically stable interface towards bone (osseointegration). The good biological properties are due to the beneficial properties of the native oxide (TiO_2) that forms on Ti when exposed to oxygen. The native titanium oxide on Ti is usually amorphous and very thin, 2-7 nm [1-3]. In addition to being stable in the physiological environment, titanium oxides increase calcium ion interactions, which are important for protein and subsequent osteoblast adhesion [4].

Enhanced bone bonding can be achieved with bioactive materials that form a stable unit with bone through a spontaneous formation of hydroxyapatite (HA) on their surface. The biomineralized HA layer acts as a bonding layer to the bone and integration at the atomic/molecular scale can develop. For this reason HA is proposed as a suitable coating material to provide stronger early fixation of uncemented prostheses. Although hydroxyapatite coatings on implants showed long-term survival [5], there are concerns about their reliability under loads. Possible ways to overcome this lack of mechanical stability could be by reinforcing the HA with metal oxides such as zirconia and alumina [6].

Apatites, as well as other calcium phosphates (CaPs), can occur in different phases, summarized in **Table 1** [7]. Most of them have been studied as biomaterials. The HA naturally occurring in bone is a multi-substituted calcium phosphate, including traces of CO_3^{2-} , F^-, Mg^{2+}, Sr^{2+}, Si^{4+}, Zn^{2+}, Li^+ etc [8, 9]. These ionic substitutions are considered to play an important role for the formation and properties of bone.

Hydroxyapatite coatings can be produced by different methods [10-19]. Early attempts used plasma spraying, which however resulted in coatings with adhesion problems. Attempts have also been made with physical vapour deposition (PVD) techniques. Both of these methods suffer from the drawback that they are line-of-sight methods, which means that coating of complex implant geometries is technically difficult. The biomimetic way to fabricate apatite coatings on implants overcomes these drawbacks. Biomimetic HA coating is, basically, a solution-based method carried out at ambient temperature mimicking body surroundings. The method allows deposition of CaP coatings on many different objects, such as sponges, cements, metal surfaces or fixation rods [20]. Biomimetic deposition of coatings also gives a possibility of co-precipitating ions, drugs, macromolecules and biological molecules together with the inorganic layer. Typically, the substrates with active surfaces are immersed in a simulated body fluid at physiological pH and temperature (approximately 37°C), and an apatite layer will automatically form, crystallize and grow on the surfaces. By varying the immersion conditions, coatings with a wide range of morphologies, thicknesses and composition can be prepared.

In this chapter, some recent developments in biomimetic HA coatings will be reviewed. In section 2 we provide an overview of different types of HA produced by biometic methods. Since biomimetic coating properties are dependent on the substrate properties, some basic properties of titanium (oxide) surfaces are described in section 3. In section 4 we briefly describe some new techniques for studying the formation and properties of biomimetic HA coatings. Sections 5 and 6 provide an overview of recent studies of HA formation on different titanium oxide surfaces, and of ion substituted biomimetic HA coatings, respectively. Finally, section 7 discusses some biological properties of biomimetic HA coatings, and in section 8 we summarize and discusses some directions for the future.

2. Selected properties of HA coatings

The standard way of producing biomimetic coatings has for a long time been based on the simulated body fluid (SBF) solutions described by Kokubo [21]. Recently, in order to improve the coating process, the composition of the solutions used for biomimetic HA coatings has been modified (**Table 2**). Except for the inorganic components, some other organic components, such as protein and lactic acid, have been added into SBF [22, 23]. The immerson temperature has also been expanded to temperatures from 4 to 65 °C [23-25]. Based on these biomimetic methods, the resulting apatite coatings will be either amorphous calcium phosphate (ACP), octacalcium phosphate (OCP) or hydroxyapatite (HA). The crystal structures of OCP and HA are shown in **Fig. 1 and 2** [26, 27]. Typical HA is a hexagonal phase, which contains two different cation sites, Ca(I) and Ca(II). A unit cell accommodates a formula unit $Ca_{10}(PO_4)_6(OH)_2$. Among the 10 cations, the 4 Ca(I)s are tightly bonded to 6 oxygens and less strongly to the other 3 oxygens, whereas the 6 Ca(II) atoms are surrounded by 7 oxygens. OCP ($Ca_8(HPO_4)_2(PO_4)_4 \cdot 5H_2O$) has a triclinic structure. Six of the Ca^{2+} ions and two of the phosphate groups are hosted in a layer (apatite layer) where they occupy almost the same positions as in HA structure, as shown in **Fig. 2**. Due to its structural features, OCP is often found as an intermediate phase during the precipitation of the thermodynamically more stable HA [26].

Bigi and his co-workers recently summarized ionic substitutions as a tool to improve the biological performance of calcium phosphate based materials [27]. Biomimetic ion substituted hydroxyapatite could therefore not only act as a bonding layer but also further strengthen the bonding and stimulate bone formation.

Investigations of the growth, boundary conditions and surface chemistry of biomimetic hydroxyapatite deposition on titanium oxide surfaces (amorphous and crystalline) can contribute to the understanding of the mechanism of the hydroxyapatite formation in vivo. Furthermore, such studies provide a means to grow different HA coatings under controlled biomimetic conditions [24].

Abbreviation	Formula	Name (mineral)	Ca/P ratio	pK_{sp} (25 °C)[a]	pH stability[a]	Occurrence in biological tissues
HA	$Ca_{10}(PO_4)_6(OH)_2$	Hydroxyapatite	1.67	116.8	9.5–12	Bone, dentin, enamel, dental calcifications, urinary stones, atherosclerotic plaques
OCP	$Ca_8H_2(PO_4)_6{\cdot}5H_2O$	Octacalcium phosphate	1.33	96.6	5.5–7.0	Dental and urinary calculi
β-TCP	$Ca_3(PO_4)_2$	β-Tricalcium phosphate (whitlokite)	1.5	28.9	[b]	Dental and urinary calculi, soft-tissue deposits, artritic cartilage, usually present as β-TCMP
α-TCP	$Ca_3(PO_4)_2$	α-Tricalcium phosphate	1.5	25.5	[b]	Not found
ACP	$Ca_x(PO_4)_y{\cdot}nH_2O$	Amorphous calcium phosphate	1.2–2.2	[c]	[b]	Soft-tissue calcifications
MCPM	$Ca(H_2PO_4)_2{\cdot}H_2O$	Monocalcium phosphate monohydrate	0.5	1.14	0–2	Not found
MCPA	$Ca(H_2PO_4)_2$	Anhydrous monocalcium phosphate	0.5	1.14	[b]	Not found
DCPD	$CaHPO_4{\cdot}2H_2O$	Dicalcium phosphate dihydrate (brushite)	1.0	6.59	2–6	Dental calculi, urinary stones chondrocalcinosis
DCPA	$CaHPO_4$	Anhydrous dicalcium phosphate (monetite)	1.0	6.90	[b]	Not found
TTCP	$Ca_4(PO_4)_2$	Tetracalcium phosphate	2.0	38–44	[b]	Not found
CDHA	$Ca_{10-x}(HPO_4)_x(PO_4)_{6-x}(OH)_{2-x}$	Calcium-deficient hydroxyapatite	1.5	85.1	6.5–9.5	Not found

[a] Data from ref. [8]
[b] Phase obtained by solid-state reaction or heat treatment of other phases [7]
[c] Cannot be measured precisely, however the following values were reported: 25.7 (pH 7.40), 29.9 (pH 6.00), 32.7 (pH 5.28) [28].

Table 1. Properties and occurrence of the biologically relevant phosphates. [7]

Ion	Na^+	K^+	Mg^{2+}	Ca^{2+}	Cl^-	HPO_4^{2-}/ $H_2PO_4^-$	SO_4^{2-}	HCO_3^-
Blood plasma[29]	142.0	5.0	1.5	2.5	103.0	1.0	0.5	27
SBF[21, 23]	142.0	5.0	1.5	2.5	148.5	1.0	0.5	4.2
PBS[24, 25, 30, 31]	145.0	4.2	0.49	0.91	143	9.6	-	-
5×SBF[32]	710	25	7.5	12.5	741	5	2.5	21
10×SBF[33]	1000	5	5	25	1065	10	-	-
HBSS[34]	141.7	5.7	0.8	1.7	145.6	0.7	0.8	4.2

HBSS: Hanks balanced salt solution

Table 2. Inorganic composition of blood plasma and different simulated body fluids (mM)

3. Surface chemistry of titanium oxide

The native titanium oxide formed during normal ambient conditions on Ti is amorphous if there is no additional treatment. In addition to the amorphous phase, three different crystalline phases of titanium dioxide exist naturally, namely rutile, anatase and brookite. **Table 3** summarizes the reported values of isoelectric point (IEP) and point-of-zero charge (PZC) for some titanium dioxides. As can be seen, for both amorphous and crystalline titanium dioxide both the IEP and PZC are in all cases lower than 7. This is very important for hydroxyapatite formation on titanium dioxide in the body simulated fluid (SBF). Because the pH of SBF is ~7.4, the lower IEP could lead to a deprotonation of the titanium oxide surface and the formation of negative Ti-O- groups in SBF. The adsorption and dissociation of water can also produce Ti-OH groups and a negative surface charge.

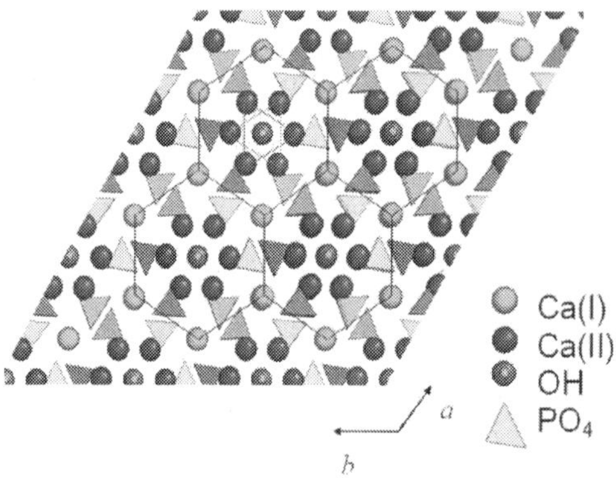

Fig. 1. HA structure along the c-axis. Black lines connect Ca(I) columns in hexagonal networks. Cyan and magenta triangles connect staggered Ca(II) atoms lying in the same plane, but at different height with respect to the c-axis.[27]

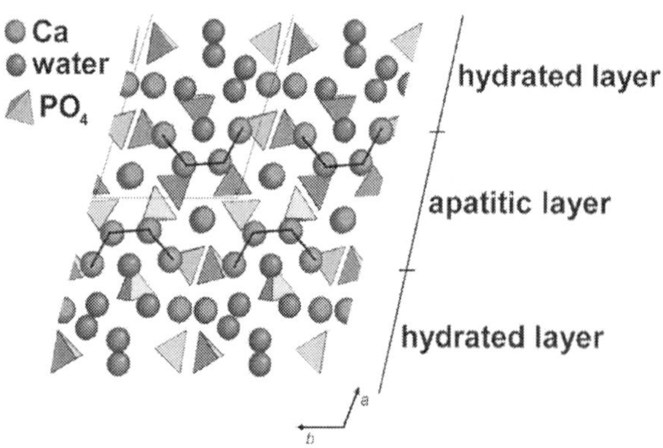

Fig. 2. OCP structure down the c-axis. The hydrated and apatitic layers are highlighted. The positions of Ca atoms connected by black lines and of the phosphate groups of the apatitic layer are very close to those found in the HA structure.[27]

Type of TiO_2	PZC	IEP
Hydrous TiO_2	5.0 [35]	5.0 [35]
Nanocrystalline	5.7 [36]	-
Anatase	6.2 [37], 6 [38]	6.2 [39], 5.6 [40]
Rutile	5.5 [38], 5.3 [37]	-

Table 3. Literature values for the point of zero charge (PZC) and iso-electric points (IEP) of TiO_2

Sol-gel derived amorphous titanium oxide [41] is not considered to be bioactive in the sense that it forms HA on its surface, despite the fact that the IEP is much lower than that of SBF. The crystalline phases of titanium dioxide, anatase and rutile, have good ability to induce hydroxyapatite formation on the surface. However, titanium dental implants with native amorphous surface oxide have shown good osseointegration and been used successfully in clinics. This means that a crystalline phase of TiO_2 is not a prerequisite for inducing hydroxyapatite formation. Uchida et al [41] have reported that the difference between amorphous and crystallized titanium oxide implied that not all Ti-OH groups, but certain types of Ti-OH groups in a specific structural arrangement, are effective in inducing apatite nucleation. The crucial part is how well structurally matched the interface between the organized hydroxylated surface and HA nuclei are, and also the surface charge.

When comparing hydroxylated 110 (anatase) and 0001 (HA) it is suggested that there are three important parts in matching their interface. (1) Hydrogen bond interaction; Ti–OH groups can form hydrogen bonds with OPO_3^{3-} on the HA (0001) surface, and also with OH^- on the HA (0001). (2) Crystal lattice matching, i.e., how the Ti–OH groups are arranged on the anatase (110) surface matching the HA (0001) (3) Stereochemical matching, which is the anatase OH- arrangement surrounding a Ca^{2+} ion along the c-axis of HA, resulting in oriented nucleation [42].

The rutile (101) surface also has a lattice match with HA (0001) [41]. The nucleation of the crystallized species and their orientation tend to be determined more by stereochemical matching than lattice matching [31]. Anatase is speculated to have a higher bioactivity than rutile, due to a better lattice match with HA and a higher acidity, as well as lower surface ζ-potential, caused by a larger number of hydroxyl groups on the surface [43]. The degree of surface acidity at a given pH is the value of the surface ζ-potential. The surface ζ-potential is lower for a more acidic surface. It has been shown that deposition of HA on anatase, at pH 7.4, is faster than on rutile at the same pH, while a less negative ζ-potential will inhibit the HA nucleation [43]. Furthermore a rise in temperature and ion concentration increases the growth rate of HA [44].

Based on the theorical considerations briefly outlined above, different chemical and physical methods have been used to improve the bioactivity of Ti based materials. In term of chemical methods, NaOH and HCl are typically used to treat the Ti surface [45]. A kind of sodium hydrogen titanate ($Na_xH_{2-x}Ti_3O_7$) is formed on the surface of titanium and its alloys after treatment in highly concentrated solutions of NaOH [45]. If this surface is subsequently treated with HCl solution, the sodium hydrogen titanate will transform into hydrogen titanate ($H_2Ti_3O_7$) [45]. The Na^+ and H^+ ions could be released from the surface via exchanging with H_3O^+ ions in the SBF to induce Ti-OH groups on the surface. However, the ability to induce hydroxyapatite formation after these treatments is relatively low. Only after such samples are further treated with heat to form rutile and anatase on the surface, can the ability of hydroxyapatite formation be improved significantly.

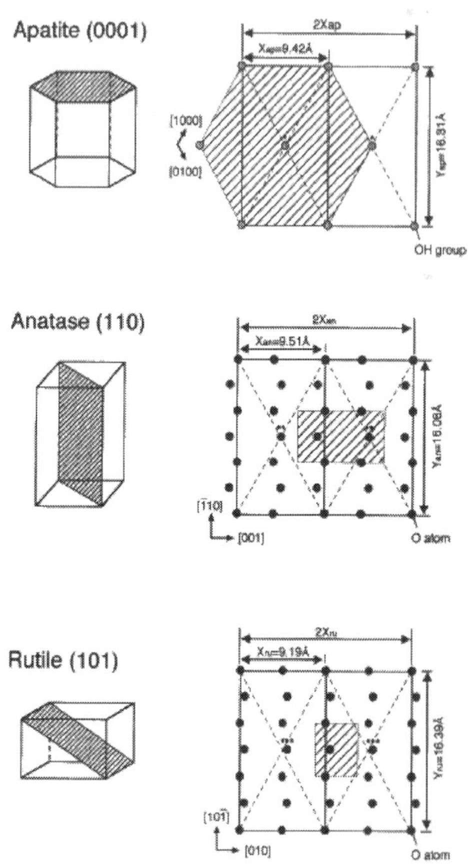

Fig. 3. Positions of hydroxyl group on (0001) plane in the hydroxyapatite crystal compared with those of oxygen on (110) plane of anatase and on (101) plane of rutile. [41]

Other methods to form or transform a crystalline titanium dioxide surface on Ti implants are important for the control of bioactivity, for examples, physical (e.g. physical vapour deposition) or heat treatment (the native amorphous surface transform into crystalline at temperature of about 300 degrees Celcius).

4. Novel techniques of interface analysis

The study of the formation and properties of biomimetic coatings requires the use of analytical techniques that can provide nanoscale information about the crystallinity, morphology and chemical composition of the coatings. In this section we briefly describe a technique that has recently been used to obtain nanoscale information about the interface between apatites and bone.

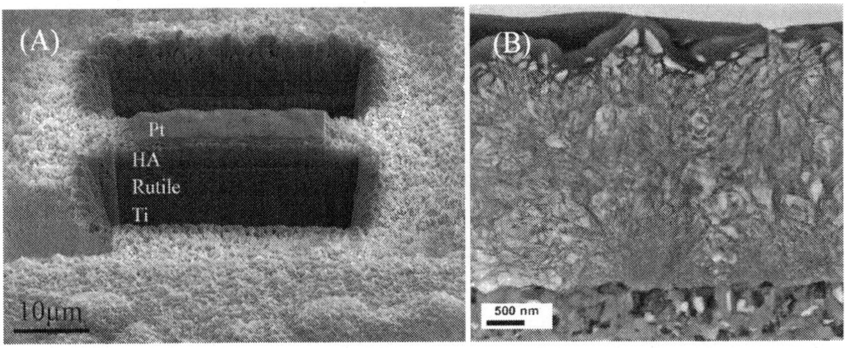

Fig. 4. (A) Preparation of a TEM sample using FIB,[46] (B) Cross-section TEM micrograph of the polycrystalline rutile TiO_2 coated with HA.[30]

Focused ion beam (FIB) microscopy has previously been used extensively in the material science community, especially in the study of semiconductor devices in the microelectronics industry [48, 49]. The FIB system scans a beam of positively charged gallium ions over the sample, similar to the electron beam in the scanning electron microscope (SEM). The ions generate sputtered neutral atoms, secondary electrons, and secondary ions. The electrons or the positively charged ions can be used to form an image. The images taken within the FIB show a different contrast than the normal SEM images, which can give additional information. More significantly it is possible to increase the beam current of the primary ion beam and use the FIB as a fine-scale micro-machining tool. Production of transmission electron microscopy (TEM) samples using focused ion beam (FIB) microscopy provides the possibility of studying interfaces with precise control of the analysis site and the ability to mill the material down to electron transparency (**Fig. 4**). This technique facilitates studies of biomaterial-tissue and coating-implants interfaces [50, 51].

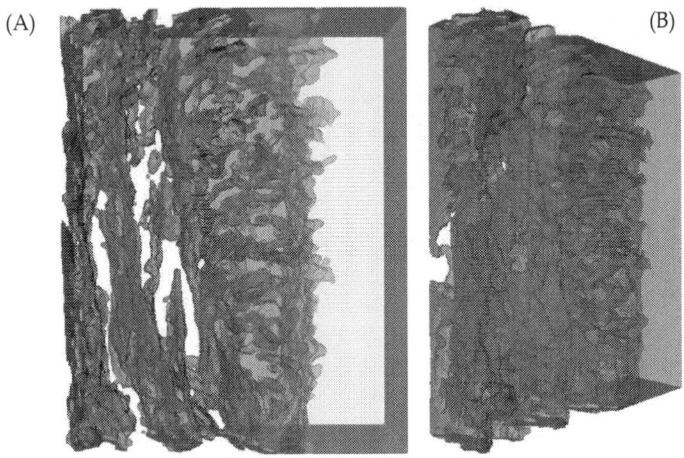

Fig. 5. Three dimensional reconstruction of the interface between human bone and a hydroxyapatite implant using Z-contrast electron tomography with FIB slice.[47]

Grandfield et al recently reported a three dimensional reconstruction of the interface between human bone and a hydroxyapatite implant using Z-contrast electron tomography with FIB slice (**Fig. 5**) [47]. Viewing this structure in three dimensions enabled observation of visualization of nanometre differences in the orientation of hydroxyapatite crystals precipitated on the implant surface in vivo versus those in the collagen matrix of bone. Insight into the morphology of biointerfaces is considerably enhanced with three-dimensional techniques.

5. Surface and interface analysis of biomimetic HA deposition on titanium oxide surfaces

Biomimetic HA deposition is mimicking the natural process of remineralization of hydroxyapatite, but without involving cellular and organic species. The surface chemistry of the substrate materials is an important factor for the coatings produced in these processes. The formation of a negatively charged surface composed with Ti-OH is a key step of inducing growth of new hydroxyapatite in a simulated body fluid, which for crystalline titanium dioxides can occur, as discussed in section 3.

No HA formation could be detected on sol-gel derived amorphous titanium oxide surfaces even after 14 days of soaking in SBF or PBS. But on both rutile and anatase HA forms readily in SBF or PBS solution. This implies that not all Ti-OH groups, but certain types of Ti-OH groups in a specific structural arrangement, are effective in inducing apatite nucleation [41, 52, 53] Nancollas explained that the surface tension of the metal oxides would influence the apatite nucleation. Uchida et al assumed the atomic arrangements in their crystal structures to be suitable for the epitaxy of apatite crystals. The good crystallographic matching is favorable to the apatite epitaxial growth along (0001) plane.

Engqvist et al has investigated some boundary conditions for HA formation on crystalline titanium oxide surfaces regarding influence of coating thickness, soaking time and soaking temperature [24]. The soaking temperature had an effect on the HA formation and

	1 h	1 day	1 week	4 weeks
4°C furnace	-	-	-	-
37°C furnace	-	HA	HA	HA
65°C furnace	-	HA	HA	HA

Table 4. HA growth for temperature versus time test matrix on oxidized rutile surfaces[24]

	1 h	1 day	1 week	4 weeks
4°C reference	-	-	-	-
37°C reference	-	-	-	-
65°C reference	-	-	HA	HA

Table 5. HA growth for temperature versus time test matrix on reference samples with native titanium oxide[24]

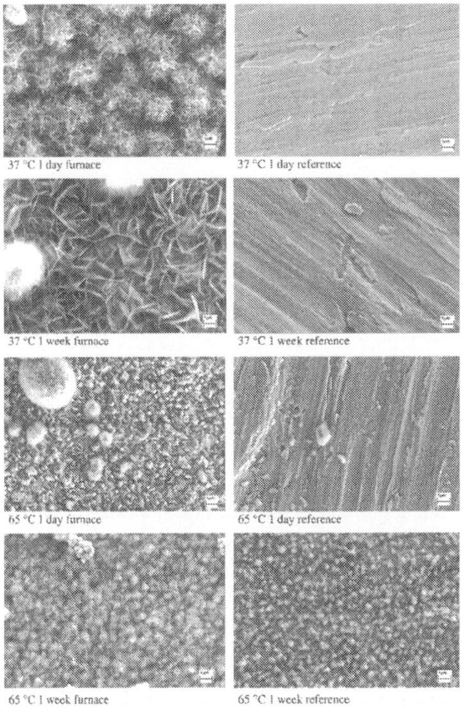

Fig. 6. SEM of HA formation at 37°C and 65°C on furnace treated samples and untreated references. None of the reference samples showed any HA growth except the 65°C immersed for 1 week [24].

growth on both rutile surfaces and native oxide on Ti substrates. Higher temperatures lead to more formation of HA. It was even possible, at 65°C, to grow HA on native titanium oxide by soaking in PBS. The coating quality was better for HA formed at 65°C compared to 37°C (**table 4 and 5, Fig. 6**).

Effects of titanium oxide PVD coating thickness (from 19 nm to 74 nm) on HA growth were also investigated [54]. All coatings were active, which is interesting from a surface modification point of view; it could well be sufficient to have very thin coatings to obtain the desired biological effect. One obvious benefit of thin coatings is the higher adhesion compared to thicker coatings. Thick coatings have higher internal stresses leading to higher probability of coating delamination. The PVD coated TiO_2 investigated was a graded bioactive coating, having a gradient by TiO_2 (~40nm), TiO_x (~70nm) and the substrate, see **Fig. 7 and 8** [54]. The adhesion to the substrate was above 1 GPa.

Because biomimetic HA coating is deposited from a supersaturated phosphate buffer solution, it shows a porous structure. So the internal strength of this coating is expected to be low, as compared to coatings prepared by sputtering methods. Forsgren et al used a scratch test to asses the adhesion of the biomimetic HA coatings [30]. This is a well established method to provide a measure of the coating-to-substrate adhesion and was found to be a useful method to test the thin HA coatings deposited on the bioactive surfaces. The critical pressure of the layer was estimated to be 2.4 ± 0.1 GPa [30].

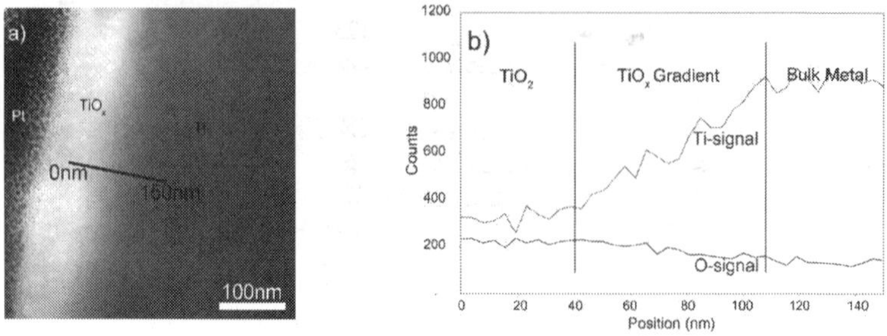

Fig. 7. (a) STEM image showing the titanium oxide layer in cross-section. The coating features are marked in the image and (b) the corresponding line profiles of Ti and oxygen over the marked line from 0 nm to 150 nm as obtained by EDS are displayed.[54]

In order to ensure coating sterility and to increase the adhesion, biomimetic hydroxyapatite (HA) coatings on titanium oxide have been heat-treated at 600 and 800°C for one hour [46]. The 600 °C heat treatment of the HA coating changed its morphology, increased its grain size and also increased the porosity. At 800 °C the coating was completely transformed to β-TCP according to XRD, see Fig.9. Fig. 10 shows that the HA crystal size increased after heat treatment, but the morphology was still porous.

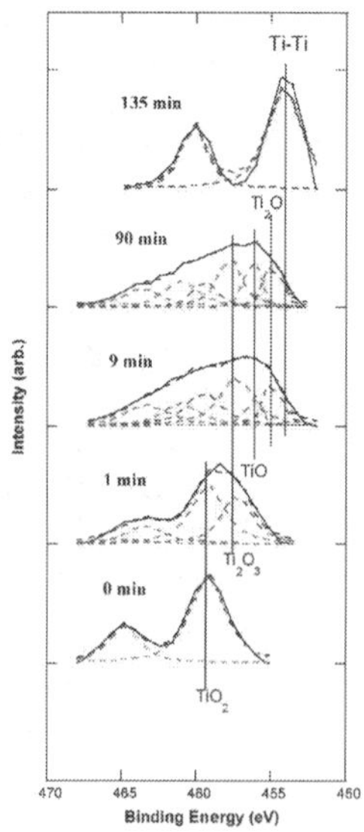

Fig. 8. XPS Ti 2p spectra (solid line) showing peak shift in titanium oxide after sputtering through the coating at the displayed times. Incorporated in the figures are curve fits, assuming Lorenzian-Gaussian Ti 2p photo peaks, to literature values [23] of binding energies for various Ti containing phases (broken lines). Vertical solid lines, indicating the binding energy of the Ti 2p3/2 peak, for TiO_2, Ti_2O_3, TiO, Ti_2O and pure Ti are also included in the figure.[54]

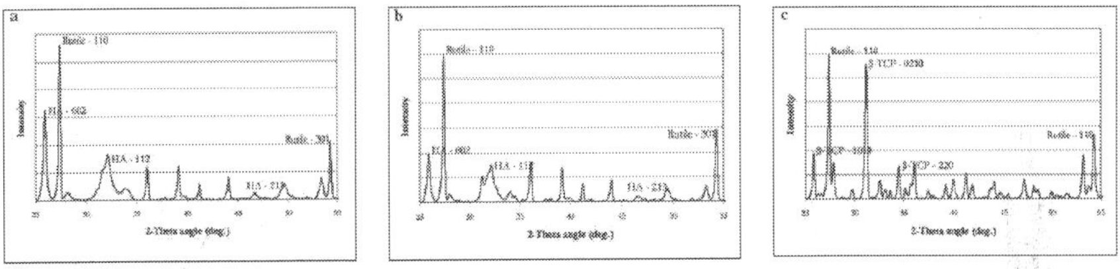

Fig. 9. XRD of biomimetic HA coating on rutile. The strongest diffraction peaks are indexed. (a) Untreated HA, (b) HA heat treated at 600 °C, (c) HA heat treated at 800 °C. [46]

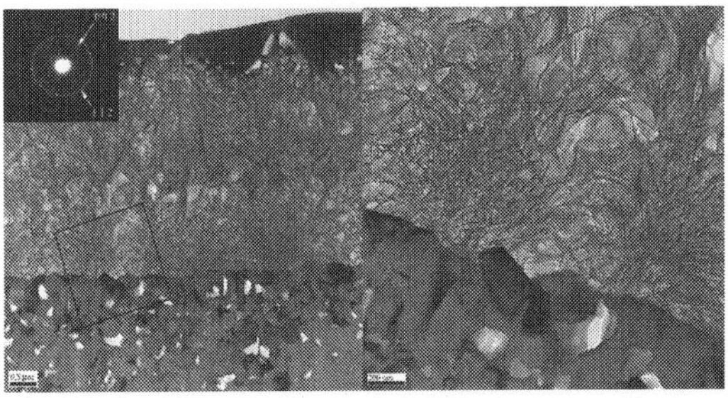

(A)

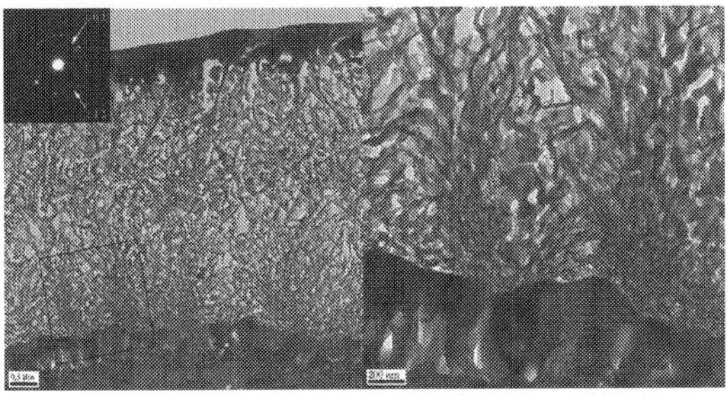

(B)

Fig. 10. TEM image of HA formed on rutile (A) and heat treated at 600 °C (B). The square shows where the right micrograph was acquired. [46]

Fundamental studies of HA growth on titanium oxide

Uchida et al showed that for certain crystallographic planes in the two ordered TiO_2 structures rutile and anatase the oxygen position match well with the hydroxyl groups in hydroxyapatite [41]. This could provide an answer why hydroxyapatite will not grow readily on amorphous TiO_2, since here the oxygen positions are not ordered. Epitaxial nucleation of hydroxyapatite on rutile is expected to occur based on the two-dimensional similarity of the two structures. Muller et al. studied the orientation of crystals in a hydroxylapatite film grown on titanium metal with a coating layer of TiH_{2-x} [55]. They found from electron diffraction that the crystallites in the film were preferentially oriented with the c axis of the hydroxyapatite directed out from the surface. The preferential orientation was limited to the outer parts of the hydroxyapatite precipitate. Hydroxyapatite crystals are plate-shaped with [001] HA normal to the plane of the plate and [100] HA within that plane [56]. When precipitated, the plates are oriented perpendicular to the substrate surface, so that the fast-growing [100] HA direction is projected outward.

Engqvist et al also reported experimental observations of early growth and growth of hydroxyapatite on single-crystal rutile substrates (100), (001), and (110) [57]. The specific crystal faces of rutile were used to study if hydroxyapatite grows differently depending on the crystal surface of rutile, and also to investigate the previously presented hypothesis of epitaxial growth of hydroxyapatite on rutile.

Table 6 shows the atomic concentrations for detected elements for an immersion series with the (110) surface. The data shows a continuous increase of the Ca and P concentrations, as well as Ca/P ratio, with immersion time. The Ca/P ratio is in all cases far below the expected for hydroxyapatite (nominal Ca/P ratio of 1.67).

	(110) ref	(110) 10 min	(110) 1 h	(110) 24 h	(001) 24 h
Ti	20.70	22.00	20.10	19.41	18.67
O	51.26	56.39	56.83	56.00	55.28
C	25.36	20.23	21.39	21.99	23.40
N	1.21	0.97	1.07	1.50	1.38
Si	1.04	0.00	0.00	0.00	0.00
Ca	0.00	0.03	0.08	0.20	0.29
P	0.00	0.41	0.53	0.91	1.01
Ca/P	n.a.	0.06	0.14	0.22	0.28

Values are mean of two measurement areas on each sample

Table 6. Relative concentrations (at.%) of elements detected in XPS analyses. Also shown are the Ca/P ratios[57]

Comparison between the (110) and (001) surfaces after 24 immersion shows higher Ca and P values for the latter. The relative intensities of the calcium and phosphate signals, as measured by time-of-flight secondary ion mass spectrometry (ToF-SIMS, see **Fig. 11**), varied for the different crystalline directions and PBS immersion times. The adsorption of calcium and phosphate ions was faster on the (001) and (100) surfaces than on the (110) surface. The measured Ca/P ratios were in all cases far below that of hydroxyapatite and other calcium phosphates, showing that no crystal formation had taken place at the surfaces after the studied immersion times.

Hydroxyapatite grown on different surfaces has fundamentally different appearances (**Fig. 12**). On the (001) surface of rutile the hydroxyapatite crystallites grow as a dense layer, with the platelike crystallites growing side by side, **Fig. 12a**. On the fast growing direction (100) HA points out from the surface. This was similar to the growth in the polycrystalline rutile, but in contrast to the growth on the (110) surface. On the (110) surface the crystallites grew in bundles. Spheres made up of several hydroxyapatite crystals were formed on the substrate surface, see **Fig. 12c**. Precipitates that had been stopped at an early stage were also studied by SEM. On the (001) surface it could be seen that underneath every upward-projecting crystallite there was another crystal lying flat on the surface, **Fig. 12b**. This could not be seen in early stages of growth on the (110) surface. Here the crystallites immediately formed spherical bundles, see **Fig. 12d**. At early stages of precipitation on the (100) surface, few and randomly oriented crystallites without the distinct plate-like shape were seen. At later stages, however, dense layers of upright crystallites were seen, **Fig. 12e and f**.

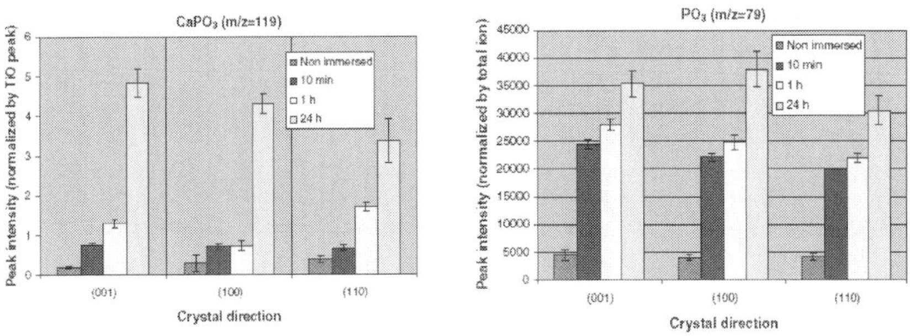

Fig. 11. Relative peak intensities $CaPO_3^+$ and PO_3^- for different crystal surfaces and PBS immersion times. The $CaPO_3^+$ Peak intensities are normalized against the TiO^+ signal from TiO_2 and the PO_3^- signal is normalized against total ion intensity. Values shown are mean ± standard deviation for three measurement areas on each sample.[57]

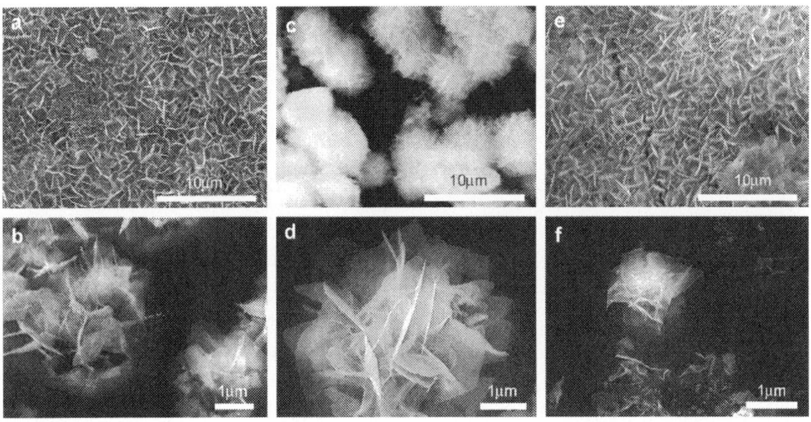

Fig. 12. Precipitation of hydroxylapatite on single-crystal substrates. (a), (c) and (e) show late stages of the precipitation process on the (001), (110) and (100) rutile surfaces, respectively. In (a) and (e) dense films of upright crystallites have formed, while in (c) the crystallites are bundled in ball-like aggregates. (b), (d) and (f) show early stages. On the (001) surface, a crystal is often seen lying flat beneath later precipitated crystals. This is not seen on the other surfaces.[31]

A good adhesion while was noted between rutile and HA at the (001) and (110) surfaces of rutile and for polycrystalline rutile, substrate-hydroxyapatite contact seemed poor at the (100) surface (**Fig. 13**). Across the whole nucleation interface in the TEM sample, the first 20 nm of the hydroxyapatite growth had the same orientation. The fast Fourier transform analysis (FFT) of the hydroxyapatite part of the micrograph (**Fig. 14**) indicated that the detected planes were (112) and (202). Thus, the [001] HA axis, which is parallel to the c axis in hydroxyapatite, is in this case oriented along the substrate surface and 11° off from the [001] rutile direction; the [100] HA was rotated about 14° away from the normal to the rutile surface. The hydroxyapatite crystals grow with their (001) HA direction along the (110)

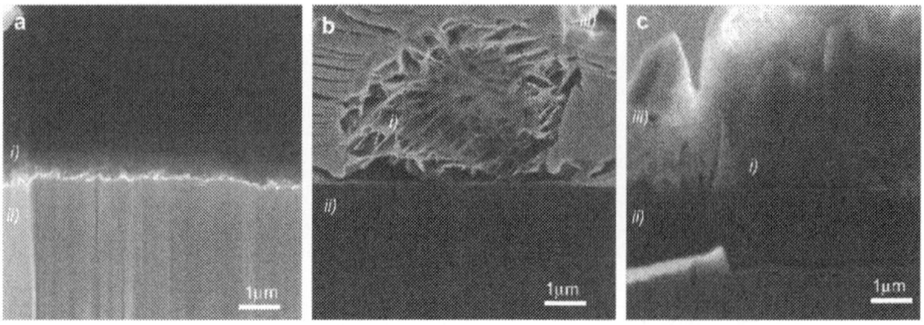

Fig. 13. SEM images recorded during the TEM sample preparation in the FIB. In the pictures (i) depicts hydroxylapatite, (ii) rutile, and (iii) the protective Pt layer deposited during the sample preparation. A solid interface is produced between the PVD-produced polycrystalline rutile surface and hydroxylapatite (a), the 001 surface and hydroxylapatite (c), and the (110) surface and hydroxylapatite (not shown). On the other hand, the interface between the (100) surface and hydroxylapatite (b) is porous and lacks good adhesion.[31]

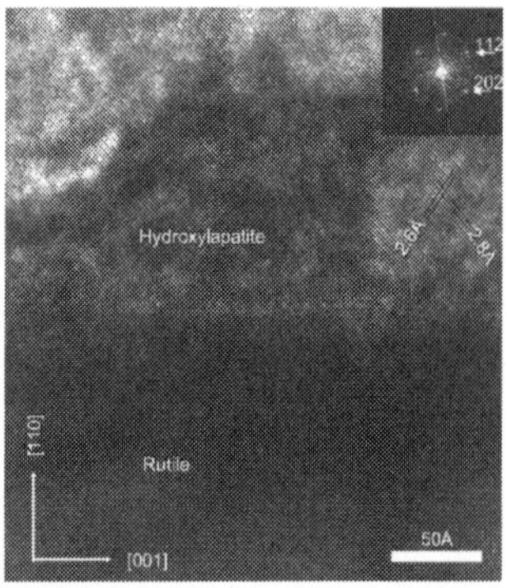

Fig. 14. On the (110) rutile surface, looking along [1–10], a 20 nm layer with the same orientation of hydroxylapatite has grown over the whole nucleation surface. From the inserted FFT, taken from that layer, the 112HA and 202HA are seen, and it can be concluded that [001] HA is oriented parallel to the substrate surface.[31]

rutile surface is an observation that seems general (**Fig. 15a and b**), which also constitute an image of the interface on the (110) surface, but instead recorded along the rutile zone axis [001].

This micrograph was taken at a lower magnification, allowing a large number of crystals to be included in the FFT calculation in order to obtain better statistics in the analysis. The FFT analysis reveals the (100) HA and equivalent to be oriented out from the surface, and thus the c axis of hydroxylapatite to be oriented along the rutile crystal face. However, as can be seen by the FFT analysis, an acceptance angle of the spread of the spots representing the direction of (100) HA is present, but no indication of ordering of (100) HA along the surface plane or of (001) HA growing out from the surface. On the (001) surface hydroxyapatite grew in another preferential direction. Contrary to the situation on the (110) surface, the FFT analysis here indicated that (100) HA and equivalent reflections are oriented along the surface (**Fig. 15c and d**). Furthermore, spots representing the (001) HA direction indicate the hydroxyapatite c axis to be oriented normal to the substrate surface.

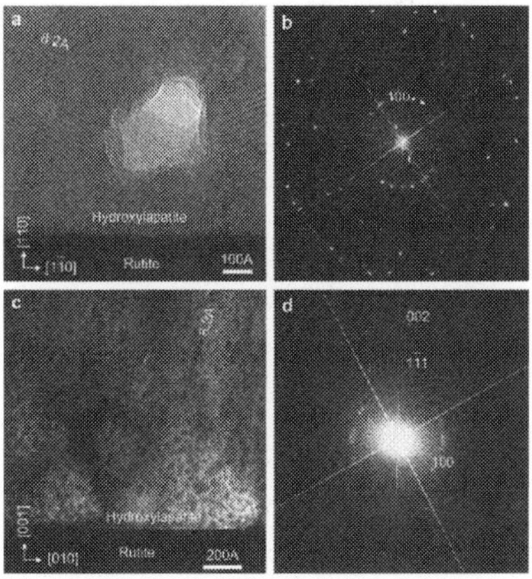

Fig. 15. (a) Micrograph recorded from the interface between hydroxylapatite and rutile (110), and (b) the corresponding FFT. The lattice fringes corresponding to the 100 spacing are indicated in the figure. In (b) it can be seen that the 100 reflection preferentially, with an acceptance angle, orders normal to the substrate surface. (c) Micrograph recorded from the interface between hydroxylapatite and rutile (001) and (d) the corresponding FFT. Judging from the FFT, the hydroxylapatite crystallites align with the c axis normal to the substrate surface, but with a directional spread of about ±25°.[31]

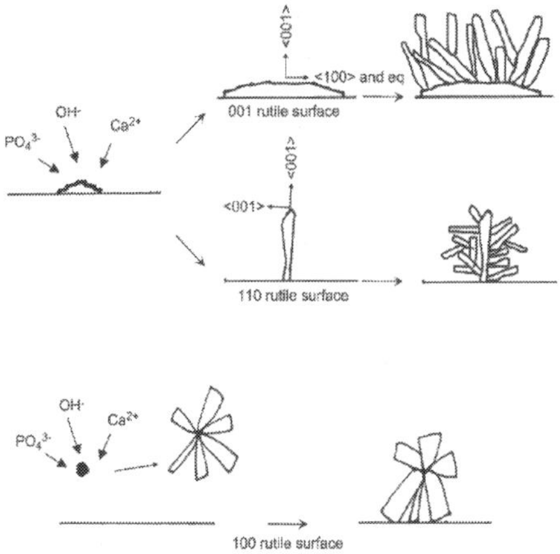

Fig. 16. Possible scenarios for the precipitation of hydroxyapatite on different rutile surfaces. [31]

Similar analysis of images taken further up in the hydroxyapatite layer, i.e., not at the interface, shows random orientation of the crystallites. Preferred orientation of the crystallites seems to be limited to the first few hundred nanometres. This explains why XRD does not reveal preferred orientation. Since the sampling volume is relatively large using this technique, the scattering from the immediate interface plays a minor role.

A possible scenario for the process of hydroxyapatite precipitation of hydroxyapatite on different rutile surfaces is shown in **Fig. 16**. At the rutile (001) surface, the hydroxyapatite nucleation seed orients so that further crystallization can proceed along the surface. At the (110) surface, the seed will nucleate so that the fast-growing directions of hydroxyapatite project out from the surface. Twin formation and dislocations in the basal layer make nucleation of additional crystals possible. The poor adhesion at the (100) rutile surface may arise if crystallites suspended in the solution form bundles that later attach to the surface. As the results, the specific orientation of the hydroxyapatite precipitate nucleus on the (001) surface leads to faster coverage of this surface compared to the (110) and (100) rutile surfaces. The preferred orientation of the precipitate is limited to the first few hundred nanometers, and the immediate interface indicated random orientation.

6. Growth of biomimetic ion doped HA on titanium oxide surfaces

Hydroxyapatite in bone is a multi-substituted calcium phosphate, including traces of CO_3^{2-}, F^-, Mg^{2+}, Sr^{2+}, Si^{4+} etc [8]. Anions can be incorporated into the sites of OH^- (type A) and PO_4^{3-} (type B) [58], and cations can be incorporated into the sites Ca^{2+} I and Ca^{2+} II [59]. These ionic substitutions play an important role in bone formation. There has been a significant research interest on the effects of CO_3^{2-}, F^-, Si^{4+} ions on the bioactivity of hydroxyapatite [60-63]. These ion substitutions not only change the composition, solubility and crystallinity of HA but also are important in cell proliferation, collagen synthesis, nuclei acid synthesis, bone development, and have pharmaceutical effects on bone regeneration. For example, strontium ranelate can reduce the incidence of fracture in osteoporotic patients.[64] The low dose administration of silicon and strontium could increase bone mass and strength by inhibiting bone resorption and augmenting bone formation.[65, 66] A local release of these trace elements at low dose is good for bone regeneration with a low drug usage compared to oral administration and injection. Silicon can increase the bone mineralization rate and enhance the osteoblast proliferation, differentiation and collagen production [62]. Fluoride, which is good for teeth, can stabilize apatite and also stimulate the osteoblast activity [61, 67]. Magnesium has been found in high concentrations in bone and cartilage tissue during the initial phases of osteogenesis, and to cause the acceleration of the nucleation kinetics of hydroxyapatite and to inhibit its crystallization process. Zn is known to be an essential trace element. It is important in the normal growth and development of the skeletal system and its deficiency is associated with a decrease in bone density [68]. Zn inhibits osteoclast differentiation and promotes osteoblast activity [69], and thus promotes bone formation.

Although biological hydroxyapatite has been used as coatings on metallic implants, there is room for improvement of this biomimetic coating in order to strengthen the implant and bone bonding and to have a stronger positive effect on new bone formation. Except for that, these ions could play their pharmaceutical functions at the same time.

Biomimietic methods for coating deposition involve mild conditions similar to those characteristic of biological environments, and allow deposition of CaP coatings on many different objects, such as metal surfaces, sponges, cements and fixation rods [70]. This is suitable for preparing the biomimetic ion substituted HA (iHA) on titanium oxide surfaces. At present, different kinds of biomimetic iHA coatings have been reported, such as CO_3^{2-}, F^-, Mg^{2+}, Zn^{2+}, Sr^{2+} Mn^{2+} and Si^{4+}. Here we will focus on the iHA coatings on titanium oxides surfaces.

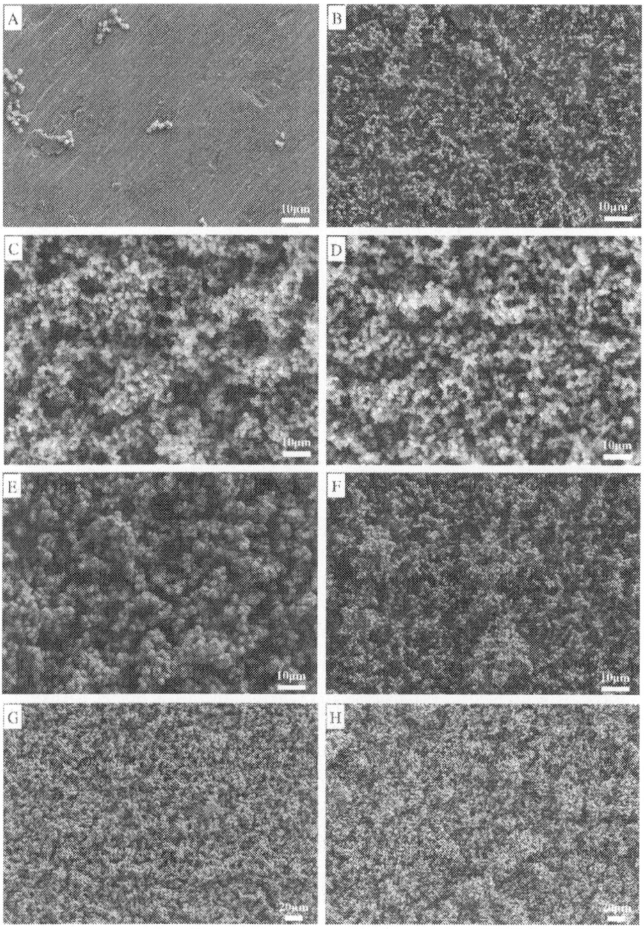

Fig. 17. SEM images of the PVD-treated titanium surface after soaking in Sr-PBS for 1 and 2 weeks. (A) 0.06 mMat 37°C for 1 week, (B) 0.6 mMat 37°C for 1 week, (C) 0.06 mM at 37°C for 2 week, (D) 0.6 mM at 37°C for 2 week, (E) 0.06 mM at 60°C for 1 week, (F) 0.6 mM at 60°C for 1 week, (G) 0.06 mM at 60°C for 2 weeks and (H) 0.6 mM at 60°C for 2 weeks.[25]

Biomimetic strontium substituted apatite coating on crystallized titanium oxide surface has been studied regarding its morphology, crystallinity, surface chemistry and composition as functions of soaking temperature and time in phosphate buffer solutions with different Sr ion concentration [25]. The increase of soaking temperature and time improved the formation rate and crystallinity of SrHA coatings, but could not greatly change the strontium content in the coating, whereas the concentration of strontium ion in the soaking medium influenced the surface composition. **Fig. 17** shows the changes of surface morphologies of SrHA coatings as functions of the concentration of Sr ion, soaking temperature and time. However, the morphology of SrHA crystals could be changed by the

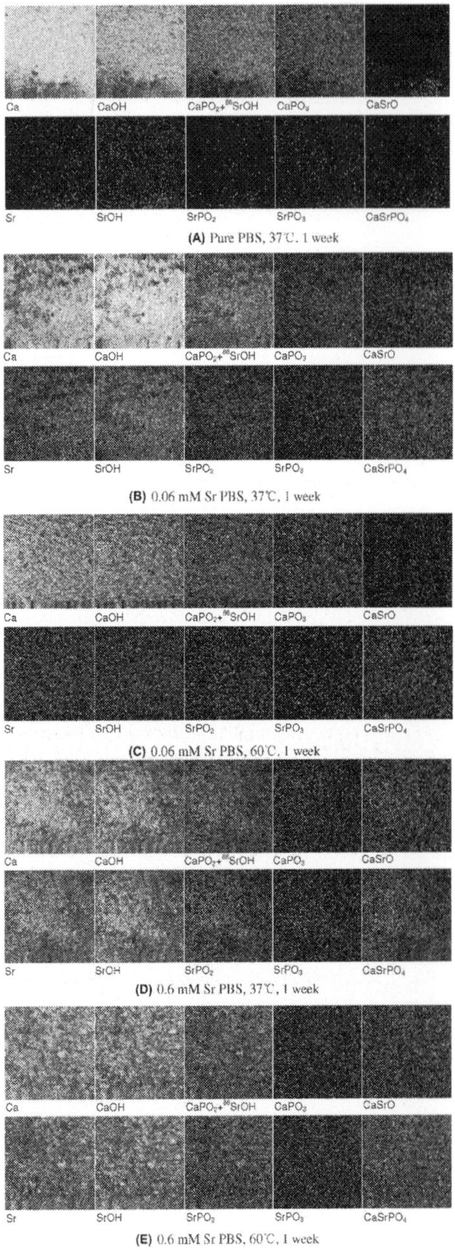

Fig. 18. TOF-SIMS ion images of the Sr-substituted apatite/titanium dioxide coating on titanium oxide [25]

soaking medium from plate-like to sphere-like [25]. Ion images obtained from ToF-SIMS analyses show homogeneous Ca and Sr distributions, indicating co-localization of the Ca and Sr ions (**Fig. 18**).

Silicon doped hydroxyapatite coating deposited on titanium oxide has been reported by Zhang and Xia et al [71, 72]. Similar morphology with biomimetic hydroxyapatite has been observed (**Fig. 19**). Cracks are also observed due to the dehydration shrinkage. The coating thickness was 5-10μm with a shear strength in the order of ~16MPa. The chemical reactions in the solution could be illustrated as following [71]:

$$H_2O + SiO_3^{2-} \rightarrow H_2SiO_4^{2-} \quad (1)$$

$$H_2SiO_4^{2-} \rightarrow H^+ + HSiO_4^{3-} \quad (2)$$

$$HSiO_4^{3-} \rightarrow H^+ + SiO_4^{4-} \quad (3)$$

$$HPO_4^{2-} \rightarrow H^+ + PO_4^{3-} \quad (4)$$

$$H^+ + HCO_3^- \rightarrow H_2O + CO_2 \uparrow \quad (5)$$

$$10Ca^{2+} + \frac{1}{3}(20-4x-y)PO_4^{3-} + xSiO_4^{4-} + yOH^- \rightarrow Ca_{10}(PO_4)_{\frac{1}{3}(20-4x-y)}(SiO_4)_x(OH)_y \downarrow \quad (6)$$

Silicon was confirmed to exist in the form of SiO_4^{4-} groups in biomimetic SiHA coating.

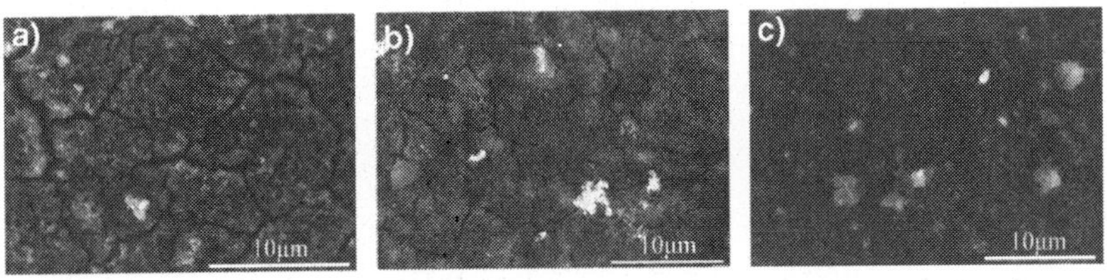

Fig. 19. SEM surface micrographs of biomimetic SiHA coatings obtained from different silicon modified Hank's balanced salt solution, (a) 1mM; (b) 5mM; (c) 100mM.[71]

6. Biological response of biomimetic HA coatings

Calcium phosphate based coatings on titanium implants are now accepted to be suitable for enhancing bone formation around implants, to contribute to cementless fixation and thus to improve clinical success at an early stage after implantation [70]. Narayanan and Kim et al summarized the interface reactions as following five steps [70].

1. Dissolution of calcium phosphate based coatings,
2. Re-precipitation of apatite,
3. Ion exchange accompanied by absorption and incorporation of biological molecules,
4. Cell attachment, proliferation and differentiation,
5. Extracellular matrix formation and mineralization.

The dissolution of HA coating is a key step to induce the precipitation of bone-like apatite on the implant surface. Because the biomimetic hydroxyapatite coatings have a low degree of crystallinity and porous structure, their solubility is higher than the for dense hydroxyapatite coatings deposited with other methods. That is bone expected to be

beneficial to early bone formation. Otherwise, rough and porous surfaces could stimulate cell attachment and formation of extra-cellular matrix [73].
The biological benefits/effects of biomimetic HA [63, 74-76] and the possibilities to use them as coatings on titanium implants for improving the biological responses have been reported. However, only a few of the developed ion-substituted and/or ion doped hydroxyapatite coatings have been tested in vitro and/or in vivo, and the improvement of the biological response due to ion substitution is thus still just a hypothesis [20, 27, 77-79]. For biomimetic SiHA coatings on heat treated titanium, Zhang et al reported higher cell proliferation on this type of deposition, and the bone ingrowth rate (BIR) was not only significantly higher than for uncoated titanium, but also significantly higher than for biomimetic hydroxyapatite coated titanium [79].

7. Conclusions

Crystallized titanium oxides induce bone-like hydroxyapatite on its surface, which can be hypothesized as an important early step for osseointegration. The understanding of mechanisms behind biomimetic HA depositions on titanium oxide surfaces could therefore contribute to increased understanding the mechanism of the osseointegration, and also provide a scientific basis for design and control of biomimetic layers for medical applications. Deposition of biomimetic hydroxyapatite on titanium oxide surfaces, acting as a bonding layer to the bone, might improve the bone-bonding ability and enhance the biological responses to bone anchored implants.

8. References

[1] Ellingsen JE, Lyngstadaas SP. Bio-implant interface: improving biomaterials and tissue reactions, CRC Press, USA.
[2] Zhou W, Zong X, Wu X, Yuan L, Shu Q, Xia Y. Plasmacontrolled nanocrystallinity and phase composition of TiO2: a smart way to enhance biomimetic response J Biomed Mat Res 2007;81A:453–464.
[3] Lausmaa J. Surface spectroscopic characterization of titanium implant materials. J Electron Spectr Related Phenom 1996;81:343-361.
[4] Ellingsen J. A study on the mechanism of protein adsorption to TiO2. Biomaterials 1991;12:593-596.
[5] Kido H, Saha S. Effect of HA coating on the long-term survival of dental implant: a review of the literature. J Long Term Eff Med Implants 1996;6(2):119-133.
[6] Hench L. Bioceramics: From concept to clinic. J Am Ceram Soc 1991;74:1487–1510.
[7] Boanini E, Gazzano M, Bigi A. Ionic substitutions in calcium phosphates synthesized at low temperature. Acta Biomater 2009; 6(6):1882-1894.
[8] Dorozhkin SV, Epple M. Biological and medical significance of calcium phosphates. Angew Chem Int Ed Engl 2002;41(17):3130-3146.
[9] Vallet-Regí M. Ceramics for medical applications. J Chem Soc, Dalton Trans 2001:97-108.
[10] Kim H, Koh Y, Li L, Lee S, Kim H. Hydroxyapatite coating on titanium substrate with titania buffer layer processed by sol-gel method. Biomaterials 2004;25:2533-2538.
[11] Montenero A, Gnappi G, Ferrari F, Cesari M, Salvioli E, Mattogno L, Kaciulis S, Fini M. Sol-gel derived hydroxyapatite coatings on titanium substrate. J Mater Sci 2000;35:2791-2797.

[12] Thian E, Khor K, Loh N, Tor S. Processing of HAcoated Ti-6Al-4V by a ceramic slurry approach: An in vitro study. Biomaterials 2001;22:1225-1232.

[13] Gledhill H, Turner I, Doyle C. Direct morphological comparison of vacuum plasma sprayed and detonation gun sprayed hydroxyapatite coatings. Biomaterials 1999;20:315-322.

[14] Inagaki M, Hozumi A, Okudera H, Yokogawa Y, Kameyama T. Improvement of chemical resistance of apatite/titanium composite coatings deposited by RF plasma spraying: Surface modification by chemical vapor deposition. Thin Solid Films 2001;382:69-73.

[15] Massaro C, Baker M, Cosentino F, Ramires P, Klose S, Milella E. Surface and biological evaluation of hydroxyapatite-based coatings on titanium deposited by different techniques. J Biomed Mater Res 2001;58:651-657.

[16] Cleries L, Fernandez-Pradas J, Morenza J. Bone growth on and resorption of calcium phosphate coatings obtained by pulsed laser deposition. J Biomed Mater Res 2000;49:43-52.

[17] Fernandez-Pradas J, Cleries L, Sardin G, Morenza J. Hydroxyapatite coatings grown by pulsed laser deposition with a beam of 355 nm wavelength. J Mater Res 1999;14:4715-4719.

[18] Yen S, Lin C. Cathodic reactions of electrolytic hydoxyapatite coating on pure titanium. Mater ChemPhys 2002;77:70-76.

[19] Kameyama T. Hybrid bioceramics with metals and polymers for better biomaterials. Bull Mater Sci 1999;22:641-646.

[20] Jalota S, Bharduri S, Tas A. Using a synthetic body fluid (SBF) solution of 27 mM HCO_3- to make bone substitutes more osteointegrative. Mater Sci Eng C 2008;28:129-140.

[21] Kokubo T, Kushitani H, Sakka S, Kitsugi T, Yamamuro T. Solutions able to reproduce in vivo surface-structure change in bioactive glass-ceramic A–W. J Biomed Mater Res 1990;24:721-734.

[22] Pasinli A, Yuksel M, Celik E, Sener S, Tas AC. A new approach in biomimetic synthesis of calcium phosphate coatings using lactic acid–Na lactate buffered body fluid solution. Acta Biomaterialia 2010;6:2282-2288.

[23] Kokubo T, Takadama H. How useful is SBF in predicting in vivo bone bioactivity? Biomaterials 2006;27:2907-2915.

[24] Lindgren M, Astrand M, Wiklund U, Engqvist H. Investigation of boundary conditions for biomimetic HA deposition on titanium oxide surfaces. J Mater Sci Mater Med 2009;20(7):1401-1408.

[25] Xia W, Lindahl C, Lausmaa J, Borchardt P, Ballo A, Thomsen P, Engqvist H. Biomineralized strontium-substituted apatite/titanium dioxide coating on titanium surfaces. Acta Biomater 2010;6(4):1591-1600.

[26] Elliot JC. Structural and chemistry of the apatites and other calcium orthophosphates. Amsterdam, Elsevier 1994.

[27] Boanini E, Gazzano M, Bigi A. Ionic substitutions in calcium phosphates synthesized at low temperature. Acta Biomater 2010;6(6):1882-1894.

[28] Onuma K, Ito A. Cluster growth for hydroxyapatite. Chem Mater 1998;10:3346-3351.

[29] Gamble J. Chemical anatomy, physiology and pathology of extracellular fluid. Cambridge, MA: Harvard University Press, 1967.

[30] Forsgren J, Svahn F, Jarmar T, Engqvist H. Formation and adhesion of biomimetic hydroxyapatite deposited on titanium substrates. Acta Biomater 2007 Nov;3(6):980-984.
[31] Lindberg F, Heinrichs J, Ericson F, Thomsen P, Engqvist H. Hydroxylapatite growth on single-crystal rutile substrates. Biomaterials 2008;29(23):3317-3323.
[32] Barrere F, van Blitterswijk CA, de Groot K, Layrolle P. Influence of ionic strength and carbonate on the Ca-P coating formation from SBFx5 solution. Biomaterials 2002;23(9):1921-1930.
[33] Tas AC, Bhaduri SB. Rapid coating of Ti6Al4V at room temperature with a calcium phosphate solution similar to 10× simulated body fluid. J Mater Res 2004;19:2742-2749
[34] Hanks JH, Wallace RE. Relation of oxygen and temperature in the preservation of tissues by refrigeration. Proc Soc Exp Biol Med 1949;71:196-200.
[35] Ottaviani MF, Ceresa EM, Visca M. Cation Adsorption at the TiO2-Water Interface. J Colloid Interf Sci 1985;108:114-122.
[36] Poznyak SK, Pergushov VI, Kokorin AI, Kulak AI, Sclapfer CW. Structure and Electrochemical Properties of Species Formed as a Result of Cu(II) Ion Adsorption onto TiO2 Nanoparticles. J Phys Chem B 1999;103:1308-1315.
[37] Malati MA, Smith AE. The Adsorption of the Alkaline Earth Cations on Titanium Dioxide. Powder Technol 1979;22:279-282.
[38] Kosmulski M. The significance of the difference in zero charge between rutile and anatase. Adv Colloid Interfac 2002;99:255-264.
[39] Vassileva E, Proinova I, Hadjiivanov K. Solid-Phase Extraction of Heavy Metal Ions on a High Surface Area Titanium Dioxide (Anatase). Analyst 1996;121:607-612.
[40] Winkler J, Marme S. Titania as a Sorbent in Normal-Phase Liquid Chromatography. J Chromatogr A 2000;888:51-62.
[41] Uchida M, Kim HM, Kokubo T, Fujibayashi S, Nakamura T. Structural dependence of apatite formation on titania gels in a simulated body fluid. J Biomed Mater Res A 2003;64(1):164-170.
[42] Mao C, Li H, Cui F, Ma C, Feng Q. Oriented growth of phosphates on polycrystalline titanium in a process mimicking biomineralization. J Cryst Growth 1999;206:308-321.
[43] Svetina M, Colombi L, Sbaizero O, Meriani S, A. D. Deposition of calcium ions on rutile (110): A first-principles investigation. Acta Mater 2001;49:2169–2177.
[44] Kim H. Ceramic bioactivity and related biomimetic strategy Current Opinion in Solid State and Materials Science 2003;7(4-5):289-299.
[45] Kokubo T. Bioceramics and their clinical applications: CRC, 2008.
[46] Forsgren J, Svahn F, Jarmar T, Engqvist H. Structural change of biomimetic hydroxyapatite coatings due to heat treatment. J Appl Biomater Biomech 2007;5(1):23-27.
[47] Grandfield K, McNally E, Palmquist A, Botton G, Thomsen P, Engqvist H. Visualizing biointerfaces in three dimensions: electron tomography of the bone–hydroxyapatite interface J R Soc Interface 2010;7:1497–1501.
[48] Phaneuf M. Applications of focused ion beam microscopy to material science specimens Micron 1999;30:277–288.

[49] Giannuzzi L, Stevie F. Introduction to Focused Ion Beams: Theory, Intrumentation, Applications and Practice. Boston: Kluwer Academic, 2004.

[50] Engqvist H, Botton GA, Couillard M, Mohammadi S, Malmström J, Emanuelsson L, Hermansson L, Phaneuf MW, Thomsen P. A novel tool for high-resolution transmission electron microscopy of intact interfaces between bone and metallic implants J Biomed Mater Res 2006;78:20-24.

[51] Forsgren J, Svahn F, Jarmar T, Engqvist H. Formation and adhesion of biomimetic hydroxyapatite deposited on titanium substrates. Acta Biomaterialia 2007;3:980-984.

[52] Wu W, Nancollas G. Kinetics of Heterogeneous nucleation of calcium phosphates on anatase and rutile Surface. J Colli Inter Sci 1998;199:206–211.

[53] Nancollas G, Wu W, Tang R. The Mechanisms of crystallization and dissolution of calcium phosphates at surfaces Glastech Ber Glass Sci 2000;73(C1):318–325.

[54] Brohede U, Zhao S, Lindberg F, Mihranyan A, Forsgren J, Stromme M, Engqvist H. A novel graded bioactive high adhesion implant coating. Applied Surface Science 2009;255:7723-7728.

[55] Muller F, Muller L, Caillard D, Conforto E. Preferred growth orientation of biomimetic apatite crystals. Journal of Crystal Growth 2007;304:464–471.

[56] Leng Y, Qu S. TEM examination of single crystal hydroxyapatite diffraction. J Mater Sci Lett 2002;21:829–830.

[57] Lindahl C, Borchardt P, Lausmaa J, Xia W, Engqvist H. Studies of early growth mechanisms of hydroxyapatite on single crystalline rutile: a model system for bioactive surfaces. J Mater Sci Mater Med 2010 Aug 1.

[58] Young RA, Mackie PE. Crystallography of human tooth enamel: initial structure refinement. Mater Res Bull 1980;15(1):17-29.

[59] Li ZY, Lam WM, Yang C, Xu B, Ni GX, Abbah SA, Cheung KMC, Luk KDK, Lu WW. Chemical composition, crystal size and lattice structural changes after incorporation of strontium into biomimetic apatite. Biomaterials 2007;28:1452-1460.

[60] Gross KA, Rodriguez-Lorenzo LM. Sintered hydroxyfluorapatites. Part I: Sintering ability of precipitated solid solution powders. Biomaterials 2004;25:1375-1384.

[61] Robinson C, Shore RC, Brookes SJ, Strafford S, Wood SR, Kirkham J. The Chemistry of Enamel Caries. Crit Rev Oral Biol Med 2000;11:481-495.

[62] Pietak A, Reid J, Stott M, Sayer M. Silicon substitution in the calcium phosphate bioceramics. Biomaterials 2007;28: 4023–4032.

[63] Landi E, Tampieri A, Belmonte MM, Celotti G, Sandri M, Gigante A, Fava P, Biagini G. Biomimetic Mg- and Mg,CO_3-substituted hydroxyapatites: synthesis charcterization and in vitro behaviour. J Euro Ceram Soc 2006;26:2593-2601.

[64] Meunier PJ RC, Seeman E, Ortolani S, Badurski JE, Spector TD, Cannata J, Balogh A, Lemmel EM, Pors-Nielsen S, Rizzoli R, Genant HK, Reginster JY The effects of strontium ranelate on the risk of vertebral fracture in women with postmenopausal osteoporosis. N Engl J Med 2004;350:459-468.

[65] Hott M dPC, Modrowski D, Marie PJ. Short-term effects of organic silicon on trabecular bone in mature ovariectomized rats. Calcified Tissue Int 1993;53:174-179.

[66] P.Ammann, V.Shen, B.Robin, MY.auras, J.P.Bonjour, R.Rizzoli. Strontium ranelate improves bone resistance by increasing bone mass and improving architecture in intact female rats. J Bone Miner Res 2004;19:2012-2020.

[67] Wang Y, Zhang S, Zeng X, Ma LL, Weng W, Yan W, Qian M. Osteoblastic cell response on fluoridated hydroxyapatite coatings. Acta Biomater 2007;3:191-197.

[68] M. Y. Role of zinc in bone formation and bone resorption. J Trace Elem Exp Med 1998;11:119-135.

[69] Moonga B, Dempster D. Zinc is a potent inhibitor of osteoclastic bone resorption in vitro. J Bone Miner Res 1995;10:453-457.

[70] Narayanan R, Seshadri SK, Kwon TY, Kim KH. Calcium Phosphate-Based Coatings on Titanium and Its Alloys. J Biomed Mater Res Part B 2008;85B:279-299.

[71] Zhang E, Zou C, Zeng S. Preparation and characterization of silicon-substituted hydroxyapatite coating by a biomimetic process on titanium substrate Surface & Coatings Technology 2009;203:1075-1080.

[72] Xia W, Lindahl C, Persson C, Thomsen P, Lausmaa J, Engqvist H. Changes of surface composition and morphology after incorporation of ions into biomimetic apatite coating. Journal of Biomaterials and Nanobiotechnology 2010:Accepted.

[73] Boyan BD, Hummert TW, Dean DD, Schwartz Z. Role of material surfaces in regulating bone and cartilage cell response. Biomaterials 1996 Jan;17(2):137-146.

[74] Landi E, Tampieri A, Celotti G, Sprio S, Sandri M, Logroscino G. Sr-substituted hydroxyapatites for osteoporotic bone replacement. Acta Biomaterials 2007;3:961-969.

[75] Thian ES, Huang J, Best SM, Barber ZH, Bonfield W. Novel silicon-doped hydroxyapatite (Si-HA) for biomedical coatings: an in vitro study using acellular simulated body fluid. J Biomed Mater Res B 2006;76:326-333.

[76] Yang L, Perez-Amodio S, de-Groot FYFB, Everts V, Blitterswijk CAv, Habibovic P. The effects of inorganic additives to calcium phosphate on in vitro behavior of osteoblasts and osteoclasts. Biomaterials 2010;31:2976-2989.

[77] Bracci B, Torricelli P, Panzavolta S, Boanini E, Giardino R, Bigi A. Effect of Mg(2+), Sr(2+), and Mn(2+) on the chemico-physical and in vitro biological properties of calcium phosphate biomimetic coatings. J Inorg Biochem 2009;103(12):1666-1674.

[78] Capuccini C, Torricelli P, Boanini E, Gazzano M, Giardino R, Bigi A. Interaction of Sr-doped hydroxyapatite nanocrystals with osteoclast and osteo-blast-like cells. J Biomed Mater Res 2009;89A:594-600.

[79] Zhang E, Zou C. Porous titanium and silicon-substituted hydroxyapatite biomodification prepared by a biomimetic process: characterization and in vivo evaluation. Acta Biomaterialia 2009;5(5):1732-1741.

21

Biomimetic Topography: Bioinspired Cell Culture Substrates and Scaffolds

Lin Wang and Rebecca L. Carrier
Northeastern University
USA

1. Introduction

In vivo, cells are surrounded by 3D extracellular matrix (ECM), which supports and guides cells. Topologically, ECM is comprised of a heterogeneous mixture of pores, ridges and fibers which have sizes in the nanometer range. ECM structures with nanoscale topography are often folded or bended into secondary microscale topography, and even mesoscale tertiary topography. For example, ECM of small intestine folds into a 3D surface comprising three length scales of topography: the centimeter scale mucosal folds, sub-millimeter scale villi and crypts, and nanometer scale topography which is created by ECM proteins, such as collagen, laminin, and fibronectin. Techniques such as photolithography, two-photon polymerization, electrospinning, and chemical vapor deposition have been utilized to recreate certain ECM topographical features at specific length scales or exactly replicate complex and hierarchical topography *in vitro*. Various *in vitro* tests have proven that mammalian cells respond to biomimetic topographical cues ranging from mesoscale to nanometer scale (Bettinger et al., 2009, Discher et al., 2005, Flemming et al., 1999). One of the most well-known effects is contact guidance, in which cells respond to groove and ridge topography by simultaneously aligning and elongating in the direction of the groove axis (Teixeira et al., 2003, Webb et al., 1995, Wood, 1988). It has also been noted that cell response to biomimetic topography *in vitro* depends on cell type, feature size, shape, geometry, and physical and chemical properties of the substrate. Questions such as whether cells respond to topographical features using the same sensory system as that used for cell-matrix adhesion; whether the size and the shape of scaffold topography may affect cell response or cell-cell interaction; whether the ECM topology plays a role in coordinating tissue function at a molecular level, other than providing a physical barrier or a support; and whether ECM topography affects local protein concentration and adhesion of cell binding proteins, are beginning to be answered.

This chapter begins by considering topography of native ECM of different tissues, and methods and materials utilized in the literature to recreate biomimetic topography on cell culture substrates and scaffolds. The influence of nanometer to sub-millimeter shape and topography on mammalian cell morphology, migration, adhesion, proliferation, and differentiation are then reviewed; and finally the mechanisms by which biomimetic topography affects cell behavior are discussed.

2. Topography of native extracellular matrix

The native ECM is comprised of fibrous collagen, hyaluronic acid, proteoglycans, laminin, fibronectin etc., which provide chemical, mechanical, and topographical cues to influence cell behavior. Extensive research has been carried out to study the effects of ECM chemistry and mechanics on cell and tissue functions. For example, ECM regulates cell adhesion through ligand binding to some specific region (e.g. RGD) of ECM molecules (Hay, 1991); the strength of integrin-ligand binding is affected by matrix rigidity (Choquet et al., 1997). Topologically, ECM is comprised of a heterogeneous mixture of pores, ridges and fibers which have sizes in the nanometer range (Flemming et al., 1999). The ECM sheet with nanoscale topography is often folded or bended to create secondary microscale topography, and even a mesoscale tertiary topography. Hierarchical organization over different length scales of topography is observed in many tissues. For example, scanning electron microscope (SEM) examination of human thick skin dermis ECM reveals surface topography over different length scales (Kawabe et al., 1985). The primary topography is composed of millimeter scale alternating wide and narrow grooves called primary and secondary grooves, respectively. Sweat glands reside in primary grooves, and topographically the bottoms of primary grooves are smoother than the bottoms of secondary grooves. The millimeter size ridges are comprised of submillimeter to several hundred micron finger-like projections: dermal papillae. The surface of each dermal papillae is covered by folds and pores approximately 10 microns in dimension. The interstitial space is composed of dermal collagen fibrils 60-70 nm in diameter forming a loose honey comb like network. The hierarchical topographies are also seen in the structure of bone, where bone structure is comprised of concentric cylinders 100 - 500 μm in diameter called osteons, which are made of 10 - 50 μm long collagen fibers (Stevens&George, 2005). The surface topography of pig small intestinal extracellular matrix, which we are working to replicate in our lab, also reveals a series of structures over different length scales (**Figure 1**). There are finger-like projections (villi) of millimeter to 400 - 500 μm scale, and well-like invaginations (crypts) 100 - 200 μm in scale. The surface of the basement membrane of villi is covered by 1 - 5 μm pores, and approximately 50 nm thick collagen fibers. These observations agree with what has been reported in the literature (Takahashi-Iwanaga et al., 1999, Takeuchi&Gonda, 2004). On the surface of rat small intestine ECM, the majority of micron-size pores are located at the upper three fourths of the villi. The pore diameter is larger in the upper villi than in the lower villi.

The basement membrane is a specialized ECM, which is usually found in direct contact with the basolateral side of epithelium, endothelium, peripheral nerve axons, fat cells and muscle cells (Merker, 1994, Yurchenco&Schittny, 1990). The surface of native tissue basement membrane presents a rich nanoscale topography consisting of pores, fibers, and elevations, which gives each tissue its unique function. Abrams *et al.* (Abrams et al., 2000) examined nanoscale topography of the basement membrane underlying the anterior corneal epithelium of the macaque by SEM, transmission electron microscopy (TEM) and atomic force microscopy (AFM) (**Figure 2**). The average mean surface roughness of monkey corneal epithelium basement membrane was between 147 and 194 nm. The surface of basement membrane is dominated by fibers with mean diameters around 77±44 nm and pores with diameters around 72±40 nm. The porosity of basement membrane is approximately 15% of the total surface area. The porous structure was postulated to have a filtering function, as well as provide conduits for penetration of subepithelial nerves into the epithelial layer.

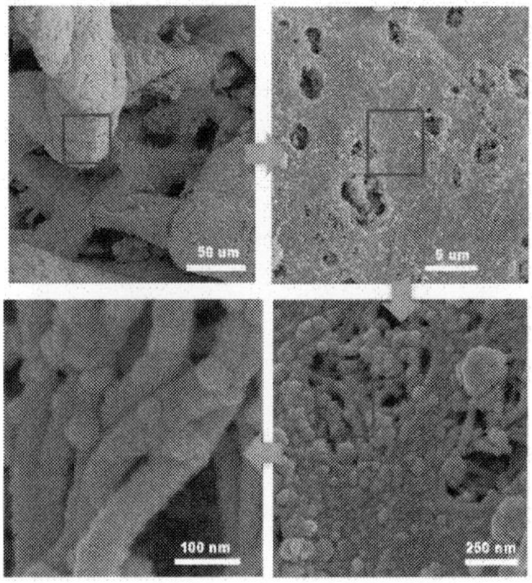

Fig. 1. Hierarchical organization of different length scale structures on the surface of pig small intestinal extracellular matrix, after removal of epithelium.

Hironaka *et al.* (Hironaka et al., 1993) examined the morphologic characteristics of renal basement membranes (i.e. glomerular, tubular, Bowman's capsule, peritubular capillary basement membrane) using ultrahigh resolution SEM (**Figure 2**). It was demonstrated that morphologically, renal basement membrane was composed of 6 - 7 nm wide fibrils forming polygonal meshwork structures with pores ranging from 4 - 50 nm. The observation of bladder basement membrane ultrastructures showed that the average thickness of bladder basement membrane is 178 nm with mean fiber diameters around 52 nm. The porous features were also found in bladder basement membrane, with mean pore diameter around 82 nm and mean inter pore distance (center to center) 127 nm (Abrams et al., 2003). In our study, it was observed that nanoscale topography of pig intestinal basement membrane was also comprised of pores and fibers (**Figure 2**) (Wang et al., 2010). Interestingly, unlilke corneal, renal, and bladder basement membrane, which often have pores around 100 nm in diameter, intestinal basement membrane has pores larger than 500 nm. Other than being perforated with 1 – 5 μm pores, the rest of the intestinal basement membrane surface is occupied by more densely packed fibers compared with corneal, renal, or Matrigel™ surfaces.

In general, ECM of native tissues possesses rich topography over broad size ranges. Length scales of topography usually range from centimeter to nanometer, and surface features of extracellular matrix often follows a fractal organization, consisting of structures comprised of repeating units throughout different levels of magnification. Most native ECM has "subunit" topography, such as papillae at the surface of dermal ECM; osteons in bone tissue; and villi and crypts at the surface of small intestine ECM, whose sizes are around 1 mm to 100 μm. The ECM surface also exhibits rich nanotopography (nanopores, and interwoven fibrils), created by ECM proteins. The size, density, and distribution of fibrils and pores are highly dependent on the source tissue (**Figure 2**) (Sniadecki et al., 2006, Stevens&George, 2005). Information on native ECM topography provides a rational basis for surface feature design of biomimetic tissue culture substrates or scaffolds.

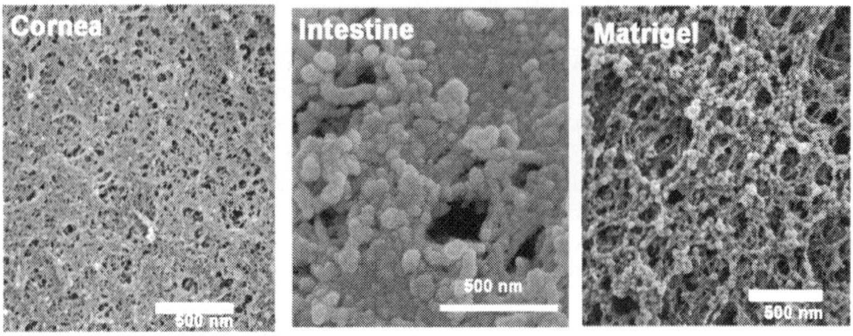

Fig. 2. Nanoscale topography and structure of basement membranes of anterior corneal epithelium (adapted with permission from Abrams et al., 2000), small intestine, and Matrigel (adapted with permission from Abrams et al., 2000)

3. Patterned cell culture substrates: fabrication methods & materials

Various methods and materials have been utilized to create 3D cell culture substrates and tissue culture scaffolds. Depending on desired 3D features as well as chemical and mechanical properties of the scaffold, a specific fabrication strategy can be selected. There are four main categories of methods reported in the literature for fabrication of a 3D cell culture substrate or scaffold: (1) methods resulting in precisely designed regular surface topographies or 3D features; (2) methods resulting in irregular topographies, such as 3D fibrils, pores, or simple increased surface nanoscale roughness; (3) methods aiming for exact replication of 3D feature of native tissue; (4) methods based on naturally derived biopolymer gels or decellularized ECM.

Micro- and nanofabrication methods, such as photolithography, electron-beam lithography, two-photon polymerization, microcontact printing and etching, have often been employed to produce surface features with controlled dimensions and specific shapes (reviewed by (Bettinger et al., 2009)). Among these techniques, photolithography is the most popular approach and is often used to generate regular surface features, such as grooves, posts, and pits. Photolithography, and other micro- nanofabrication techniques are typically fine-tuned for silicon, silicon oxide, polycrystalline silicon, and other inorganic systems such as titanium. Therefore, either these inorganic materials, such as silicon or titanium, or organic polymers replicas of inorganic master molds have been utilized as cell culture substrates to study the effect of topography on cell behavior (Reviewed by (Bettinger et al., 2009)). Organic polymers used in this manner include poly (dimethylsiloxane), polystyrene, poly(methyl methacrylate), polycarbonate, and poly(ethylene glycol), as well as biodegradable polymers such as poly (ε-caprolactone), poly(L-lactic acid), poly(glycolic acid), and poly(L-lactic-co-glycolic acid). Some more recently developed techniques, such as multiphoton lithography, are capable of fabricating much more complex 3D topographies than simple groove, post or pit arrays. For example, it was reported that layer-by-layer stereolithography was able to create free-form complicated 3D constructs: a layer of 400 mg/ml bovine serum albumin (BSA) was deposited and photocrosslinked by exposed to patterned UV light, and repeated many times to incrementally build a 3D structure. The

resolution of multiphoton lithography is around 0.1 - 0.5 μm, which is in a similar range as soft lithography (Nielson et al., 2009).
Electrospinning processes are able to create 3D scaffolds comprised of non-woven fibrous networks with fiber diameters ranging from tens of nanometers to microns (Liang et al., 2007). Synthetic polymers, such as polyamides, polylactides, cellulose derivatives, and water soluble polyethyleneoxide; natural polymers, such as collagen (type I, II, III), elastin, silk fibrin, and chitosan; and copolymers of either synthetic or natural polymers can be adapted to eletrospinning processes (Liang et al., 2007). Fiber diameter, morphology, porosity, and biological properties of electrospun scaffolds can be modified via copolymerization or adjusting electrospinning conditions. Traditional electrospinning processes are only capable of creating nanofibers with radom orientations; however, perfectly aligned fiber scaffolds can be obtained via modification of fiber collection methods (Liang et al., 2007). Techniques such as fiber bonding (unwoven mesh), solvent casting/particulate leaching, gas foaming and phase separation/emulsification have been utilized to produce porous scaffolds (Mikos&Temenoff, 2000). Porous structure allows cells to penetrate into the scaffold and facilitates nutrient and waste exchange of cells located deep inside of constructs. One fiber bonding technique creates porous constructs by soaking polymer (e.g., PGA) fibers in another polymer (e.g., PLLA) solution, evaporating the solvent, heating the polymer mixture above the melting point, and finally removing one polymer through dissolving in an organic solution (e.g. methylene chloride). This method can result in a polymer (PGA) foam with porosities as high as ~ 80% (Mikos et al., 1993a). The solvent casting/particulate leaching process involves the use of a water soluble porogen. First polymer (e.g., PLLA, PLGA) is dissolved in an organic solvent (e.g., methylene chloride) and then mixed with porogen (e.g. NaCl). After evaporating the solvent, the salt crystals inside the polymer/salt composite are removed by leaching in water, resulting in a porous polymer scaffold. The pore size and pore density can be controlled by the amount and size of salt crystal (Mikos et al., 1993b). The gas foaming method utilizes gas as a porogen, where a polymer (e.g., PGA, PLLA, PLGA) is exposed to high pressure gas (e.g., CO_2) for a long period of time (e.g., 72 h), and then the pressure is rapidly reduced to atmospheric pressure, resulting in a polymer scaffold with porosties up to 93% (Mooney et al., 1996). Phase separation/emulsification methods create porous scaffolds based on the concepts of phase separation rather than incorporation of a porogen (Mikos&Temenoff, 2000). For example, Whang *et al.* (Whang et al., 1995) dissolved PLGA in methylene chloride and then added water into the PLGA solution to form an emulsion. The mixture was cast into a mold and freeze-dried to remove water and methylene chloride, resulting in a scaffold with high porosities (up to 95%) but relatively small pore size (< 40 μm). In addition to generating fibrillous or porous scaffolds utilizing techniques such as electrospinning, particulate leaching, and gas foaming; irregular surface topography can also be fabricated by abrading. For example, Au *et al.* (Au et al., 2007) created rough polyvinyl carbonate surface by abrading the surface with 1 - 80 μm grain size lapping paper. The resulting surface had V-shaped abrasions with peak to peak widths from 3 - 13 μm, and depths from 140 - 700 nm.
Other methods, such as chemical vapor deposition (CVD), conformal-evaporated-film-by-rotation (CEFR), and deposition in supercritical fluid (Cook et al., 2003, Martín-Palma et al., 2008, Pfluger et al., 2010, Wang et al., 2005) have been utilized to precisely replicate the complex and irregular hierarchical topography from a biological sample over several length scales. Pfluger *et al.* (Pfluger et al., 2010) reported precise replication of the complex

topography of pig small intestinal basement membrane using plasma enhanced CVD of biocompatible polymer: poly(2-hydroxyethyl methacrylate) (pHEMA) (**Figure 3**). A pHEMA film was generated via introducing a mixed vapor of precursor: 2-hydroxyethyl methacrylate, and initiator: tert-butyl peroxide, into a CVD chamber to react with a cross-linker: ethylene glycol diacrylate, when exposed to an Argon plasma. Chemical vapor deposited pHEMA is able to replicate villus (100 - 200 μm in height, 50 - 150 μm in diameter), crypt (20 - 50 μm in diameter), and pore (1 - 5 μm in diameter) structures on the surface of intestinal basement membrane; the thickness of pHEMA coating is around 1 μm. Cook *et al.* (Cook et al., 2003) demonstrated replication of the surface features of butterfly wings using controlled vapor-phase oxidation of silanes. Hydrogen peroxide was evaporated and reacted with gaseous silane creating silica primary clusters, which have extraordinary flow properties and are able to creep into small gaps on the surface of a biological specimen. After the deposition of silica, biological specimen was removed by calcination at 500°C. This method was able to generate a 100 - 150 nm thick replica, which reproduced nanometer scale (~ 500 nm) features on the surface of a biological sample. Martin-Palma *et al.* (Martín-Palma et al., 2008) created a 0.5 - 1 μm thick chalcogenide glass ($Ge_{28}Sb_{12}Ge_{60}$) replica of fly eyes using oblique angle deposition (OAD) technique while rapidly rotating the specimen (**Figure 3**). The OAD technique is based on directing a vapor towards a substrate with a trajectory of atoms not parallel to the substrate normal. Wang *et al.* (Wang et al., 2005) replicated the surface features of pollen grains and cotton fiber from ~100 nm scale upwards (**Figure 3**). The replica was fabricated by dissolving titanium isopropoxide precursor in supercritical CO_2, and then depositing on the surface of a biological specimen. The adsorbed precursor then reacted with water molecules and hydroxyl groups on the surface of the biological sample, resulting in the condensation of titanium at the interface. Finally, the biological specimen embedded inside the titanium coating was removed by calcination.

Decellularized tissue and organs are another type of three dimensional scaffold used for tissue engineering/regenerative medicine applications (Gilbert et al., 2006). ECM from a variety of tissues, including heart valves, blood vessels, skin, nerves, skeletal muscle, tendons, ligaments, small intestinal submucosa, urinary bladder, and liver, have been isolated, decellularized, and then used as cell cutlure scaffolds (reviewed by (Gilbert et al., 2006)). The decellularized ECM often retains biologically functional molecules and three dimensional organization of native ECM, therefore provide a favorable environment for tissue regeneration (Badylak, 2004). Physical, chemical, enzymatic, or combined methods are utilized to decellularize tissue. The physical methods involve agitation, sonication, mechanical massage, pressure, and freezing and thawing. The chemical methods include alkaline and acid treatments, non-ionic detergents (e.g. Triton X-100), ionic detergents (e.g. Triton X-200), Zwitterionic detergents (e.g. CHAPS), tri(n-butyl)phosphate, hypotonic and hypertonic treatment, and chelating agents (e.g. EDTA). Enzymes, such as trypsin, endonucleases, and exonucleases, are also often utilized in decellularization processes (Gilbert et al., 2006). A general approach to decellularization begins with lysis of the cell membrane using physical treatments or incubation with ionic detergent solution, followed by enzymatic treatment to dissociate cellular components from ECM, and removal of cytoplasmic and nuclear cellular components using detergent (Gilbert et al., 2006). Simple hydrogels made of natural polymers, such as ECM components: collagen, elastin, fibrin, hyaluronic acid, and basement membrane extract (e.g. Matrigel™); as well as materials

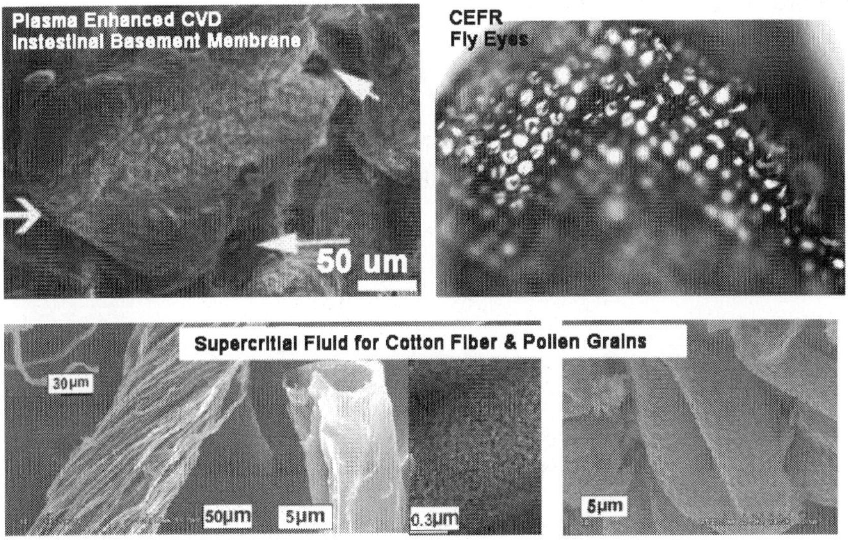

Fig. 3. Precise replication of biological structures: replication of small intestinal basement membrane utilizing plasma enhanced chemical vapor deposition (CVD) of poly(2-hydroxyethyl methacrylate) (adapted with permission from Pfluger et al., 2010); chalcogenide glass ($Ge_{28}Sb_{12}Ge_{60}$) replication of fly eyes by conformal-evaporated-film-by-rotation technique (CEFR) (adapted with permission from Martin-Palma et al., 2008) ; titanium replication of cotton fiber and pollen grains utilizing supercritical CO_2 (adapted with permission from Wang et al., 2005).

derived from other biological sources: alginate, agarose, chitosan, and silk fibrils, are also utilized for three dimensional cell culture (reviewed by (Lee&Mooney, 2001, Tibbitt&Anseth, 2009)). Collagen is an abundant ECM protein; it forms gels by changing the temperature or pH of its solution (Butcher&Nerem, 2004, Raub et al., 2007); these gels can be further cross-linked by glutaraldehyde or diphenylphosphoryl azide. Gelatin is a derivative of collagen that can also form gels when the temperature of its solution changes. Hyaluronate is one of the ECM glycosaminoglycans; it can form gels by covalently cross-linking with various hydrazide derivatives, and be degraded by hyaluronidase (Pouyani et al., 1994, Vercruysse et al., 1997). Fibrin can be collected from blood, and forms gels by the enzymatic polymerization of fibrinogen at room temperature in the presence of thrombin (Ikari et al., 2000).

Hydrogels can also be formed from synthetic polymers, such as poly(ethylene glycol), poly(vinyl alcohol), poly(2-hydroxy ethyl methacrylate), and polyethylene glycol (PEG). Morphologically, hydrogels are highly porous and have loosely packed fibers. Cells cultured on 3D hydrogel scaffolds can be encapsulated inside the hydrogel scaffold by mixing cell suspension with hydregel solution and then solidifying, instead of seeding directly on the surface of the hydrogel. The stiffness of hydrogel can be adjusted by varying gel concentration or introducing cross-linking agent.

4. Effect of substrate pattern on cell behavior (morphology, migration, adhesion, proliferation, and differentiation)

Cell shape, migration, and adhesion can be influenced by surface topography of a substrate. Sub-micron to nanometer scale topographies are smaller than the size of a cell and in the similar size range as topography created by ECM proteins, such as collagen, fibronectin, and laminin fibers. This size range of substrate topography may influence cell behavior at the cellular level. Sub-millimeter scale topographies are in the similar range as tissue subunits, such as small intestinal crypt-villus units, osteons of bone, and dermal papillae. As tissue subunits often contain tens to hundreds of cells, sub-millimeter scale topography might influence group cell behavior by affecting cell-cell contact, cell-cell signaling, and other regulation among cells. In the following section, the effect of sub-micron to nanometer scale topography, as well as sub-millimeter scale topography on cell behavior is discussed. Relatively speaking, most studies in the literature pertaining to effect of substrate topography are performed in systems lacking multiple aspects of physiological conditions, utilizing impermeable substrates made of polymer or inorganic materials, such as polydimethylsiloxane, silicon, and titanium oxide. These studies are typically focused on short term effects (culture time equal to or less than 7 days), mostly on cell morphology; the scale of topography is generally limited to cellular to subcellular length scale, and shape of topography is often restricted to simple features such as grooves and ridges. Therefore, more biologically relevant or more biomimetic systems and longer cell culture time might be required to study the effect of substrate topography on cell behavior.

4.1 Cellular and subcellular (ten micron to nanometer) length scale topography

A large body of work has reported that cellular and subcellular length scale topographic features play an important role in affecting cell morphology, migration, and adhesion to substrates. Groove pattern is the most commonly studied pattern type; in general cells have been observed to align along grooves or ridges. Wood *et al.* (Wood, 1988) cultured fin mesenchymal explants on quartz substrates patterned with grooves of 1 - 4 μm width, 1.1 μm depth, and 1 - 4 μm spacing, and found groove topography directed and facilitated mesenchymal cell migration away from explants. Cells were aligned parallel to grooves and migrated 3 - 5 fold faster than those on flat surfaces. Cells attached to the ridge region were able to spread from one ridge to another by bridging the groove. However, not all cells prefer aligning along groove axes; cell reaction to groove topography depends on cell type. Rajnicek *et al.* (Rajnicek et al., 1997) cultured central nerve system neurons (embryonic Xenopus spinal cord and embryonic rat hippocampus neurons) on quartz surfaces patterned with regular grooves (14 - 1100 nm in depth; 1, 2, and 4 μm in width, 1 μm spacing). The preferred direction of neurite spreading depended on cell type and dimension of the groove. Spinal neurons extended their neurites along grooves, while hippocampus neurons extended their neurites perpendicular to shallow, narrow grooves and parallel to deep, wide ones. Similarly, Webb et al. (Webb et al., 1995) cultured oligodendrocyte progenitors, rat optic nerve astrocytes, rat hippocampal and cerebellar neurons on quartz substrates patterned with regular and irregular 1 - 4 μm wide and 0.1 - 1.2 μm deep grooves and 0.13 - 8 μm ridges coated with 0.01% poly-D-lysine. When cultured on the surface grated with ~100 nm wide and 100 - 400 nm deep grooves and ridges, hippocampal and cerebellar granule cell neurons extended their neurites perpendicular to the grooves.

Cells cultured on substrates patterned with cellular and subcellular scale topography were also reported to synthesize more cell adhesion molecules (e.g., fibronectin (Fn)) than those cultured on flat surfaces. For example, Chou *et al.* (Chou et al., 1995) found that human fibroblasts secreted 2-fold more ECM Fn when cultured on surfaces patterned with V-shaped grooves (3 μm in depth, 6 μm in width, and 10 μm in spacing). Manwaring *et al.* (Manwaring et al., 2004) studied rat meningeal cell alignment and ECM protein distribution while cultured on Fn (20 μg/ml) coated polystyrene surfaces patterned with irregular grooves with average roughness ranging from 50 nm to 1.6 μm. Nanometer-scale groove topography affected both meningeal cell alignment and the alignment of cell-deposited ECM; the alignment increased with increasing surface roughness.

Cellular and subcellular scale topography affects cell adhesion on substrates, and the influence depends on shape of pattern (e.g., grooves, pits) and cell types. For example, groove topography enhanced human corneal epithelial cell adhesion. Karuri *et al.* (Karuri et al., 2004) seeded SV40 human corneal epithelial cells on silicon surfaces patterned with 400 - 4000 nm wide grooves and incubated cells for 24 hours. Cells attached to silicon substrates were then transferred to a flow chamber, in which cells were exposed to different levels of sheer stress. It was found that cells were most adherent to surfaces patterened with smaller features; there were more cells attached to surfaces patterned with 400 nm grooves compared to surfaces patterned with grooves larger than 400 nm when cells were subjected to the same sheer force. Cukierman *et al.* (Cukierman et al., 2001) compared human foreskin fiboblast morphology, migration, and adhesion when cultured on 3D ECM deposited by NIH-3T3 fibroblasts with those of cells cultured on the same substrate, but mechanically compressed into 2D. In this experiment, the composition and nano-scale fibrillous topography of 3D ECM is the same as 2D ECM; the only differences between these two substrates are the reduction of thickness from ~ 5 μm to < 1 μm, and the increase in local ECM concentration. Cell adhesion on 3D ECM was 10 fold higher than on 2D ECM 10 minutes after plating; the elongation of cells on 3D ECM was 3 fold higher than on 2D ECM 5 hours after plating. Interestingly, the difference in cell elongation disappeared after 18 hours. The migration of cells on 3D ECM was slightly slower than on 2D ECM. Kidambi *et al.* (Kidambi et al., 2007) cultured 3T3 fibroblasts, Hela cells, and primary hepatocytes on surfaces of PDMS substrates patterned with micro-well arrays (1.25 - 9 μm in diameter, 2.5 μm in depth, and 18 μm well center to center distance) coated with polyelectrolyte multilayers (10 layers of sulfonated poly(styrene)/poly-(diallyldimethylammonium chloride)). Micron-well topography was found to inhibit cell attachment. The number of cells adherent to patterned surfaces was lower than that to smooth surfaces. The attached cell number decreased with increase of well diameters.

Cytoskeletal organization and adhesion to substrate alter the way in which cells sense and respond to the environment, and hence affect cell proliferation and differentiation (Ingber, 1997). Rajnicek *et al.* (Rajnicek et al., 1997) found that neurite growth of central nerve system neurons (embryonic Xenopus spinal cord and embryonic rat hippocampus neurons) was enhanced by groove patterns, and proliferation rate was greater when cells were orientated in a preferred direction. Green *et al.* (Green et al., 1994) studied the growth rate of human abdomen fibroblasts (CCD-969sk) cultured on silicone surfaces patterned with 2, 5, or 10 μm rectangular pit or pillar arrays for up to 12 days. Cells were observed to be more sensitive to small size topography (i.e. 2 and 5 μm features) instead of 10 μm pits or pillars. 2 and 5 μm pillar features enhanced fibroblast proliferation as compared with the same size pit feature and flat surfaces. Dalby *et al.* (Dalby et al., 2007) cultured human mesenchymal stem cells (MSCs) and osteoprogenitors on polymethylmethacrylate (PMMA) embossed with 120 nm diameter, 100 nm depth , and 300 nm center to center spacing pits arranged as a square array, hexagonal array, or random (with different randomness) array for 21 or 28 days. Both osteoprogenitors and MCSs exhibited bipolar morphology on planar surface, and formed dense bone nodule-like aggregates on substrates patterned with random pit array topography. Osteoprogenitors on surfaces patterned with mild random pit arrays (a few pits slightly out of alignment) also expressed raised levels of bone-specific extracellular matrix proteins: osteopontin and osteocalcin. MSCs on surfaces with mild random pit arrays exhibited osteogenic gene up-regulation (11 out of 101 genes tested). Huang *et al.* (Huang et al., 2006) grew murine myoblasts on poly(dimethylsiloxane) (PDMS) surfaces patterned with grooves 10 μm wide, 10 μm apart, and 2.8 μm deep, or poly(L-lactide) (PLLA) scaffolds with either well-aligned or randomly arranged 500 nm wide fibers. Both micron-scale grooves and nanofibers inhibited cell proliferation over the first 2 days in culture. 10 μm groove topography promoted myotube elongation by 40%, while 500 nm nanofibers enhanced myotube length by 180% after 7 days. The inhibition of cell proliferation during early culture and the promotion of myotube assembly in late culture suggested that micropatterned surfaces may enhance cell cycle exit of myoblasts and differentiation into myotubes, and that myoblasts were more sensitive to nanometer scale topography than micron-scale topography. The reduction in cell proliferation by culturing on surfaces patterned with subcellular scale topography was also observed by Yim *et al.* (Yim et al., 2005). They cultured bovine pulmonary artery smooth muscle cells (SMC) on poly(methyl methacrylate) (PMMA) and poly(dimethylsiloxane) (PDMS) surfaces patterned with 700 nm wide and 350 nm deep grooves and found that SMCs cultured on patterned surfaces incorporated significantly lower BrdU than cells cultured on flat surfaces during 4 hours of incubation. Den Braber *et al.* (Den Braber et al., 1995) cultured fibroblasts from ventral skin on PDMS substrates patterned grooves 2 - 10 μm wide, 2 - 10 μm spaced, and 0.5 μm deep grooves. No effect of surface topography on cell proliferation was observed. These observations suggest that the effect of subcellular scale topography on cell behavior is highly dependant on cell type, shape and size of the pattern, and possibly the physical and chemical properties of the substrate material.

4.2 Tissue subunits (submillimeter) scale topography

Subunit scale topography has also been found to affect cell morphology, adhesion, proliferation, and differentiation. However, compared with cellular and subcellular scale topography, the effect of subunit scale topography is more subtle. Dunn *et al.* (Dunn&Heath, 1976) cultured chick embryonic heart fibroblasts on the surface of cylindrical fibers with diameters ranging from 50 to 350 μm. After 24 hours of cultivation, it was found that cell nuclei preferred to orient along the fiber axis, and the shape of aligned cell nuclei are related to fiber diameter: the smaller the diameter, the higher the axis width to cross axis width ratio. However, the effect of cylindrical topography on cell nuclei alignment disappeared when fiber diameter was bigger than 200 μm. Brunette et al. (Brunette et al., 1983) studied outgrowth of human gingival explants on a titanium surface etched with trapezoid shape grooves (groove upper width 130 μm and lower width 60 μm, ridge width 10 μm). The direction of outgrowth was strongly guided by the grooves. Interestingly, cells preferred to reside inside grooves instead of on top of ridges, which might be due to the width of ridges being much smaller than the width of grooves (10 μm vs. 130 μm). The above studies suggested that subunit scale grooves might also provide guidance for cell migration; however, this may occur through different mechanisms than for cells aligned on surfaces patterned with submicron to nanometer scale grooves. In another study, Dunn *et al.* (Dunn&Heath, 1976) cultivated chick heart ventricle explants on surfaces of prisms with different ridge angles (i.e. 179°, 178°, 176°, 172°, 166° and 148°). It was found that abrupt change in surface orientation inhibited cell migration or changed the cell migration direction from perpendicular to the ridge to either parallel or away from the ridge; ridges with angles less than 166° inhibited cells from crossing ridges. Further investigation of microfilament arrangement inside of cells spanned across ridges suggested that the majority of microfilaments terminated when they encountered a ridge, and a new set microfilaments formed at the other side of the ridge, oriented in a completely different direction. Mata *et al.* (Mata et al., 2002) investigated human connective tissue progenitor cell spreading and colony formation on a PDMS substrate patterned with C-shape microgrooves (11 μm deep, 45 μm wide, separated by 5 μm wide ridge). Cells were cultured for 9 days, and the size, shape, and cell density of cell colonies were studied. Colony area of cells grown on patterned surfaces was half the average size as that of cells on flat surfaces; however, the cell density was two times higher than on flat surfaces. The groove topography affected progenitor cell colony alignment and elongation; most cell colonies extended and spread within and along the grooves. SEM images also showed that cells located at the curvy bottom of the groove didn't attach conformally to the concave surface; instead they spanned across the concave bottom. Mrksich *et al.* (Mrksich, 2000) fabricated a polyurethane substrate patterned with V-shape grooves (25 or 50 μm in width, 25 or 50 μm in spacing). The groove region was coated with protein adhesive self-assembled monolayers (SAM), and the ridge region was coated with non-adhesive SAMs, or vice versa. Fn was then adsorbed to the surfaces, and bovine capillary endothelial (BCE) cells were seeded and cultured for 3 days. Cells were found only to attach to Fn adsorbed regions. SEM images of cell spreading suggested that cells located in grooves were more elongated, less spread, and had more distinctive protrusions than those located on plateau ridges. Similar to what was found when culturing human connective tissue progenitor cells inside 45 μm wide C-shape grooves, BCE didn't attach conformally to sharp V-shape bottoms of the grooves. Instead, they spanned across them. In general, the submillimeter scale convex topography, such as the surface of a cylindrical fiber, or a surface of a prism, prevents cell migrating in a direction tangential to a curvy surface or perpendicular to a ridge; the concave topography, such as a C-shape, U-shape, or V-shape groove, induces cells to take a "short-cut" by spanning across the bottom of grooves instead of spreading conformally to the surface. Concave submillimeter topography restricts cell spreading, as cells located inside of grooves spread slower than cells on plateau ridges.

Effect of subunit scale topography on cell proliferation and differentiation has also been studied, and in general it has been found that subunit scale topography has no or very little effect on cell proliferation and differentiation. Mata *et al.* (Mata et al., 2002) cultured human connective tissue progenitor cells on PDMS substrates patterned with C-shape microgrooves (11 μm deep, 45 μm wide, separated by 5 μm wide ridge) for 9 days; cells were stained for alkaline phosphatase (ALP) afterwards. The ALP staining suggested the microgroove topography did not affect the differentiation of progenitor cells into an osteoblastic phenotype. Lack of effect of substrate surface topography on cell differentiation was also observed by Charest *et al.* (Charest et al., 2007). In their study, primary and C2C12 myoblasts were grown on surfaces of polycarbonate substrates patterned with 5 - 75 μm wide and 5 μm deep groove or pit arrays, and covalently coated with fibronectin. The level of sarcomeric myosin expression (marker of myogenic differentiation) was examined 50 hours after seeding for primary myoblasts and 102 hours after seeding for C2C12 myoblasts. Surface topography had no effect on sarcomeric myosin expression and cell density. The lack of effect of sub-millimeter scale topography on cell proliferation and differentiation may be due to the fact that proliferation and cell differentiation is only sensitive to nanometer to several micron scale topography, but not topographies in ten- to hundred-micron scales as mentioned in previous section (section 4.1). However, not all cell types are insensitive to ten- to hundred-micron scale topography; thus, the modulation of cell phenotype by surface topography may be cell type specific. For example, Pins *et al.* (Pins et al., 2000) cultivated human epidermal keratinocytes on type I collagen membranes patterned with sub-millimeter scale channels (40 to 310 μm wide), which presented a similar topography as the invaginations found in native skin basal lamina. Cells grown on patterned substrates were shown to form differentiated and stratified epidermis. Zinger *et al.* (Zinger et al., 2005) grew MG63 osteoblast-like cells on titanium substrates patterned with both micron-scale cavities 100, 30 and 10 μm in diameter and sub-micron-scale roughness (Ra = 0.7 μm). PGE_2 levels of cells were dependent on dimensions of micron-scale cavities. 100 μm cavities enhanced osteoblast growth, while sub-micron-scale roughness induced cell differentiation and TGF-β1 production. Liao *et al.* (Liao et al., 2003) cultivated neonatal rat osteoblasts on PDMS substrates patterned with pyramid arrays (23 μm in height and a square base with the length of each side being 33 μm). The patterned PDMS substrates were either exposed to oxygen plasma to increase surface hydrophilicity, or left untreated. The pyramid topography enhanced osteoblast differentiation. Cells grown on hydrophilic patterned substrates formed the most mineralized and alkaline phosphatase (ALP) positive nodules and expressed the highest ALP activities.

5. Theories of mechanisms

In vivo, cells grow on or inside ECM; the molecular composition, mechanical properties, and topography of ECM affect cell behavior (Reviewed by (Geiger et al., 2001)). Most adherent cells' adhesion to ECM is mediated by integrins, which are a family of transmembrane proteins responsible for signal transduction between ECM and cytoskeleton (Reviewed by (Roskelley et al., 1995) (Clark&Brugge, 1995)). Integrins interact with the actin cytoskeleton at the cell interior (Geiger et al., 2001). Cell proliferation and differentiation is a synergic response to growth factors and adhesive cues, where cell adhesion is usually mediated by integrins. The topography and morphology of cell culture substrates might affect cell adhesion ligand distribution and local concentration; the manner of cell surface receptor (integrin) interaction with ligands (3D configuration); the expression and function of cell adhesion integrins; spatial distribution of cells, which might affect cell-cell contacts and signaling; local mechanical stress, etc., all of which might eventually affect cell phenotype. Teixeira *et al.* (Teixeira et al., 2003) reported that a higher percentage of human corneal epithelial cells elongated along micron-scale grooves when cultured in serum containing medium than serum-free medium on surfaces of patterned silicon oxide. As serum contains cell adhesion proteins which can adsorb to cell culture surfaces prior to cell adhesion, this observation suggests that surface topography affects the distribution of cell adhesion proteins (ligands) and their local concentration. Stevens *et al.* (Stevens&George, 2005) postulated that nanoscale features, such as micropores, microfibers and nanofibers, may affect the adsorption, conformation, and local distribution of integrin binding proteins, changing the availability and local concentration for interacting with integrins. The presence of surface topography might increase local ligand concentration and lead to clustering of integrin, in turn activating focal adhesion kinase, which is a prerequisite process for cell migration (Kornberg et al., 1991, Sieg et al., 1999). For example, it was reported that HepG2 cells formed membrane projections and focal adhesions in the middle of the cell ventral surface when cells were cultured on poly(glycolic-co-lactic)acid (PGLA) surfaces patterned with 0.92 to 3.68 μm pores; meanwhile no membrane projections and focal adhesions were observed when cells were cultured on flat PGLA surfaces (Ranucci&Moghe, 2001). Subcellular scale pores might locally create a reservoir of cell culture medium containing high concentration of adhesion ligands, hence inducing the formation of focal adhesions in the middle of cells instead of at the cell periphery. In addition, the formation of membrane projections suggested the possible non-homogenous distribution of adhesion ligands on the patterned surface, which may require cells to generate protrusions to reach out to places having higher ligand concentration. Interestingly, similar size micro-pillar topography was reported to inhibit the formation of focal contacts. Lim *et al.* (Lim et al., 2004) cultured retinal pigment epithelial cells on polydimethylsiloxane (PDMS) substrates patterned with 5 μm in diameter and 5 μm in spacing pillar arrays. The focal contact formation and actin filament assembly were interrupted by pillars. The subcellular scale topology might also increase the scaffold surface area, which in turn increases the total amount of integrin adsorption on the surface of scaffolds. On the other hand, subscellular topology likely modulates the interfacial forces that guide the cytoskeletal organization (Stevens&George, 2005).

Substrate surface topography affects cell morphology. One of the most well-known phenomena, described extensively above, is contact guidance: cells orient and elongate themselves parallel to instead of perpendicular to groove or cylindrical fiber axes. The smallest feature reported to induce contact guidance is 70 nm wide ridges (Teixeira et al., 2003). It has been proposed that actin microfilaments (Dunn&Heath, 1976, Dunn&Brown, 1986, Heidi Au et al., 2007), focal contacts (Ohara&Buck, 1979), and microtubules (Oakley&Brunette, 1993) are vital for cell adhesion. Cells spreading on grooved substrates develop cytoskeletal polarity before orienting themselves, suggesting alignment of either microtubules, microfilaments, focal contacts, or all of the above, leading to cell alignment (Oakley&Brunette, 1993). Focal adhesion and actin filament alignment along micron-scale grooves and ridges was observed in fibroblasts (Den Braber et al., 1995). Actin filament assembly was found to be critical for orientation and elongation of cardiomyocytes along abrasions, as cell alignment disappeared when actin polymerization was inhibited (Heidi Au et al., 2007). It was postulated that the tension generated by actin stress fibers is necessary for the focal adhesion formation (Chrzanowska-Wodnicka&Burridge, 1996); in other words, the alignment of microfilaments leads to the orientation of focal contacts. However, fibroblasts have been reported to form aligned microtubules first, followed by forming aligned focal contacts and then well-aligned actin filaments. Interestingly, microtubules preferred to concentrate and align inside grooves, while focal contacts and actin filaments formed and concentrated on tops of ridges (Oakley&Brunette, 1993). Another possible mechanism of forming aligned focal contacts along ridges may be physical restriction. A focal contact is oval shaped, 2-5 μm in its major axis (Geiger et al., 2001), and 250 - 500 nm in its minor axis (Ohara&Buck, 1979), suggesting that a 2-5 μm wide ridge is required for focal contact formation in the direction perpendicular to the ridge. If a ridge is narrower than 2-5 μm, a focal contact must orient itself parallel to the ridge to be able to fit, which causes cells to orient in the direction along ridges. This assumption is supported by some observations; for example, the percentage of human corneal epithelial cell aligned along ridges decreased when the width of ridges exceeded 2 μm (Teixeira et al., 2003).

Other than groove and ridge topography, cylindrical fibers have also been found to control cell orientation: cells preferred elongating and extending along the long axis of a fiber rather than bending around a fiber (Dunn&Heath, 1976). It was postulated that contact guidance on cylindrical fibers and the resistance of cells to bend around a curved surface might be due to the fact that straight actin filaments are not able to assemble in a bent state (Dunn&Heath, 1976, Dunn, 1991, Rovensky&Samoilov, 1994, Rovensky Yu&Samoilov, 1994). This theory might also explain the phenomenon of cells preferring to span across concave or discontinuous surface features rather than spreading conformally on substrates. For example, Mata *et al.* (Mata et al., 2002) found that when cells were cultured on a PDMS surface patterned with C-shape microgrooves (11 μm deep, 45 μm wide, separated by 5 μm wide ridges), cells located at the curved bottom of the groove spanned across the bottom. Rat liver epithelial IAR cells and fetal bovine trachea epithelial FBT cells were also found to resist bending around a cylindrical surface (12-13 or 25 μm radii), instead of elongating along the axis (Rovensky Yu&Samoilov, 1994). SEM of cross-section of human corneal epithelial cells attached on a patterned silicon oxide surface suggested that lamellipodia of epithelial cells were not able to adhere to the bottom of 330 nm wide, 150 nm and 600 nm deep grooves, but spanned across grooves (Teixeira et al., 2003). Actin filament elongation and extension might be temporally interrupted or inhibited in circumstances where continuity of the actin filament may be disrupted by abrupt bending of the cytoplasm. However, some research suggests that formation and alignment of actin filaments and focal contacts might not be the driving force for cell contact guidance on patterned surfaces for some cell types. For example, Webb *et al.* (Webb et al., 1995) observed high alignment of oligodendrocytes and oligodendrocyte-type 2 astrocyte progenitors on surfaces patterned with submicron size grooves; however, no high-order F-actin cytoskeletal networks were observed. On the other hand, extensive organization of F-actin into stressed fibers and cables was detected among aligned astrocytes. The presence of surface topography might also create a physical barrier for cell-cell contact, or restrict available spreading area for cells, which then influences cell morphology. Direct cell-cell contact has been found to promote cell proliferation; for expamle, smooth muscle cells or endothelial cells contacted with one or more neighbor cells have significantly higher growth rates than single cells without contacts (Nelson&Chen, 2002)

The alteration of cell morphology was reported to affect cell proliferation and phenotype. For instance, the commitment of human mesenchymal stem cells (hMSCs) to adipocyte or osteoblast phenotype was regulated by cell shape: the widely spread and flattened hMSCs underwent osteogenesis, while round and unspread hMSCs underwent adipogenesis (Mcbeath et al., 2004). Folkman *et al.* (Folkman&Moscona, 1978) found that the shape of mammalian cells (i.e. bovine endothelial cells, WI-38 human fetal lung fibroblasts, and A-31 cells) is tightly coupled to DNA synthesis. Extremely flat shaped cells incorporate ~ 30 fold more ^{3}H-thymidine than spheroidal conformation cells, suggesting much more active DNA synthesis of extensively spread cells. However, in this paper cell shape was modulated by varying the substrate adhesiveness. The spheroidal cells had much lower adhesion to surfaces than flat shape cells, therefore, it was hard to uncouple the effects of cell shape and adhesion on DNA synthesis. Cukierman *et al.* (Cukierman et al., 2001) also observed the enhancement of BrdU incorporation (one of characteristics for S-phase cells) among most elongated fibroblasts, which were cultured on a 3D ECM deposited by NIH-3T3 fibroblasts. Furthermore, they found that the cell-matrix adhesion mechanism was affected by the substrate z dimensional topography. The overlapping of the focal and fibrillar adhesions was observed among cells cultured on a 3D ECM, whereas focal and fibrillar adhesions were found presenting at different locations on cell membrane when cultured on a 2D ECM with the same composition except the lack of z dimension. The focal adhesions anchor actin filaments and mediate strong adhesion of cells to the matrix; where fibrillar adhesions are associated with ECM fibrils and responsible for fibronectin generation (reviewed by (Geiger et al., 2001)). Narrowed integrin usage (i.e. involvement in only adhesion rather than adhesion and spreading, as observed on 2D surfaces) among fibroblasts cultured on 3D substrates was also observed, and the sensing of and reaction to z dimensional topography was $\alpha5$ integrin dependent (Cukierman et al., 2001). Wang *et al.* (Wang et al., 1998) reported a bidirectional cross-modulation of β-1 integrin and epidermal growth factor receptor signaling through mitogen activated protein kinase pathway in human mammary epithelial cells when cultured in 3D Matrigel™ (basement membrane from Englebreth-Holm-Swarm tumors), which didn't occur in 2D cultures. The above observations suggest that in 3D culture cell surface integrins such as β-1 and α-5 have different function or regulate different cellular processes compared with cells cultured on a 2D substrate. It was also postulated that surface topography might lead to local restriction or redistribution of cell membrane proteins such as ion channels, which might cause cytoskeletal reorganization, or vice versa. The change of cytoskeleton was also reported to be able to regulate ion channel distribution on the cell surface; Levina *et al.* (Levina et al., 1994) found that the disruption of cortical cytoskeleton in the growing tip of the oomycete affected ion channel distribution.

Reaction of cells to surface topography is cell type dependent. This is possibly related to the fact that *in vivo* different types of cells are exposed to different 3D environments. For example, epithelial cells are often highly polarized and in direct contact with 3D basement membrane via their basolateral sides, while fibroblasts often found in connective tissues are surrounded by 3D ECM, and adapt to a specific 3D matrix. When cultured *in vitro* on patterned surface with similar 3D patterns as native ECM, cells might react as *in vivo*. In the Xenopus spinal cord, sensory ganglion neurons extend along longitudinally alined Rohon-Beard neurons and aligned longitudinal channels (~0.6 μm to 3 μm wide) sandwiched between Rohon-Beard neurons and neighboring neuroepithelial cells (Nordlander&Singer, 1982). In hippocampus, neurites often exhibit perpendicular contact guidance on parallel arrays of pre-existing neurites (Hekmat et al., 1989). When cultured *in vitro* on a quartz surface patterned with grooves (14 - 1100 nm in depth; 1,2, and 4 μm in width, 1 μm spacing), Xenopus spinal cord neurons extended their neurites along grooves, while hippocampus neurons extended their neurites perpendicular to shallow, narrow grooves (Rajnicek et al., 1997). *In vivo,* the diameter of a 7-day-old rat optic nerve axon is approximately 0.19 ± 0.5 μm in diameter (Webb et al., 1995), and *in vitro* it was observed that rat optic nerve astrocytes aligned along ~ 1 μm wide and ~ 1 μm deep grooves. Meanwhile, it was also found that cells became less sensitive to groove topography when the size of

groove features increased to several microns, which supports the theory that cells would be most sensitive to substrate topography having the size close to *in vivo* features.
Surface topography might also play a role in confining cell movement and migration, and delaying cell spreading. For example, Teixeira *et al.* (Teixeira et al., 2003) utilized time-lapse microscopy to plot human corneal epithelial cell centroid trajectories on silicon oxide surfaces patterned with 400 nm deep grooves over a 10 hour period. It was also found that centroids of cells on patterned surface were more stationary compared with cells on flat surfaces. The intestinal crypt-like well topography (50 μm in diameter and 120 μm in depth) was found to delay intestinal epithelial Caco-2 cell spreading for up to 2 days (Wang et al., 2009).

6. Conclusions

ECMs of native tissues possess unique, intricate, and often fractal topography ranging from submillimeter to nanometer scale. In the native state, cells are surrounded or in direct contact with 3D matrix, which guides cell migration, modulates cell adhesion, alters cytoskeletal organization, and affects cell phenotype. In vitro studies have documented that nanometer to submillimeter scale biomimetic topographical features influenced cell behavior, suggesting that topography of ECM plays an important role in regulating cell behavior, such as cell morphology, alignment, adhesion, migration, proliferation, and differenitation. The influence of topological cues depends on cell type, shape, and size of topographical feature; the more biomimetic topography induced more *in vivo* like cell phenotype. Relatively speaking, the majority of studies have been done using synthetic materials as cell culture scaffolds, focusing on simple topographical features (e.g. grooves and ridges) with sizes in single cell or subcellular scale (nanometer to tens micron) range and short periods of cultivation. In order to fully understand the role of ECM topography on cellular behavior and tissue function, chemically, mechanically, and physiologically more biomimetic cell culture substrates need to be fabricated. Information pertaining to the influence of topography on cell behavior will benefit rational design of tissue engineering scaffolds and *in vitro* cell model development.

7. References

Abrams, G., A. et al. (2003). Ultrastructural basement membrane topography of the bladder epithelium. *Urological Research,* Vol.31, No.5, 341-346, 0300-5623

Abrams, G. A. et al. (2000). Nanoscale topography of the basement membrane underlying the corneal epithelium of the rhesus macaque. *Cell and Tissue Research,* Vol.299, No.1, 39-46, 0302-766X

Badylak, S. F. (2004). Xenogeneic extracellular matrix as a scaffold for tissue reconstruction. *Transplant immunology,* Vol.12, No.3-4, 367-377, 0966-3274

Bettinger, C. J. et al. (2009). Engineering substrate topography at the micro- and nanoscale to control cell function. *Angewandte Chemie (International ed. in English),* Vol.48, No.30, 5406-5415, 1433-7851

Brunette, D. M. et al. (1983). Grooved titanium surfaces orient growth and migration of cells from human gingival explants. *Journal of Dental Research,* Vol.62, No.10, 1045-1048, 0022-0345

Butcher, J. T.&Nerem, R. M. (2004). Porcine aortic valve interstitial cells in three-dimensional culture: Comparison of phenotype with aortic smooth muscle cells. *The Journal of Heart Valve Disease,* Vol.13, No.3, 478-486, 0966-8519

Charest, J. L. et al. (2007). Myoblast alignment and differentiation on cell culture substrates with microscale topography and model chemistries. *Biomaterials,* Vol.28, No.13, 2202-2210, 0142-9612

Choquet, D. et al. (1997). Extracellular matrix rigidity causes strengthening of integrin-cytoskeleton linkages. *Cell,* Vol.88, No.1, 39-48, 0092-8674

Chou, L. et al. (1995). Substratum surface topography alters cell shape and regulates fibronectin mrna level, mrna stability, secretion and assembly in human fibroblasts. *Journal of Cell Science,* Vol.108, No.4, 1563-1573, 0021-9533

Chrzanowska-Wodnicka, M.&Burridge, K. (1996). Rho-stimulated contractility drives the formation of stress fibers and focal adhesions. *The Journal of Cell Biology,* Vol.133, No.6, 1403-1415, 0021-9525

Clark, E.&Brugge, J. (1995). Integrins and signal transduction pathways: The road taken. *Science,* Vol.268, No.5208, 233-239, 0193-4511

Cook, G. et al. (2003). Exact replication of biological structures by chemical vapor deposition of silica. *Angewandte Chemie International Edition,* Vol.42, No.5, 557-559, 1521-3773

Cukierman, E. et al. (2001). Taking cell-matrix adhesions to the third dimension. *Science,* Vol.294, No.5547, 1708-1712, 0193-4511

Dalby, M. J. et al. (2007). The control of human mesenchymal cell differentiation using nanoscale symmetry and disorder. *Nature materials,* Vol.6, No.12, 997-1003, 1476-1122

den Braber, E. T. et al. (1995). Effect of parallel surface microgrooves and surface energy on cell growth. *Journal of Biomedical Materials Research,* Vol.29, No.4, 511-518, 0021-9304

Discher, D. E. et al. (2005). Tissue cells feel and respond to the stiffness of their substrate. *Science,* Vol.310, No.5751, 1139-1143, 0193-4511

Dunn, G. A.&Heath, J. P. (1976). A new hypothesis of contact guidance in tissue cells. *Experimental Cell Research,* Vol.101, No.1, 1-14, 0014-4827

Dunn, G. A.&Brown, A. F. (1986). Alignment of fibroblasts on grooved surfaces described by a simple geometric transformation. *Journal of Cell Science,* Vol.83, 313-340, 0021-9533

Dunn, G. A. (1991). How do cells respond to ultrafine surface contours? *Bioessays,* Vol.13, No.10, 541-543, 0265-9247

Flemming, R. G. et al. (1999). Effects of synthetic micro- and nano-structured surfaces on cell behavior. *Biomaterials,* Vol.20, No.6, 573-588, 0142-9612

Folkman, J.&Moscona, A. (1978). Role of cell shape in growth control. *Nature,* Vol.273, No.5661, 345-349, 0028-0836

Geiger, B. et al. (2001). Transmembrane crosstalk between the extracellular matrix--cytoskeleton crosstalk. *Nature reviews. Molecular cell biology,* Vol.2, No.11, 793-805, 1471-0072

Gilbert, T. W. et al. (2006). Decellularization of tissues and organs. *Biomaterials,* Vol.27, No.19, 3675-3683, 0142-9612

Green, A. M. et al. (1994). Fibroblast response to microtextured silicone surfaces: Texture orientation into or out of the surface. *Journal of Biomedical Materials Research,* Vol.28, No.5, 647-653, 1097-4636

Hay, E. D. (1991). *Cell biology of extracellular matrix,* Plenum Press, 0306439514, New York

Heidi Au, H. T. et al. (2007). Interactive effects of surface topography and pulsatile electrical field stimulation on orientation and elongation of fibroblasts and cardiomyocytes. *Biomaterials,* Vol.28, No.29, 4277-4293, 0142-9612

Hekmat, A. et al. (1989). Small inhibitory cerebellar interneurons grow in a perpendicular orientation to granule cell neurites in culture. *Neuron,* Vol.2, No.2, 1113-1122, 0896-6273

Hironaka, K. et al. (1993). Renal basement membranes by ultrahigh resolution scanning electron microscopy. *Kidney international,* Vol.43, No.2, 334-345, 0085-2538

Huang, N. F. et al. (2006). Myotube assembly on nanofibrous and micropatterned polymers. *Nano letters,* Vol.6, No.3, 537-542, 1530-6984

Ikari, Y. et al. (2000). A1-proteinase inhibitor, α1-antichymotrypsin, or α2-macroglobulin is required for vascular smooth muscle cell spreading in three-dimensional fibrin gel. *Journal of Biological Chemistry,* Vol.275, No.17, 12799-12805, 0021-9258

Ingber, D. E. (1997). Tensegrity: The architectural basis of cellular mechanotransduction. *Annual review of physiology,* Vol.59, 575-599, 0066-4278

Karuri, N. W. et al. (2004). Biological length scale topography enhances cell-substratum adhesion of human corneal epithelial cells. *Journal of Cell Science,* Vol.117, No.15, 3153-3164, 0021-9533

Kawabe, T. T. et al. (1985). Variation in basement membrane topography in human thick skin. *The Anatomical Record,* Vol.211, No.2, 142-148, 1552-4892

Kidambi, S. et al. (2007). Cell adhesion on polyelectrolyte multilayer coated polydimethylsiloxane surfaces with varying topographies. *Tissue Engineering,* Vol.13, No.8, 2105-2117, 1076-3279

Kornberg, L. J. et al. (1991). Signal transduction by integrins: Increased protein tyrosine phosphorylation caused by clustering of beta 1 integrins. *Proceedings of the National Academy of Sciences of the United States of America,* Vol.88, No.19, 8392-8396, 0027-8424

Lee, K. Y.&Mooney, D. J. (2001). Hydrogels for tissue engineering. *Chemical Reviews,* Vol.101, No.7, 1869-1880, 0009-2665

Levina, N. et al. (1994). Cytoskeletal regulation of ion channel distribution in the tip-growing organism saprolegnia ferax. *Journal of Cell Science,* Vol.107, No.1, 127-134, 0021-9533

Liang, D. et al. (2007). Functional electrospun nanofibrous scaffolds for biomedical applications. *Advanced Drug Delivery Reviews,* Vol.59, No.14, 1392-1412, 0169-409X

Liao, H. et al. (2003). Response of rat osteoblast-like cells to microstructured model surfaces in vitro. *Biomaterials,* Vol.24, No.4, 649-654, 0142-9612

Lim, J.-M. et al. (2004). Retinal pigment epithelial cell behavior is modulated by alterations in focal cell-substrate contacts. *Investigative ophthalmology & visual science,* Vol.45, No.11, 4210-4216, 0146-0404

Manwaring, M. E. et al. (2004). Contact guidance induced organization of extracellular matrix. *Biomaterials,* Vol.25, No.17, 3631-3638, 0142-9612

Martín-Palma, R. J.&et al. (2008). Replication of fly eyes by the conformal-evaporated-film-by-rotation technique. *Nanotechnology,* Vol.19, No.35, 355704, 0957-4484

Mata, A. et al. (2002). Analysis of connective tissue progenitor cell behavior on polydimethylsiloxane smooth and channel micro-textures. *Biomedical Microdevices,* Vol.4, No.4, 267-275, 1387-2176

McBeath, R. et al. (2004). Cell shape, cytoskeletal tension, and rhoa regulate stem cell lineage commitment. *Developmental Cell,* Vol.6, No.4, 483-495, 1534-5807

Merker, H.-J. (1994). Morphology of the basement membrane. *Microscopy Research and Technique,* Vol.28, No.2, 95-124, 1097-0029

Mikos, A. G. et al. (1993a). Preparation of poly(glycolic acid) bonded fiber structures for cell attachment and transplantation. *Journal of Biomedical Materials Research,* Vol.27, No.2, 183-189, 1097-4636

Mikos, A. G. et al. (1993b). Laminated three-dimensional biodegradable foams for use in tissue engineering. *Biomaterials,* Vol.14, No.5, 323-330, 0142-9612

Mikos, A. G.&Temenoff, J. S. (2000). Formation of highly porous biodegradable scaffolds for tissue engineering. *Journal of Biotechnology,* Vol.3, No.2, 0168-1656

Mooney, D. J. et al. (1996). Novel approach to fabricate porous sponges of poly(-lactic-co-glycolic acid) without the use of organic solvents. *Biomaterials,* Vol.17, No.14, 1417-1422, 0142-9612

Mrksich, M. (2000). A surface chemistry approach to studying cell adhesion *Chemical Society reviews,* Vol.29, 267-273, 0306-0012

Nelson, C. M.&Chen, C. S. (2002). Cell-cell signaling by direct contact increases cell proliferation via a pi3k-dependent signal. *FEBS Letters,* Vol.514, No.2-3, 238-242, 0014-5793

Nielson, R. et al. (2009). Microreplication and design of biological architectures using dynamic-mask multiphoton lithography. *Small,* Vol.5, No.1, 120-125, 1613-6829 (Electronic)

Nordlander, R. H.&Singer, M. (1982). Spaces precede axons in xenopus embryonic spinal cord. *Experimental Neurology,* Vol.75, No.1, 221-228, 0014-4886

Oakley, C.&Brunette, D. (1993). The sequence of alignment of microtubules, focal contacts and actin filaments in fibroblasts spreading on smooth and grooved titanium substrata. *Journal of Cell Science,* Vol.106, No.1, 343-354, 0021-9533

Ohara, P. T.&Buck, R. C. (1979). Contact guidance in vitro. A light, transmission, and scanning electron microscopic study. *Experimental Cell Research,* Vol.121, No.2, 235-249, 0014-4827

Pfluger, C. A. et al. (2010). Biocompatibility of plasma enhanced chemical vapor deposited poly(2-hydroxyethyl methacrylate) films for biomimetic replication of the intestinal basement membrane. *Biomacromolecules,* Vol.11, No.6, 1579-1584, 1525-7797

Pins, G. D. et al. (2000). Microfabrication of an analog of the basal lamina: Biocompatible membranes with complex topographies. *The FASEB Journal,* Vol.14, No.3, 593-602, 0892-6638

Pouyani, T. et al. (1994). Novel hydrogels of hyaluronic acid: Synthesis, surface morphology, and solid-state nmr. *Journal of the American Chemical Society,* Vol.116, No.17, 7515-7522, 0002-7863

Rajnicek, A. et al. (1997). Contact guidance of cns neurites on grooved quartz: Influence of groove dimensions, neuronal age and cell type. *Journal of Cell Science,* Vol.110, No.23, 2905-2913, 0021-9533

Ranucci, C. S.&Moghe, P. V. (2001). Substrate microtopography can enhance cell adhesive and migratory responsiveness to matrix ligand density. *Journal of Biomedical Materials Research,* Vol.54, No.2, 149-161, 1552-4965

Raub, C. B. et al. (2007). Noninvasive assessment of collagen gel microstructure and mechanics using multiphoton microscopy. *Biophysical journal,* Vol.92, No.6, 2212-2222, 0006-3495

Roskelley, C. D. et al. (1995). A hierarchy of ecm-mediated signaling regulates tissue-specific gene-expression. *Current Opinion in Cell Biology,* Vol.7, No.5, 736-747, 0955-0674

Rovensky, Y. A.&Samoilov, V. I. (1994). Morphogenetic response of cultured normal and transformed fibroblasts, and epitheliocytes, to a cylindrical substratum surface. Possible role for the actin filament bundle pattern. *J Cell Sci,* Vol.107, No.5, 1255-1263, 0021-9533 (Print)

Rovensky Yu, A.&Samoilov, V. I. (1994). Morphogenetic response of cultured normal and transformed fibroblasts, and epitheliocytes, to a cylindrical substratum surface. Possible role for the actin filament bundle pattern. *Journal of Cell Science,* Vol.107 No.5, 1255-1263, 0021-9533

Sieg, D. J. et al. (1999). Required role of focal adhesion kinase (fak) for integrin-stimulated cell migration. *Journal of Cell Science,* Vol.112 No.16, 2677-2691, 0021-9533

Sniadecki, N. J. et al. (2006). Nanotechnology for cell-substrate interactions. *Annals of Biomedical Engineering,* Vol.34, No.1, 59-74, 0090-6964

Stevens, M. M.&George, J. H. (2005). Exploring and engineering the cell surface interface. *Science,* Vol.310, No.5751, 1135-1138, 1095-9203 (Electronic)

Takahashi-Iwanaga, H. et al. (1999). Porosity of the epithelial basement membrane as an indicator of macrophage-enterocyte interaction in the intestinal mucosa. *Archives of histology and cytology,* Vol.62, No.5, 471-481, 0914-9465

Takeuchi, T.&Gonda, T. (2004). Distribution of the pores of epithelial basement membrane in the rat small intestine. *The Journal of veterinary medical science,* Vol.66, No.6, 695-700, 0916-7250

Teixeira, A. I. et al. (2003). Epithelial contact guidance on well-defined micro- and nanostructured substrates. *Journal of Cell Science,* Vol.116, No.10, 1881-1892, 0021-9533

Tibbitt, M. W.&Anseth, K. S. (2009). Hydrogels as extracellular matrix mimics for 3d cell culture. *Biotechnology and bioengineering,* Vol.103, No.4, 655-663, 1097-0290

Vercruysse, K. P. et al. (1997). Synthesis and in vitro degradation of new polyvalent hydrazide cross-linked hydrogels of hyaluronic acid. *Bioconjugate Chemistry,* Vol.8, No.5, 686-694, 1043-1802

Wang, F. et al. (1998). Reciprocal interactions between beta1-integrin and epidermal growth factor receptor in three-dimensional basement membrane breast cultures: A different perspective in epithelial biology. *Proceedings of the National Academy of Sciences of the United States of America,* Vol.95, No.25, 14821-14826, 0027-8424

Wang, L. et al. (2009). Influence of micro-well biomimetic topography on intestinal epithelial caco-2 cell phenotype. *Biomaterials,* Vol.30, No.36, 6825-6834, 0142-9612

Wang, L. et al. (2010). Synergic effects of crypt-like topography and ecm proteins on intestinal cell behavior in collagen based membranes. *Biomaterials,* Vol.31, No.29, 7586-7598, 0142-9612

Wang, Y. et al. (2005). Replication of biological organizations through a supercritical fluid route. *Chemical communications,* Vol.21, No.23, 2948-2950, 1359-7345

Webb, A. et al. (1995). Guidance of oligodendrocytes and their progenitors by substratum topography. *Journal of Cell Science,* Vol.108, No.8, 2747-2760, 0021-9533

Whang, K. et al. (1995). A novel method to fabricate bioabsorbable scaffolds. *Polymer,* Vol.36, 837-842, 0032-3861

Wood, A. (1988). Contact guidance on microfabricated substrata: The response of teleost fin mesenchyme cells to repeating topographical patterns. *Journal of Cell Science,* Vol.90, No.4, 667-681, 0021-9533

Yim, E. K. F. et al. (2005). Nanopattern-induced changes in morphology and motility of smooth muscle cells. *Biomaterials,* Vol.26, No.26, 5405-5413, 0142-9612

Yurchenco, P. D.&Schittny, J. C. (1990). Molecular architecture of basement membranes. *FASEB Journal,* Vol.4, No.6, 1577-1590, 0892-6638

Zinger, O. et al. (2005). Differential regulation of osteoblasts by substrate microstructural features. *Biomaterials,* Vol.26, No.14, 1837-1847, 0142-9612

22

Bioengineering the Vocal Fold: A Review of Mesenchymal Stem Cell Applications

Rebecca S. Bartlett, MA and Susan L. Thibeault, Phd
University of Wisconsin-Madison
United States

1. Introduction

The vocal folds are a remarkably unique tissue in the body, in that they can produce vibration at rates between 100-1000 hertz throughout the course of a day (Guimaraes & Abberton, 2005; Hunter et al., 2006). When this robust tissue is disrupted by scarring associated with vocal fold lesion excision, carcinoma, radiation, trauma, or inflammatory disease, the associated degradation in vocal quality can be devastating. More than half of individuals with voice disorders attribute their dysphonia as having a negative impact on their social interactions, career and mental health (Smith et al., 1995). Traditional surgical treatments and voice therapy have been suboptimal for improving the dysphonia and fatigue associated with vocal fold scarring (Hansen & Thibeault, 2006). Over the past decade, a number of promising pre-clinical studies targeted at vocal fold regeneration using mesenchymal stem cells (MSCs) have been completed. As nearly all of the dedicated stem cell investigation has been completed in vitro and in animal models, there exists a great opportunity for innovation and landmark work in the future of this field. Our intention is to present the therapeutic interventions explored in the literature to date for mesenchymal stem cell (MSC) based approaches for vocal fold regeneration, in order to inform optimal approaches of the future.

2. Key aspects of vocal fold function

2.1 Basic cellular constitution of the vocal mucosa

The vocal folds have a defined multilayered structure; whereby the vocal mucosa, made up of the epithelium, basement membrane zone and superficial lamina propria, is anchored to the underlying intermediate and deep layers of the lamina propria and thyroartenoid muscle. The vocal mucosa vibrates during phonation and is the most common site for injury and scarring. As such, the anatomical target of the majority of bioengineered constructs for the larynx is the vocal mucosa. The lamina propria is home to fibroblasts, myofibroblasts and macrophages, and the epithelium contains epithelial cells and some dendritic cells that gain entry via the basement membrane zone (Catten et al., 1998). Due to their abundance and the utility of their unique functions, the two cell types of primary interest for vocal fold tissue engineers are epithelial cells and vocal fold fibroblasts. The vocal folds are covered by stratified squamous epithelium, which serves as a protective barrier against chemical, pathogenic and mechanical insults (Sivasankar et al., 2010; Mogi et al., 1979; Gray & Titze, 1988; Gipson et al., 1995; Johnston et al., 2003). Laryngeal epithelial cells also help maintain local hydration, which is essential for healthy voice production (Fisher et al., 2001). The most abundant cell type in the lamina propria is the vocal fold fibroblast. These cells are largely evenly spread throughout the depth of the tissue (Catten et al, 1998). During a wound healing response, vocal fold fibroblasts migrate to the site of injury and remodel the tissue by generating extracellular matrix (ECM) (Hirano et al., 1999).

2.2 Basic ECM constitution of the vocal mucosa

The ECM profile determines the biomechanical properties of vocal fold tissue, which, in turn, influences vocal quality (Thibeault et al., 2002). Vocal fold scarring can be identified by the fibrotic conversion of the native ECM (Benninger et al., 1996). While this later phase in injury and repair processes is innate, it can have a deleterious effect on vocal quality by altering the viscoelasticity of the tissue. As such, vocal fold bioengineers must utilize cell sources, scaffolds, and growth factors that will remodel ECM profiles to mimic the viscoelasticity of healthy tissue. Accurate measurement of the elastic properties of vocal fold mucosa is difficult due to its small size and difficult to access location. Investigators have used various models (cadaveric human larynges, *in vivo* and *ex vivo* canine larynx, etc) and techniques (nerve stimulation, parallel plate rheometry, indentation, etc), and have reported a range of shear moduli results (Hirano, 1981; Chhetri et al., 2010).

The layered structure of vocal fold tissue can be defined by its relative constituent makeup; the vocal fold mucosa is primarily composed of ECM, and the underlying thyroartenoid is largely composed of cells (Gray et al., 2000b). The robust ECM of the vocal fold mucosa is made up of fibrous proteins (i.e., collagens, elastins), interstitial proteins (i.e., hyaluronic acid, decorin, fibromodulin, decorin, versican) and other molecules such as lipids and carbohydrates.

The fibrous proteins of the vocal fold ECM have traditionally received a large amount of attention, as they contribute significantly to viscoelasticity. Collagens provide tensile strength to vocal fold tissue. The lamina propria hosts collagen type I, II and III and the basement membrane zone contains type IV and VII (Gray, et al., 1993; Mossallam, et al., 1986; Courey, et al., 1996; Gray, 1991). Elastins afford vocal tissue the ability to be stretched and then return to its original shape. The interstitial proteins are found between the collagens and elastins, and provide a variety of functions to the tissue. The large size, porous quality and high water content of hyaluronic acid (HA) are thought to offset the chronic vibration associated with phonation via shock absorption (Gray et al., 1999). HA also affects the viscosity of tissue, as a higher content corresponds to a higher tissue viscosity. Decorin and fibromodulin also have a role in wound healing, as they are able to bind to collagen and regulate fibril synthesis (Gray, et al., 1999). Versican has an ability to bind water molecules and plays a role as a space-filler in the lamina propria (Gray, 2000b).

ECM remodeling in the vocal folds is a finely coordinated, complex process, which is not yet fully understood. Further investigation into how to modulate this process following injury is warranted.

3. Therapeutic interventions explored to date

Reference	MSC type	Cell Therapy Length	Model	Scaffold	Growth factor	Outcomes
Quinchia-Johnson et al., 2010	BM MSCs (murine)	4 weeks	18 rats	HA hydrogel	-	Improved ECM and TGF-β1 production, and increased hyaluronan metabolism over 3 other treatment combinations
Hertegård et al., 2006a	BM MSCs (human)	4 weeks	10 rabbits	-	-	Improved tissue viscoelasticity and reduced collagen type 1 in treated folds
Kanemaru et al., 2005	BM MSCs (murine)	8 weeks	4 rats	-	-	MSCs differentiated into cells + for epithelial and muscle markers
Kanemaru et al., 2003	BM MSCs (canine)	8 weeks	8 dogs	1% HCl atelo-collagen	-	2/8 dogs had granulation and 2/8 dogs had atrophic changes on untreated, scarred fold, while none of the treated vocal folds showed signs of damage
Svensson et al., 2010	BM MSCs (human)	12 weeks	11 rabbits	-	-	Improved tissue viscoelasticity and reduced collagen type I in treated folds
Lee et al, 2006	ASCs (canine)	24 weeks	10 dogs	atelo-collagen	-	Less granulation tissue and atrophic changes in the treated folds

Table 1. Animal models for vocal fold regeneration using MSCs

3.1 Cells

MSCs have many favorable characteristics, including an ability to migrate to a site of injury and to encourage proliferation and differentiation of progenitor cells. They have also been shown to exert control over the microenvironment via secretion of growth factors and matrix remodeling (Caplan, 2007; Uccelli et al., 2007). There is evidence that the activity of T-lymphocytes, B-lymphocytes, and natural killer cells can be inhibited by MSCs, which suggests their potential allogeneic use without risk of immune response (Le Blanc & Ringden, 2007; Rasmussen et al., 2007). Interestingly, bone marrow derived mesenchymal stem cells (BM MSCs), adipose derived mesenchymal stem cells (ASCs) and human vocal fold fibroblasts found in the lamina propria demonstrate similar immunophenotypic properties, differentiation potential and cell surface markers (Long et al., 2009; Puissant et al., 2005; Hanson et al., 2010). This shared cell surface profile included a positive expression for MSC markers (i.e., CD29, CD44, CD73, CD90 and CD105) and a negative expression for hematopoietic stem cell markers (i.e., CD14, CD31, CD34, CD45). Additionally, BM MSCs and ASCs have been shown to differentiate down epithelial and fibroblast lineages (Kanemaru et al., 2005; Long et al., 2009; Ohno et al., 2009). Collectively, these findings support the use of BM MSCs and ASCs in future vocal fold regeneration interventions. Further inquiry distinguishing the utility of these two cell sources is necessary, as there have been no *in vivo* reports directly comparing them in laryngeal research.

There have been a few reports of injecting MSCs directly into the vocal fold, without a scaffold or soluble factors, in order to encourage regeneration following injury (see Table 1). These *in vivo* animal models have generally used a common investigative paradigm, which involves first creating a lesion unilaterally or bilaterally in the membranous portion of the vocal fold. After a period of days to weeks which allows the mature scar to form, the investigator then injects the cell therapy into the scarred region. Outcomes are determined with morphological assessment to characterize the anatomical structure of the tissue, rheometric analysis to determine the tissue's viscoelasticity, and/or with gene or protein expression levels to analyze extracellular matrix component production.

Measures of tissue biomechanics may be the most meaningful outcome to report in vocal fold literature, as viscoelasticity is known to significantly affect voice quality and patient outcomes. Thus, rheometric assessment is becoming an important functional measure in laryngeal literature. Improved viscoelastic measures have been reported for vocal folds treated with BM MSCs alone in a rabbit model (Hertegård et al., 2006a; Svensson et al., 2010).

Improved tissue morphology (less granulation tissue, less rough vocal fold edge) has been reported in injured vocal folds treated with BM MSCs as compared with controls, over a recovery periods lasting from four and twelve weeks (Hertegård et al., 2006a; Kanemaru et al., 2005, Svensson et al., 2010). Figure 1 demonstrates the resolution of one dog's granuloma and rough vocal fold morphology over a 24 week recovery period.

Protein and gene expression analysis can provide useful information about signaling pathways and ECM production. The literature to date has focused largely on the expression and some quantification of the ECM components known to be involved with wound healing, such as collagen, fibronectin, and hyaluronic acid. A reduction in collagen I content (Hertegård et al., 2006a, Svensson et al., 2010) and an increase in TGF-β1 production (Quinchia-Johnson et al., 2010) have been reported in vocal folds injected with BM MSCs alone versus scarred, untreated controls. Additionally, it has been found *in vitro* that a co-culture of ASCs and scar fibroblasts (SF) had decreased collagen production levels and

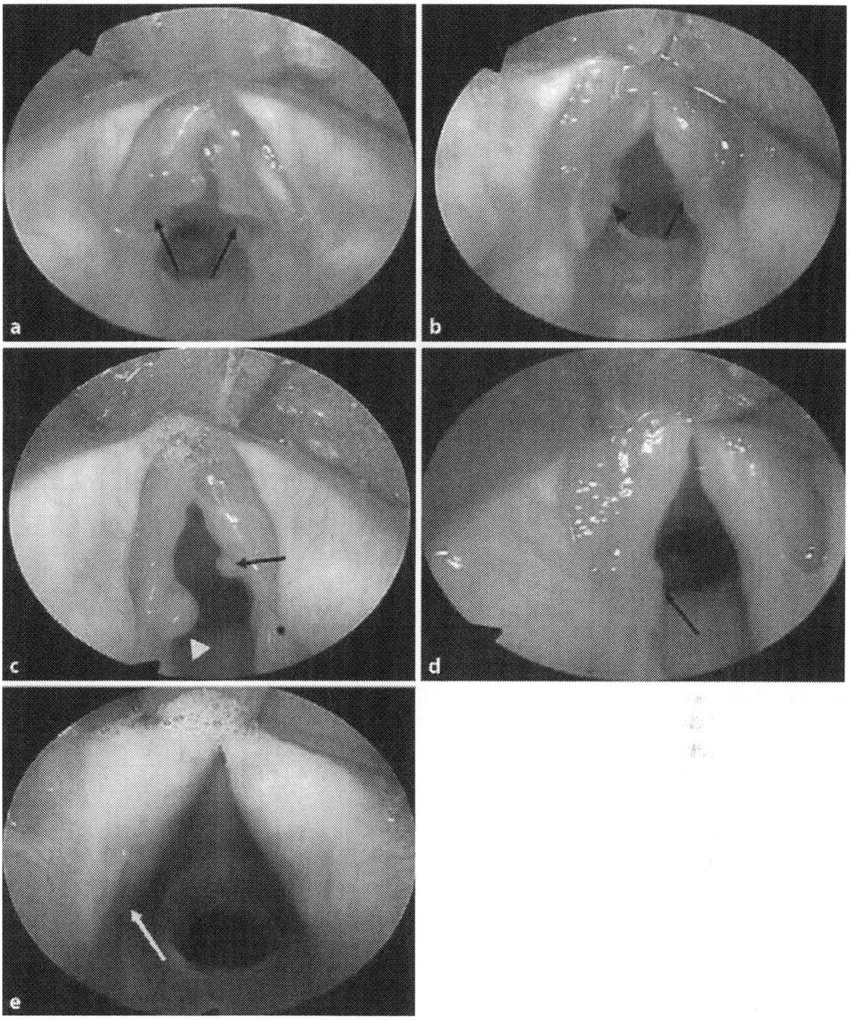

Fig. 1. Reprinted from *Cells Tissues and Organs,* Vol. 184/No. 3-4. Lee., B.Y., Wang, S.G., Lee, J.C., Jung, J.S., Bae, Y.C., Jeong, H.J., Kim, H.W., Lorenz, R.R. The prevention of vocal fold scarring using autologous adipose tissue-derived stromal cells, pp. 198-204, (2006), with permission from S Karger AG, Basel. Improved vocal fold morphology was observed in the scarred, treated right vocal fold, as compared with the scarred, untreated left vocal fold. *a:* On day 4, bilateral vocal fold lesions (see arrows) were created via electrocautery. *b*: On day 14, edema noted in right vocal fold, with irregular vocal mucosa noted in left vocal fold. *c:* On day 28, granuloma was larger on the left than on the right. *d:* On day 57, right-sided granuloma has resolved, but left-sided granuloma remains. *e:* During week 24, the authors noted the appearance of scarring in the left vocal fold, but not in the right vocal fold.

SF proliferation rates when compared with SFs in monoculture (Kumai et al., 2009). These data suggest that BM MSCs and ASCs support an anti-fibrotic profile when exposed to a scar environment. Further protein and gene expression investigation is needed to uncover signaling pathways that may allow future bioengineers to control these processes.
An optimal cell source to remediate vocal fold scarring and promote regeneration would be non-immunogenic, remain viable amidst significant vibration, migrate to the site of injury, encourage remodeling of ECM to reduce the fibrotic scar profile and efficiently differentiate into vocal fold fibroblasts and epithelial cells. To date, a handful of initial studies have indicated the therapeutic potential of injecting BM MSCs or ASCs alone for vocal fold regeneration, but further characterization using the above criteria may prove useful. Investigation using pluripotent cells (embryonic stem cells, induced pluripotent stem cells) and MSCs isolated from other sources (i.e., spleen, thymus, umbilical cord blood, amniotic fluid and dental pulp) may also be considered.

3.2 Scaffolds without cells

Scaffold materials have long been used in injection laryngoplasty procedures by otolaryngologists for the treatment of patients with vocal fold paresis, paralysis or anatomical defects. In this treatment, the biomaterial/scaffold is primarily used as a bulking agent to push the affected vocal fold toward midline and allow for a closer physical approximation during phonation. Synthetic materials (silicone, polytetrafluoroethylene-Teflon, polyhydroxyethylmethacrylate) have largely been eschewed for clinical use because of their propensity for foreign body response, migration of material and non-biodegradability (Ejnell et al., 1984; Nakayama et al., 1993). These materials have been replaced in the clinic by more degradable biomaterials, such as collagen matrix (Kriesel et al., 2002) and fat (McCulloch et al., 2002; Lo Cicero et al., 2008). These materials have viscoelastic properties more similar to vocal mucosa than the previous injectables. Additionally, the site of injection has changed from the thyroartenoid muscle to the lamina propria.
Interestingly, it has recently reported that abdominal adipose tissue harvested for clinical use as a fat injection contains a local population of MSCs. These stem cells have a high proliferative potential and the ability to differentiate down multiple lineages (Lo Cicero et al., 2008). These data suggest that a resident MSC population in vocal fold fat injections may contribute to long-term graft survival, which is suspected to occur in 55-100% of patients (McCulloch et al., 2002; Lo Cicero et al., 2008).
Commercially available composite materials have also been commonly used in clinic, such as Gelfoam paste (Schramm et al., 1978), Cymetra (Milstein et al., 2005), calcium hydroxylapatite (Rosen et al., 2007), Restylane and Hylaform (Hertegard et al., 2006b). While these materials have all been reported to improve vocal function, they are not traditionally thought to grow and remodel the tissue, as many of them biodegrade in the body. Resorption is an advantage for patients with temporary vocal fold pathology and for those interested in a short-term trial, but it is a significant limitation for patients that are interested in long-term treatment, as they can necessitate repeated injections.
A promising line of research is the investigation of gels and hydrogels as vocal fold injectables, as they may offer greater potential for vocal fold regeneration and improved viscoelastic properties over current scaffold materials. To date, hydrogels have primarily been HA based (Duflo et al., 2006a, Duflo et al., 2006b, Jia et al., 2004) and collagen based (Hahn et al., 2006). Figure 2 demonstrates the distinct rheometric measurements obtained from four treatment groups that included a semi-synthetic gel matrix (Thibeault et al., 2009).

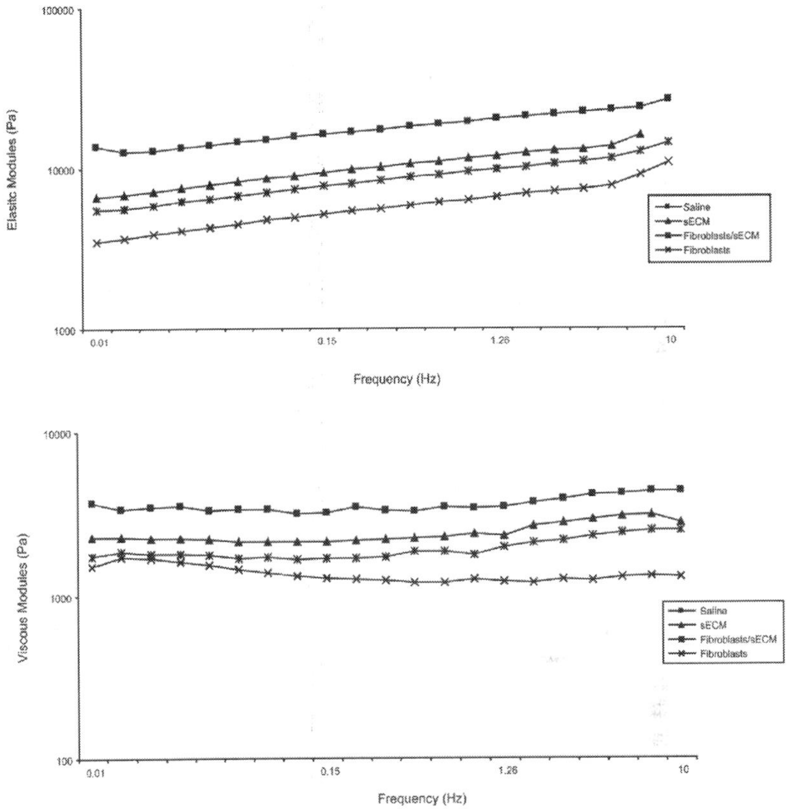

Fig. 2. Reprinted from *Tissue Engineering Part A*, Vol. 15/No. 7, Thibeault, S.L., Klemuk, S.A., Smith, M.E., Leugers, C., Prestwich, G. In vivo comparison of biomimetic approaches for tissue regeneration of the scarred vocal fold, 1481-1487, (2009), with permission from Mary Ann Liebert, Inc. Using a stress-controlled rheometer, the authors were able to demonstrate distinct elastic and viscous moduli associated with the four treatment groups.

Decellularized xenogeneic matrices derived from porcine small intestine, urinary bladder and bovine vocal fold tissue have also been investigated as potential laryngeal scaffolds (Ringel et al., 2006; Xu et al., 2007). In this model, the tissue is decellularized, leaving the potential for ECM-based repair of native via release of endogenous growth factors and activation of local cells.

3.3 Scaffolds with cells

There are many well characterized biomaterials used for injection laryngoplasty, though, only a few substances (i.e., HA based hydrogels, atelocollagen, fibrin) have been investigated for use as scaffolds in vocal fold MSC based therapies (Long et al., 2009; Kanemaru et al., 2003; Lee et al., 2010; Quinchia-Johnson et al., 2010; Ohno et al., 2009).

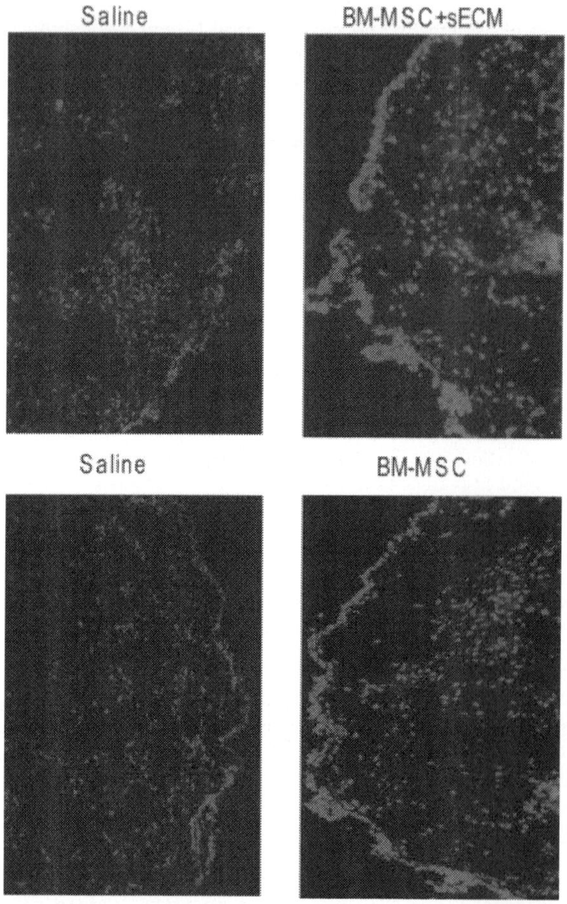

Fig. 3. Reprinted from *The Laryngoscope*, Vol. 120/No. 3, Quinchia-Johnson, B.H., Fox, R., Chen, X., Thibeault, S.L. Tissue regeneration of the vocal fold using bone marrow mesenchymal stem cells and synthetic extracellular matrix injections in rats, pp. 537-545, (2010), with permission from John Wiley and Sons (publisher). More BM MSCs tagged with green fluorescent protein (shown in red) remain in the tissue 30 days postinjection for the combination therapy than the cells alone condition.

HA based hydrogels have been shown to be noninflammatory, nonimmunogenic and biocompatible, as well as have significant shock absorption ability. Carbylan-GSX (a thinly-modified semisynthetic GAG derived of HA mixed with a thiolated gelatin, and cross linked with polyethylene glycol), has viscoelastic properties similar to vocal mucosa when injected *in vivo* (Duflo et al., 2006a). When encapsulated in Extracel, BM MSCs maintained a high viability (96% or better), and were able to sustain their cell growth over a three day period (Duflo et al., 2006b). They remained alive 30 days post injection (See Fig. 3). In addition, this construct injected *in vivo* produced an ECM profile more supportive of wound healing (i.e., increased expression of fibronectin and pro-collagen III) than a cells only approach and the control condition (Quinchia-Johnson et al., 2010).

Atelocollagen, a biomaterial found in a few recent reports, is derived from calf dermis and can be degraded *in vivo* by endogenous collagenase at a slower rate than collagen scaffolds. It can be used for tissue engineering purposes in an unmodified form (Lee et al., 2006), made into a sponge (Ohno et al., 2009) or into a gel (Kanemaru et al., 2003). Adherence of cells to the material is an important criterion for potential scaffold biomaterials. Approximately 20% of BM MSCs initially adhered to an atelocollagen sponge *in vitro,* with significant proliferation noted on days 3 and 5 (Ohno et al., 2009). The authors credited the cellular entry to the large pore size. BM MSCs labeled with a fluorochrome and seeded within a 1% hydrochloric acid atelocollagen gel were found to have "good proliferation" *in vitro* (Kanemaru et al., 2003). Similarly, " a large number" of fluorochrome-labeled cells were observed in canine vocal folds eight weeks after having been injected with ASCs within an atelocollagen scaffold (Lee et al., 2006). Despite this, atelocollagen has the distinct disadvantage of being an animal derived substance, which brings with it the threat of immune response activation or transmission of an endogenous retrovirus.

A third reported scaffold biomaterial for vocal fold stem cell applications is fibrin. Long et al. (2009, 2010) was able to demonstrate *in vitro* that a fibrin-based construct seeded with ASCs have good physical integrity and handling characteristics, slow degradation patterns and an ability to support cell viability. Recent findings demonstrate that these constructs have the elastic modulus and collagen orientation similar to native vocal mucosa, and are able to withstand oscillation when sutured onto an excised cadaveric larynx on top of pipe through which air can flow (Long et al., 2010). See Figure 4.

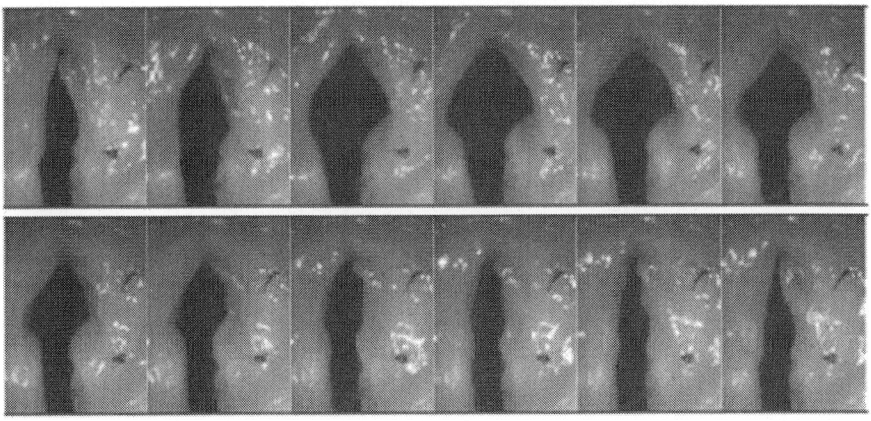

Fig. 4. Reprinted from *Otolaryngology-Head and Neck Surgery,* Vol. 142 / No. 3, Long, J.L., Neubauer, J., Zhang Z., Zuk, P., Berke, G.S., Chhetri, D.K. Functional testing of a tissue-engineered vocal fold cover replacement, 438-440, 2010, with permission from Elsevier. Native vocal fold cover of cadaveric larynx has been replaced with a tissue engineered construct and vibrated with air from an underlying pipe. Arrows mark the edges of the construct. The top of images is the anterior commissure. These images were captured with a high speed camera.

An optimal scaffold for stem cell applications for vocal fold regeneration would be noninflammatory, nonimmunogenic, encourage adherence and viability of resident cells, support appropriate cell-cell signaling, biodegrade at an acceptable rate, remain intact during investigator handling, as well as be able to sustain vocal fold vibration. The scaffold materials listed previously have demonstrated some of these attributes in animal models, but applications in conjunction with stem cell approaches is scant, currently. There exists a great opportunity to advance vocal fold regeneration strategies by finding an optimal scaffold to deliver cells and growth factors.

3.4 Growth factor delivery

To date, the delivery of only a few growth factors, including epidermal growth factor (EGF) fibroblast growth factor (FGF) and hepatocyte growth factor (HGF) have been investigated within MSC-based therapies for vocal fold regeneration. All of this work has been completed *in vitro*.

The effect of soluble signaling has been used to examine the differentiation potential of ASCs. A bilayered, three dimensional construct was created *in vitro* by seeding ASCs within fibrin hydrogels, and once gelation was complete, additional ASCs were added directly on top. When EGF, FGF and retinoic acid were added to the media surrounding these constructs, it was found that EGF encouraged differentiation of ASCs into epithelial cells more efficiently than the other soluble signals (Long et al., 2009). The authors found that the cells on the top, epithelial-like surface stained positive for E-cadherin and cytokeratin 8, epithelial phenotype markers. It was found that these cells differentiated along this lineage only when they had an air interface and exposure to EGF. Interestingly, the authors hypothesized that mechanotransduction may have also played a role in differentiation, as the cells were cultured on a matrix with similar stiffness to the lamina propria. The cells on the inside of the hydrogel stained positive for vimentin, a cytoskeletal protein expressed by cells of mesenchymal origin. It should be noted that during the two week culture period, the epithelial cells did not form a confluent layer, suggestive of reduced efficiency of differentiation and proliferation of epithelial cells.

HGF is known to have strong anti-fibrotic activity, and has been investigated in the voice literature as a stand-alone injection to remediate vocal fold scarring in an animal model (Hirano et al., 2004). In this study, the HGF treated vocal folds had improved rheometric measurements and less collagen deposition than the scarred, untreated vocal folds. In the MSC literature, HGF has been implicated as being secreted by ASCs and encouraging an anti-fibrotic extracellular matrix profile when they are in co-culture with scar fibroblasts (Kumai, 2009). Following vocal fold scarring, ASCs and scar fibroblasts (SF) were isolated from male ferrets, and then co-cultured in a variety of conditions to investigate their relationship with HGF. In order to demonstrate that HGF was one of the growth factors implicated in reducing the production of collagen, a neutralization assay was used. Following four days of co-culture of ASCs and SFs with an anti HGF antibody in the medium, the SFs had significantly higher amounts of collagen secretion than in the control condition. This condition did not affect HA secretion, and thus it was concluded that the HGF secreted by ASCs encourages the anti-fibrotic profile of SFs by downregulating collagen production, but not by upregulating HA production. Additionally, the authors suggested that a tissue engineering construct delivering HGF through ASCs to the vocal fold microenvironment rather than through an exogenous agent is preferable because of the slow release associated with having residency in the tissue and the potential activation of concurrent endogenous facilitatory factors. So, while there have been few studies of introducing growth factors exogenously to tissue engineering for vocal fold regeneration, endogenous growth factors are often thought to be present.

4. Future directions

4.1 Bioreactors

Bioreactors provide *ex vivo* mechanical stimulation that mimics a specific tissue's microenvironment for cells in media. With regard to laryngeal research, bioreactors can provide a unique model for studying the effects of vibration (similar to phonation) on cells in a controlled environment. For the custom designed bioreactors currently used in this line of research, frequency, amplitude and duration of vibration and tension of the substrate which cells are adherent to can often be programmed according to the experimental question of interest. There are many potential applications of this technology, including examination of the effects of dosage of vibration on cells of various laryngeal diseases, investigation of scar fibroblast activity at varying time intervals post laryngeal surgery (to inform recommendations about when to resume voicing post-operatively) and to compare the effects different laryngeal configurations during phonation on healing (to mimic different voice therapies at the cellular level), etc.

While there have been several reports of the effects of stem cell therapies on ECM production, few studies have investigated the mechanisms for encouraging specific vocal fold ECM profiles. Bioreactors may provide a mode of inquiry toward these ends. Interestingly, recent literature suggests that fibroblasts are able to convert mechanical stimuli into ECM modifications, and thereby induce tissue remodeling via mechanotransduction (Ingber, 2006). Recent voice research using bioreactors have found significant vibration induced changes in the ECM profile. For example, human dermal fibroblasts vibrated in hydrogels for periods of five and ten days demonstrated increased expression of HA synthase 2, decorin and fibromodulin (Kutty & Webb, 2010). Human laryngeal fibroblasts vibrated for periods between 1-21 days showed an increased production of fibronectin and collagen type I (Wolchok et al., 2009). Finally, human vocal fold fibroblasts vibrated for 6 hours showed an upregulation of fibronectin and HA-associated genes (Titze et al., 2004). Comparison of the ECM produced by multiple cell types exposed to vibration that mimics phonation may help scientists determine an optimal cell source for vocal fold bioengineering.

Currently bioreactors provide a research model, but in the future they may be utilized in therapeutic inventions. It may be found that cells can be primed in a bioreactor to create an optimal ECM profile before they are implanted into an organism with scarring or other vocal pathology. The use of bioreactors is a promising line of research that could shape future tissue regeneration approaches.

5. Conclusion

The regenerative potential of vocal fold tissue is a topic that is currently being investigated by an increasing number of teams internationally. While the literature to date has merely scratched the surface of the basic parameters involved in laryngeal tissue engineering, there is great opportunity for advancement of the knowledge base with the advent of high throughput experimental techniques, systems biology approaches and their associated statistical analysis. These developments allow for more efficient and comprehensive assessments of cell/scaffold interactions and ECM production profiles. Current themes in the literature include morphological and rheological outcomes of cell based therapies and how to use scaffolds and bioreactors to encourage optimal ECM regeneration. Future topics may include how to encourage efficient differentiation into epithelial cells via signaling mechanisms, how to engineer confluent and distinct layers that mimic normal vocal fold anatomy, how to induce angiogenesis that will be able to withstand vibration without hemorrhage and how to innervate the tissue.

6. Acknowledgements

The authors would like to acknowledge the National Institute of Deafness and Other Communication Disorders-R01 DC4336 for supporting this work.

7. References

Benninger, M.S., Alessi, D., Archer, S, Bastian, R., Ford, C., Koufman, J. (1996). Vocal fold scarring: current concepts and management. *Otolaryngology- Head Neck Surgery,* Vol.115, No. 5, (Nov 1996) 474-482, 0194-5998

Caplan, A. (2007). Adult mesenchymal stem cells for tissue engineering versus regenerative medicine. *Journal of Cellular Physiology,*Vol. 213, No. 2, (Nov 2007) 341-7, 0021-9541

Catten, M., Gray, S.D., Hammond, T.H., Zhou, R., Hammond, E. (1998). Analysis of cellular location and concentrations in vocal fold lamina propria. *Otolaryngology- Head Neck Surgery,* Vol., 118, No.5, (May 1998) 663-667, 0194-5998

Chhetri, D.K., Zhang, Z., Neubauer, J. (2010). Measurement of young's modulus of vocal folds by indentation. *Journal of Voice,* article in press

Courey, M., Shohet, J., Scott, M., Ossoff, R. (1996). Immunohistochemical characterization of benign laryngeal lesions. *Annals of Otology, Rhinology & Laryngology,* Vol. 105, No.7, (July 1996) 525-531, 0003-4894

Duflo, S., Thibeault, S.L., Li, W., Shu, X.Z., Prestwich, G.D. (2006a). Vocal fold tissue repair *in vivo* using a synthetic extracellular matrix. *Tissue Engineering,* Vol. 12, No.8, (Aug 1996) 2171-2179, 2152-4955

Duflo, S., Thibeault, S.L., Li, W., Shu, X.Z., Prestwich, G.D. (2006b). Effect of a synthetic extracellular matrix on vocal fold lamina propria gene expression in early wound healing. *Tissue Engineering,* Vol. 12, No. 11, (Nov 2006) 3201-3207, 2152-4955

Ejnell, H., Mansson, I., Blake, B., Stenborg, R. (1984). Laryngeal obstruction after Teflon injection. *Acta Laryngologica,* Vol. 98, No. 3-4, (Sept-Oct 1984) 374-379, 1758-5368.

Fisher, K.V., Telser, A., Phillips, J.E., Yeates, D.B. (2001). Regulation of vocal fold transepithelial water fluxes. *Journal of Applied Physiology,* Vol. 91, No. 3, (Sept 2001) 1401-1411, 8750-7587

Gipson, I.K., Spurr-Michaud, S.J., Tisdale, A.S., Kublin, C., Cintron, C., Keutmann, H. (1995). Stratified squamous epithlelial produce mucin-like glycoproteins. *Tissue and Cell,* Vol. 27, No. 4, (Aug 1995) 397-404, 0040-8166

Gray, S.D., Titze, I. (1988). Histologic investigation of hyperphonated canine vocal cords. *The Annals of Otology, Rhinology and Laryngology,* Vol. 97, No. 4, (July-Aug 1988) 381-8, 0003-4894

Gray, S. D. (1991) Basement membrane zone injury in vocal nodules. *Vocal Fold Physiology Conference,* pp. 21-28, Singular Publishing Group, San Diego

Gray, S.D., Hirano, M., Sato, K. (1993). Molecular and cellular structure of vocal fold tissue, In: *Vocal fold physiology: frontiers of basic science, 1st ed.,* Titze, I. (Ed.), 1-34., Singular Publishing, 1870332997, San Diego

Gray, S.D., Titze, I., Chan, R., Hammond, T.H. (1999). Vocal fold proteoglycans and their influence on biomechanics. *The Laryngoscope,* Vol. 109, No. 6, (June 1999) 845-854, 1531-4995

Gray, S.D. (2000a). Cellular physiology of the vocal folds. *Otolaryngologic Clinics of North America,* Vol. 33, No. 4 (Aug 2000), 679-697, 0030-6665

Gray, S.D., Titze, I., Alipour, F., Hammond, T.H. (2000b). Biomechanical and histologic observations of vocal fold fibrous proteins. *Annals of Otology, Rhinology & Laryngology,* Vol. 109, No. 1, (Jan 2000) 77-84, 0003-4894

Guimaraes, I., Abberton, E. (2005). Fundamental frequency in speakers of Portuguese for different voice samples. *Journal of Voice,* Vol. 19, No. 4, (Dec 2005) 592-606, 0892-1997

Hahn, M.S., Teply, B.A., Stevens, M.M., Zeitels, S.M., Langer, R. (2006). Collagen composite hydrogels for vocal fold lamina propria restoration. *Biomaterials,* Vol. 27, No. 7, (Mar 2006), 1104-1109, 0142-9612

Hansen, J.K., Thibeault, S.L. (2006). Current understanding and review of the literature: vocal fold scarring. *Journal of Voice,* Vol. 20, No. 1, (March 2006) 110-120, 0892-1997

Hanson, S., Kim., J., Quinchia-Johnson, B., Bradley, B., Breunig, M., Hematti, P., Thibeault, S. (2010). Characterization of mesenchymal stem cells from human vocal fold fibroblasts. *The Laryngoscope,* Vol. 120, No. 3, (March 2010) 546-551, 1531-4995

Hertegård, S., Cedervall, J., Svensson, B., Forsberg, K., Maurer, F.H.J., Vidovska, D., Olivius, P., Ahrlund-Richter, L., Le Blanc, K. (2006a). Viscoelastic and histologic properties in scarred rabbit vocal folds after mesenchymal stem cell injection. *The Laryngoscope,* Vol. 116, No. 7, (July 2006) 1248-1254, 1531-4995

Hertegård, S., Dahlqvist, A., Goodyer, E. (2006b). Viscoelastic measurements after vocal fold scarring in rabbits—short-term results after hyaluronan injection. *Acta Otolaryngologica,* Vol. 126, No. 7, (July 2006b) 758-763, 0365-5237

Hirano, M. (1981). Structure of the vocal fold in normal and disease states. Anatomical and physical study. *ASHA Rep;* 11:11-30, 1981

Hirano, M., Sato, K., Nakashima, T. (1999). Fibroblasts in human vocal fold mucosa. *Acta Oto-Laryngologica,* Vol. 119, No. 2, (Mar 1999) 271-276, 1758-5368

Hirano, S., Bless, D.M., Rousseau, B., Welham, N., Montequin, D., Chan, R.W., Ford, C.N. (2004). Prevention of vocal fold scarring by topical injection of hepatocyte growth factor in a rabbit model. *The Laryngoscope,* Vol. 114, No. 3, (Mar 2004) 548-556, 1531-4995

Hunter, E.J., Svec, J.G., Titze, I.R. (2006). Comparison of the produced and perceived voice range profiles in untrained and trained classical singers. *Journal of Voice,* Vol. 20, No. 4, (Dec 2006) 513-526, 0892-1997

Ingber, DE. (2006). Cellular mechanotransduction: putting all the pieces together again. *The FASEB Journal,* Vol. 20, No. 7, (May 2006) 811-827, 0892-6638

Jia, X., Burdick, J.A., Kobler, J., Clifton, R.J., Rosowski, J.J., Zeitels, S.M., Langer, R. (2004). Synthesis and characterization of in situ cross-linkable hyaluronic acid-based hydrogels with potential application for vocal fold regeneration. *Macromolecules,* Vol. 37, No. 9, (Apr 2004), 3239-3248, 1874-3439

Johnston, N., Bulmer, D., Ross, P.E., Axford, S.E., Pearson, J.P., Dietmar, P.W., Panetti, M., Pignatelli, M, Koufman, J.A. (2003). Cell biology of laryngeal epithelial defenses in health and disease: further studies. *Annals of Otology, Rhinology Laryngology,* Vol. 112, No. 6, (Jun 2003) 481-491, 0003-4894

Kanemaru, S., Nakamura, T., Omori, K., Kojima, H., Magrufov, A., Yiratsuka, Y., Hirano, S., Ito, J., Shimizu, Y. (2003). Regeneration of the vocal fold using autologous mesenchymal stem cells. *Annals of Otology, Rhinology & Laryngology,* Vol. 112, No. 11, (Nov 2003) 915-920, 0003-4894

Kanemaru, S., Nakamura, T., Yamashita, M., Magrufov, A., Kita, T., Tamaki, H., Tamura, Y., Iguchi, F., Kim, T.S., Kishimoto, M., Omori, K., Ito, J. (2005). Destiny of autologous bone marrow-derived stromal cells implanted in the vocal fold. *Annals of Otology, Rhinology & Laryngology,* Vol. 114, No. 12, (Dec 2005) 907-912, 0003-4894

Kriesel, K., Thibeault, S.L., Chan, R.W., Suzuki, T., Van Groll, P.J., Bless, D.M., Ford, C.N. (2002). Treatment of vocal fold scarring: rheological and histological measures of homologous collagen matrix. *Annals of Otology, Rhinology and Laryngology,* Vol. 111, No. 10, (Oct 2002) 884-889, 0003-4894

Kumai, Y., Kobler, J.B., Park, H., Lopez-Guerra, G., Karajanagi, S., Herrera, V., Zeitels, S. (2009). Crosstalk between adipose-derived stem/stromal cells and vocal fold fibroblasts in vitro. *The Laryngoscope,* Vol. 119, No. 4, (Mar 2009), 799-805, 1531-4995

Kutty, J.K. & Webb, K. (2010). Vibration stimulates vocal mucosa-like matrix expression by hydrogel-encapsulated fibroblasts. *Journal of Tissue Engineering and Regenerative Medicine,* Vol. 4, No. 1, (Jan 2010) 62-72, 1932-6254

Le Blanc, K., Ringden, O. (2007). Immunomodulation by mesenchymal stem cells and clinical experience. *Journal of Internal Medicine,* Vol. 262, No. 5, (Nov 2007) 509-525, 1539-3704

Lee., B.Y., Wang, S.G., Lee, J.C., Jung, J.S., Bae, Y.C., Jeong, H.J., Kim, H.W., Lorenz, R.R. (2006). The prevention of vocal fold scarring using autologous adipose tissue-derived stromal cells. *Cells, Tissues and Organs,* Vol. 184, No. 3-4, (2006) 198-204, 1422-6405

Lo Cicero, V.L., Montelatici, E., Cantarella, G., Mazzola, R., Sambataro, G., Rebulla, P., Lazzari, L. (2008). Do mesenchymal stem cells play a role in vocal fold fat graft survival? *Cell Proliferation,* Vol. 41, No. 3, (Jun 2008), 460-473, 0960-7722

Long, J.L., Zuk, P., Berke, G.S., Chhetri, D.K. (2009). Epithelial differentiation of adipose-derived stem cells for laryngeal tissue engineering. *The Laryngoscope,* Vol. 120, No. 1, (Jan 2010), 125-131, 1531-4995

Long, J.L., Neubauer, J., Zhang, Z., Zuk, P., Berke, G.S., Chhetri, D.K. (2010). Functional testing of a tissue-engineered vocal fold cover replacement. *Otolaryngology-Head and Neck Surgery,* Vol. 142, No. 3, (Mar 2010) 438-440, 0194-5998

McCulloch, T.M., Andrews, B.T., Hoffman, H.T., Graham, S.M., Karnell, M.P., Minnick, C. (2002). Long-term follow-up of fat injection laryngoplasty for unilateral vocal cord paralysis. *The Laryngoscope,* Vol. 112, No. 7, (Jul 2002) 1235-1238, 1531-4995

Milstein, C.F., Akst, L.M., Hicks, M.D., Abelson, T.I., Strome, M. (2005). Long-term effects of micro-ionized alloderm injection for unilateral vocal fold paralysis. *The Larygoscope,* Vol.115, No. 9, (Sept 2005) 1691-1696, 1531-4995

Mogi, G., Watanabe, N., Maeda, S. Umehara, T. (1979). Laryngeal secretions: an immunochemical and immunohistological study. *Acta Oto-laryngologica*, Vol. 87, No. (1-2), (Jan-Feb 1979) 129-141, 0365-5237

Mossallam, I., Kotby, M., Ghaly, A., Nassar, A., Barakah, M. (1986). Histopathological aspects of benign vocal fold lesions associated with dysphonia. In: *Vocal fold histopathological: a symposium, 1st ed.*, Kirchner J., (Ed.), pp. 65-80, College Hill Press, San Diego

Nakayama, M., Ford, C.N., Bless, D.M. (1993). Teflon vocal fold augmentation: failures and management in 28 cases. *Otolaryngology-Head and Neck Surgery*, Vol. 109, No. 3 Pt 1, (Sept 1993), 493-498, 0194-5998

Ohno, S., Hirano, S., Tateya, I., Kanemaru, S., Umeda, H., Suehiro, A., Kitani, Y., Kishimoto, Y., Kojima, T., Nakamura, T., Ito, J. (2009). Atelocollagen sponge as a stem cell implantation scaffold for the treatment of scarred vocal folds. *Annals of Otology, Rhinology & Laryngology*, Vol. 118, No. 11, (Nov 2009) 805-810, 0003-4894

Puissant, B., Barreau, C., Bourin, P., Clavel, C., Corre, J., Bousquet, C., Taureau, C., Cousin, B., Abbal, M., Laharrague, P., Penicaud, L, Casteilla, L., Blancher, A. (2005). Immunomodulatory effect of human adipose tissue-derived adult stem cells: comparison with bone marrow mesenchymal stem cells. *British Journal of Haematology*, Vol. 129, No. 1, (Apr 2005) 118-129, 0007-1048

Quinchia-Johnson, B.H., Fox, R., Chen, X., Thibeault, S.L. (2010). Tissue regeneration of the vocal fold using bone marrow mesenchymal stem cells and synthetic extracellular matrix injections in rats. *The Laryngoscope*, Vol. 120, No. 3, (Mar 2010) 537-545, 1531-4995

Rasmussen, I., Uhlin, M., Le Blanc, K., Levitsky, V. (2007). Mesenchymal stem cells fail to trigger effector functions of cytotoxic T lymphocytes. *Journal of Leukocyte Biology*, Vol. 82, No. 4, (Oct 2007) 887-893, 0741-5400

Ringel, R.L., Kahane, J.C., Hillsamer, P.J., Lee, A.S., Badylak, S.F. (2006) The application of tissue engineering procedures to repair the larynx. *Journal of Speech, Language and Hearing Research*, Vol. 49, No. 1, (Feb 2006), 194-208, 1558-9102

Rosen, C.A., Gartner-Schmidt, J., Casiano, R., Anderson, T.D., Johnson, F., Reussner, L., Remacle, M., Sataloff, R.T., Abitbol, J., Shaw, G., Archer, S., McWhorter, A. (2007). Vocal fold augmentation with calcium hydroxyapatite. *Otolaryngology-Head and Neck Surgery*, Vol. 136, No. 2, (Feb 2007) 198.e1-198e.12, 0194-5998

Schramm, V.L., May, M., Lavorato, A.S. (1978). Gelfoam paste injection for vocal cord paralysis: temporary rehabilitation of glottic incompetence. *The Laryngoscope*, Vol. 88, No. 8, (Aug 1978) 1268-1273, 1531-4995

Sivasankar, M., Erickson, E., Rosenblatt, M., Branski, R. (2010) Hypertonic challenge to porcine vocal folds: effects on epithelial barrier function. *Otolaryngology-Head and Neck Surgery*, Vol. 142, No. 1, (Jan 2010) 79-84, 0194-5998

Smith, E., Gray, S., Verdolini, K, Lemke, J. (1995). Effects of voice disorders on quality of life. *Otolaryngology-Head and Neck Surgery*, Vol. 113, No. 2, (Aug 1995) 121, 0194-5998

Svensson, B., Nagubothu, R.S., Cedervall, J., Le Blanc, K.L., Ahrlund-Richter, L., Tolf, A., Hertegård, S. (2010). Injection of human mesenchymal stem cells improves healing of scarred vocal folds: analysis using a xenograft model. *The Laryngoscope*, Vol. 120, No. 7, (Jul 2010) 1370-1375, 1531-4995

Thibeault, S.L., Gray, S.D., Bless, D.M., Chan, R.W., Ford, C. (2002). Histologic and rheologic characterization of vocal fold scarring. *Journal of Voice,* Vol. 16, No. 1, (Mar 2002) 96-104, 0892-1997

Thibeault, S.L., Klemuk, S.A., Smith, M.E., Leugers, C., Prestwich, G. (2009). In vivo comparison of biomimetic approaches for tissue regeneration of the scarred vocal fold. *Tissue Engineering Part A,* Vol. 15, No. 7, (Jul 2009), 1481-1487, 2152-4947

Titze, I.R., Hitchcock, R.W., Broadhead, K., Webb, K., Li, W., Gray, S.D., Tresco, P.A. (2004). Design and validation of a bioreactor for engineering vocal fold tissues under combined tensile and vibrational stresses. *Journal of Biomechanics,* Vol. 37, No. 10, (Oct 2004) 1521-1529, 0021-9290

Uccelli, A., Pistoia, V., Moretta, L. (2007). Mesenchymal stem cells: a new strategy for immunosuppression? (2010). *Trends in Immunology,* Vol. 28, No. 5, (May 2010) 219-226, 1471-4906

Wolchok, J.C., Brokopp, C., Underwood, C.J., Tresco, P.A. (2009). The effect of bioreactor induced vibrational stimulation on extracellular matrix production from human derived fibroblasts. *Biomaterials,* Vol. 30, No. 3, (Jan 2009) 327-335, 0142-9612

Xu, C.C., Chan, R.W., Tirunagari, N. (2007). A biodegradable, acellular xenogeneic scaffold for regeneration of the vocal fold lamina propria. *Tissue Engineering,* Vol. 13, No. 3, (Mar 2007), 551-566, 1937-3368

23

Design, Synthesis and Applications of Retinal-Based Molecular Machines

Diego Sampedro, Marina Blanco-Lomas,
Laura Rivado-Casas and Pedro J. Campos
Departamento de Química, Unidad Asociada al C.S.I.C., Universidad de La Rioja
Spain

1. Introduction

Progress of mankind has always been related to the development and construction of new machines. In the last decades, science and technology have been involved in a race to increase the capacity of novel machines as well as in a progressive miniaturization of their parts. Further efforts to design and construct machines at the nanometer scale will lead to new and exciting applications in medicine, energy and materials. However, until now every attempt to build artificial systems at the molecular level with complex functions pales beside the Nature's molecular machines at work. Myosin and kinesin enzymes responsible of muscle contraction, ATP synthase and cellular transport are all examples of Nature's ability to provide living systems with complex machinery whose structures and detailed mechanisms we are just starting to unveil. Thus, by learning from Nature, we will be able to make use of the excellent properties refined by slow evolution.

When we mimic Nature, we try to duplicate some of the features found in biological systems using synthetic analogues. Taking natural molecular machines as a starting point, we will try to design, synthesize and explore biomimetic artificial machines. Located at the interface between biology, physics and chemistry, the task of mimicking Nature's results will need combined efforts from different disciplines and the use of every possible tool from theoretical calculations to advanced synthetic chemistry and structural characterization.

In this chapter we will briefly review some of the better-known natural molecular machines as an inspiration for the design of biomimetic artificial machines. Specifically, the structure and function of the retinal molecular machine will be discussed. Taking the Nature's work as a starting point, we will specify some of the requirements to build efficient molecular machines, such as controlling the motion at the molecular level and the energy supply. We will use these concepts to design a set of retinal-based biomimetic chemical switches. Comparison between the synthetic and biological structures allows to gather a better understanding of both systems together with some suggestions for further improvements. Some practical applications will also be presented together with an outlook for the near future.

2. Why mimic Nature's work?

Science ability to design, build and manipulate devices of increasing complexity has allowed mankind to reach and occupy every corner of Earth. We are now able to fly through air and to cleave through the waves. We have developed new materials with enhanced properties. We have built machines capable of performing complex functions. However, we should bear in mind that Nature had solved most of these problems time ago (Ball, 2001). Even more, Nature solutions are usually more complex, elegant and efficient that the human equivalents. For example, some natural materials are designed to be hard and strong enough to protect living organisms, such as those forming shells and bones (Smith, 1999). Beyond their excellent mechanical properties (Wainwright, 1982), these materials are usually the most economic choice from a biological point of view, thus allowing the living organism to save energy and components for other important biological functions. Mankind has taken advantage of natural materials, but always has tried to emulate or improve Nature's design. For instance, silk is one of the strongest natural fibers. It is made up of the aminoacid series Gly-Ser-Gly-Ala forming beta-sheets with hydrogen bonds between chains. The high proportion of glycine allows the fibers to be strong and resistant to stretching. Thousands of years ago, Chinese recognized the remarkable properties of silk and tried to emulate them looking for an artificial silk (Kaplan & Adams, 1994). However, it wasn't until 1890's when the first artificial silk (viscose) was produced from cellulose. With the emerge of bionics in the 20th century, research on systems based upon or similar to those of living organisms allowed new types of bioengineered devices. A rapid growth in interest followed on learning how living systems achieve high degrees of organization, synthesize materials with exceptional properties and develop complex devices to interact with the environment.

Scientists have drawn their bioinspiration in two main ways. On one hand, a biological system could be used in a synthetic system as is. Using this approach, the system's functionality is transferred to an artificial construction in order to use its properties in a new way, even completely diverse from its original one (Willner 2002). For instance, DNA has been employed in recent years for new and exotic uses, very different from its biological role such as using selective bonds between complementary DNA sequences to link particles to surfaces. On the other hand, Nature's work can be emulated trying not only to use or understand how biological systems work, but also to use them in artificial devices with new and improved properties (Sarikaya & Aksay, 1993; Mann, 1996). Taking biological systems as a starting point, scientists try to identify the key factors behind their structure and function to build new systems with different, improved or more controllable properties.

Nature has also developed great examples of efficient machinery. Over millions of years of refinement, living organisms show a number of biomechanical machines much more capable than our synthetic prototypes. Responsible of innumerable biological processes, these biomolecular motors and machines are nanoscale versions of macroscopic machines that we use every day. From these biomolecular machines, we could learn how to efficiently design our own versions of nanoscopic devices. Our goal could be to mimic Nature at first and, why not, try to improve the properties of these systems or at least to adapt them to our specific needs. In the next section we will briefly present some natural machines. Learning how these machines work, we will be able to design and build biomimetic artificial machines exploiting the slow evolutionary Nature's work.

3. Natural molecular motors

The way macroscopic machines and motors are regarded can be extended to a molecular level (Balzani et al., 2008). In the last 50 years, Nanotechnology has advanced in the study of machines at the microscopic grade, which are constructed by a "bottom-up" approach.

However, different examples of nanoscale machinery can be found in Nature. Specifically, cells house hundreds of different molecular machines and motors, each of them specialized for a particular function. These nanomachines are primarily composed of proteins, nucleic acids and other organic molecules. In order to work, energy is needed, so these natural molecular machines and motors convert chemical energy stored in chemical bonds or gradients across membranes into mechanical energy. They are involved in a multitude of essential biological processes, such as transport of cations (*i.e.* H^+, Ca^+, K^+), synthesis of ATP, and muscle contraction. In the following paragraphs, different examples of natural molecular machines and motors are described.

3.1 Natural metal ion channels

Cells require the passage of cations such as Na^+, Ca^+ and K^+, across their membranes, so they can be distributed to their components. However, this process is prevented by the existence of membranes that protect the contents of cells. Therefore, cation transfer has to take place either by carriers or through ion channels. Carriers are hosts molecules that are embedded in the membrane and help cations to go through the membrane by means of complexation. The rate of this transport mechanism is relatively slow, because it is limited by diffusion. On the other hand, ion channels are membrane proteins that form aqueous ion-conduction pathways through the center of the protein and expand the cell membrane so the ions can move across. These protein channels are found to transport ions faster than a carrier. As an example of a natural ion channel, the mechanism of a light driven proton pump, bacteriorhodopsin, a membrane protein of the halophilic microorganism *Halobacterium salinarum* is described below (Subramaniam & Henderson, 2000; Kühlbrandt, 2000).

Bacteriorhodopsin, consists of seven membrane-spanning helical structures linked by short loops on either side of the cell membrane. It also contains one molecule of a linear pigment called retinal that is covalently attached to the protein via a protonated Schiff base. The retinal chromophore, which will be further studied in section 3.5, suffers an isomerization from all-*trans* to 13-*cis* upon illumination. This structural change is used by the Schiff base to push a single proton through the seven-helix bundle, from the inside of the cell to the extracellular medium, being subsequently reprotonated from the cytoplasm. Therefore, in this particular movement, the retinal chromophore acts as a valve inside of the cell membrane of this organism.

3.2 ATP synthase

As it was stated before, energy is required in order for the molecular machines and motors to work. They are usually fueled by the energy stored in cells. Two of the most common energy repositories of cells are in the phosphate bonds of nucleotides, generally ATP (adenosine triphosphate), and in transmembrane electrochemical gradients. Synthesis of ATP is carried out by the enzyme ATP synthase, which is a natural rotary motor that uses both kinds of the energy sources mentioned above (Metha et al., 1999). This protein is a multidomain complex consisting of two units attached to a common shaft: a hydrophobic proton channel (F_0) embedded in the mitochondrial membrane and a hydrophilic catalytic unit (F_1) protruding into the mitochondria. The complex can be thought of as two rotary motor units coupled together. The F_1 motor uses free energy of ATP hydrolysis to rotate in one direction whereas the F_0 motor uses the energy stored in a transmembrane electrochemical gradient to turn in the opposite direction. The F_1F_0-ATP synthase is reversible;

whereas the full enzyme complex can synthesize or hydrolyze ATP, F_1 in isolation only hydrolyzes it. This depends on the driven force of the movement. When F_0 takes over, which is the normal situation, it drives the F_1 motor in reverse producing the synthesis of ATP from ADP and inorganic phosphate. However, when F_1 motor controls the rotation, it drives the F_0 motor in reverse, becoming an ion pump that moves ions across the membrane against the electrochemical gradient. Rotation of F_1 was demonstrated by directly observing the motion of a fluorescent actin filament specifically bound to the rotor element (Noji et al., 1997). Also, discrete 120° rotations were observed under low ATP concentrations and with actin filaments of variable length (Yasuda et al., 1998). Moreover, they estimated the work required to rotate the actin filament against viscous load to be as much as 80 pN nm, which is approximately the free energy liberated by a single ATP hydrolysis under physiological conditions. Therefore, they concluded that the F_1-ATPase could couple nearly 100% of its ATP-derived energy into mechanical work, so it was considered a really efficient motor.

3.3 Kinesin and myosin

Linear-like movements are essential in Nature, because they are related to intracellular trafficking, cell division and muscle contraction (Goodsell, 1996; Howard, 2001). Therefore, one of the main classes of biomolecular motors is linear motors. These are organic molecules or molecular assemblies which move in a linear fashion along a track of some kind. The first type of linear motor is a processive motor, which is constantly in contact with the track it moves along. Processive motors are exemplified by the kinesin protein super-family that moves along microtubules (Schliwa & Woehlke, 2001). RNA polymerase, which synthesizes new RNA from a single strand RNA template (Gelles & Landick, 1998), and DNA helicase, which translates along and unwinds DNA in preparation for new DNA synthesis (Lohman et al., 1998), are also linear processive motors.

In addition to processive motors, there are also non-processive motors, which detach from the track and subsequently re-attach, and therefore can be seen as hopping along the track instead of walking. Non-processive linear motors include myosin (Yildiz et al., 2003), which binds to actin filaments and generates the contractile force in muscle tissue (Irving et al., 1992), as well as the dynein protein family that transports cargo along microtubules in the opposite direction to kinesin (Taylor & Holwill, 1999).

Conventional kinesin is a protein assembly whose total size is approximately 80nm. It is composed of two larger protein chains, which are involved in microtubule binding, mobility, ATP hydrolysis and protein dimerization, as well as two smaller protein chains, which regulate heavy chain activity and binding to cargo. Kinesin transports cargo along microtubules, self assembled from monomeric proteins, using a walking-like motion with 8 nm steps (Svoboda et al., 1993). Each of these steps is coupled to the hydrolysis of an ATP molecule, which provides the chemical energy for motion (Coy et al., 1999). It moves with a high speed of about 1.8 $\mu m\ s^{-1}$, and can move against loads of 6 pN. Kinesin is one of the most widely studied motor proteins, and it can be easily modified by genetic engineering and incorporated into a variety of synthetic systems. Microtubules may be bound to a substrate while retaining their structure and function (Turner et al., 1995). Then, molecules functionalized with kinesin can be shuttled along the tracks by the addition of ATP (Diez et al., 2003). It is possible to align microtubules by fluid flow, allowing the kinesin-powered cargo to move in a directional fashion.

The term myosin refers to at least 14 classes of proteins, each containing actin-base motors. Myosin is composed of two large heads, containing a catalytic unit for ATP hydrolysis,

connected to a long tail (Metha et al., 1999). Myosin II (skeletal muscle myosin) provides the power for all our voluntary motion (running, walking, etc.) and involuntary muscles (*i.e.* beating heart). In muscle cells, many myosin II molecules combine by aligning their tails, each staggered relative to the next. These muscle cells are also filled with filaments of actin (helical polymers), which are used as a ladder on which myosin climbs. The head groups of myosin extend from the surface of the resulting filament like bristles in a bottle brush. The bristling head groups act independently and provide the power to contract muscles. They reach from the myosin filament to a neighboring actin filament and become attached to it. Breakage of an ATP molecule then forces the myosin head into a radically different shape. It bends near the center and drags the myosin filament along the actin filament. This results in the power stroke of muscle contraction. In a rapidly contracting muscle, each myosin head may stroke five times a second, each stroke moving the filament approximately 10 nm. Besides muscle contraction, myosin II is also involved in several forms of cell movement, including cell shape changes, cytokinesis, capping of cell surface receptors, and retraction of pseudopods (Spudich, 1989). Myosin II shares many structural features with kinesin. Both use ATP to move along their respective tracks, but as it was said in previous paragraphs, myosin II is a non-processive motor, which means that a single molecule cannot move along its track for large distances so organized ensembles of molecules can move their track at higher speeds. Myosin is thought to undergo a conformational change when it binds to actin, resulting in a "working stroke."
The myosin-actin system can also be used to produce the same effect as the one described for kinesin (Harada et al., 1997). As myosin is larger than kinesin, and actin filaments are more flexible than microtubules, more freedom is allowed in the design of synthetic systems.

3.4 Other molecular machines

In addition to linear and rotary motors, Nature has devised many other types of nanomachines, such as:

- Springs: The spasmoneme supra-molecular spring is an example of a biological version of a spring (Mahadevan & Matsudaira, 2000). Thanks to the binding and removal of calcium these filaments cause a reversible contraction and extension that is used by the organism for his protection.
- Hinges: Some proteins, such as the maltose-binding protein, have been found to undergo hinge-like conformational changes when binding a ligand. As a result, a very sensitive maltose sensor can be constructed *in vitro* (Benson et al., 2001).
- Spindles: The mechanism that some viruses use for packaging their DNA into the viral capsid is analogous to a spindle used for spinning yarn.
- Electrostrictive materials: Presin is a motor protein that resides in the inner ear, whose shape responds to changes in electrical potential across membranes (Liberman et al., 2002). Prestin's electroselective mechanism is responsible for sound amplification and results in a 1000-fold enhacement of sound detection.

3.5 Retinal chromophore

One of the most remarkable examples in Nature of a molecular motor is the retinal chromophore of rhodopsin, which suffers a *cis-trans* photoisomerization during the process of vision (Kandori et al., 2001). Rhodopsin, is a photoreceptor protein (a visual pigment), which is located in the rod visual cells responsible for twilight vision. Rhodopsin has 11-*cis* retinal as its chromophore (Figure 1), which is embedded inside a single peptide transmembrane protein called opsin. The role of rhodopsin in the signal transduction cascade of vision is to activate transducin, a heterotrimeric G protein, upon absorption of light (Hofmann & Helmreich, 1996). Rhodopsin (opsin), a member of G-protein coupled receptor family, is composed of 7-transmembrane helices. The 11-*cis* retinal forms the Schiff base linkage with a lysine residue of the 7th helix (Lys296 in the case of bovine rhodopsin), and the Schiff base is protonated, which is stabilized by a negatively charged carboxylate (Glu113 in the case of bovine rhodopsin). The bionone ring of the retinal is coupled with hydrophobic region of opsin through hydrophobic interactions (Matsumoto & Yoshizawa, 1975). Thus, the retinal chromophore is fixed by three kinds of chemical bonds in the retinal binding pocket of rhodopsin.

In the absence of visible light, retinal presents a *cis* conformation between its carbons 11 and 12. However, when 11-*cis*-retinal absorbs visible light (λ between 400-700 nm), photoisomerization of this double bond takes place to give a *trans* conformation. Picosecond time-resolved spectroscopy of 11-*cis* locked rhodopsin analogs reveals that the *cis-trans* isomerization of the retinal chromophore is the primary reaction in the process of vision, and it is followed by a conformational change in the rhodopsin protein, which generates an electric impulse that reaches the brain, so objects and images can be perceived.

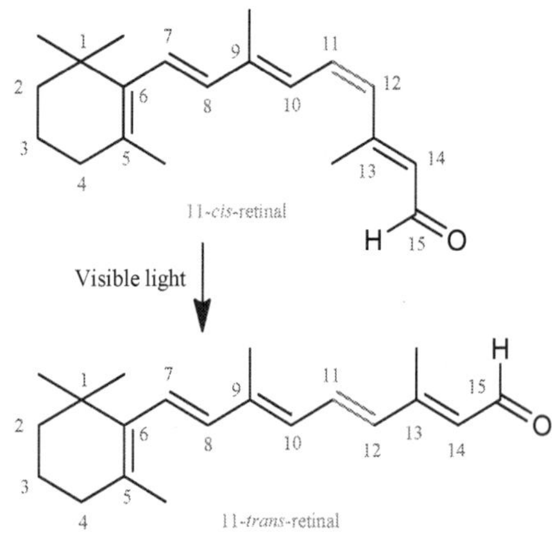

Fig. 1. Chemical structure of the retinal chromophore in rhodopsin

It is known that the *cis-trans* isomerization is highly efficient in rhodopsin (quantum yield, Φ_{isom}= 0.67, Dartnall, 1967), which is essential to make twilight vision highly sensitive. In fact, a human rod cell can respond to a single photon absorption. Such an efficient photoisomerization of the retinal chromophore is characteristic in the protein environment of rhodopsin, being in contrast to the rhodopsin chromophore in solution. This indicates that the protein environment facilitates the isomerization.

In order to mimic Nature's molecular machines, the molecular structure of the retinal chromophore may be used as a pattern for the design of new prototypes of molecular motors, whose movement is based on *cis-trans* photoisomerizations. Therefore, molecular motors that work efficiently may be obtained.

4. Artificial molecular machines

As stated before, two different approaches can be adopted in order to design practical biomimetic molecular machines. The first approximation is to introduce natural molecular machines, such as those shown in section 3, into artificial devices. This way, new hybrid machinery could be built combining the efficiency of natural machines with new applications and uses of these hybrid devices. In fact, several examples of this approach have already been developed (Steinberg-Yfrach et al., 1998; Soong et al., 2000; Hess et al., 2004). The other possibility is to use the natural systems as an inspiration and starting point, trying to adjust their properties to specific needs or even trying to improve their performance. In order to design efficient artificial molecular machines, some key factors should be considered. For instance, some basic questions such as size, medium of operation, type of motion and time scale, to cite a few should be carefully considered in the design. Especially important is the energy supply to make the machine work. In this section we will summarize some of these factors.

4.1 Basic concepts

Molecular machines (both natural or artificial) are devices designed to accomplish a specific function. This function is achieved by converting energy into mechanical work. Molecular devices operate via electronic or nuclear rearrangement that have to be controlled beyond the Brownian motion (Astumian, 2005).

As explained in previous paragraphs, different types of motion may be performed by the machine components (oscillatory, linear, rotatory,...). Therefore, the machine should be carefully designed in order to maximize the desired movement while minimizing other competitive motions that would diminish efficiency of the machine. For instance, rotary movement might be achieved using rotations around covalent bonds.

However, not only is important to control the movement of the components of the machine, but also to monitor this movement. In order to achieve this, the electronic or nuclear rearrangements should cause a change in a physical or chemical property that could be measured. In particular, we will see later how the use of light is especially convenient as it can be used both to operate the machine and to monitor the state of the system.

Moreover, a machine capable of cyclic process will be much easier to control and operate. In the case of devices unable to repeat the operation, an external stimulus different from the energy input, should be used to reset the system. This will clearly contribute to slow down the machine operation and increase the complexity of the system. On the other hand, a machine that can operate in a cyclic way could become autonomous, which means that it would keep operating in a constant environment as long as the energy source is still available. Most of the natural machines are autonomous while the majority of artificial devices need a reset. This is one of the main advantages of natural devices that artificial analogues should try to mimic.

Finally, the time scale of the process is also relevant. The time of operation of a molecular machine depends on the type of rearrangement, the components involved and the medium surrounding the machine. The time scale can range from picoseconds to seconds. Thus, other properties such as the type of motion and the property to be monitored should also be in a similar time scale.

4.2 Energy supply

A key factor in the design of efficient molecular machines is the energy supply. As said before, molecular machines act through rearrangements caused by suitable stimuli that eventually convert energy into mechanical work. The nature of these stimuli determines not only the chemical nature of the machine, but also the type of motion and the control of the movement (Balzani, 2008). As we have seen in the previous section, most of natural machines are activated by chemical stimuli. Proton concentration, ion gradients or interaction with molecules can affect (either activating or deactivating) the machine's operation. However, for a machine activated by chemical energy, it has to be considered also the need for an effective removal of waste products formed during the machine's operation. This fact implies serious limitations in the design and function of artificial molecular machines based on chemical stimuli (Khramov et al., 2008).

Perhaps the simplest stimulus to activate a machine is temperature. For example, the activity of an enzyme can be seriously affected by a temperature increase causing small conformational changes (Min et al., 2005). However, using heat as the energy supply has some serious drawbacks as it is quite difficult to control (both in terms of time and location) and heat dissipates quite rapidly.

Even though it is difficult to employ mechanical forces as an adequate stimulus in artificial systems, this kind of energy supply can be observed in natural devices. For instance, the sense of hearing and touch rely on the effect of mechanical forces.

The ability of electrochemical inputs to produce endergonic and reversible reaction has also been exploited in order to design devices activated by these inputs (Kaifer & Gómez-Kaifer, 1999). Therefore, heterogeneous electron transfer processes can be used to operate molecular machines with some advantages, such as the absence of waste products to remove and the allowance of electrodes of a very efficient interface between the molecular-level device and the macroscopic world.

Finally, light is probably the most advantageous stimulus as it lacks most of the drawbacks shown by other types of energy inputs. There are no waste products, it is easily controlled by modern optical apparatus, it shows high temporal and spatial resolution with the use of lasers, and precise selection of wavelength allows the selective operation of the device in complex media. Photochemical inputs can be used at the same time to operate and control the machine motion, which facilitates both the design and function of the device. To be more specific, probably the simplest and most used type of reaction to activate a light-driven molecular device is an isomerization reaction.

5. Retinal-based molecular switches

We have seen in previous sections how the combination of advanced synthesis, supramolecular chemistry, surface science and molecular biology can provide exciting opportunities toward the development of smart molecular materials and machines (Feringa, 2007). In this section we will review some of the work done on the artificial molecular switches based in the retinal chromophore, one of the best natural examples of efficient molecular machinery.

5.1 Basic features and design

Molecular switches and motors are essential components of artificial molecular machines. In fact, switchable molecular systems are molecules which respond to external stimuli and constitute several examples of how simple concepts can be built upon to yield properties with a very wide range of applications. In 1999, a biarylidene molecule was synthesized that uses chemical energy to activate and bias a thermally induced isomerization reaction, and thereby achieve unidirectional intramolecular rotary motion. This one was the first example of a molecular motor able to do photo-induced isomerizations repetitive and unidirectional. (Komura et al., 1999).

Many advances have occurred from that moment in order to improve the performance of these nanostructures (Vicario et al., 2006). Special emphasis is given to the control of a range of functions and properties, including luminescence, self-assembly, motion, color, conductance, transport, and chirality. Currently, the design and preparation of molecular switches, *i.e.* molecules that can interconvert among two or more states, based on photochemical *cis/trans* isomerization constitute an attractive research target to obtain novel materials for nanotechnology (Amendola, 2001; Drexler, 1992; Balzani et al., 2008). Indeed, switches based on the photoisomerization of the azobenzene chromophore have been already used to control ion complexation (Shinkai et al., 1983), electronic properties (Jousselme et al., 2003) and catalysis (Cacciapaglia et al., 2003) or to trigger folding/unfolding of oligopeptide chains (Bredenbeck et al., 2003). Most remarkably, a sophisticated application of the above principle led to the preparation of light-driven molecular rotors (Feringa, 2001) where chirality turned out to be an essential feature to impose unidirectional rotation. In these systems helical bis-arylidene scaffolds featuring a single exociclyc double bond have been employed to achieve photo-induced unidirectional rotary motion. Thanks to the structural changes in these compounds, the rotational velocity is now comparable with those natural ones (*i.e.* ATP-synthase, see section 3). Among the most natural amazing examples is the *cis / trans* isomerization of retinal chromophore (rhodopsin protein) in the process of vision (Figure 2) (Gennadiy et al., 2005).

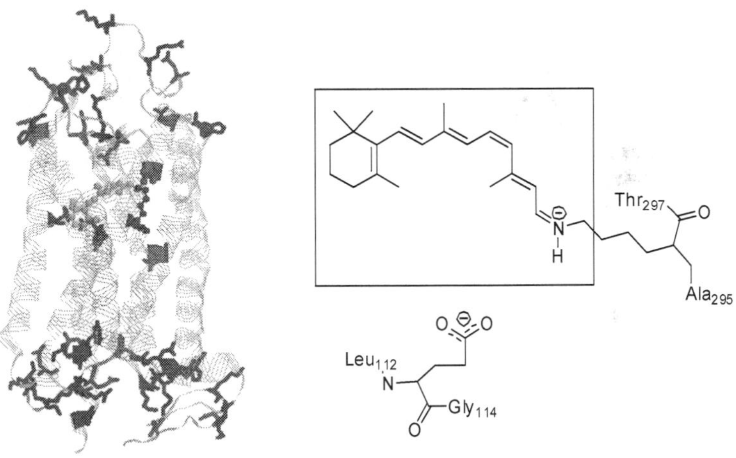

Fig. 2. Rhodopsin protein and retinal chromophore.

As said before, rhodopsin (Rh) is a red-coloured protein due to the 11-*cis*-retinal. The chromophore is bound to the hydrophobic core of the molecule, causing its absorption maximum at approximately 380 nm. The chromophore is covalently linked to Lys296 in bovine rhodopsin through a protonated Schiff base (PSB11, Teller et al., 2001). The process of vision takes places due to the cis-trans isomerization which is activated by photons of visible light (400-700 nm). This molecular movement triggers an electric impulse to the brain in femtoseconds. Due to the high efficiency of retinal *in vivo* isomerization, it has been comprehensively studied and used as a model to the design of many light driven molecular switches. While it has been established that the efficiency of the PSB11 isomerization reaction is enhanced by the complex protein environment, an interesting modification is to design a non-natural protonated Schiff base (PSB) capable of replicating in solution the properties of the protein-embedded chromophore. Thus, PSBs of polyenals constitute a class of light-driven switches selected by biological evolution that provide a useful model for the development of artificial light driven molecular switches or motors.

In spite of the increasing interest in these systems, few works of switches based in this mechanism have appeared in literature. In 2004, a new family of retinal-based molecular switches was designed and synthesized (Sampedro et al., 2004). These molecular systems based in the retinal chromophore included an *N*-alkylated pirroline (NAP) moiety and presented some of the features of an efficient light-driven molecular switch (Figure 3).

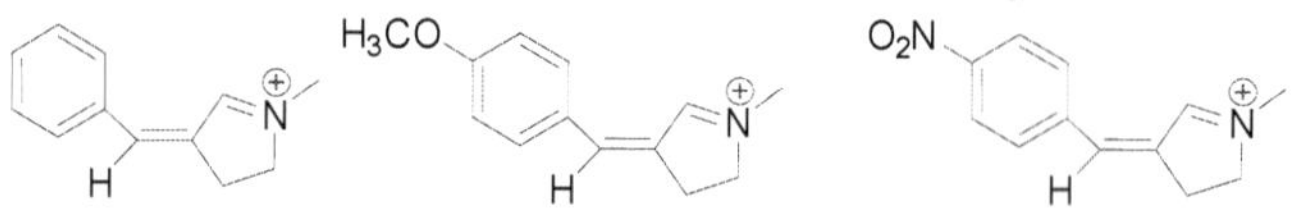

Fig. 3. *N*-alkylated pirroline (NAPs) molecular switches.

NAPs and other derivates are "chimerical" switches that incorporate into the Feringa's biarylidene skeleton a protonated or alkylated Schiff base function that could potentially replicate the dynamics of the PSB11 isomerization in Rh. One of the characteristic features of these compounds is the quaternization of nitrogen atom, searching for a similarity to the retinal chromophore *in vivo*. However, one of the principal problems of NAP switches is their low quantum yield (6×10^{-3}). This result is due to the fact that some energy is not used in the photoisomerization process, but in the isomerization of other bonds different from the central double bond. In general an effective light-driven molecular switch should optimize their performance in order to use all the light energy in a mechanical, controlled way.

Thus, among other important features, an efficient molecular switch must have in its structure a double bond capable of selective photoisomerization in the presence of other bonds. Using the retinal chromophore as a starting point and inspiration, the challenge is to design and synthesize systems that can act as light-driven molecular switches.

5.2 Synthesis

A set of molecular switches with the NAPs substructure was synthesized using the following route (Figure 4):

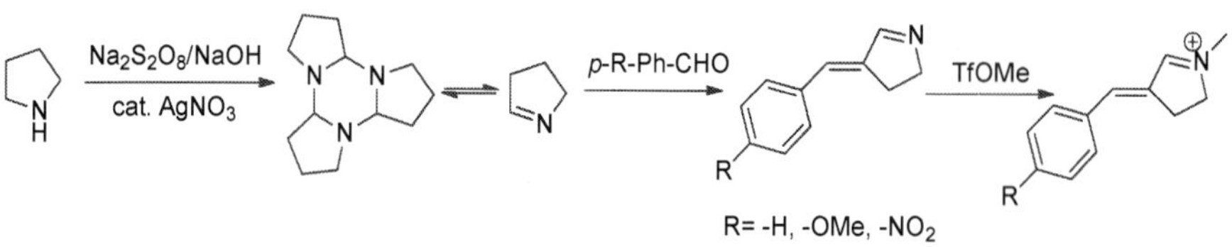

Fig. 4.

The main drawback of these compounds is the presence of different bonds able to isomerize. Due to this, the quantum yield of isomerization around the central double bond is quite low. In order to solvent this problem, a new type of compound with an *N*-alkylated fluorenylidene-pyrroline (NAFP) substructure was designed. Isomerization in these compounds is selective as only the C=C central bond can rotate. Besides, the extended conjugated π system allows for absorption bands in the visible (Figure 5, Rivado-Casas et al., 2009).

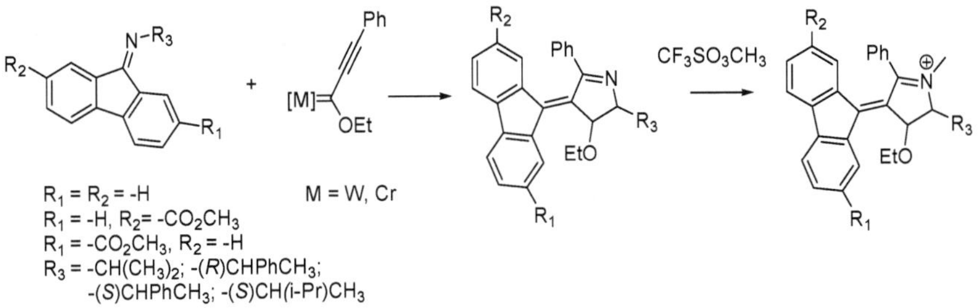

Fig. 5. NAFP light-driven molecular switches.

This new family satisfies some of the features of an ideal molecular switch:

i. selective isomerization (five-membered rings block competitive isomerizations);
ii. high quantum yield;
iii. linking points present in the molecule.

Using NAFPs it is possible to achieve biomimetic light-driven switches where the absorption maximum of an unsubstituted system has been red-shifted by >50 nm with respect to that of the NAPs and rotation is now easily achieved by using visible light.

The new structures are one type of biomimetic light-driven *Z/E* molecular switches that constitute an attractive alternative (*e.g.* with higher polarity and reduced molecular size) to the previously used azobenzene switch. It should be noted that the *cis/trans* nomenclature used in the case of the retinal chromophore becomes ambiguous when referring to NAFPs. In this case the use of the *Z/E* terminology is necessary, but both refer to the same isomerization reaction. Another advantage was the synthesis of chiral molecular switches potentially acting as molecular motors. Moreover, the chiral compounds constitute one of the first examples of a potential light-driven biomimetic single molecule motor whose $Z \rightarrow E$ and $E \rightarrow Z$ rotation direction are ultimately determined by the absolute configuration of the stereogenic centre.

A different group of switches with an N-alkylated indanylidene-pyrroline (NAIP) moiety were also synthesized (Lumento et al., 2007). These compounds display in solution properties similar to the Rh-embedded PSB11 (Figure 6).

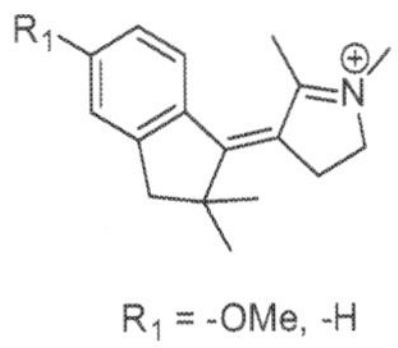

Fig. 6. NAIP molecular switches.

All these compounds (NAPs, NAFPs y NAIPs) show features that in some cases clearly improve those shown by the most popular azobenzenes. Activation may be achieved using low-energy vision light (NAFPs), the length of the indane-pyrroline framework is shorter and may be more easily integrated in a biological compound, such as in a peptide backbone, and they all have good photochemical and mechanical properties. Therefore, they are appropriate candidates to act as molecular light driven switches.

5.3 Properties

Retinal-based switches incorporate into the biarylidene skeleton a protonated or alkylated Schiff base function that could potentially replicate the dynamics of the PSB11 isomerization in Rh. This protein features a S_1 lifetime of 150 fs, a S_0 transient (photorhodopsin) appearance time of 180 fs, and a primary photoproduct (bathorhodopsin) appearance time of 6 ps (Wang et al., 1994). This ultrafast reaction time scale and vibrational coherence suggests that the reaction occurs without intermediates along the reaction path. These intermediates could divide the proton energy up and so it would decrease the efficiency of the switch. In an efficient switch, the reaction path from the excited state happens without any intermediate, and the excited reactive quickly fall over to the product state.

NAIP derivates have been shown, through a highly interdisciplinary research effort (Sinicropi et al., 2008) to be photochromic compounds completing its $Z \rightarrow E$ and $E \rightarrow Z$ photocycle in picoseconds, a few orders of magnitude faster than the fastest known biarylidene (≈ 6 miliseconds for a half-cycle, Vicario et al., 2006). This is in agreement with a reaction path where the formation of the photoproduct takes place without any intermediate, as in the case of the retinal chromophore *in vivo*. Thus, these biomimetic switches constitute very efficient compounds as they show limited energy redistribution and fast isomerization. Also, these compounds show high thermal interconversion barriers (>40 kcal/mol). These barriers indicate that the *E*- and *Z*- forms will no thermally interconvert at room temperature.

The high efficiency of this photoreaction is a clear improvement over switches based on azobenzene. In rhodopsin, the photoisomerization of the native 11-*cis*-retinal chromophore to its *all-trans* form occurs with a 0.67 quantum yield (Dartnall, 1967). This value is larger than the 0.25 value measured for the same chromophore in ethanol solution (Becker, 1988) and also larger than the approximately 0.39 value measured for the photoisomerization of *trans*- and *cis*- azobenzene, respectively (Bortolus & Monti, 1979). However, the quantum yields measured for NAFPs (0.5) are much closer to retinal chromophore *in vivo*. This behaviour is also in agreement with a reaction path without intermediates.

One of the most remarkable properties of NAFPs is that these switches display absorption maxima in the near visible region (Rivado-Casas et al., 2009). Specifically, they have an absorption maximum of *ca*. 400 nm that is red-shifted compared to the NAPs derivates (Lumento et al., 2007). This displacement is due to the replacement of the pyrroline unit of NAPs with moieties displaying an expanded π system. This constitutes a clear improvement over previous results and makes NAFP retinal-based molecular switches interesting candidates for technological applications.

NAFP switches show also high stability, both thermal and photochemical. In fact, the degree of photodegradation was assessed irradiating the switches. It was found that the ^{1}H-NMR spectrum remained unaltered after long times (>24 hours), showing that the photochemical decomposition of these molecules is minimal.

To summarize:

i. these switches are suitable for applications in highly polar environments while azobenzene derivates are neutral with limited dipole-moment values;
ii. the length of the indane (or fluoren-pyrroline) framework is shorter that those of azobenzenes and may be more easily integrated, for instance, in a peptide backbone.
iii. the photoisomerization of these switches happens in picoseconds (10^3 times faster than azobenzene);
iv. their quantum yield is closer to retinal.

5.4 Applications

The use of light to trigger changes in molecular systems has great importance in biochemistry and medicine (Gorostiza & Isacoff, 2008). Systems based on the reversible photoreactions of diarylethenes have advanced the area of "smart" materials. Their potential use as components of molecular electronics, optical memories and variable-transmission filters has been well documented (Irie, 2000). Their appeal is based on the fact that light can be tuned to reversibly and specifically trigger optical and electronic changes such as colour, emission and refractive index in materials that contain this versatile molecular architecture.

What are the potential applications of molecular switches, motors and machines is a question asked frequently in the context of future technology based on (molecular) nanoscience. A glance at the myriad of molecular machines on biology and the fascinating diversity of processes is perhaps the best testimony to the prospects ahead. The first examples of molecular motors and switches at work have already been reported (Browne & Feringa, 2006; Kay et al., 2007; Stoddart, 2001; Harada, 2001). The fascinating idea of casting single molecules capable to convert light energy into "mechanical" motion prompted chemists to develop, in different contexts, systems capable of undergoing light-driven structural changes.

In fact, molecular switches based on photochemical *Z/E* isomerization have been employed in different contexts to convert light energy into "mechanical" motion at molecular level (Sauvage, 2001). In basically all applications, the induced motion results in a permanent or transient conformational change of a molecular scaffold bounded to the switch. The spatial asymmetry (*i.e.* the chirality) of the molecular framework of NAFPs, NAIPs and NAPs determinates the direction (either clockwise or anticlockwise) of the $E \rightarrow Z$ and $Z \rightarrow E$ conformational changes leading, after sequential abortion of two photons, to a complete 360° rotation.

One of the uses of these systems is their union to more complex structures. In fact, the analysis and modulation of the conformation and function of biomolecules (*e.g.* ion transport (Lougheed et al.,2004), protein folding (Fierz et al., 2007), cell signalling (Cordes et al., 2006) and cell adhesion (Schütt et al., 2003) with photochromic switches is an area of increasing interest (Duvage & Demange, 2003). Among the photoisomerizable subunits for the photomodulation of secondary structure elements in peptides and proteins, photosensitive ω-amino acids are highly promising candidates. ω-Amino acids are non-protein amino acids in which amino and acid groups are in opposite sides of a chain (Figure 7).

For instance, hemithioindigo ω-amino acids (HTI) have shown favourable properties to use in biological systems (Cordes at al., 2007). Photoswitchable amino acids can be used to reversibly activate and deactivate a bioactive compound, and are therefore valuable diagnostic instruments to study complex living systems using light. In fact, the structure of biomolecules

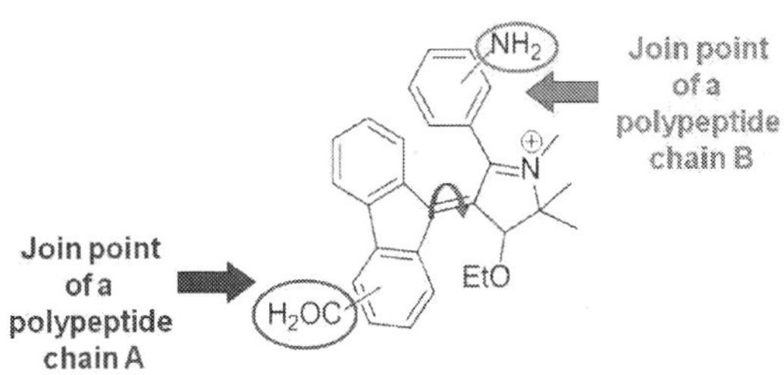

Fig. 7. Use of NAFP switches for protein photomodulation.

can be modified in a defined way using light, which opens a variety of fascinating new applications in biology and medicine. The potential use of this strategy has been demonstrated and has been already used to control physiological processes in living organisms (Szobata et al., 2007), to activate or modify the expressions of enzymes or to regulate their biological function. Rapid structural changes can also be induced in small bio-molecules allowing direct experimental studies of the initial processes in protein folding (Schrader et al., 2007).

6. Conclusions and outlook

Through this chapter we have reviewed some natural machines and what we can learn from them in order to design and build our versions of artificial machines. Improving Nature's work is clearly a huge task, but we should not relinquish this intention. A careful exploration of natural machines will lead not only to valuable information on how to design efficient nanoscopic devices, but also will help us to understand how these natural machines work, their advantages and weak points. However, we should bear in mind that biomimetism is more than a slight resemblance to a natural structure. In Nature, the look or structure of biomolecular machine, or any chemical structure in general, is far from being important. Any natural structure responds to the necessity of survival of an organism. Thus, design and synthesis are always subordinated to the accomplishment of this task without any unnecessary expense. Bioinspiration will help us to rapidly improve our nanomachinery, but also the design and construction of new nanoscopic devices and machines will facilitate our understanding of these fascinating examples of natural engineering.

Although the application of retinal-based switches and derivates to the construction of rotary motors will require further research work, computational and spectroscopic data indicate that their photoisomerization dynamics replicates the behaviour of the PSB11 in Rh.

A particularly challenging issue is the control of molecular motion as the performance of the motor will be essential in powering future nanoscale machines. The controlled directional movement along a trajectory, the use of molecular motors as transporters for molecular cargo, the construction of motor-powered nanomachines and devices that can perform several mechanical functions and the design of smart switchable surfaces are just a few of the developments that can be envisioned in the near future.

It is evident that this whole field is still in its infancy and offers a wide range of opportunities for molecular design and discovery.

7. Acknowledgements

We thank the MICINN, Comunidad Autónoma de La Rioja and Universidad de La Rioja for financial support.

8. References

Amendola, V. *Structure & Bonding*, Springer, Berlín, 2001.

Astumian, R. D. *Proc. Natl. Acad. Sci. U.S.A.*, 2005, *102*, 1843.

Ball, P. *Nature* 2001, *409*, 413.

Balzani, V.; Venturi, M.; Credi, A. *Molecular Devices and Machines. Concepts and Perspectives for the Nanoworld*, Wiley-VCH, Weinheim, 2008.

Becker, R. S. *Photochem. Photobiol.* 1988, *48*, 369.

Benson, D.E.; Conrad, D.W.; de Lorimier, R.M.; Trammell, S.A.; Hellinga, H.W. *Science*, 2001, *293*, 1641.
Bortolus, P.; Monti, S. *J. Phys. Chem.*, 1979, *83*, 648.
Bredenbeck, J.; Helbing, J.; Sieg, A.; Schrader, T.; Zinth, W.; Renner, C.; Behrendt, R.; Moroder, L.; Wachtveilt, J.; Hamm, P. *Proc. Natl. Acad. Sci. U.S.A.*, 2003, *100*, 6452.
Browne, W. R.; Feringa, B. L. *Nat. Nanotechnol.*, 2006, *1*, 25.
Cacciapaglia, R.; Stefano, S. D.; Mandolini, L. *J. Am. Chem. Soc.*, 2003, *125*, 2224.
Cordes, T.; Heinz, B.; Regner, N.; Hoppmann, C.; Schrader, T. E.; Summerer, W.; Rück-Braun, K.; Zinth, W. *Chem. Phys. Chem.*, 2007, *8*, 1713.
Cordes, T.; Weinrich, D.; Kempa, S.; Riesselmann, K.; Herre, S.; Hoppmann, C.; Rück-Braun, K.; Zinth, W. *Chem. Phys. Lett.*, 2006, *428*, 167.
Coy, D.L.; Wagenbach, M.; Howard, J. *J. Biol. Chem.*, 1999, *274*, 3667.
Dartnall, H. *Visio Res.* 1967, *8*, 339.
Diez, S.; Reuther, C.; Dinu, C.; Seidel, R.; Mertig, M.; Pompe, W.; Howard, J. *Nano Lett.*, 2003, *3*, 1251.
Drexler, K. E. *Nanosystems: Molecular Machinery, Manufacturing and Computation*, John Wiley & Sons, New York, 1992.
Duvage, C.; Demange, L. *Chem. Rev.*, 2003, *103*, 2475.
Feringa, B. L. *Acc. Chem. Res.*, 2001, *34*, 504.
Feringa, B. L. *J. Org. Chem.*, 2007, *72*, 6635.
Fierz, B.; Satzger, H.; Root, C.; Gilch, P.; Zinth, W.; Kiefhaber, T. *Proc. Natl. Acad. Sci. U.S.A.*, 2007, *104*, 2163.
Gelles, J.; Landick, R. *Cell*, 1998, *93*, 13.
Gennadiy, M.; Ying, C.; Yusuke, T.; Bill, W.; Jiang-Xing, M. *Proc. Natl. Acad. Sci.*, 2005, *102*, 12413.
Goodsell, D.S. *Our Molecular nature: The Body's Motors, Machines, and Messages*, 1996, Copernicus, New York.
Gorostiza, P.; Isacoff, E. *Science*, 2008, *322*, 395.
Harada, Y.; Noguchi, A.; Kishino, A.; Yanagida, T. *Biophys. J.*, 1997, *72*, 1997.
Harada, A. *Acc. Chem. Res.*, 2001, *34*, 456.
Hess, H.; Bachand, G. D.; Vogel, V. *Chem. Eur. J.* 2004, 10, 2110
Hofmann, K.P.; Helmreich, E. J. M. *Biochim. Biophys. Acta*, 1996, *1286*, 285.
Howard, J. *Mechanics of Motor Proteins and Cytoskeleton*, 2001, Sindauer Associates, Sunderland.
Irie, M. *Chem. Rev.*, 2000, *100*, 1685.
Irving, M.; Lombardi, V.; Piazzesi, G.; Ferenczi, M.A. *Nature*, 1992, *357*, 156.
Jousselme, B.; Blanchard, P.; Gallego-Planas, N.; Delaunay, J.; Allain, M.; Richomme, P.; Levillain, E.; Roncali, J. *J. Am. Chem. Soc.*, 2003, *125*, 2888.
Kaifer, A. E.; Gómez-Kaifer, M. *Supramolecular Electrochemistry*, Wiley-VCH, Weiheim, 1999.
Kandori, H.; Shichida, Y.; Yoshizawa, T. *Biochem. (Moscow)*, 2001, *66*, 1197.
Kaplan,D. ; Adams, W. W. *Silk Polym.; ACS Symp. Ser.* 1994, *544*, 2.
Kay, E. R.; Leigh, D. A.; Zerbetto, F. *Angew. Chem. Int. Ed.*, 2007, *46*, 72.
Khramov, D.M.; Rosen, E. L.; Lynch, V. M.; Bielawsky, C. W. *Angew. Chem. Int. Ed.* 2008, *47*, 2267.
Komura, N.; Zijistra, R. W. J.; van Delden, R. A.; Harada, N.; Feringa, B. L. *Nature*, 1999, *401*, 15.
Kühlbrandt, W. *Nature*, 2000, *406*, 569.
Liberman, M.C.; Gao, J.; He, D.Z.Z.; Wu, X.; Jia, S.; Zuo, J. *Nature*, 2002, *419*, 300.
Lohman, T.M.; Thorn, K.; Vale, R.D. *Cell*, 1998, *93*, 9.
Lougheed, T.; Borisenko, V.; Henning, T.; Rück-Braun, K.; Wooley, G. A. *Org. Biomol. Chem.*, 2004, *2*, 2798.
Lumento, F.; Zanirato, V.; Fusi, S., Busi, E.; Latterini, L.; Elisei, F.; Sinicropi, A.; Andruniów, T.; Ferré, N.; Basosi, R.; Olivucci, M. *Angew. Chem. Int. Ed.*, 2007, *47*, 414.

Mahadevan, L.; Matsudaira, P. *Science*, 2000, *288*, 95.
Mann, S. *Biomimetic Materials Chemistry*, VCH, New York, 1996
Matsumoto, H.; Yoshizawa, T. *Nature*, 1975, *258*, 523.
Metha, A.D.; Rief, M.; Spudich, J.A.; Smith, D.A.; Simmons, R.M. *Science*, 1999, *283*, 1689.
Min, W.; English, B. P.; Luo, G.; Cherayil, B. J.; Kou, C.; Xie, X. S. *Acc. Chem. Res.* 2005, *38*, 923.
Noji, H.; Yasuda, R.; Yoshida, M.; Kinosita Jr., K. *Nature*, 1997, *386*, 299.
Piermattei, A.; Karthikeyan, S.; Sijbesma, R. P. *Nat. Chem.* 2009, *1*, 133.
Rivado-Casas, L.; Sampedro, D.; Campos, P. J.; Fusi, S.; Zanirato, V.; Olivucci, M. *J. Org. Chem.*, 2009, *74*, 4666.
Rivado-Casas, L.; Campos, P. J.; Sampedro, D. *Organometallics*, 2010, 29, 3117.
Sampedro, D.; Migani, A.; Pepi, A.; Busi, E.; Basosi, R.; Latterini, L.; Elisei, F.; Fusi, S.;
Ponticelli, F.; Zanirato, V.; Olivucci, M. *J. Am. Chem. Soc.*, 2004, *126*, 9349.
Sarikaya, M. and I. A. Aksay, *Biomimetics: Design and processing of Materials*, American Institute of Physics, College Park, 1993
Sauvage, J.-P. *Molecular Machines and Motors*, Springer-Verlag, Berlín, London, 2001.
Schliwa, M.; Woehlke, G. *Nature*, 2001, *411*, 424.
Schrader, T. E.; Schreier, W. J.; Cordes, T.; Koller, F. O.; Babitzi, G.; Denschlag, R.; Renner, C.; Dong, S. L.; Löweneck, M.; Moroder, L.; Tavan, P.; Zinth, W. *Proc. Natl. Acad. Sci. U.S.A.*, 2007, *104*, 15729.
Schütt, M.; Krupka, S. S.; Alexander, G.; Milbradt, D.; Deindl, S.; Sinner, E.-K.; Oesterhelt, D.; Renner, C.; Moroder, L. *Chem. Biol.*, 2003, *10*, 487.
Shinkai, S.; Minami, T.; Kusano, Y.; Manabe, O. *J. Am. Chem. Soc.*, 1983, *105*, 1851.
Sinicropi, A.; Martin, E.; Ryasantsev, M.; Helbing, J.; Briand, J.; Sharma, D.; Léonard, J.; Haacke, S.; Canizzo, A.; Chergui, M.; ZAnirato, V.; Fusi, S.; Santoro, F.; Basosi, R.; Ferré, N.; Olivucci, M. *Proc. Natl. Acad. Sci. U.S.A.*, 2008, *105*, 17642.
Smith,B.L.; Schaffer, T.E.; Viani, M.; Thompson, J. B.; Frederick, N. A.; Kindt, J.; Belcher, A.; Stucky, G. D.; Morse, D. E.; Hansma, P. K. *Nature* 1999, *399*, 761.
Soong, R. K.; Bachand, G. D; Neves, H. P.; Olkhovets, A. G.; Craighead, H. G.; Montemagno, C. D. Science, 290, 1555.
Spudich, J.A. *Cell Regul.*, 1989, *1*,1.
Steinberg, G.; Rigaud, J.L.; Durantini, E. N.; Moore, A. L.; Gust, D.; Moore, T. A.; *Nature*, 1998, 392, 479.
Stoddart, J. F. *Acc. Chem. Res.*, 2001, *34*, 410.
Subramaniam, S.; Henderson, R. *Nature*, 2000, *406*, 653.
Svoboda, K.; Schmidt, C.F.; Schnapp, B.J.; Block, S.M. *Nature*, 1993, *365*, 721.
Szobata, S.; Gorosita, P.; Del Bene, F.; Wyart, C.; Fortin, D. L.; Kolstad, K. D.; Tulythan, O.;
Volgraf, M.; Numano, R.; Aaron, H. L.; Scoot, E. K.; Kramer, R. H.; Flannery, J.; Baier, H.; Trauner, D.; Isacoff, E. *Neuron*, 2007, *54*, 535.
Taylor, H.C.; Holwill, E.J. *Nanotechnology*, 1999, *10*, 237.
Teller, D. C.; Okada, T.; Behnke, C. A.; Palczewski, K.; Stenkamp, R. E. *Biochemistry*, 2001, *40*, 7761.
Turner, D.C.; Chang, C.Y.; Fang, K.; Bradow, S.L.; Murphy, D.B. *Biophys. J.*, 1995, *69*, 2782.
Vicario, J.; Walko, M.; Meetsma, A.; Feringa, B. L. *J. Am. Chem. Soc.*, 2006, *128*, 5127.
Wainwright, S. A. *Mechanical Design in Organisms*, Princeton University Press, Princeton, 1982.
Wang, Q.; Schoenlein, R.W.; Petenau, L. A.; Mathies, R. A.; Shnak, C. V. *Science*, 1994, *266*, 422.
Willner, I. *Science* 2002, *298*, 2407.
Yasuda,R.; Noji, H.; Kinosita Jr., K.; Yoshida, M. *Cell*, 1998, *93*, 1117.
Yildiz, A.; Forkey, J.N.; McKinney, S.A.; Ha, T.; Goldman, Y.E.; Selvin, P.R. *Science*, 2003, *300*, 2061.

24

Development and Experiments of a Bio-inspired Underwater Microrobot with 8 Legs

Shuxiang Guo[1,2], Liwei Shi[1] and Kinji Asaka[3]
[1]*Faculty of Engineering, Kagawa University, 2217-20 Hayashi-cho, Takamatsu, Kagawa*
[2]*Harbin Engineering University, 145 Nantong Street, Harbin, Heilongjiang*
[3]*Kansai Research Institute, AIST, 1-8-31 Midorigaoka, Ikeda, Osaka 563*
[1,3]*Japan*
[2]*China*

1. Introduction

In recent two decades, research of underwater microrobots developed at a high speed. They can be widely applied in the field of underwater monitoring operations including pollution detection, video mapping, and exploration of unstructured underwater environments. Based on the underwater monitoring, this kind of microrobot is of great interest for cleaning the micro pipeline in the radiate area, getting samples from the seabed for archeology or mining, and so on (Kim et al., 2005; Behkam & Sitti, 2006; McGovern et al., 2008). For example, some underwater robots with screw propellers have been developed. However, the electromagnetic structure of traditional motors is difficult to shrink. So, motors are rarely found in this sort of application (Zhang et al., 2006a; Wang et al., 2008), and special actuator materials are used instead. As a result, many kinds of smart materials, such as ionic polymer metal composite (IPMC), piezoelectric elements, pneumatic actuator, shape memory alloy, which can be used as artificial muscles, have been reported (Heo, 2007; Park et al., 2007). Although problems such as electrical leakage, water safety, physical bulk, and high stiffness persist in real applications, these smart materials have been widely used as actuators to develop new type of microrobot.

Ionic polymer metal composite (IPMC) is an innovative material made of an ionic polymer membrane chemically plated with gold electrodes on both sides. Its actuation characteristics, such as suitable response time, high bending deformation and long life, have significant potential for the propulsion of underwater microrobots. Flexible IPMC propulsion blades operating at low driving voltages provide many new possibilities for underwater locomotion applications (Lee & Kim, 2006; Nakadoi & Yamakita, 2006; Dogruer et al., 2007; Punning et al., 2007; Liu et al., 2008). They have been widely used on soft robotic actuators such as artificial muscles, as well as on dynamic sensors (Guo et al., 2008b; Ye et al., 2008).

Now, many kinds of underwater microrobots have been developed using IPMC actuators as artificial muscles to propel the robots back and forth. They are widely used in swimming microrobots as oscillating or undulating fins where fast response is required (Jung et al., 2003; Guo et al., 2004; Kamamichi, 2006; Guo et al., 2007; Brunetto et al., 2008). IPMC actuators are also used for underwater bipedal walking microrobots (Kamamichi et al., 2003; Guo et al., 2006; Yim et al., 2007), and a kind of ion-conducting polymer gel film microleg with two DOF has been developed (Zhang et al., 2006c). In addition, a six-legged insect-inspired underwater walking microrobot has also been described (Zhang et al., 2006d). For the six-legged one, the driving forces on the left and right sides are different because of the device's asymmetry. It has difficulty maintaining a straight path when walking forward. Because its centre of gravity and centre of rotation are not the same, it cannot be positioned precisely, and it consumes a lot of energy while rotating. In addition, the six-legged device cannot perform the movements required to dive or surface. With the aim of creating a compact structure with efficient and precise locomotion, we first developed a biomimetic underwater microrobot with eight IPMC actuators as legs to provide better performance in walking and rotating.

The remainder of this paper consists of five parts. Firstly, we described the design of the biomimetic leg shown in Figure 2. Secondly, we proposed a new type of microrobot with three DOF shown in Figure 4, including its walking, rotating, and floating mechanisms. Thirdly, we evaluated the mechanical behavior of the IPMC actuator, analyzed the forces applied to the four driving legs and simulated the walking speed. Fourthly, we developed the prototype microrobot and carried out experiments to measure its walking and rotating speeds on underwater flat. And the last is our conclusions.

2. The biomimetic locomotion

Each leg of a stick insect is composed of a coxa, a femur, a tibiae, and a tarsus. The tarsus is also called foot, and does not contribute to the movements. The coxa offers the foot one DOF motion in the direction of movement. The femur and the tibiae offer the foot a 2-DOF motion to enable it to find a reliable foothold together in the swing-search phase and touch the ground and support the body while moving in the stance phase, as shown in Figure 1. (Zhang et al., 2006a; Zhang et al., 2006b; Zhang et al., 2006d)

Based on the walking motion of the stick insect, a stick insect inspired biomimetic locomotion prototype using two IPMC actuators is developed, as shown in Figure 2. The actuator in vertical direction is called the driver. The actuator in the horizontal direction is called the supporter. The free end of the driver is the foot. The driver and supporter are controlled by two channels of square wave signals, with the same frequency. The driver and supporter can bend along Tra.2 and Tra.1 respectively. The phase of supporter is 90 degrees delayed than that of driver, so that driver and supporter can cooperate with each other in clawing motion as shown in Figure 3, where the swing-search phase is from (a) to (d) and the stance phase is from (d) to (e) (Zhang et al., 2006c; Zhang et al., 2006d).

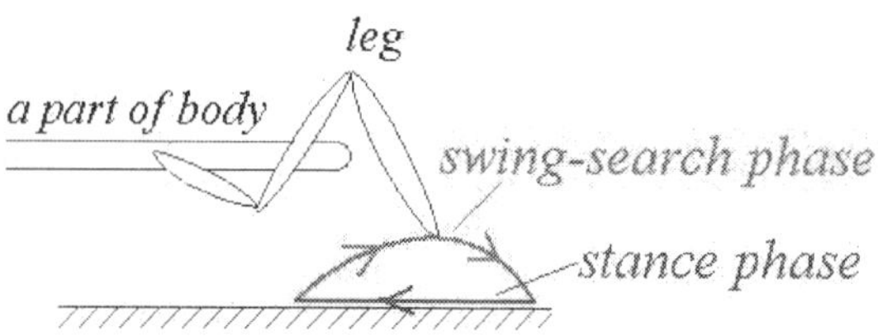

Fig. 1. Two phases in stick insect walking

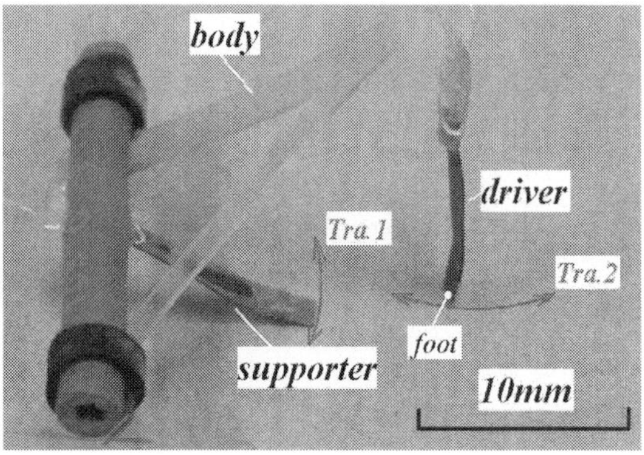

Fig. 2. The prototype of the biomimetic locomotion

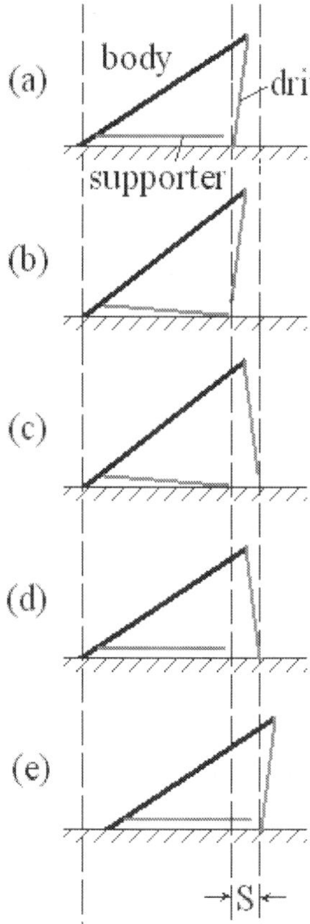

Fig. 3. One step cycle of the biomimetic locomotion

3. Proposed Eight-legged Microrobot

3.1 Proposed Eight-legged Microrobot Structure

Using this locomotion, we had previously developed several microrobots (Zhang et al., 2006a; Zhang et al., 2006d). As shown in Figure 4, both of them have six IPMC actuators on plastic film body, which are divided into two groups, the drivers are from A to C, and the supporters are the others.

Walker-1 can not only walk in 3 straight lines, but also rotate around its symmetric axis. Its disadvantage is that its moving motion is inefficient because one driver always resists forward moving limited by its structure(Zhang et al., 2006d). For the Walker-2, the drivers and the supporters are on both sides of a rectangle film body. However, the driving forces on the left and right sides are different because of the device's asymmetry. So, it has difficulty maintaining a straight path when walking forward. Because its centre of gravity and centre of rotation are not the same, it cannot be positioned precisely, and it consumes a lot of energy while rotating. In addition, it cannot perform the movements required to dive or surface with a stable gesture for its asymmetry.

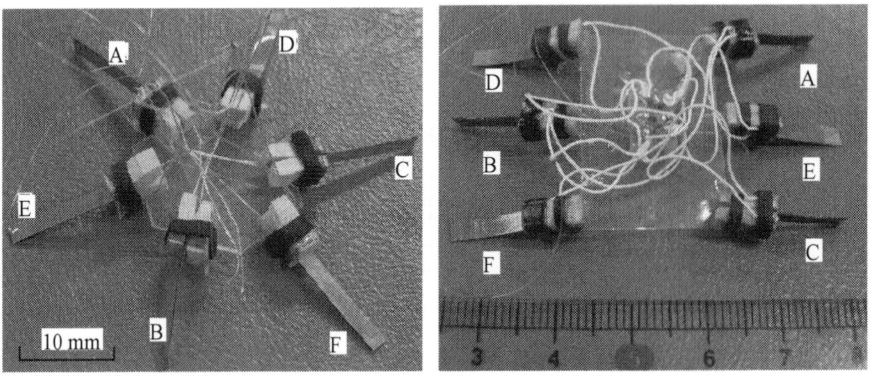

Walker-1 Walker-2

Fig. 4. Photos of previously developed six-legged biomimetic microrobots

To inherit the advantages of previously developed microrobots and overcome their disadvantages, we proposed a new biomimetic microrobot with a centrosymmetric structure around which the eight legs are symmetrically distributed, as shown in Figure 5 and Figure 6. It is 33 mm long, 56 mm wide, and 9 mm high. It has eight IPMC actuators designated A through H. Actuators A, B, C, and D are the drivers, and their bending directions are shown in Figure 7. The other four actuators are supporters. The actuators are all 11 mm long, 3 mm wide, and 0.2 mm thick. The distance between two adjacent drivers or between a driver and a supporter is 10 mm (Guo et al. 2008a; Guo et al. 2009).

The biomimetic microrobot is capable of walking, rotating, and floating. Table 1 lists the control strategies for crawling.

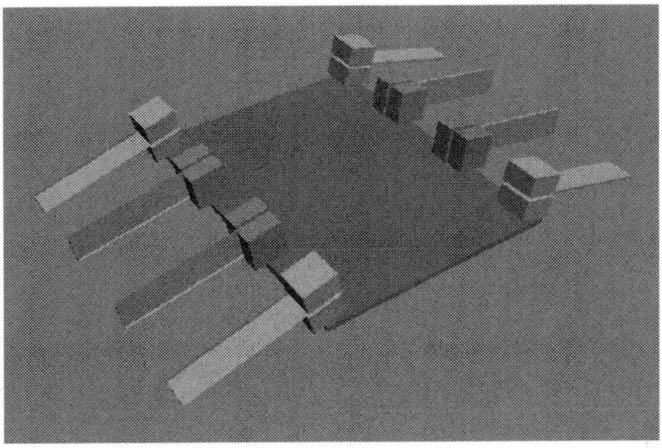

Fig. 5. Proposed eight-legged biomimetic microrobot

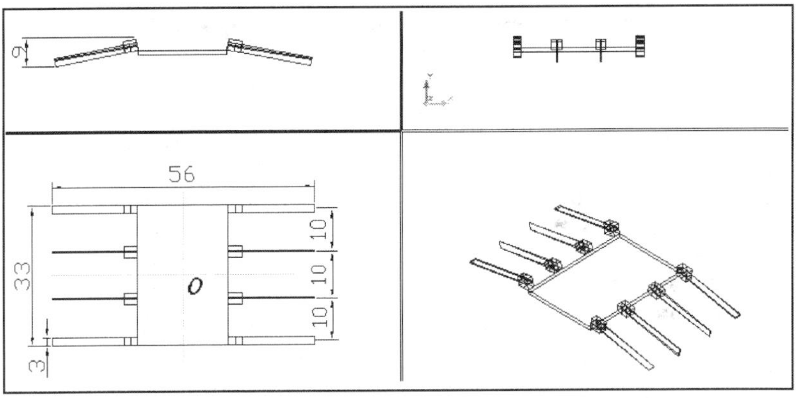

Fig. 6. Proposed microrobot structure

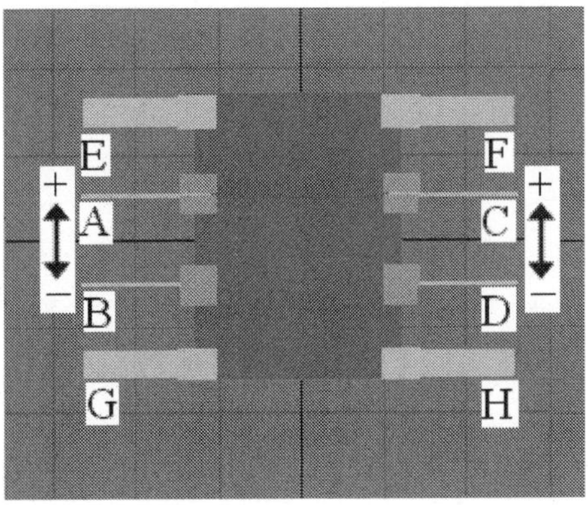

Fig. 7. Bending directions for the four drivers

Motions	A	B	C	D
Walking forward	+	+	+	+
Walking backward	-	-	-	-
Rotating in clockwise	+	+	-	-
Rotating in counter clockwise	-	-	+	+

A, B, C, and D stand for the drivers, as shown in Fig. 7. "+" and "-" mean the drivers bending forward and backward, respectively.

Table 1. Control strategies for crawling locomotion

3.2 Crawling motion mechanism

The drivers and supporters are driven at the same oscillating frequency. When crawling, the phase of the supporters lags that of the four drivers by 90°. Each step cycle of the walking motion can be separated into four periods as shown in Figure 8:

1. From d to a, the supporters lift the body up, and the drivers are off the ground.
2. From a to b, the drivers bend forward.
3. From b to c, the supporters bend upward far enough so that they are off the ground, while the drivers in contact with the ground support the body.
4. From c to d, the drivers bend backward in the propulsion stroke, and the body is pushed forward (Guo et al., 2008a).

During periods (1), (2), and (3), the drivers are off the ground and move to another foothold point with the help of the supporters. In period (4), the drivers push the body forward.

The walking speed is determined by the displacement of the drivers and the frequency of the control signal. Because the four drivers are distributed symmetrically on both sides of the structure and they have the same size and mass, the four drivers support equivalent loads and drag forces. Therefore, the four drivers experience the same displacement for the same applied input voltage. The deflections of all the drivers are equal, and they experience the same displacement in each step. The walking speeds on each side of the structure are the same. Suppose that the displacement of the actuator without a payload is d_0, and the microrobot can move forward with a displacement of d in one step cycle. Because of the payload or water resistance, a decrease Δd in the displacement of the drivers cannot be ignored. Equation (1) describes the relationship between d_0 and d, and Eq. (2) describes the walking speed, where v is the average speed and f is the frequency of the input signal.

$$d = d_0 - \Delta d \tag{1}$$

$$v = (d_0 - \Delta d) \times f \tag{2}$$

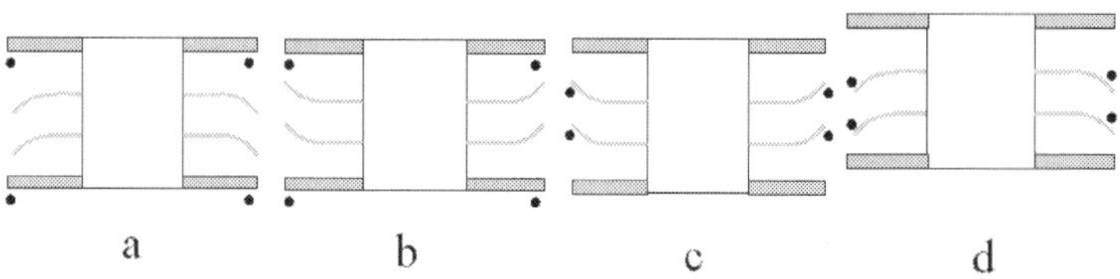

Fig. 8. One step cycle of walking forward. The • marks indicate which legs contact the ground.

3.3 Rotating motion mechanism

Figure 9 shows the example of counter-clockwise rotation. From c to d, the drivers push the body to rotate. In the other periods, the drivers are pushed up by the supporters to prepare for the next stroke (Guo et al., 2008b).

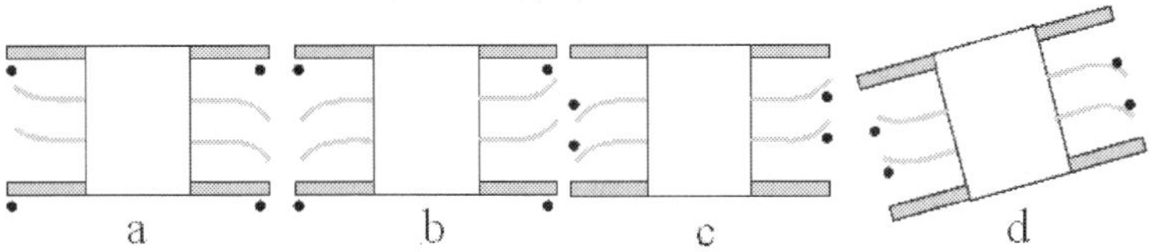

Fig. 9. One step cycle of the rotating motion. The • marks indicate which legs contact the ground.

The speed of the rotating motion is determined by the angle of the driver in one cycle and the frequency of the step, as shown in Figure 10 (a). The device can rotate by an angle of θ in one step cycle, as shown in Eq. (3).

$$\theta = \frac{L}{R} = \frac{2L}{D} \tag{3}$$

Where L is the length of the rotating arc, R is the radius of the rotating rotundity, and D is the diameter, as shown in Figure 10 (a) and Figure 10 (c). The diameter D could be calculated using Eq. (4).

$$D = \sqrt{(10+d)^2 + (56-2\Delta l)^2} \tag{4}$$

Where d is the displacement of the driver in the stance phase and Δl stands for the displacement decrease of the IPMC actuator, as shown in Eq. (5).

$$\Delta l = l - l_s \tag{5}$$

Where l is the length of IPMC actuator, l *and* ls are shown in Figure 10 (b). Based on the geometry theorem, we can get the Eq. (6).

$$|\mathrm{AN}| \times |\mathrm{BN}| = |\mathrm{CN}| \times |\mathrm{DN}| \tag{6}$$

From the Figure 10 (b), r is the bending radius of the IPMC actuator, $|\mathrm{AN}| = |\mathrm{BN}| = ls$, $|\mathrm{CN}| = d/2$, $|\mathrm{DN}| = |2r - d/2|$, so ls can be calculated as shown in Eq. (7).

$$l_s = \sqrt{\frac{d}{2} \times \left|2r - \frac{d}{2}\right|} \tag{7}$$

According to Eq. (3), Eq. (4), Eq. (5), and Eq. (7), the device can rotate by an angle of θ in one step cycle, as shown in Eq. (8).

$$\theta = \frac{L}{R} = \frac{2L}{D} = \frac{2L}{\sqrt{(10+d)^2 + \left[56 - 2\left(l - \sqrt{\frac{d}{2} \cdot \left|2r - \frac{d}{2}\right|}\right)\right]^2}} \tag{8}$$

Equation (9) gives the rotating speed. Here, because the rotating arc $L \approx d$, we can approximate L by d in Eq. (9). The ω and f are the rotating speed and the frequency, respectively. Figure 10 (a) shows that the structure's centre of rotation is at point O, which is also the structure's centre of symmetry. Because the eight legs are symmetrically distributed around the centre of symmetry of the centrosymmetric structure and because the eight legs have the same size and mass, the centre of symmetry is also the centre of gravity. Thus, the centre of rotation of the microrobot is its centre of gravity. In addition, because the oscillating directions of the four drivers are close to perpendicular to the radius of rotation, the eight-legged device has a larger torsion angle than did the previous six-legged version.

$$\omega = \theta * f = \frac{2(d_0 - \Delta d)}{\sqrt{(10+d)^2 + \left[56 - 2\left(l - \sqrt{\frac{d}{2} \cdot \left|2r - \frac{d}{2}\right|}\right)\right]^2}} f \tag{9}$$

3.4 Floating motion mechanism

The water around the surface of the IPMC actuators is electrolysed by decreasing the frequency of the applied voltage to 0.3 Hz. The buoyancy of the microrobot can be controlled by the resulting change in volume to make it float upwards, remain neutrally buoyant, or sink downwards. Table 2 lists the control strategies for the floating motion.

Conditions	Floating motions
$\rho g(V + \Delta V) < mg$	sinking downward
$\rho g(V + \Delta V) = mg$	suspended
$\rho g(V + \Delta V) > mg$	floating upward

ρ is the density of water, g is the acceleration of gravity, V is the volume of the microrobot, ΔV is the volume of the bubbles, and mg is the weight of the microrobot.

Table 2. Control strategies of floating locomotion

4. Theoretical dynamic performance analysis

4.1 Tip displacements of IPMC without payloads

Figure 8 shows one step cycle for forward motion. The microrobot can move a distance of d during one step cycle. We measured the displacement of one IPMC actuator by applying different signals to simulate the theoretical crawling speed of the microrobot as shown in Figure 11. The IPMC actuator was 14 mm long, 3 mm wide, and 0.2 mm thick. The actuator was driven by a PC equipped with a digital-to-analogue converter card, and the deflection of the IPMC was measured by a laser displacement sensor. The laser sensor was used to translate the displacement to a voltage, and then the voltages were recorded and translated to the PC using an oscilloscope.

Because the actuator was designed for use in a water tank, the relationship between the tip distance and the laser senor voltage was different from that relationship in air. This means that the laser sensor must first be calibrated for use in water (Guo et al, 2009). Figure 12 shows the tip displacements of the actuator recorded experimentally for different frequencies and voltages. These results show that the tip displacement decreased as the frequency increased. Therefore, the microrobot had a top walking speed, and the theoretical walking speed could be calculated using equation (2).

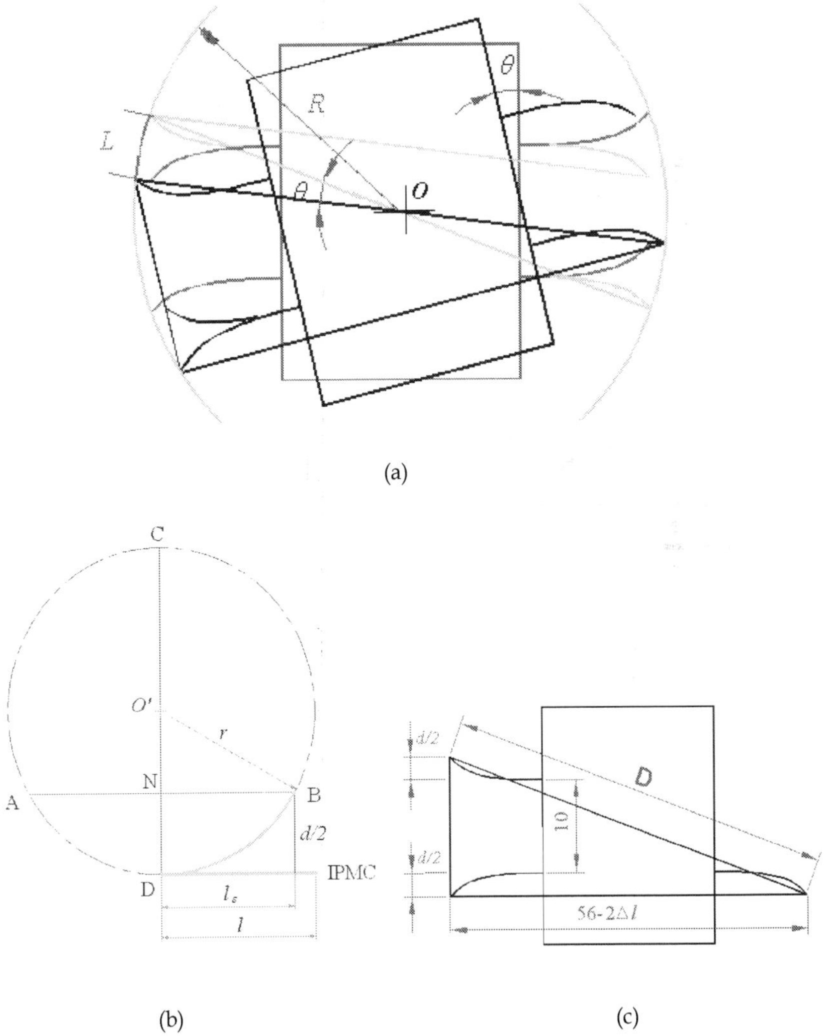

Fig. 10. Efficiency of the driver during rotating motion

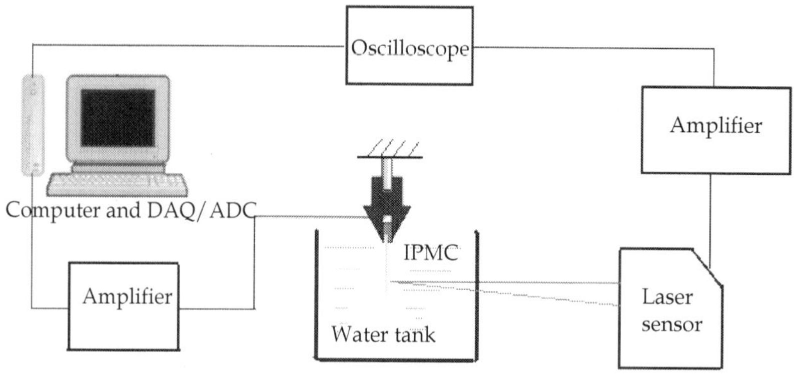

Fig. 11. Displacement measuring system

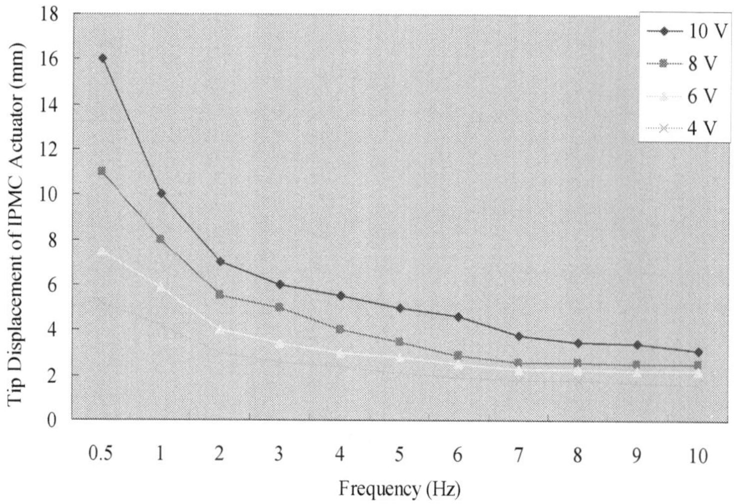

Fig. 12. Tip displacements (d_0) of the IPMC actuator

4.2 Equivalent beam modeling

The IPMC beam actuator can be modelled as a supported cantilever beam as shown in Figure 13 (Cilingir et al., 2008; Pugal et al., 2008; Stoimenov et al., 2008; Mbemmo et al., 2008). When the microrobot crawling, the forces applied to one leg are shown in Figure 14, where q is the surface tension of the IPMC actuator and F is the resultant force of friction and water resistance to one leg. According to the cantilever beam theory, the relationship between the deformation curvature $1/\rho(x)$ and mechanical moment M is shown in the equation (10).

$$\frac{1}{\rho(x)} = \frac{M(x)}{EI} \tag{10}$$

Where E is the elastic modulus for IPMC in hydrated conditions and I is the moment of inertia for the equivalent cantilever beam. Mechanical moment M, produced duo to IPMC bending is a function of applied forces.
Also, according to curvature equation (11) of deflection curve, we can get the equation (12).

$$\frac{1}{\rho(x)} = -\frac{\frac{d^2w}{dx^2}}{\left[1+(\frac{dw}{dx})^2\right]^{3/2}} \tag{11}$$

$$\frac{\frac{d^2w}{dx^2}}{\left[1+(\frac{dw}{dx})^2\right]^{3/2}} = -\frac{M(x)}{EI} \tag{12}$$

For the small deflection, equation (12) is simplified as shown in equation (13), which is approximately expressed.

$$\frac{d^2w}{dx^2} = -\frac{M(x)}{EI} \tag{13}$$

The tip displacement generated by the surface tension q in one direction, can be defined as w_q. So, the tip displacement in two directions $d_0 = 2w_q$ can be calculated in equation (14).

$$d_0 = 2\times w_q = 2\times\frac{qx^2}{24}(-4lx+6l^2+x^2) = 2\times\frac{ql^4}{8EI} = \frac{ql^4}{4EI} \tag{14}$$

The tip displacement generated by the resultant force F in one direction, can be defined as w_F. So, the tip displacement in two directions $\Delta d = 2w_F$ can be calculated in equation (15). As a result, the resultant deflection d can be obtained from equation (16).

$$\Delta d = 2\times w_F = 2\times(-\frac{Fx^3}{6EI}+\frac{Flx^2}{2EI}) = \frac{2Fl^3}{3EI} \tag{15}$$

$$d = d_0 - \Delta d = 2\times(w_q - w_F) = d_0 - \frac{2Fl^3}{3EI} \tag{16}$$

In order to calculate the w_F, the IPMC bending stiffness EI can be calculated from experiments and equation (17) respectively.

$$I = \frac{b\cdot h^3}{12} \tag{17}$$

The elastic modulus E for IPMC in hydrated conditions is measured with the value of about 83 MPa (Park et al., 2007). With cross dimension of 0.2×3mm, the moment of inertia for the IPMC can be obtained about 2.0×10^{-3} mm^4. Then the bending stiffness is calculated as 166.0 mN·mm^2. For one leg, the force F is the friction, as shown in equation (18).

$$F = \mu_s N \tag{18}$$

Where N is the positive pressure between the leg and the bottom of water tank, and μ_s is the static friction coefficient. According to the materials of IPMC and the hard steel bottom, we choose μ_s=0.30 in our experiments. With the weight of 1.63 g in air and cubage of 0.79 cm^3, the weight of the microrobot in water can be calculated as 0.84 g, N=0.84 g. So, the force F of one leg can be obtained about 8.232 mN. With the length of leg l=11 mm, the force F= 0.6175 mN, and the bending stiffness of the leg EI=166.0 mN·mm^2, the displacement decreases of IPMC drivers Δd can be evaluated as 3.301 mm and the walking speeds can be calculated by equation (2). The simulated results are shown in Figure 15.

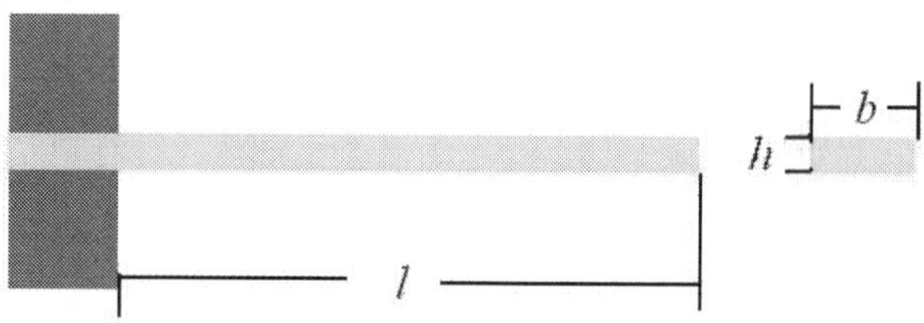

Fig. 13. Equivalent cantilever beam for an IPMC actuator

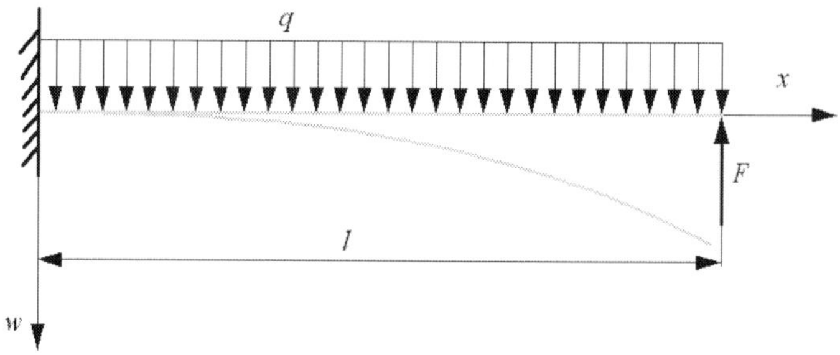

Fig. 14. Forces and deflection of IPMC actuator in w direction

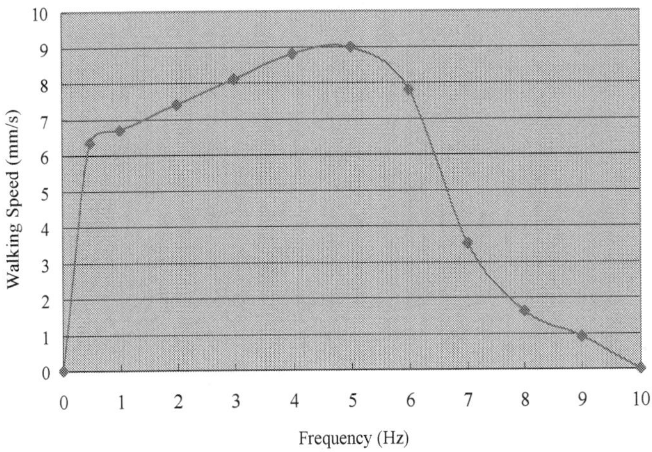

Fig. 15. Theoretical walking speed (10 V)

5. Prototype microrobot and experiments

5.1 Prototype eight-legged microrobot

Figure 16 shows the prototype of the eight-legged microrobot. It has eight actuators fixed on a film body with wood clips. The control signals are transmitted by enamel-covered wires 300 mm long with a copper diameter of 0.03 mm. The wires are soft enough that the resistance can be ignored.

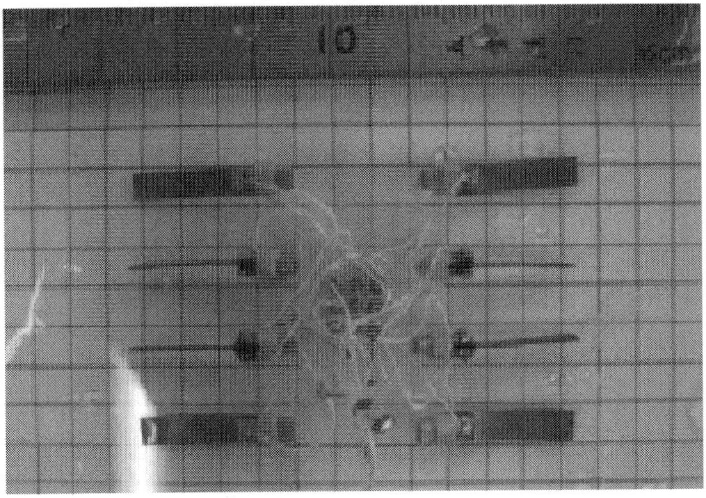

Fig. 16. Prototype eight-legged underwater microrobot

5.2 Walking experiment on underwater flat surface

To evaluate walking locomotion, we carried out an experiment on an underwater plastic surface. We recorded the times required to walk a distance of 50 mm using different applied signal voltages and frequencies. The experiment was repeated 10 times for every set of control signals to determine the average speed on the flat surface. The experimental results described in Figure 17 show that the walking speed was nearly proportional to the input voltage, and a top speed of 8.3 mm/s was obtained with a control signal of 10 V and 5 Hz. We compared the experimental value with the theoretical value with a control signal of 10 V, as shown in Figure 18. From the comparison, we could see that the experimental results approached the theoretical results very well. The displacement of the IPMC actuator would be less in real applications due to slippage and short response time at high frequencies. Therefore, some differences between the theoretical and experimental results still exist.

5.3 Rotating experiment on underwater flat surface

We also investigated the rotating motion on the same underwater plastic surface. We recorded the times for rotating through 90° under the influence of different voltages and frequencies of the control signal, and calculated the average angular velocity for 10 repetitions of the same experiment. The experimental results described in Figure 19 show that the angular velocity was nearly proportional to the input voltage, and a top angular rotation speed of 11.86°/s was obtained for a voltage of 10 V and a frequency of 5 Hz.

5.4 Floating experiment

To test floating locomotion, we set the frequency of the applied voltage to 0.15 Hz to electrolyse the water around the IPMC surface. When the input voltage was cut off while the microrobot was floating upward, the microrobot gradually stopped moving upward and then started to sink. The maximum upward floating speed was 4 mm/s with a voltage of 10 V as shown in Figure 20.

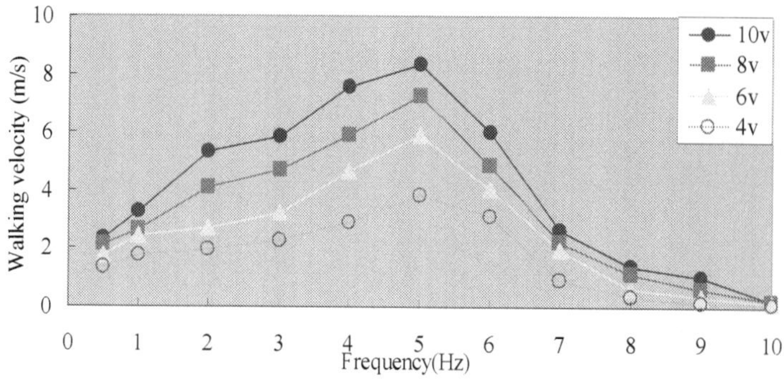

Fig. 17. Experimental walking speed results (10 V)

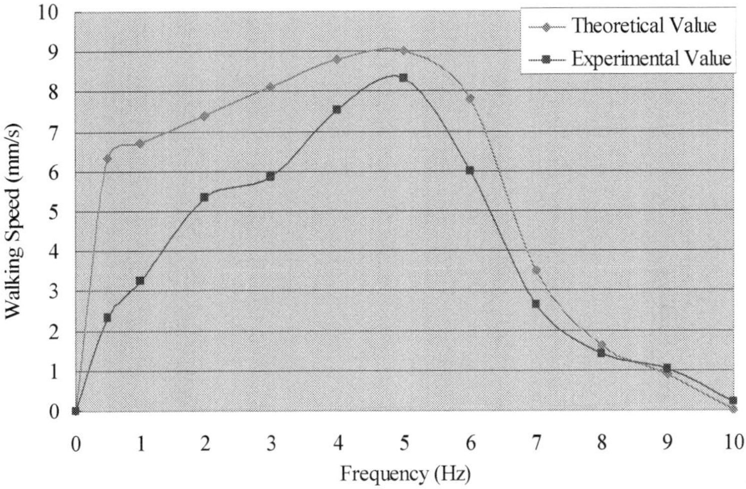

Fig. 18. Relationship between theoretical and experimental walking speeds (10 V)

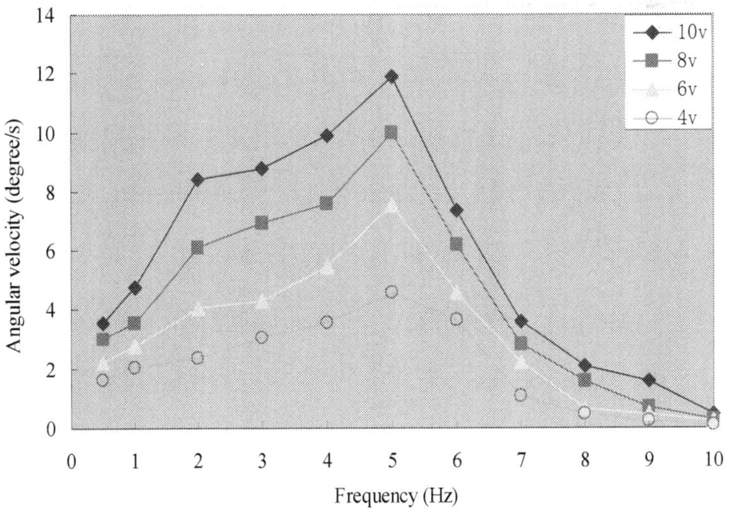

Fig. 19. Experimental angular velocity results during rotation

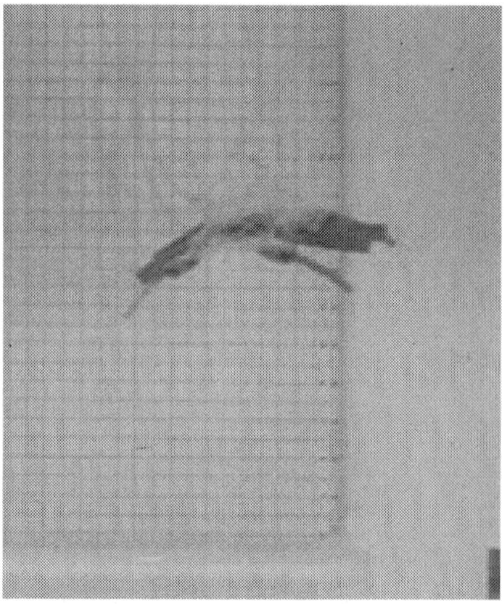

Fig. 20. Floating motion of the eight-legged microrobot

6. Conclusions

To resolve the problem of the asymmetry in previous six-legged microrobots, we proposed a new type of underwater microrobot with eight IPMC actuators distributed symmetrically around the microrobot's centre of symmetry. We evaluated the walking, rotating, and floating mechanisms of this proposed robot. Then, we evaluated the mechanical behavior of the IPMC actuator, analyzed the forces applied to the four driving legs and simulated the walking speed. We also constructed a prototype of the eight-legged microrobot and conducted experiments to measure its walking speed and angular velocity without payloads. Its walking and rotating speeds were faster than those of the previous six-legged version. We also made the microrobot dive and surface by electrolysing the water around the IPMC surface. Controlling the electrolysis process and thus the buoyancy of the microrobot was difficult, so the vertical motion of the device could not be controlled very well. In the following research, we developed a jellyfish-type microrobot to improve the floating motion.

7. Acknowledgment

This research is supported by Kagawa University Characteristic Prior Research Fund 2010.

8. References

Behkam, B. & Sitti, M. (2006). Design methodology for biomimetic propulsion of miniature swimming robots, Journal of Dynamic Systems, Measurement, and Control, Vol.128, Issue 1, 2006, 36-43.

Brunetto, P.; Fortuna, L.; Graziani, S. & Strazzeri, S. (2008). A model of ionic polymer–metal composite actuators in underwater operations, Journal of Smart Material and Structures, 17, 2008, 025-029.

Cilingir, H.; Menceloglu, Y. & Papila, M. (2008). The effect of IPMC parameters in electromechanical coefficient based on equivalent beam theory, Journal of Electroactive Polymer Actuators and Devices (EAPAD), Proc. of SPIE Vol. 6927, 2008, 69270L.

Dogruer, D.; Tiwari, R. & Harvesters, K. (2007). Ionic Polymer Metal Composites as Energy Harvesters, Journal of Electroactive Polymer Actuators and Devices (EAPAD), Proc. of SPIE Vol. 6524, 2007, 65241C.

Guo, S.; Okuda, Y. & Asaka, K. (2004). Development of a Novel Type of Underwater Micro Biped Robot with Multi DOF, Proceedings of the fourteenth of International offshore and polar engineering conference, vol. II, 2004, 284-289.

Guo, S.; Okuda, Y.; Zhang, W.; Ye, X. & Asaka, K. (2006). The Development of a Hybrid Underwater Micro Biped Robot, Journal of Applied Bionics and Biomechanics, Vol.3, No.3, 2006, 143-150,.

Guo, S.; Shi, L. & Asaka, K. (2008a). IPMC Actuator-based an Underwater Microrobot with 8 Legs, Proceedings of 2008 IEEE International Conference on Mechatronics and Automation, Japan, 2008, 551 - 556.

Guo, S.; Shi, L. & Asaka, K. (2008b). IPMC Actuator-Sensor based a Biomimetic Underwater Microrobot with 8 Legs, Proceedings of the IEEE International Conference on Automation and Logistics, China, 2008, 2495-2500.

Guo, S.; Shi, L.; Asaka, K. & Li, L. (2009). Experiments and Characteristics Analysis of a Bio-inspired Underwater Microrobot, Proceedings of the 2009 IEEE International Conference on Mechatronics and Automation, China, 2009, 3330-3335.

Guo, S.; Shi, L.; Ye, X. & LI, L. (2007). A New Jellyfish Type of Underwater Microrobot, Proceedings of the 2007 IEEE International Conference on Mechatronics and Automation, China, 2007, 509-514.

Heo, S. (2007). Effect of an artificial caudal fin on the performance of a biomimetic fish robot propelled by piezoelectric actuators, Journal of Bionic Engineering, 4(3), 2007, 151 - 158.

Jung, J.; Kim, B.; Tak, Y. & Park, J. (2003). Undulatory Tadpole Robot (TadRob) using ionic polymer metal composite (IPMC) actuator, Proceedings of the IEEE/RSJ Intl. Conference on Intelligent Robots and Systems, 2003, 2133-2138.

Kamamichi, N. (2006). A snake-like swimming robot using IPMC actuator/sensor, Proceedings of the 2006 IEEE International Conference on Robotics and Automation, 2006, 1812 - 1817.

Kamamichi, N.; Kaneda, Y.; Yamakita, M.; Asaka, K. & Luo, Z. (2003). Biped Walking of Passive Dynamic Walker with IPMC Linear Actuator, SICE Annual Conference in Fukui, 2003, 212-217.

Kim, B.; Kim, D.; Jung a, J. & J. Park. (2005). A biomimetic undulatory tadpole robot using ionic polymer–metal composite actuators, Journal of Smart Material and Structures, 14, 2005, 1579-1585.

Kim, S.; Lee, I. & Kim, Y. (2007). Performance enhancement of IPMC actuator by plasma surface treatment, Journal of Smart Material and Structures, 16, 2007, N6-N11,.

Lee, S. & Kim, K. (2006). Muscle-like Linear Actuator Using an Ionic Polymer-Metal Composite and Its Actuation Characteristics, Journal of Smart Structures and Materials: Electroactive Polymer Actuators and Devices (EAPAD), Proc. of SPIE Vol. 6168, 2006, 616820.

Liu, S.; Lin, M. & Zhang, Q. (2008). Extensional Ionomeric Polymer Conductor Composite Actuators with Ionic Liquids, Journal of Electroactive Polymer Actuators and Devices (EAPAD), Proc. of SPIE Vol. 6927, 2008, 69270H.

Mbemmo, E.; Chen, Z.; Shatara, S. & Tan, X. (2008). Modeling of biomimetic robotic fish propelled by an ionic polymer-metal composite actuator, Proceedings of the IEEE International Conference on Robotics and Automation, 2008, 689-694.

McGovern, S. T.; Spinks, G. M.; Xi, B.; Alici, G.; Truong, V. & Wallace, G. G. (2008). Fast bender actuators for fish-like aquatic robots, Proceedings of SPIE Vol. 6927, 2008, 69271L.

Nakadoi, H. & Yamakita, M. (2006). Integrated Actuator-Sensor System on Patterned IPMC Film: Consideration of Electoric Interference, Proceedings of SI2006 International Conference, 2006.

Park, I. ; Kim, S.; Kim, D. & Kin, K. (2007). The Mechanical Properties of Ionic Polymer-Metal pomposites, Journal of Electroactive Polymer Actuators and Devices (EAPAD), Proc. of SPIE Vol. 6524, 2007, 65241R.

Pugal, D.; Kasemagi, H.; Kruusmaa, M. & Aabloo, A. (2008). An Advanced Finite Element Model of IPMC, Journal of Electroactive Polymer Actuators and Devices (EAPAD), Proc. of SPIE Vol. 6927, 2008, 692711.

Punning, A.; Kruusmaa, M. & Aabloo, A. (2007). Surface resistance experiments with IPMC sensors and actuators, Journal of Sensors and Actuators, A 133, 2007, 200–209.

Stoimenov, B.; Rossiter, J.; Mukai, T. & Asaka, K. (2008). Frequency response of anisotropic ionic polymer metal composite (IPMC) transducers, Journal of Electroactive Polymer Actuators and Devices (EAPAD), Proc. of SPIE Vol. 6927, 2008, 69270K.

Wang, Z.; Hang, G.; Li, J.; Wang, Y. & Xiao, K. (2008). A micro-robot fish with embedded SMA wire actuated flexible biomimetic fin, Journal of Sensors and Actuators, A 144, 2008, 354–360.

Ye, X.; Su, Y.; Guo, S. & Wang, L. (2008). Design and Realization of a Remote Control Centimeter-Scale Robotic Fish, Proceedings of the 2008 IEEE/ASME International Conference on Advanced Intelligent Mechatronics, China, 2008, 25-30.

Yim, W.; Lee, J. & Kim, K. (2007). An artificial muscle actuator for biomimetic underwater propulsors, Journal of Bioinspiration and Biomimetics. 2, 2007, S31–S41.

Zhang, W.; Guo, S. & Asaka, K. (2006a). A New Type of Hybrid Fish-like Microrobot, International Journal of Automation and Computing, Vol.3, No.4, 2006, 358-365.

Zhang, W.; Guo, S. & Asaka, K. (2006b). Characteristics Analysis of a Biomimetic Underwater Walking Microrobot, Proceedings of the 2006 IEEE International Conference on Robotics and Biomimetics, Kuming, China, 2006, 1600-1605.

Zhang, W.; Guo, S. & Asaka, K. (2006c). Development of a novel type of an underwater microrobot with biomimetic locomotion, Journal of Applied Bionics and Biomechanics. Woodhead Publishing, Limited, Vol.3, No.3, 2006, 245-252.

Zhang, W.; Guo, S. & Asaka, K. (2006d). Development of an underwater biomimetic microrobot with both compact structure and flexible locomotion, Journal of Microsystem Technologies, DOI 10.1007：s00542-006-0294-9, 2006.